W0043067

Atlas of
Bone Marrow Pathology

Current Histopathology

Consultant Editor
Professor G. Austin Gresham, TD, ScD, MD, FRCPath.
Professor of Morbid Anatomy and Histology, University of Cambridge

Volume Fifteen

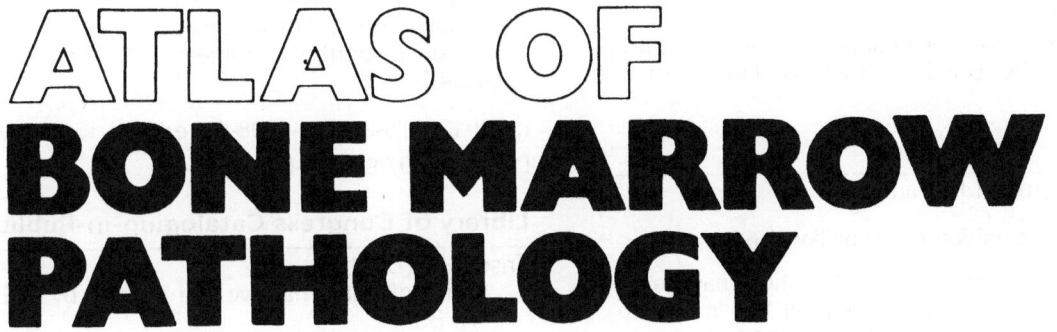

ATLAS OF BONE MARROW PATHOLOGY

BY

B. FRISCH
Institute of Haematology
Ichilov Hospital and
Sackler Faculty of Medicine, Tel-Aviv University
Israel

R. BARTL
Bone Marrow Diagnosis
Dept. of Internal Medicine "Innenstadt",
University of Munich
FRG

Immunohistology on cryostat sections in collaboration with **Dr C. SCHMID**,
Institute of Pathologic Anatomy, University of Graz, Austria.
Studies on paraffin-embedded biopsies in collaboration with **Dr N. HURWITZ**,
Institute of Pathology, Kaplan Hospital, Rehovoth, Israel.

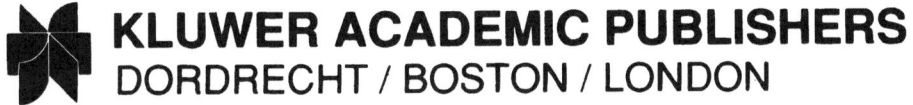

KLUWER ACADEMIC PUBLISHERS
DORDRECHT / BOSTON / LONDON

Distributors

for the United States and Canada: Kluwer Academic
Publishers, PO Box 358, Accord Station, Hingham, MA
02018-0358, USA
for all other countries: Kluwer Academic Publishers Group,
Distribution Center, PO Box 322, 3300 AH Dordrecht,
The Netherlands

Copyright

© 1990 by B. Frisch and R. Bartl

Softcover reprint of the hardcover 1st edition 1990

All rights reserved. No part of this publication may be
reproduced, stored in a retrieval system, or transmitted in
any form or by any means, electronic, mechanical,
photocopying, recording or otherwise, without prior
permission from the publishers, Kluwer Academic
Publishers BV, PO Box 17, 3300 AA Dordrecht, The
Netherlands.

Published in the United Kingdom by Kluwer Academic
Publishers, PO Box 55, Lancaster, UK.

Kluwer Academic Publishers BV incorporates the
publishing programmes of D. Reidel, Martinus Nijhoff, Dr
W. Junk and MTP Press.

Typeset and originated by Speedlith Photolitho Ltd.,
Longford Trading Estate, Thomas Street, Stretford,
Manchester M32 0JT

Bound by Butler and Tanner Ltd., Frome and London

British Library Cataloguing in Publication Data

Frisch, B. (Bertha)
  Atlas of bone marrow pathology.
  1. Man. Bone marrow. Diseases
  I. Title II. Bartl, R. (Reiner) III. Series
  616.4'1

ISBN-13: 978-94-010-6808-6   e-ISBN-13: 978-94-009-0717-1

DOI: 10.1007/978-94-009-0717-1

Library of Congress Cataloging-in-Publication Data

Frisch, B. (Bertha)
  Atlas of bone marrow pathology / by B. Frisch,
  R. Bartl.
    p. cm. — (Current histopathology ; v. 15)
  Includes bibliographical references.

  1. Bone marrow — Histopathology — Atlases.
  I. Bartl, R. (Reiner) II. Title III. Series.
  [DNLM: 1. Bone Marrow Diseases — atlases. W1
CU788JBA v. 15 / WH 17 F917a]
RC645.7.F74 1989
616.4'1 — dc20
DNLM/DLC
for Library of Congress   89-20102
                                                CIP

Contents

Current Histopathology Series

Consultant Editor's Note

At the present time books on morbid anatomy and histo-pathology can be divided into two broad groups: extensive textbooks often written primarily for students and mono-graphs on research topic.

This takes no account of the fact that the vast majority of pathologists are involved in an essentially practical field of general diagnostic pathology providing an important service to their clinical colleagues. Many of these pathologists are expected to cover a broad range of disciplines and even those who remain solely within the field of histopathology usually have single and sole responsibility within the hospital for all this work. They may often have no chance for direct discussion on problem cases with colleagues in the same department. In the field of histo-pathology, no less than in other medical fields, there have been extensive and recent advances, not only in new histochemical techniques but also in the type of specimen provided by new surgical procedures.

There is a great need for the provision of appropriate information for this group. This need has been defined in the following terms:-

1. It should be aimed at the general clinical pathologist or histopathologist with existing practical training, but should also have value for the trainee pathologist.
2. It should concentrate on the practical aspects of histopathology taking account of the new techniques which should be within the compass of the worker in a unit with reasonable facilities.
3. New types of material, e.g. those derived from endo-scopic biopsy should be covered fully.
4. There should be an adequate number of illustrations on each subject to demonstrate the variation in appearance that is encountered.
5. Colour illustrations should be used wherever they aid recognition.

The present concept stemmed from this definition but it was immediately realized that these aims could only be achieved within the compass of a series, of which this volume is one. Since histopathology is, by its very nature, systemized, the individual volumes deal with one system or where this appears more appropriate with a single organ.

Examination of bone marrow is no longer the sole province of the haematologist. Samples of marrow are frequently sent for histological examination and need to be treated in various ways to provide maximum informa-tion. This volume deals with the processing and interpret-ation of bone marrow biopsies. This is a rapidly developing field as techniques such as marrow transplantation are being used in many centres. The book is an essential aid for histopathologists and haematologists concerned with bone marrow interpretation.

G. Austin Gresham
Cambridge

Introduction

Examination of the bone marrow has always been, and to a large extent still is, within the domain of the haematologist. This is because smears of bone marrow aspirates together with peripheral blood films and results of other tests and investigations provided the information on which the clinical diagnosis was based.

Recently, the widespread availability of both improved biopsy needles and techniques for processing has greatly increased the number of routinely taken bone biopsies and placed the examination of bone marrow biopsy sections also in the field of histopathology – so that this Atlas is one of the *Current Histopathology* series. Therefore, the haematologist and the histopathologist now complement each other in the interpretation of bone marrow smears, imprints and sections, thus utilizing all available information and expertise to arrive at a diagnosis.

An attempt has been made in this Atlas to provide fairly comprehensive coverage of the areas in which examination of bone biopsy sections has proved useful. Clearly, bone biopsies have been more frequently taken in some disorders – such as the lymphoproliferations and the myeloproliferations – so that the chapters devoted to these subjects are much longer than those on other topics.

Examples of histochemistry and immunohistology using monoclonal antibodies have been included, indicating some of the diagnostic possibilities offered by these up-to-date techniques whose application will undoubtedly increase in the future.

After lengthy discussions and enquiries, the conclusion was reached that the magnifications of most of the illustrations could be omitted without detracting from the usefulness of the Atlas. The magnifications used are indicated in Fig. 1.25. In addition, not every detail specifically indicated in a figure or its legend is necessarily mentioned in the text; and often a range of observations is illustrated and in these cases the legends are self-explanatory.

This Atlas is directed to haematologists and to histopathologists and to anyone interested in the investigation and understanding of the human bone marrow.

Acknowledgements

The authors wish to thank all doctors who referred patients or sent biopsies, as well as the technical staff of the laboratories and of the photographic units.

We are indebted to Mrs A. Nachum for secretarial help and for typing the manuscript and to Dr N. Hurwitz for critical reading of the manuscript.

We would like to express our appreciation and gratitude to the editor Mr Phil Johnstone for his help and advice at every step in the process of producing this volume.

Biology, Structure and Components of Normal Bone Marrow

In recent years there has been a great increase in the number of bone marrow biopsies (BMB) taken for three major reasons: the introduction of plastic embedding which obviates the necessity of decalcification, improvements in needles for taking the biopsies, and thirdly, it has become apparent that much diagnostic information may be obtained. Consequently, indications for taking BMB have increased especially in internal medicine, oncology and osteology, as well as in haematology. This is attested to by the increasing number of texts and articles that have appeared over the past two decades[1-22].

Since BMB may be obtained from patients at all ages the differences in skeletal structure and bone marrow in different bones, and the age-related alterations in both osseous and haematopoietic components, must be taken into account. Moreover, there is an intimate and inseparable relationship between marrow and bone, and functional disturbances in the one almost invariably affect the other[23-25]

The anterior and posterior iliac crests are the preferred sites from which BMB are obtained under local anaesthesia (Fig. 1.1). In addition, BMB are taken under radiological guidance and/or general anaesthesia from almost any skeletal area depending on the diagnostic requirements[26,27]. But when dealing with pathology of the haematopoietic system the preferred site is generally the ilium.

The anterior iliac crest is the site of choice for large BMB taken with the electric drill or for transilial, horizontal biopsies obtained with a wide-bore manual trephine (Fig. 1.2)[28-30]. The majority of BMB are taken with an 11 or 8 gauge trephine (2 or 3 mm width) from the posterior iliac crest. Their length varies greatly – up to 4–5 cms (Figs 1.3 and 1.4). This is because the needle is pushed between the two cortices and therefore there is no danger to the patient even when a long biopsy core is removed. In addition, large bone biopsies provide the possibility of performing multiparameter studies (Figs 1.5–1.7). In both the authors' laboratories the undecalcified biopsies are embedded in methyl-methacrylate and sections cut at 2–4 μm are stained by Giemsa, H&E, toluidine blue, PAS, Prussian blue, Ladewig and Gomori's stain as previously described[31,32]. Unless otherwise stated the illustrations in this atlas are of Giemsa-stained sections of plastic-embedded biopsies.

Biology of Bone Marrow

In addition to local skeletal differences such as in thickness of cortex and in trabecular width and density, and the topography of haematopoietic marrow in relation to age and possibly sex, the fact that the bone marrow is the organ which produces the mature blood cells must also be taken into account. All formed elements of the circulating blood have a finite life span and are constantly replenished by the bone marrow (Fig. 1.9)[33,34]. Therefore, the haematopoietic marrow itself is not a static organ and, within the confines of its bony cage, it can expand or contract as required by means of an increase or decrease in the proportion of adipose tissue present, as well as by changes in the microcirculation.

The term marrow cellularity, as generally used by haematologists, refers to the actively producing compartment and does *not* include the fat cells. Hence, a hypocellular or aplastic marrow is one in which the haematopoietic compartment has been partially or completely replaced by fat cells.

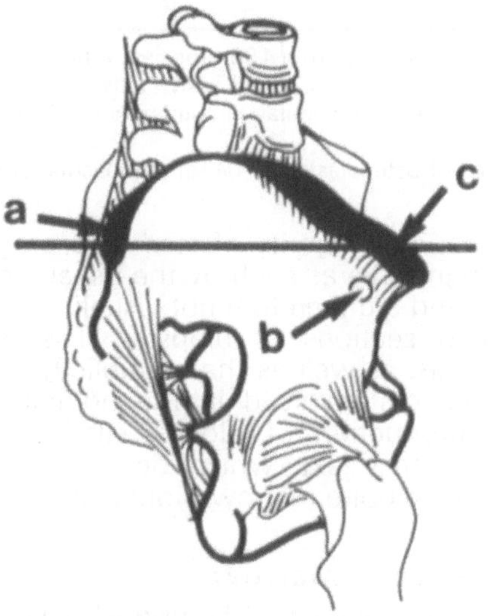

Fig. 1.1 Representation of lateral aspect of the pelvic bone; sites for different iliac crest biopsies: (**a**) Jamshidi or other manual trephine, such as the Islam needle (posterior iliac spine); (**b**) Bordier or other needle for transilial, horizontal biopsies (anterior iliac spine); (**c**) electric drill (anterior iliac crest) – thick horizontal line for orientation of the horizontal plane of the pelvis

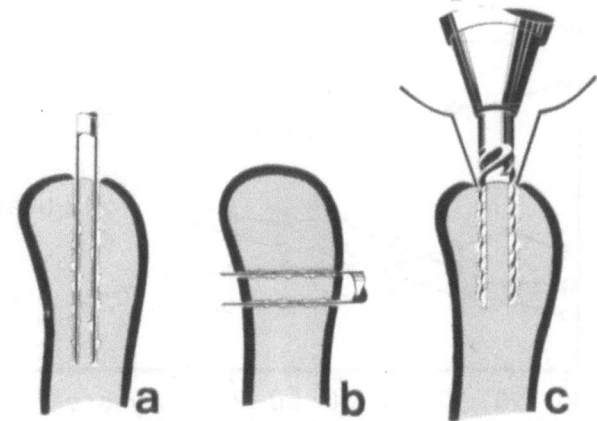

Fig. 1.2 Schematic representation of iliac crest: (**a**) 'vertical' biopsy, taken perpendicularly with the needle inserted between the two layers of compact, cortical bone; (**b**) transilial biopsy, taken horizontally to include both outer and inner compacta of the anterior ilium, **a** and **b**: biopsies taken with manual trephine only; (**c**) biopsy taken with electric drill, anterior ilium only.

Different bone marrow biopsy instruments used by haematologists: (**a**) Jamshidi needle or manual trephine, 2 or 3 mm core diameter, (**b**) Bordier or other transilial needle, 8 mm core diameter; (**c**) electric drill, 4 mm core diameter

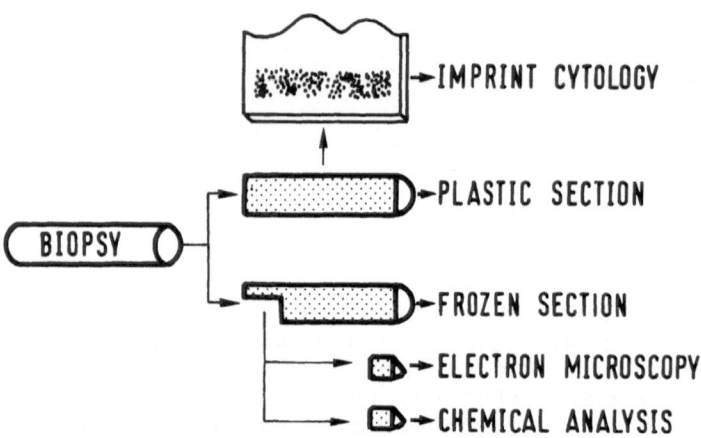

Fig. 1.6 Possibilities for processing biopsies: after cutting the biopsy, one half is used for plastic or paraffin histology and the other half is used for imprints (cytological details), cryostat sections (rapid diagnosis, immunohistology and histochemistry), EM and other techniques (chemical analysis)

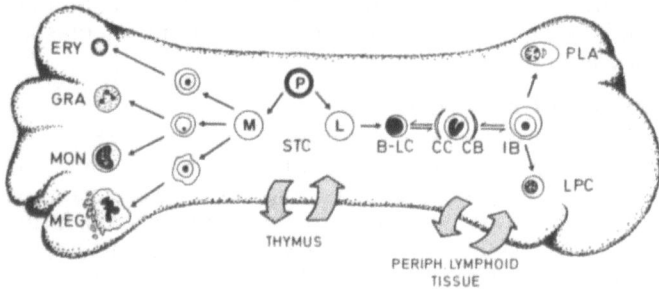

Fig. 1.9 Myeloid and lymphoid cell lines in the bone marrow: pluripotent stem cells (P) are recruited in the bone marrow for myeloid (M) differentiation, through the mediation of cell-specific 'poietins' and of the 'haematopoietic inductive microenvironment'. The differentiation of B lymphocytes (B-LC) to functional immunoglobulin-producing cells (PLA and LPC) proceeds in the peripheral lymphatic tissues. Pluripotent cells which have migrated from the marrow and settled in the thymus differentiate into T lymphocytes. STC = Stem cells; ERY = erythropoiesis; MON = monopoiesis; MEG = megakaryopoiesis; CB/CC = centroblastic/centrocytic cells; IB = immunoblast

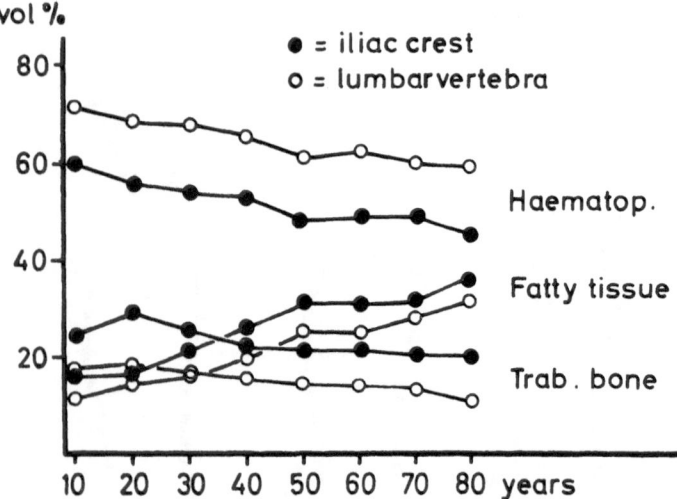

Fig. 1.10 Histomorphometric data from bone marrow biopsies, taken from the iliac crest (●) and lumbar vertebra (○) correlated with age (150 autopsy cases, non-haematological and non-osseous disorders)

A continuous supply of precursor cells is provided by the pluripotent stem cell compartment capable of self-renewal and also having the ability to differentiate into the progenitor cells committed to erythro-, granulo-, mono-, and megakaryopoiesis. The bone marrow is also a site for lymphopoiesis and maturation of plasma cells[35],

Table 1.1 Components in section of normal bone marrow biopsy

Bone
  Periosteal tissues
  Cortical bone
  Cancellous bone
  Endosteal cells
  Osteoblasts – osteoclasts – osteocytes

Haematopoiesis
  Erythroid precursors
  Myeloid precursors
  Megakaryocyte precursors

Stroma
  Fat cells
  Fibroblasts, fibres
  Blood vessels
  Histiocytes and variants
  Macrophages (+ iron)
  Lymphoid cells
  Plasma cells
  Mast cells

Table 1.2 Histomorphometry of bone and bone marrow[a]

Variables	Mean value (SD)		Dimension
Haematopoietic tissue	40	(9)	Vol %
Fatty tissue	28	(8)	
Trabecular bone	26	(5)	
Osteoid	0.3	(0.2)	
Sinusoids	4.5	(2.1)	
Lymphocytes (diffuse)	20	(12)	/mm²
Mast cells	2	(1)	
Megakaryocytes	8	(4)	
Macrophages			
(containing iron)	16	(10)	
Plasma cells	21	(18)	
Lymphoid nodules[b]	2		%
Arteries	3	(4)	/100 mm²
Arterioles	26	(18)	
Capillaries	101	(61)	
Sinusoids	1700	(825)	
Osteoblastic index (OB)[c]	5	(5)	%
Osteoclastic index (OC)[d]	4	(3)	/100 mm

[a] These values are derived from 158 biopsies of healthy individuals
[b] When present (seen more in older individuals)
[c] OB = percentage of trabecular circumference covered by cuboidal osteoblasts
[d] OC = number of osteoclasts per 100 mm trabecular circumference

however, the vast majority of stem and progenitor cells are not recognizable as such by the usual morphological techniques, and are therefore not visualized on smears of aspirates and sections of biopsies. The dynamics of haematopoiesis, as well as the multiplicity of interacting regulatory factors involved in the normal (as well as abnormal) production of blood cells[36,37], are beyond the scope of this text, which deals with the clinical interpretation of bone marrow biopsy findings.

The Normal Bone Marrow

The various components of the normal bone and marrow are listed in Tables 1.1 and 1.2, and the quantitative age-related changes in Fig. 1.10. A typical bone marrow biopsy section is illustrated in Fig. 1.11 and some of the variations that may be encountered are shown in Figs 1.11–1.18.

The most important pitfalls in histological diagnosis are: (1) histological variation within the biopsy (a) sub-

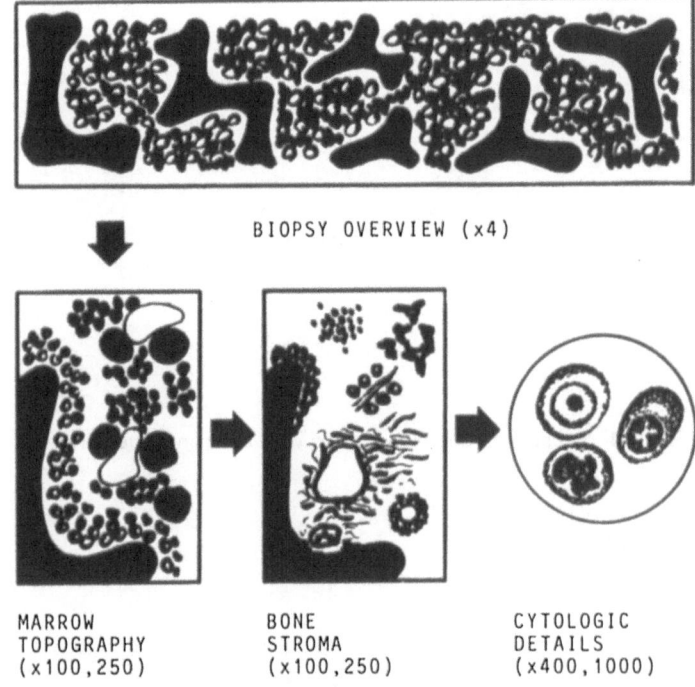

BIOPSY OVERVIEW (x4)

MARROW
TOPOGRAPHY
(x100,250)

BONE
STROMA
(x100,250)

CYTOLOGIC
DETAILS
(x400,1000)

Fig. 1.25 Evaluation of biopsy section for bone marrow report: overview of bone and marrow, architecture of marrow, topography of haematopoiesis, bone marrow stroma and cytological details. The magnifications given are those used for the photomicrographs in this text

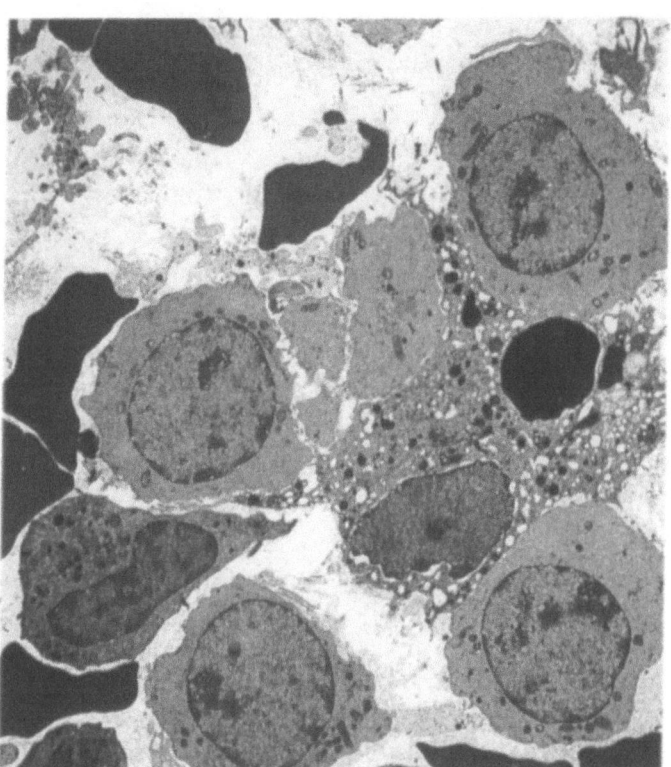

Fig. 1.31 Early erythroblasts around a macrophage. EM × 7000

cortical hypoplasia (Figs 1.11 and 1.12); (b) alternating fatty and hyperplastic areas in deeper parts of the biopsy and accumulation of one cell type in single intertrabecular areas (Figs 1.13–1.18); (2) non-representative tangentially taken biopsies (Figs 1.19–1.21); (3) presence of misleading artefacts – displaced pieces of epidermis, skeletal muscles, periosteal tissues, cartilage or bone, or blood and clots within the biopsy (Figs 1.22 and 1.23). Moreover, changes in haematopoietic cells due to technical factors should also be recognized – for example, swelling or shrinkage due to inadequate fixation, dehydration or impregnation with plastic embedding medium, and inadequate staining.

Diagnostic Evaluation

A systematic survey is made, beginning with a scan of the whole biopsy section at low power and ending with examination at high power, under oil if necessary, of individual cells and structures (Fig. 1.25). Though this text is concerned with haematopoietic tissue it is important to consider the bone and marrow together as a single system, because alterations in the one are almost invariably accompanied by changes in the other.

Topography and Bone Marrow Architecture

Haematopoiesis takes place in the extravascular marrow compartment. Early myeloid precursors occupy the paratrabecular regions close to the endosteal surface as well as the peri-arteriolar regions, while the more mature granulocytic cells are found in the central marrow areas (Figs 1.26–1.35). Erythroid islands and megakaryocytes are situated close to the sinusoids in the centres of the intertrabecular spaces (Figs 1.26–1.35). There are obviously many individual variations in the quantitative and qualitative distribution of the precursors of erythrocytes, granulocytes and megakaryocytes in the bone marrow. This topographic arrangement may be altered in hyperplastic and hypoplastic bone marrows and when osseous changes are present – such as trabecular osteopenia (osteoporosis).

Erythropoiesis

The erythron (Figs 1.29–1.30) consists of a cluster of erythroblasts at various maturational stages around a reticular cell (macrophage) whose long cytoplasmic processes extend between the red cell precursors (Fig. 1.31). This macrophage usually contains stainable iron and haemosiderin and some cellular and nuclear debris. It appears to play a supporting role in normal red cell production. Rarely, normoblasts in the process of extruding their nuclei may be observed, or normoblast nuclei within the cytoplasm of reticular cells or macrophages.

Myeloid precursors

Myeloblasts, promyelocytes, myelocytes, metamyelocyte bands and segmented forms of neutrophils, eosinophils and basophils are all seen in sections of the bone marrow. Some are illustrated in Figs 1.32–1.37.

Mast cells

Mast cells are thought to develop from the same precursors which produce the basophilic leucocytes[35]. They may be found adjacent to endothelial cells of sinusoids, at the endosteal surface, at the periosteum, in the walls of small arteries, scattered in the marrow and at the edges or within lymphoid aggregates or nodules. Mast cells may be oval or spindle-shaped, resembling fibroblasts, with only few cytoplasmic granules (Figs 1.38–1.40). Small aggregates of histiocytes and mast cells (fibrohistiocytic lesions) may be found occasionally; their significance is not known; they may be increased in infections, perhaps associated with stimulation of endothelial cells; or occur as a reaction to some drugs.

Monocytes, macrophages, and iron-containing reticular cells

Monocytes belong to the myeloid cell line but are not often identified as they are readily confused with granulocytic precursors having oval to kidney-shaped vesicular nuclei

(Continued on p. 18)

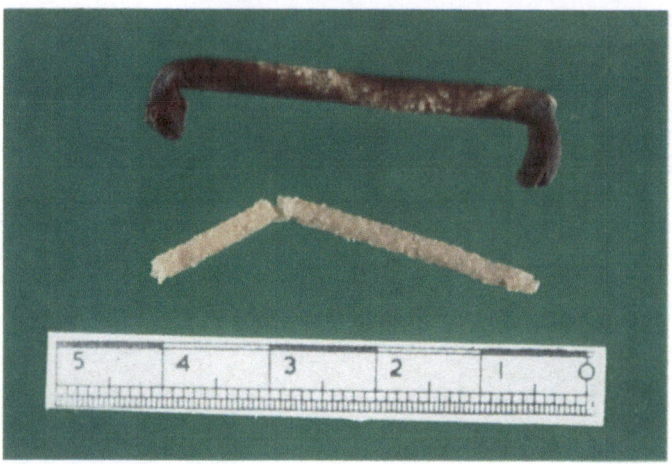

Fig. 1.3 Two biopsies taken with the manual trephine from the posterior ilium

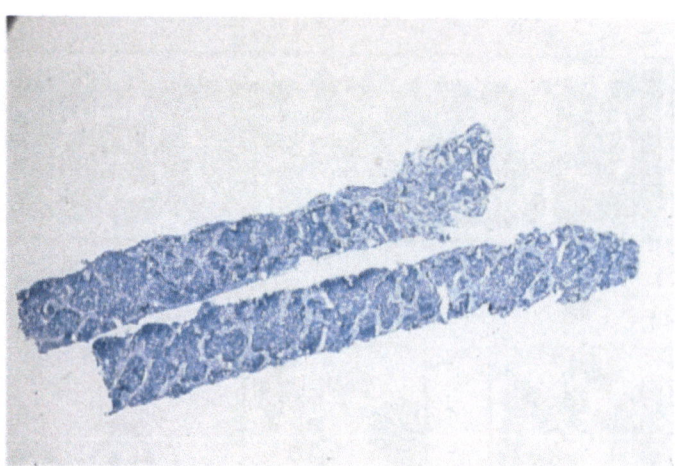

Fig. 1.4 Sections of one biopsy taken with the manual trephine

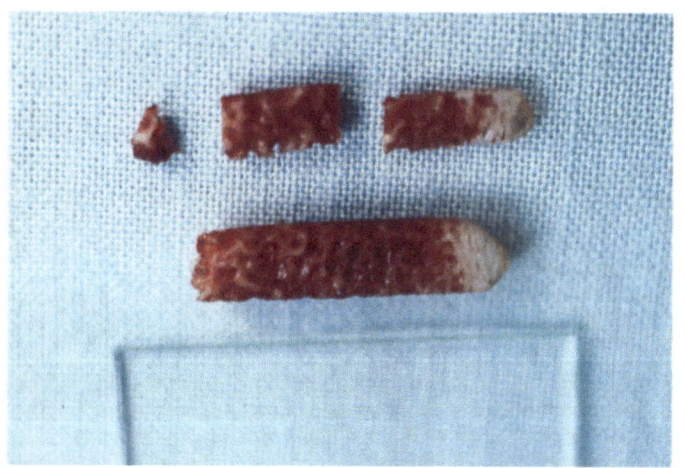

Fig. 1.5 Biopsy, 4 mm width, taken vertically with the electric drill as in Fig. 1.2, cut to enable multiparameter studies

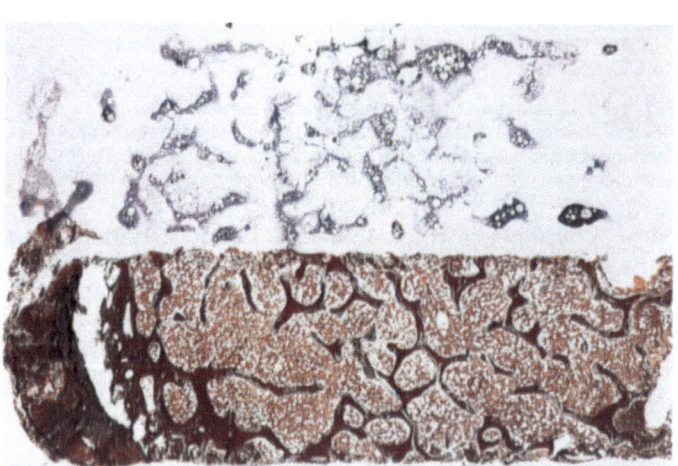

Fig. 1.7 Biopsy imprint for 'aspirate' cytology and section on the same slide, stained by Gomori's reticulin stain

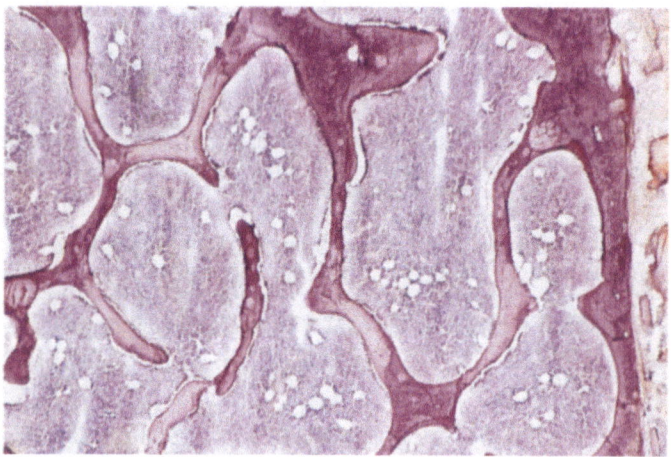

Fig. 1.8 Cryostat section, stained by H&E; note relatively good preservation of structure

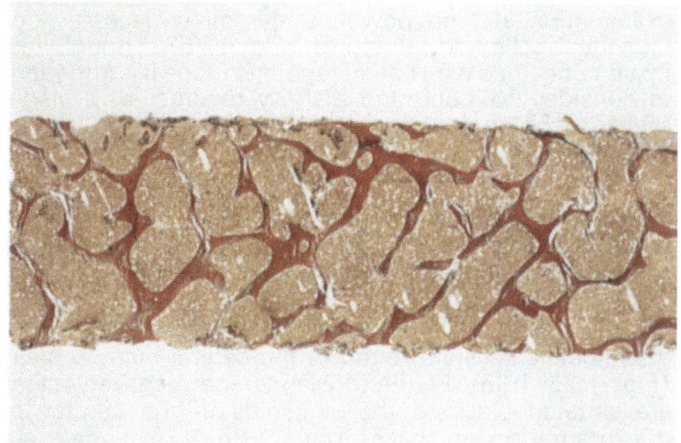

Fig. 1.9 Myeloid and lymphoid cell lines in the bone marrow: pluripotent stem cells (P) are recruited in the bone marrow for myeloid (M) differentiation, through the mediation of cell-specific 'poietins' and of the 'haematopoietic inductive microenvironment'. The differentiation of B lymphocytes (B-LC) to functional immunoglobulin-producing cells (PLA and LPC) proceeds in the peripheral lymphatic tissues. Pluripotent cells which have migrated from the marrow and settled in the thymus differentiate into T lymphocytes. STC = Stem cells; ERY = erythropoiesis; MON = monopoiesis; MEG = megakaryopoiesis; CB/CC = centroblastic/centrocytic cells; IB = immunoblast

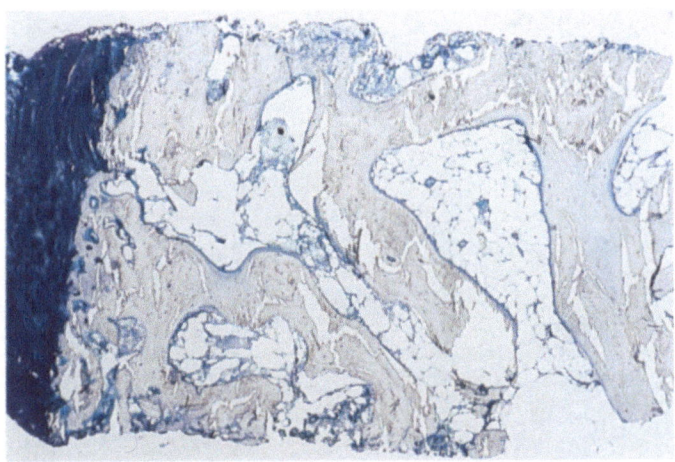

Fig. 1.12 Periosteal tissues, cortical bone and subcortical marrow consisting of fat cells in bone biopsy of 60-year-old patient without haematological disorders

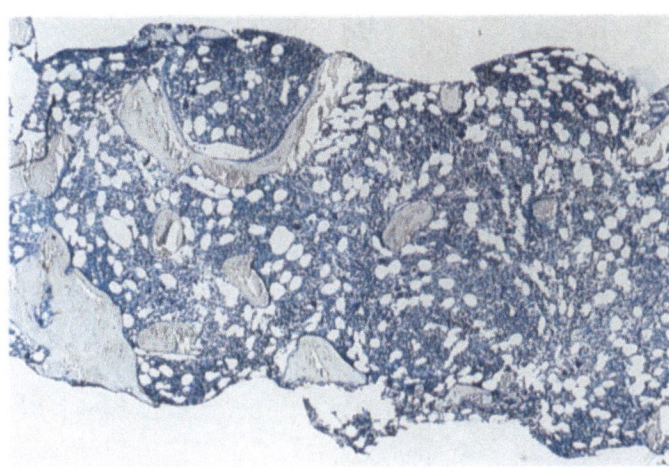

Fig. 1.13 Deeper part of the same biopsy as in Fig. 1.11, normocellular bone marrow. Note progressive decrease in trabecular network and thickness of the ossicles

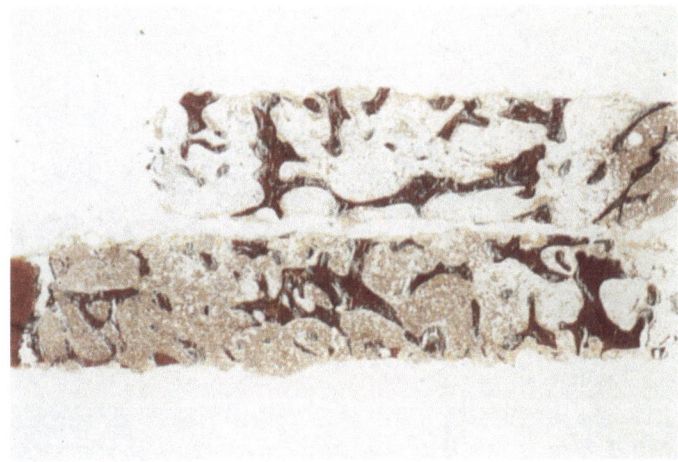

Fig. 1.14 Shows patchy replacement by fat cells in different parts of the biopsy, alternating with cellular areas. Gomori

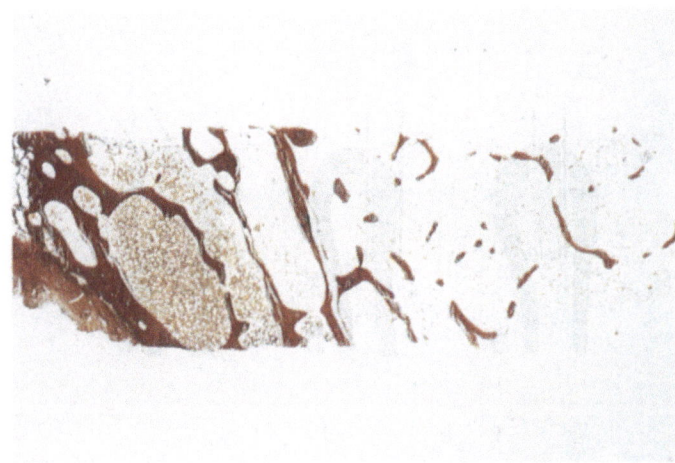

Fig. 1.15 Subcortical haematopoiesis with fatty replacement in deeper areas. Gomori

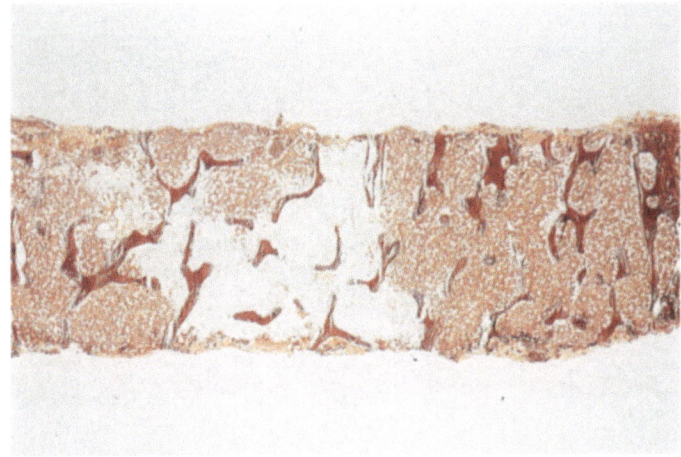

Fig. 1.16 Area of fatty marrow alternating with hypercellular areas. Gomori

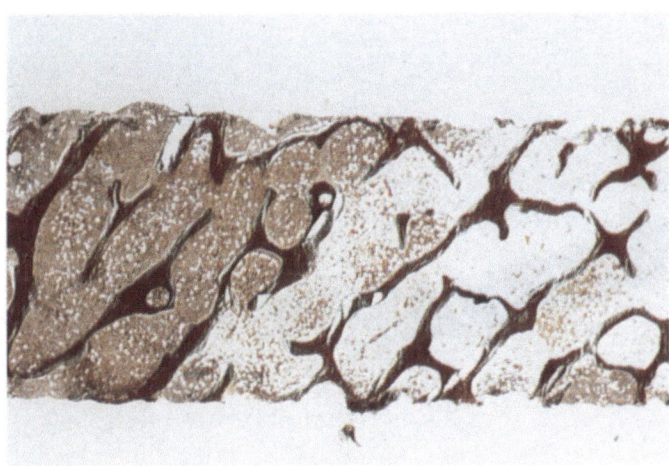

Fig. 1.17 Variations in bone marrow cellularity. Gomori

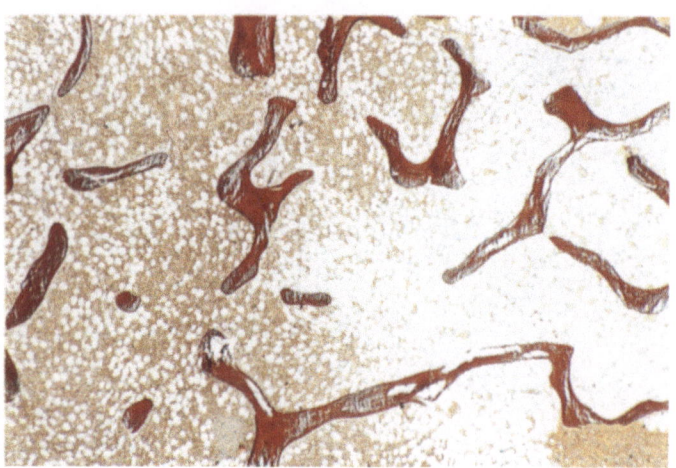

Fig. 1.18 Section showing transition between normal and hypocellularity. Gomori

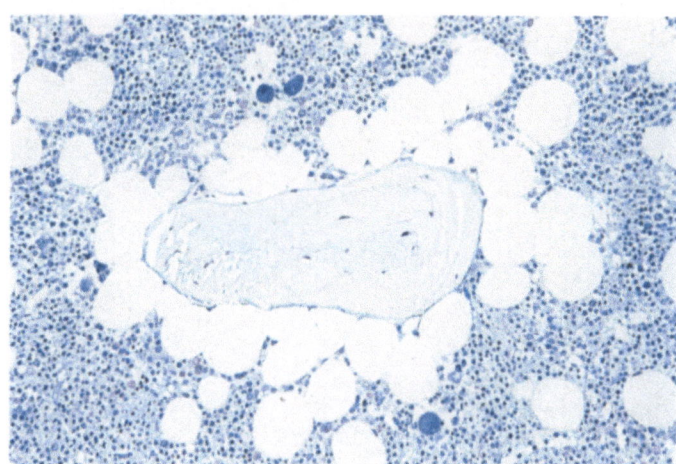

Fig. 1.19 Paratrabecular layers of fat cells with cellular bone marrow between them

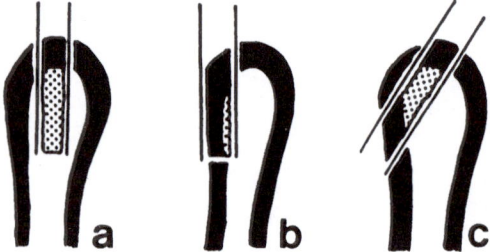

Fig. 1.20 Variations encountered in the biopsy sections, due to the angle or direction of the biopsy needle: (**a**) vertical and between the cortical plates of the ilium; (**b**) vertical, but including one cortex instead of the cancellous bone between the cortices; (**c**) tangential, thereby penetrating the cortical bone twice

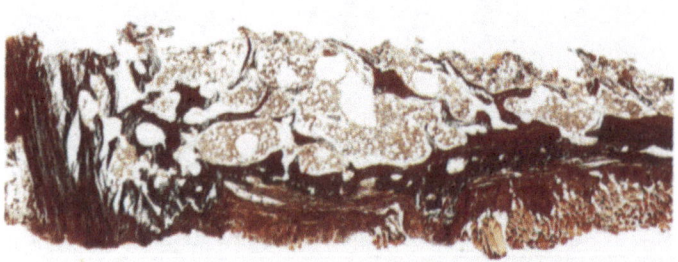

Fig. 1.21 Tangentially taken biopsy containing disproportionate amounts of periosteal tissues and cortical bone and only subcortical (possibly non-representative) bone marrow. Gomori

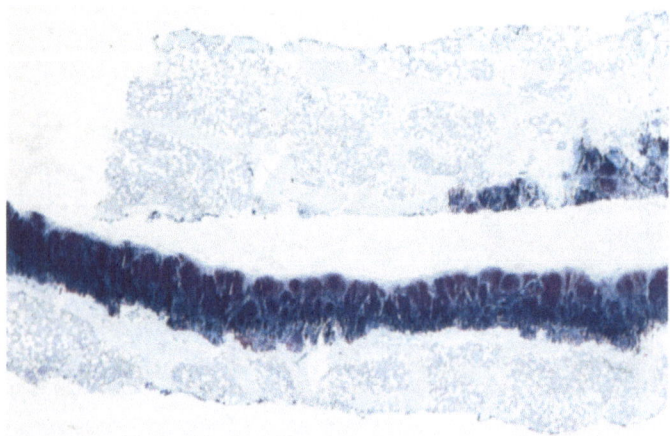

Fig. 1.22 Tangential biopsy including a layer of cartilage and only a small amount of bone marrow.

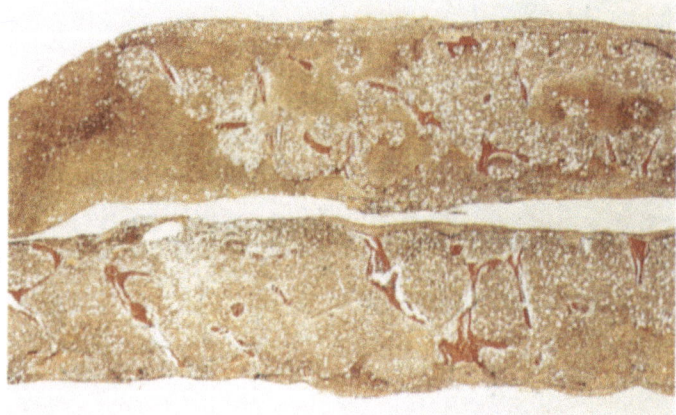

Fig. 1.23 Bone biopsy containing areas of haemorrhage and surrounded by blood. Gomori

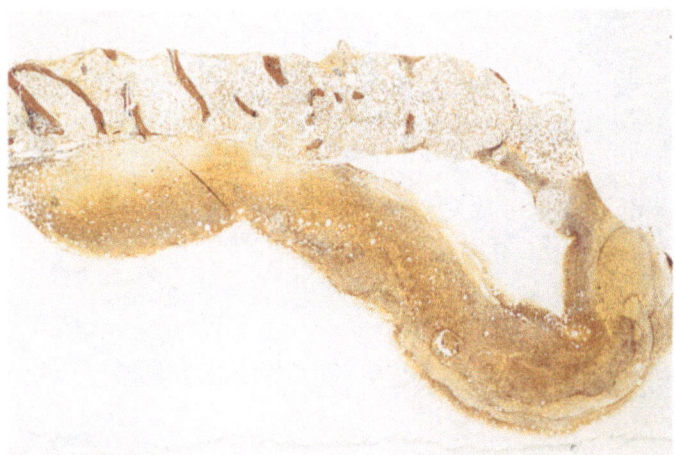

Fig. 1.24 Half of this apparently long biopsy consists of blood clot. Gomori

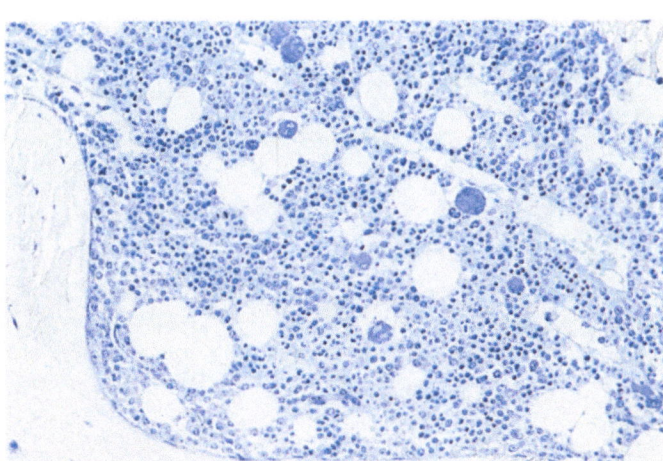

Fig. 1.26 Topography of normal bone marrow in a marrow space, paratrabecular area

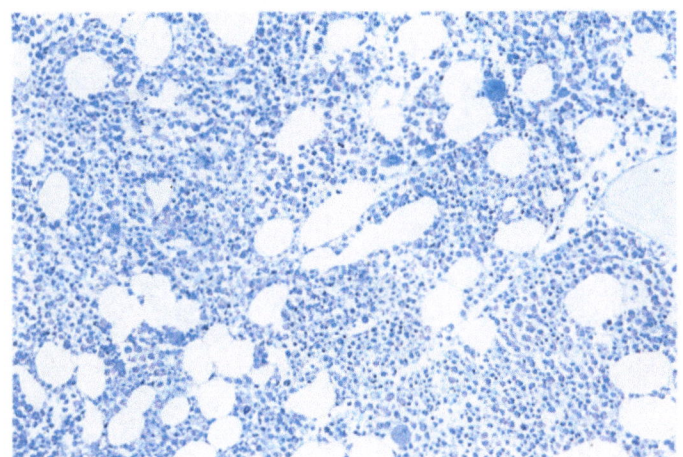

Fig. 1.27 Topography of normal bone marrow, central area

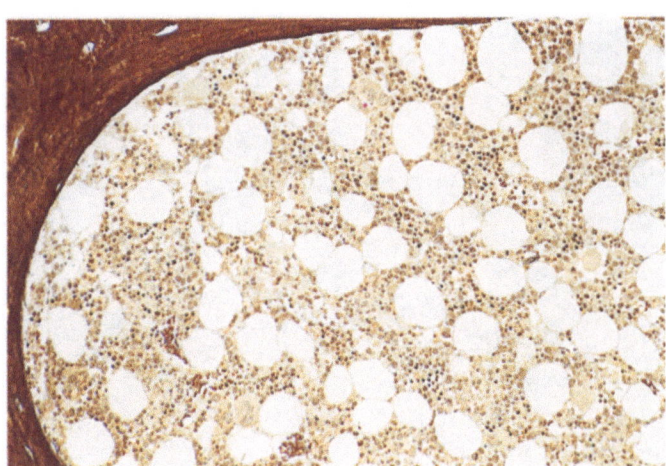

Fig. 1.28 Normal cellular bone marrow. Gomori, few fibres present

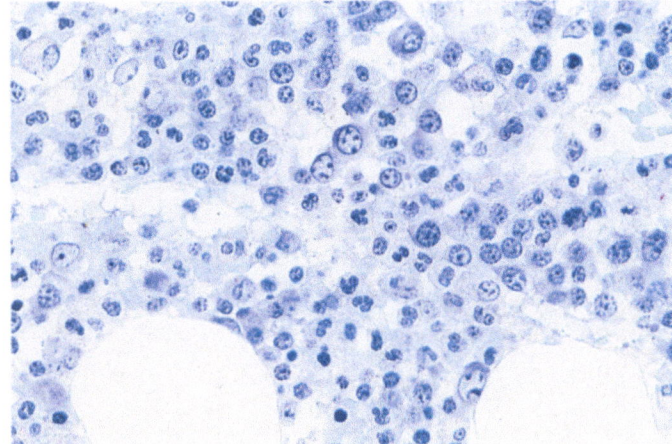

Fig. 1.29 Granulopoiesis at different maturational stages, and erythropoiesis, centre right side

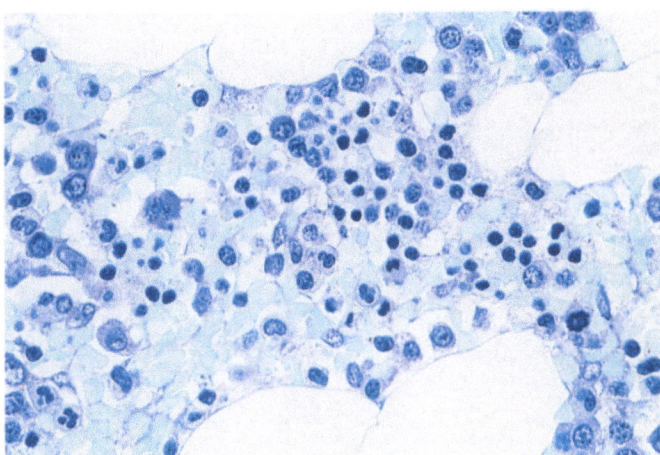

Fig. 1.30 Eythropoiesis in central marrow area, on right

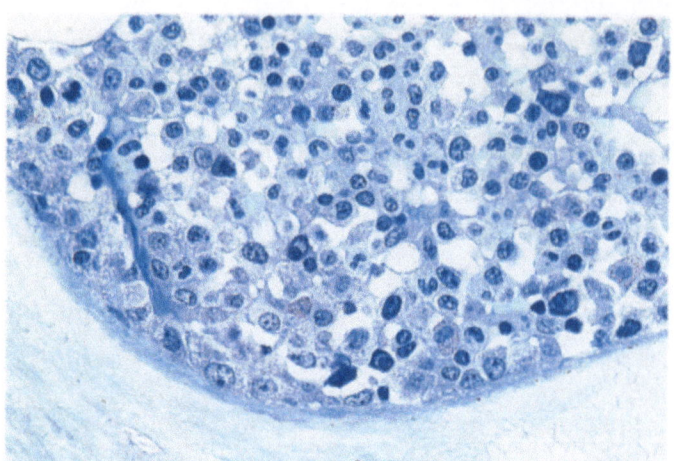

Fig. 1.32 Paratrabecular granulopoiesis. Note promyelocytes at endosteal surface

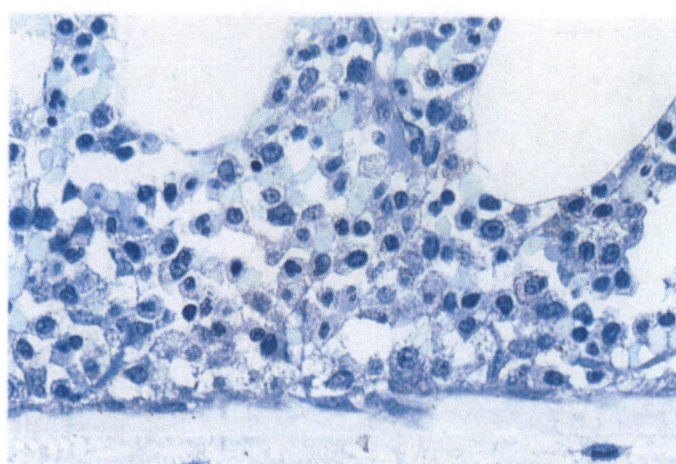

Fig. 1.33 Narrow granulopoietic seam at trabecular surface

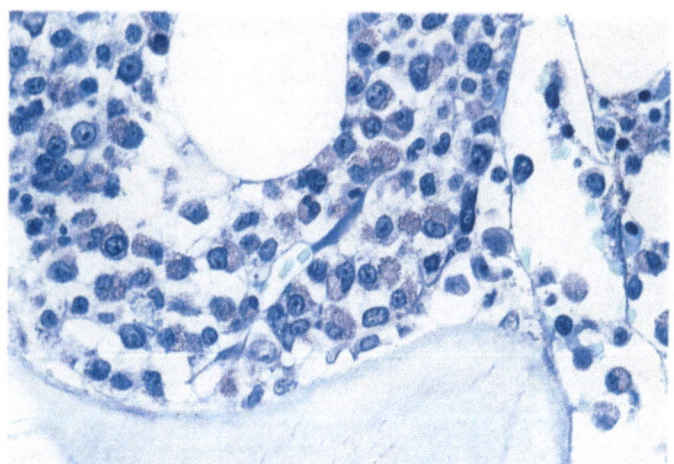

Fig. 1.34 Granulopoiesis, predominantly eosinophilic

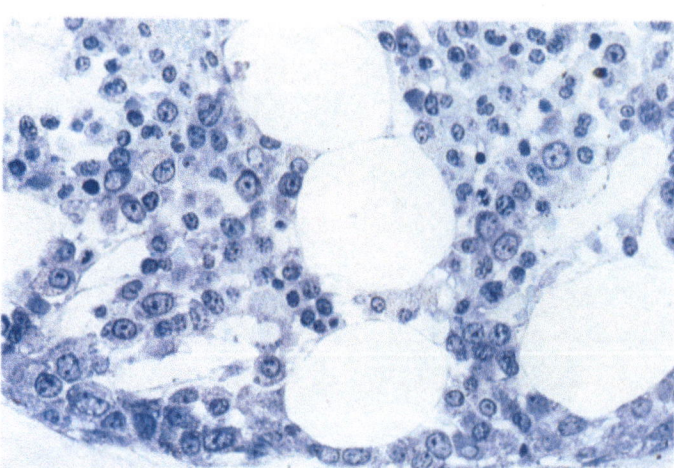

Fig. 1.35 Immature precursors of granulopoiesis extending from endosteal surface into marrow space

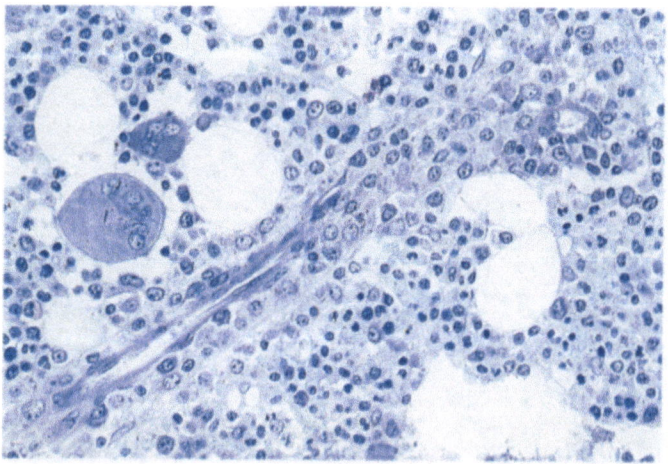

Fig. 1.36 Arteriole surrounded by immature myeloid cells. Note megakaryocytes at left and erythropoiesis at right and lower centre

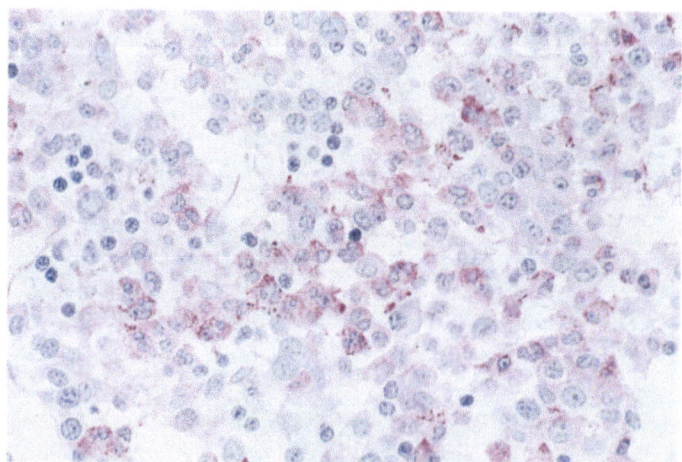

Fig. 1.37 Bone biopsy section stained by PAS for glycoproteins; note reaction in myeloid elements, none in the erythroid cells

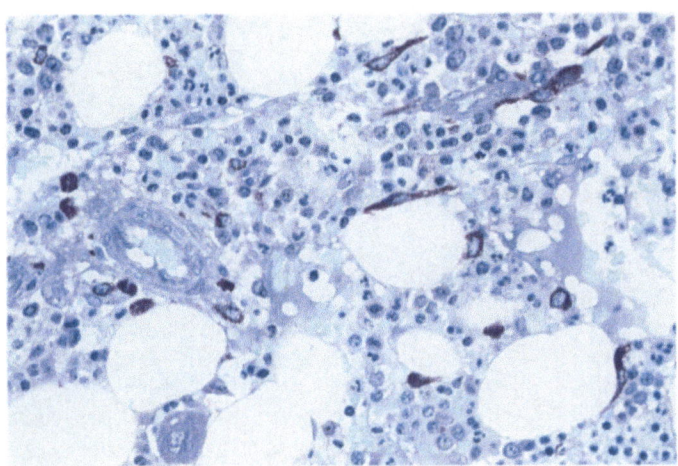

Fig. 1.38 Note elongated fibroblast-like mast cells among haematopoietic cells

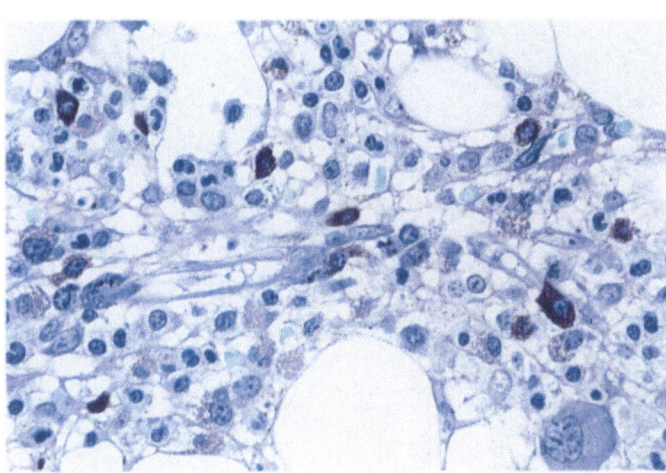

Fig. 1.39 Mast cells in marrow interstitium and around a capillary

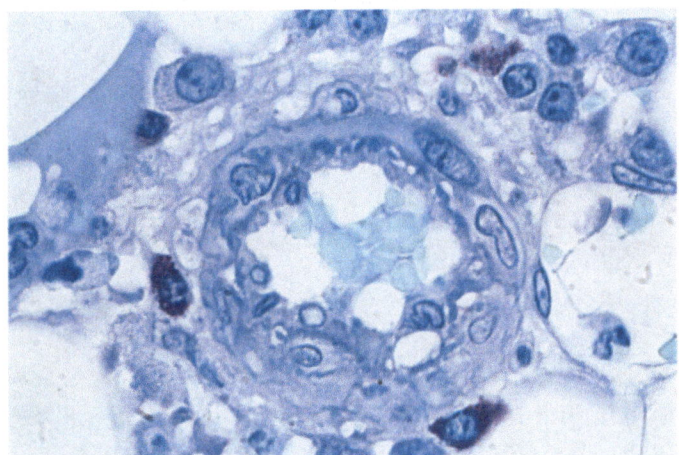

Fig. 1.40 Periarteriolar mast cells

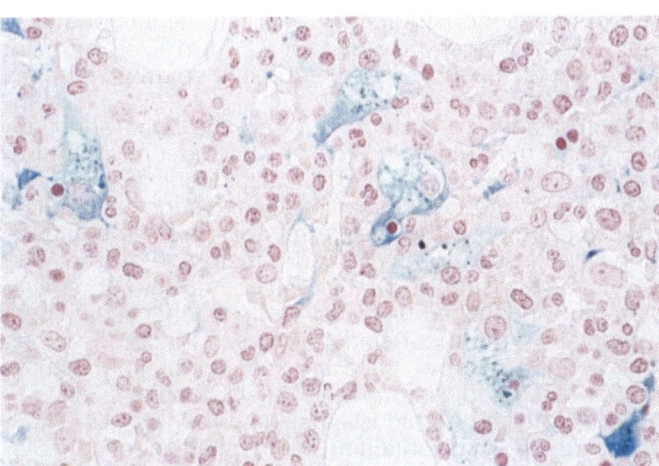

Fig. 1.41 Bone biopsy section stained by Prussian blue for demonstration of distribution and quantity of iron-containing cells in normal bone marrow

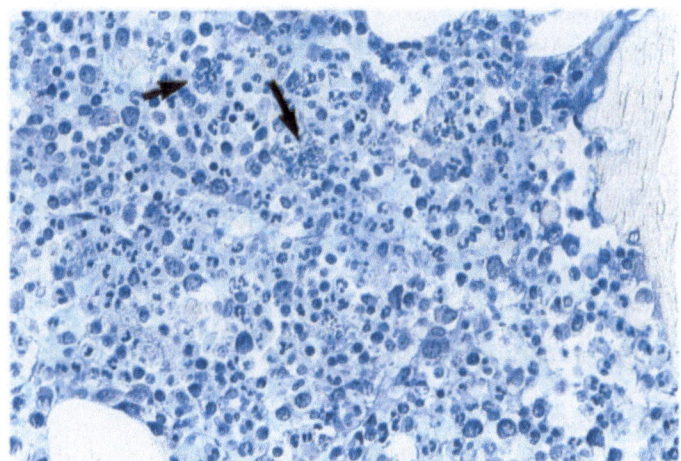

Fig. 1.42 Macrophages containing cellular debris (arrowed)

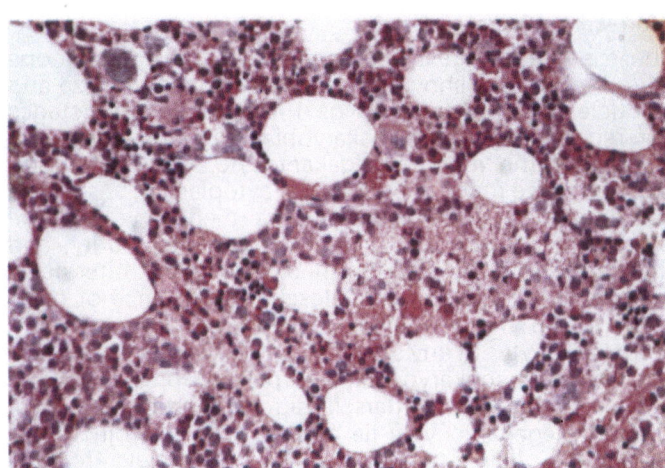

Fig. 1.44 Paraffin-embedded bone biopsy of patient with myeloid hyperplasia and numerous macrophages, PAS

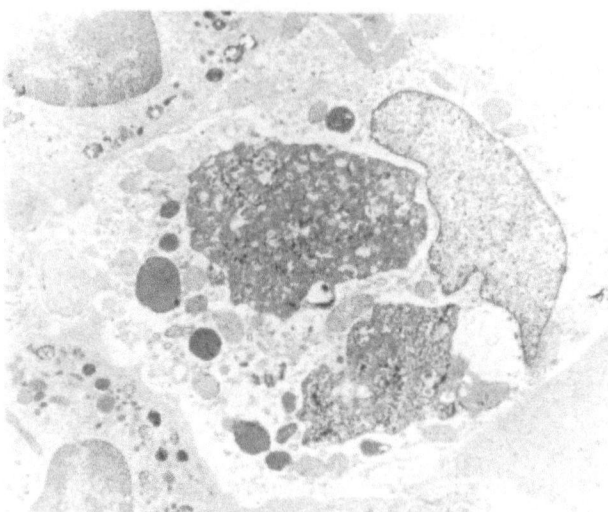

Fig. 1.43   Macrophage containing cellular debris. EM × 20 000

and abundant cytoplasm with variable granulation. They are recognized in greater quantities in immune histology than in conventional paraffin- or plastic-embedded sections. Macrophages may be derived from fixed reticular cells, from precursors of the granulocyte–monocyte series or from mature monocytes.

Macrophages (or histiocytes) may be large and their cytoplasm may contain iron, haemosiderin, granules, vacuoles, lipid, cellular and nuclear debris (Figs 1.41–1.48). These monocyte–macrophage–histiocytic (reticular) cells comprise the system responsible for the elimination of senescent red cells and the storage of iron. The iron is demonstrable by the Prussian blue or similar technique and the ferritin by immunohistochemistry. There is generally a good correlation between the two[38]. In the normal bone marrow there are iron-containing macrophages scattered among the haematopoietic cells – especially near erythroid islands – and the fat cells. There are about 16 iron-containing macrophages (or reticular cells) per mm^2 of bone marrow. Lipomacrophages, foam cells, 'Gaucher' cells or pseudo-Gaucher cells, and sea-blue histiocytes are also thought to develop out of reticular, adventitial, or even endothelial cells. Epithelioid and giant cells are presumed to be derived from the monocyte series by endomitosis, by fusion or by coalescence (Figs 1.44–1.48).

Megakaryocytes

These are the largest cells present in the normal bone marrow, but they show considerable variation in size and in nuclear configuration (Figs 1.49–1.61). Three stages are recognized: the megakaryoblast, the pro-megakaryocyte and the mature megakaryocyte. On progression through these maturational stages cytoplasmic basophilia decreases, so that in the mature megakaryocyte the cytoplasm is eosinophilic with variable granularity, and three zones may be distinguished: perinuclear, intermediate and marginal[39]. Emperipolesis (the presence of other cells within megakaryocyte cytoplasm) may occur in megakaryocytes of any size, but is more frequent in mature ones, when megakaryocyte hyperplasia is present, and in myeloproliferative disorders. Its significance is not known. Mature megakaryocytes lie adjacent to, or project into, the lumina of sinusoids into which the platelets are shed and/or the megakaryocytes migrate.

Lymphocytes

Lymphoid cells belong to the normal marrow population, are dispersed singly among haematopoietic and fat cells, or in aggregates or lymphoid nodules which may be found

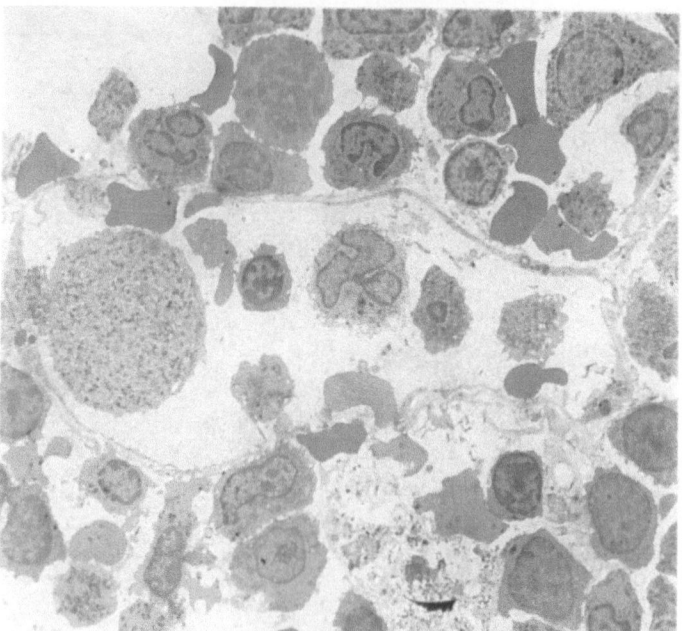

Fig. 1.58   Portion of megakaryocyte cytoplasm jutting into sinusoidal lumen. EM × 5000

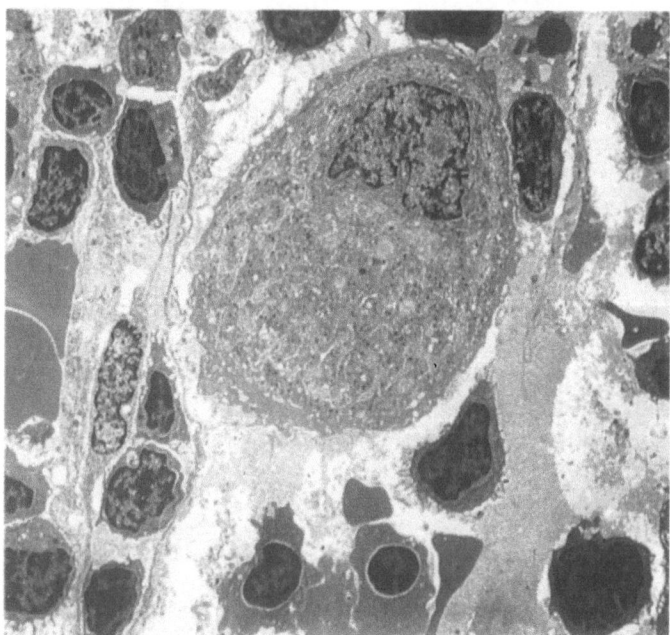

Fig. 1.59   Mature megakaryocyte in sinus. EM × 7000

in 1% to over 40% of bone biopsies, particularly in the older age groups (Figs 1.62 and 1.63). Four types have been described: (1) nodules with germinal centres, (2) sharply demarcated nodules, (3) nodules with irregular borders, (4) small aggregates of lymphoid cells (Figs 1.64–1.73). Though there is generally no difficulty in recognizing lymphoid cells in sections of plastic-embedded biopsies, immunohistology is required for identification of T and B cells and for quantitative estimates of lymphoid cells in the bone marrow (Fig 1.74)[40].

Plasma Cells

These represent the final maturational stage of the B lymphocyte; this process possibly takes place in the bone marrow as well as in other tissues (Fig 1.75). Plasma cells lie in close apposition to walls of small blood vessels but may also be found singly and in groups of two or three scattered among the haematopoietic elements (Fig 1.76–1.79).

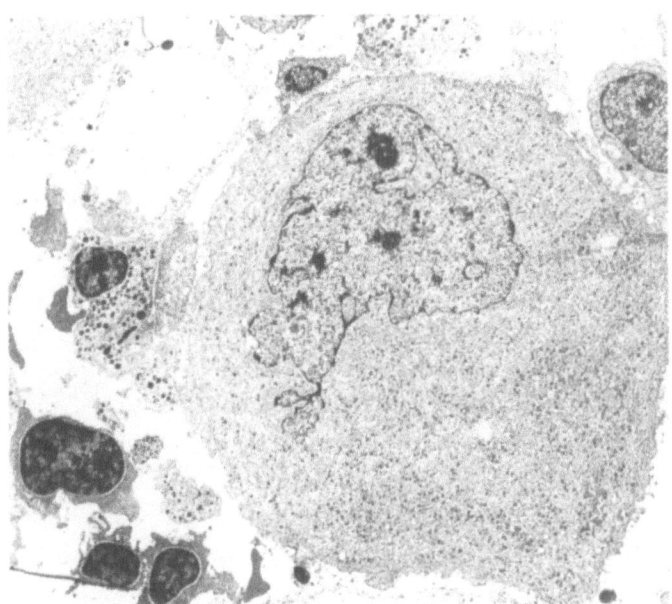

Fig. 1.60 Configuration of megakaryocyte nucleus and platelet fields in cytoplasm of mature megakaryocyte. EM × 20 000

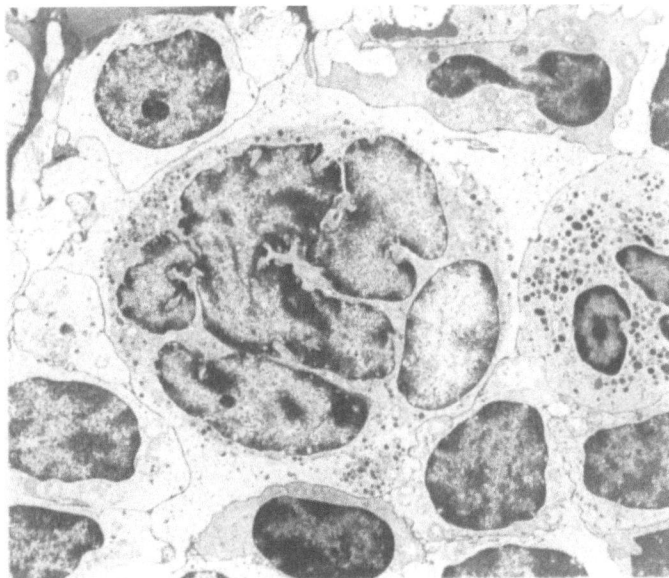

Fig. 1.61 Senescent megakaryocyte with naked nucleus. EM × 25 000

Bone marrow stroma

This forms the framework which supports the extravascular haematopoietic compartment and constitutes the bone marrow haematopoietic microenvironment[41-47]. It consists of reticular cells, fat cells, fibroblasts and their fibrils, the network of blood vessels and sinusoids. The close association between the mesenchymal elements – the endothelium of blood vessels, the endosteal lining cells, osteoblasts and osteoclasts, reticular cells and macrophages – has induced much speculation and experimental work on their possible origins and capabilities of transformation.

The normal bone marrow contains few fibres (Fig. 1.80), found mainly in apposition to blood vessels and endosteum (Figs 1.81–1.84). The medullary arteries, accompanied by nerve fibres (Figs 1.85 and 1.86), enter through the cortical bone (Fig. 1.87 and 1.88) and branch within the trabeculae and the marrow (Figs 1.89 and 1.90), forming arterioles and capillaries which lead into the sinusoids (Figs 1.91 and 1.92) and which in turn drain into the periosteal veins (Figs 1.93–1.97). At any one time, some of these sinusoids may be collapsed and

therefore difficult to identify in ordinary sections. The expansion and contraction of the vascular system, together with increases or decreases in fat cells, accompany the fluctuations in the amount of haematopoietic tissue within the rigid bony cage of which the marrow is capable. This contributes to the great variety in amount and proportion of haematopoietic tissue and fat cells seen in the 'normal' range in sections of bone biopsies. Moreover, there is also considerable variability in the apparent amount of stromal elements present. The components of the bone marrow stroma are usually more readily seen in marrows with a greater proportion of fat cells to haematopoietic tissue and in pathological conditions. Nerves are rarely found in the bone marrow; one is illustrated in Figs 1.85 and 1.86.

Bone Cells

These include the flat endosteal cells which line the subcortical and trabecular surfaces, and which often appear to become higher, and more cuboidal when they merge with osteoblasts (Figs 1.98–1.101)[48,49]. They are also frequently contiguous with osteoclasts and endothelial cells. The osteoblasts are the bone cells which form the matrix which is subsequently ossified, and during this process some are trapped within the bone and converted into osteocytes (Figs 1.102–1.106). These form an interconnected network both within the bone and to its surface, by means of their long cytoplasmic extensions bnwithin the canaliculi. The osteoclasts, the bone-resorbing cells, are thought to arise from precursors of a haematopoietic cell line, while osteoblasts develop from precursors of the bone marrow stroma[50].

Osteoclasts may be uni-, bi-, tri- or multinuclear (Figs 1.107–1.111); they are generally elongated and are found on or near the surface of a bone, often next to osteoblasts or endothelial cells. When multinucleated they may become even larger than megakaryocytes. The cytoplasm is pink and may contain granules or vacuoles. The ruffled border seen in the electron microscope is not visible in the light microscope (Figs 1.112–1.114).

Histomorphometry

With the introduction of semi-automatic and of computerized systems for the quantitation of bone marrow compartments and elements, as well as of bone and dynamic parameters of osseous remodelling, histomorphometry has gained in popularity[51]. However, it is not generally required for the interpretation and diagnosis of bone

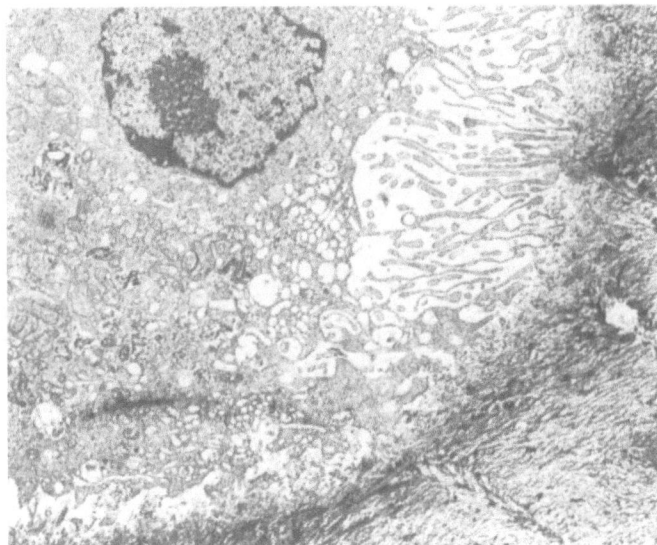

Fig. 1.112 Active osteoclast in erosion cavity. Note ruffled membrane. EM × 20 000

(Continued on p. 31)

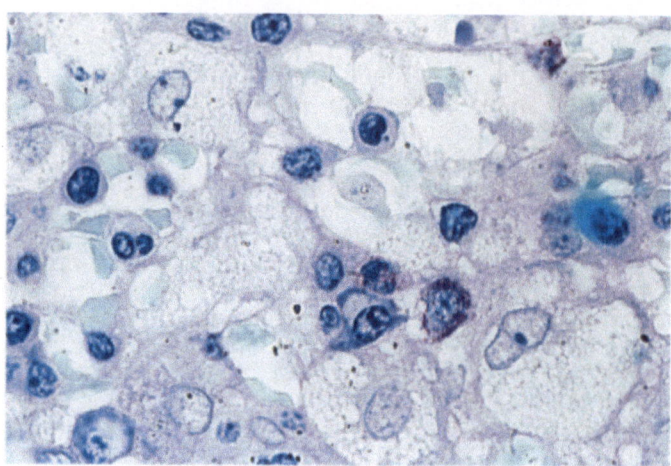

Fig. 1.45   Aggregate of lipomacrophages

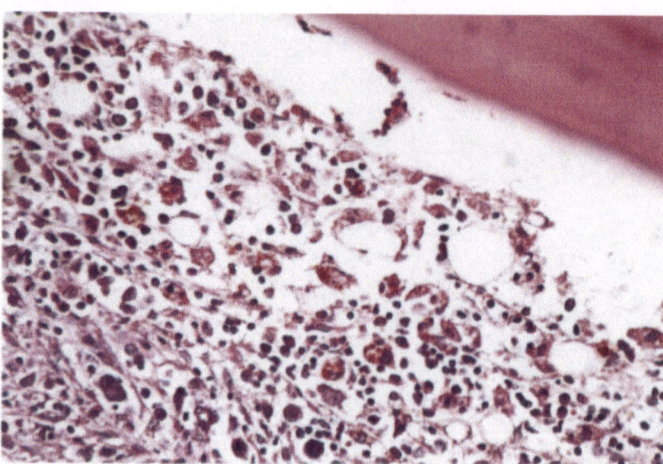

Fig. 1.46   Section of paraffin-embedded bone biopsy of patient with Hodgkin's disease with marrow involvement. Note numerous macrophages, PAS and Hodgkin cell, lower right

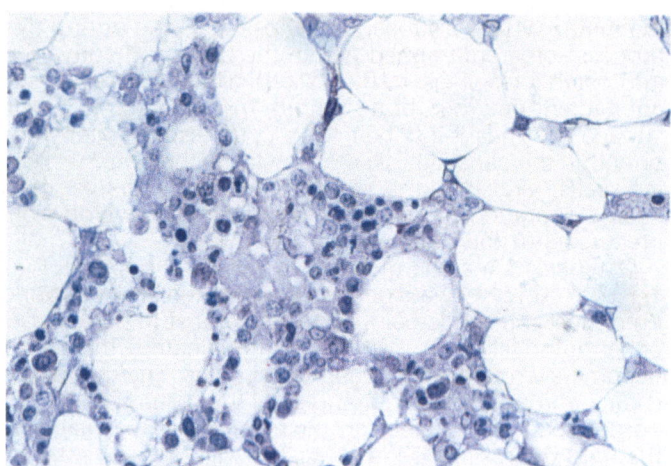

Fig. 1.47   Macrophage aggregate in hypocellular bone marrow

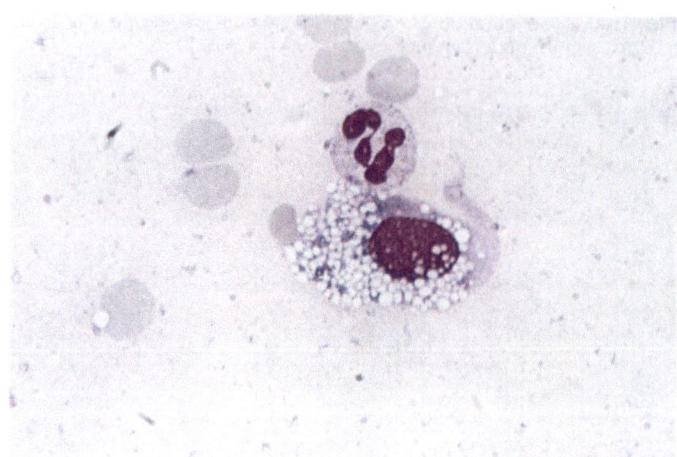

Fig. 1.48   Vacuolated foam cell in smear of bone marrow aspirate

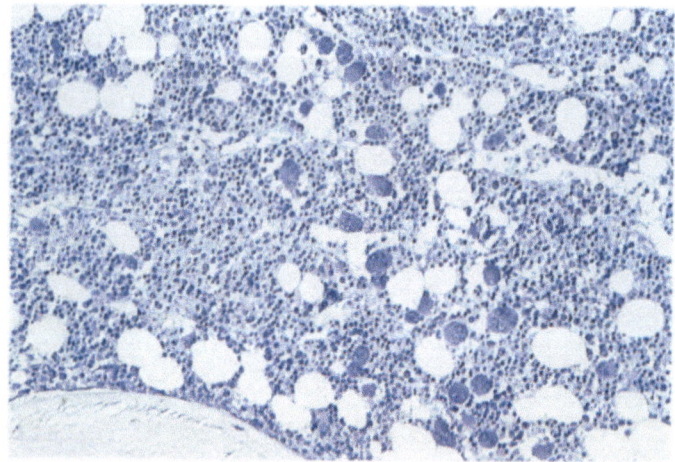

Figs 1.49 to 1.57   These figures illustrate range in megakaryocyte size, shape and nuclear configuration that may be encountered in normal bone marrows; note also variations in quantity

Fig. 1.49   Overview of megakaryocytes in marrow space

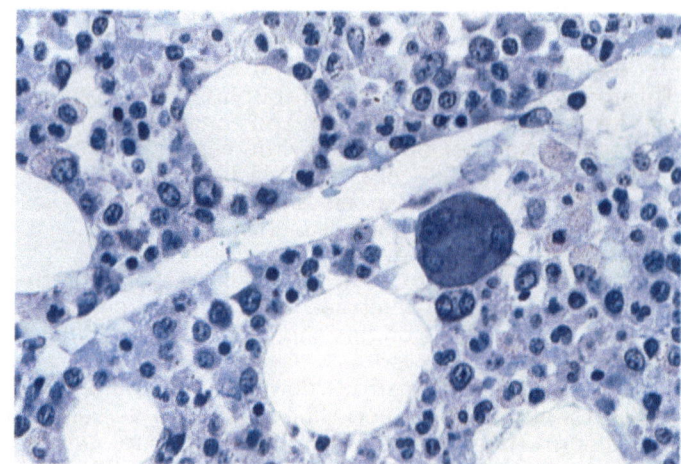

Fig. 1.50   Megakaryocyte adjacent to a small sinusoid

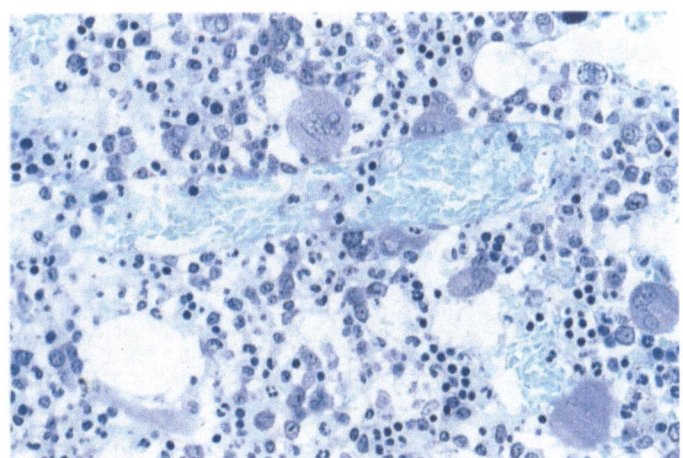

Fig. 1.51 Megakaryocytes at sinusoidal endothelium

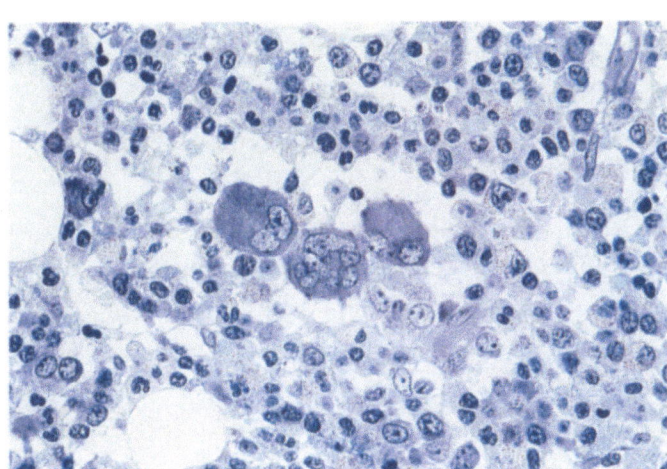

Fig. 1.52 Maturing megakaryocytes in interstitium

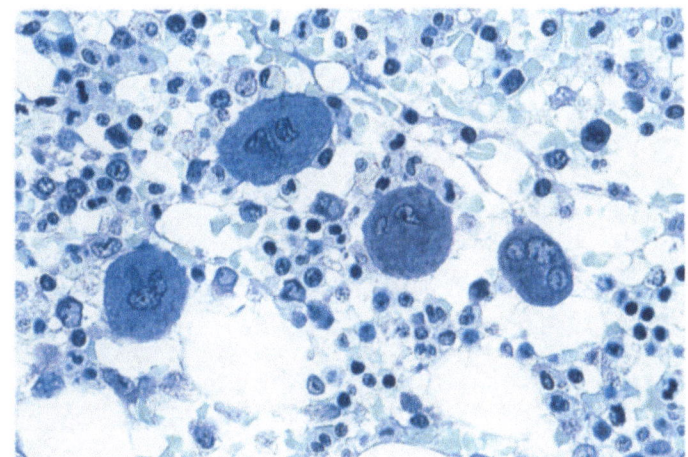

Fig. 1.53 Note range in nuclear configuration

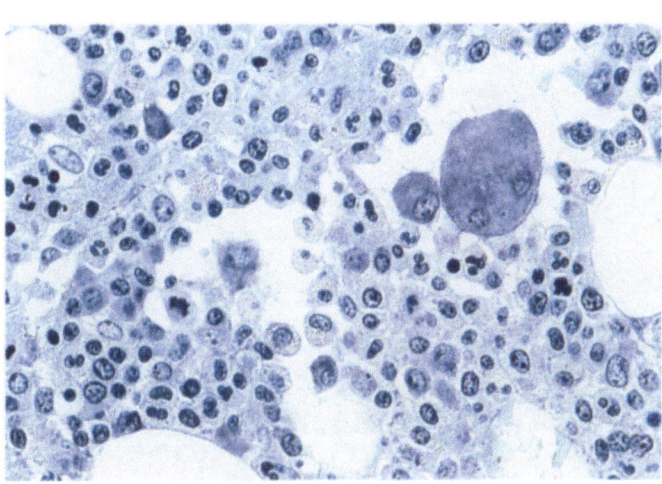

Fig. 1.54 Range in megakaryocyte size

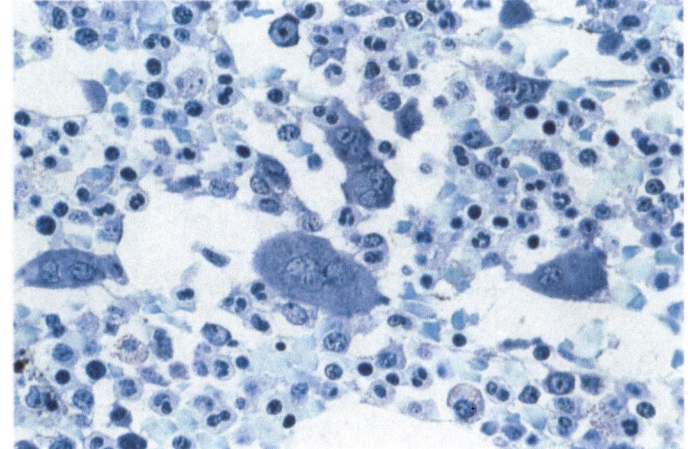

Fig. 1.55 Cluster of small megakaryocytes

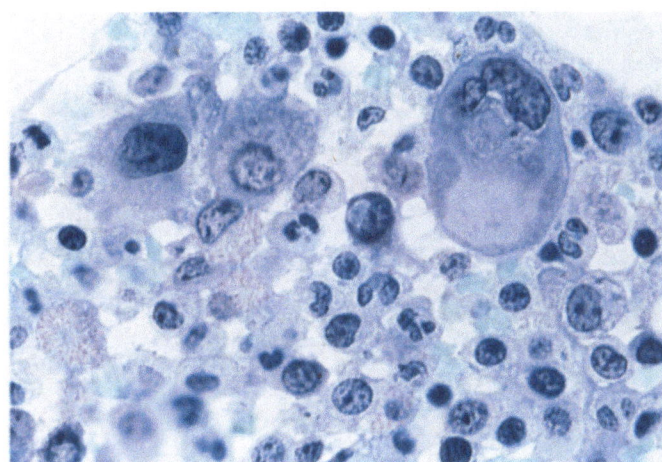

Fig. 1.56 Variably stained areas in megakaryocyte cytoplasm

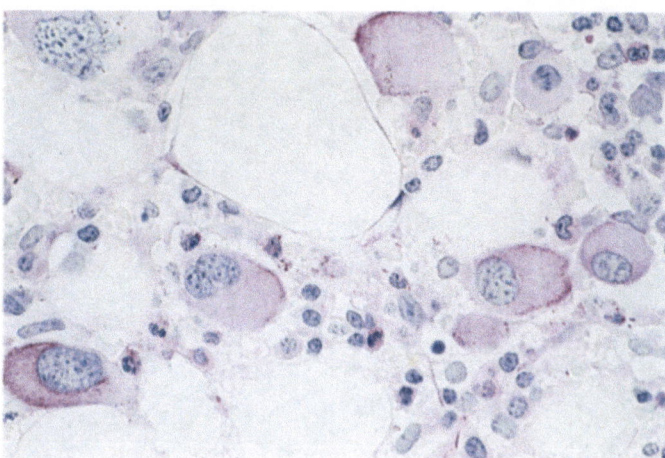

Fig. 1.57   Bone biopsy section stained by PAS; megakaryocytes show a variable reaction from pink cytoplasm to dark red intracellular granules

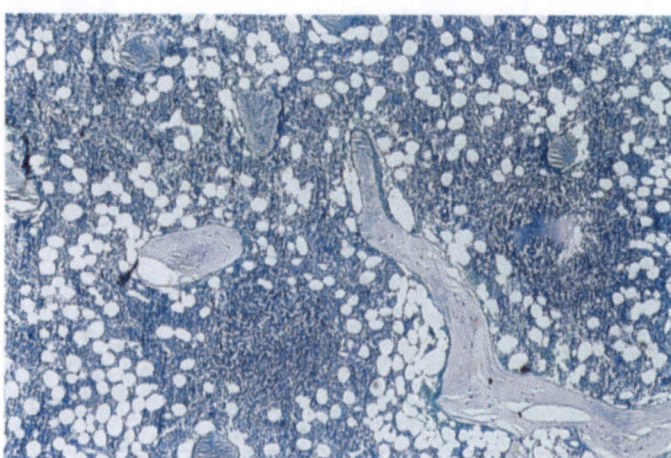

Figs 1.62–1.74   These figures illustrate the range of lymphoid tissues that may be seen in bone biopsies of individuals without any disorders affecting the haematopoietic or lymphopoietic systems

Fig. 1.62   Lymphoid nodules in normocellular bone marrow

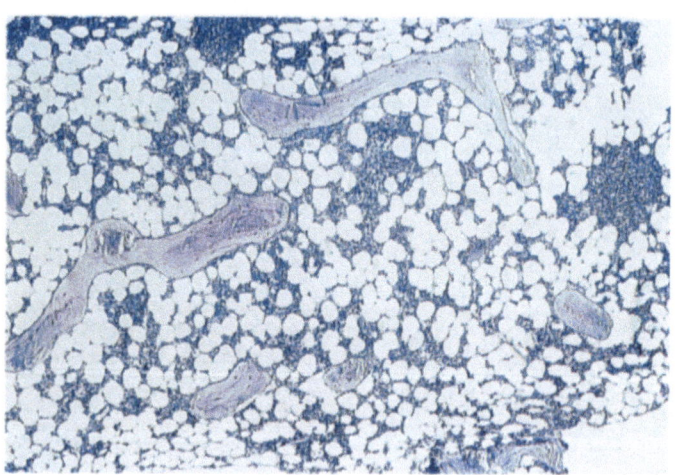

Fig. 1.63   Lymphoid nodules in hypocellular bone marrow

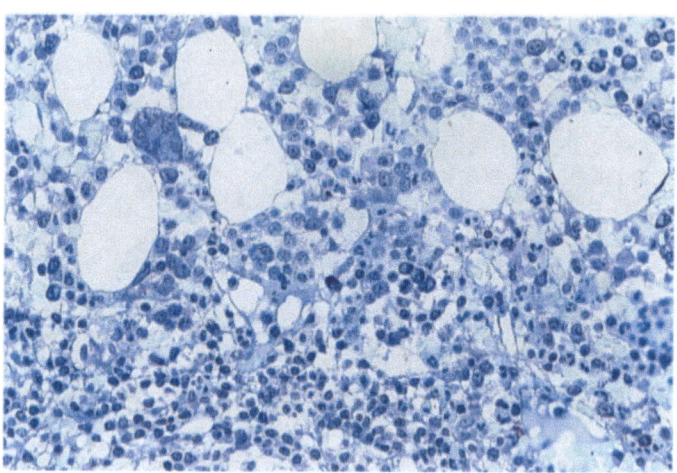

Fig. 1.64   Interstitial lymphoid cells in the bone marrow

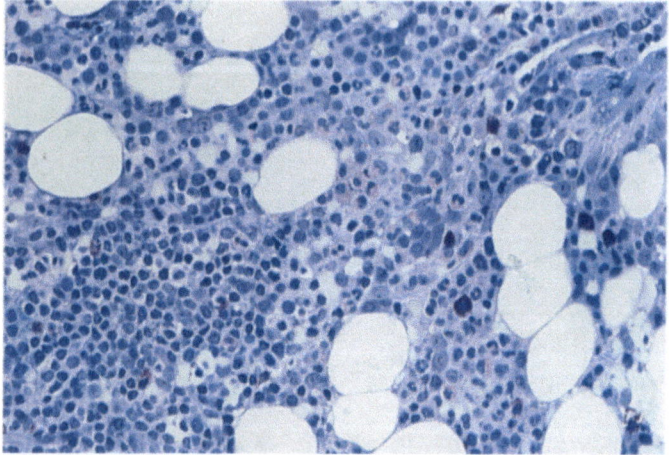

Fig. 1.65   Lymphoid cell aggregate easily identified in plastic histology (lower left)

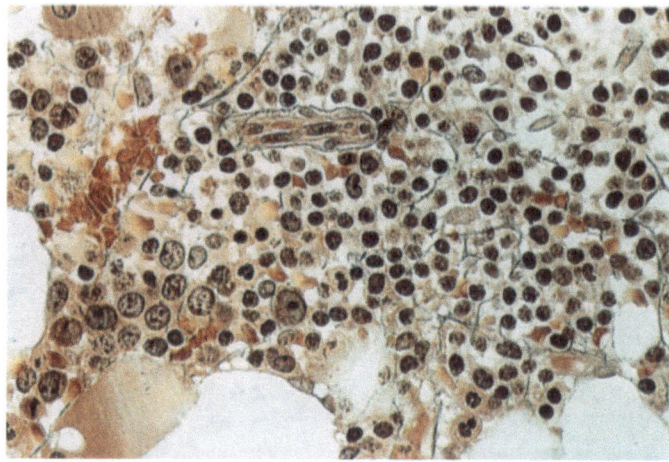

Fig. 1.66   Very small lymphoid nodule with delicate reticular fibre network. Gomori

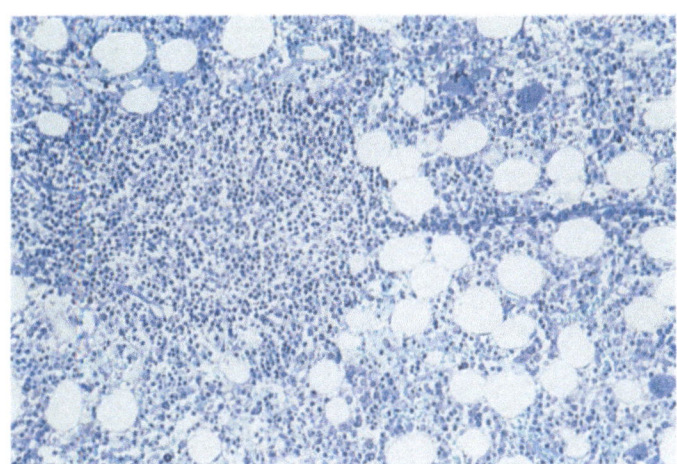

Fig. 1.67 Large lymphoid nodule. Note capillary with plasma cells

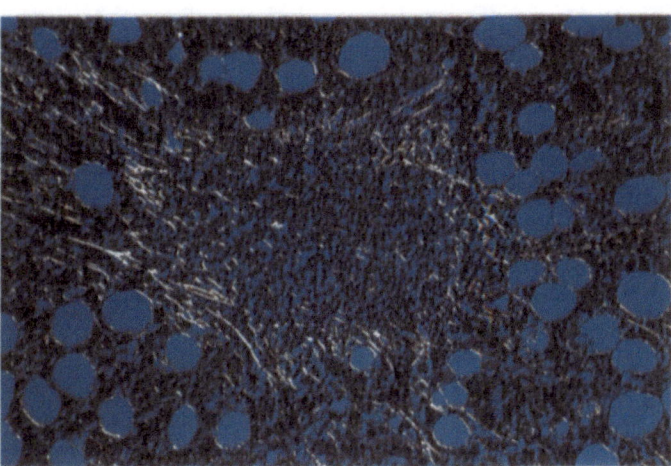

Fig. 1.68 Lymphoid aggregate in normal bone marrow. Gomori, polarized light

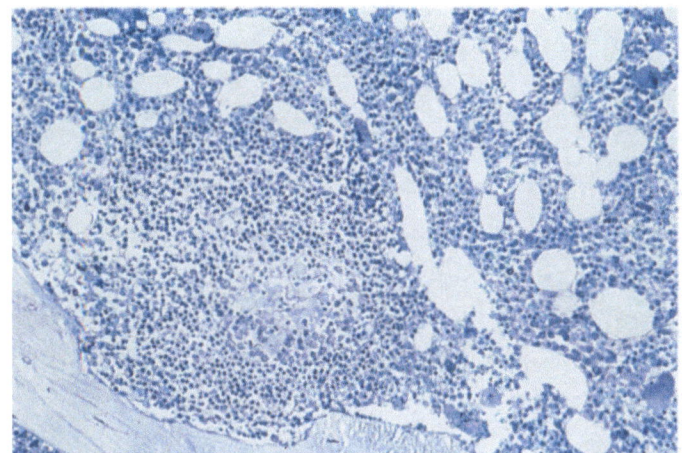

Fig. 1.69 Paratrabecular lymphoid nodule with epithelioid cells in centre

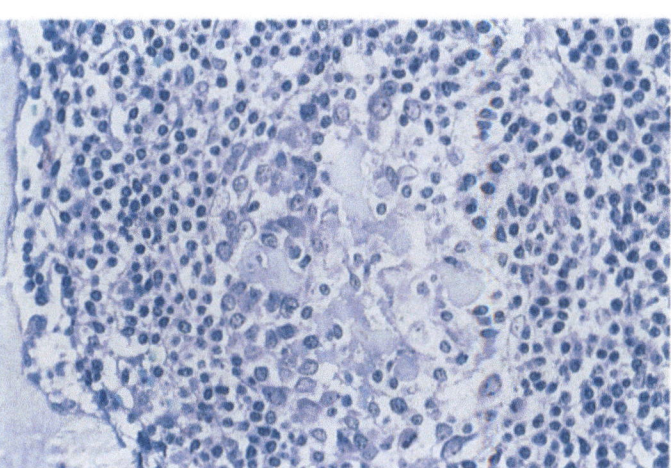

Fig. 1.70 Higher magnification of Fig. 1.69 to illustrate epithelioid cells. Note erosion of bone (at left) in both figures

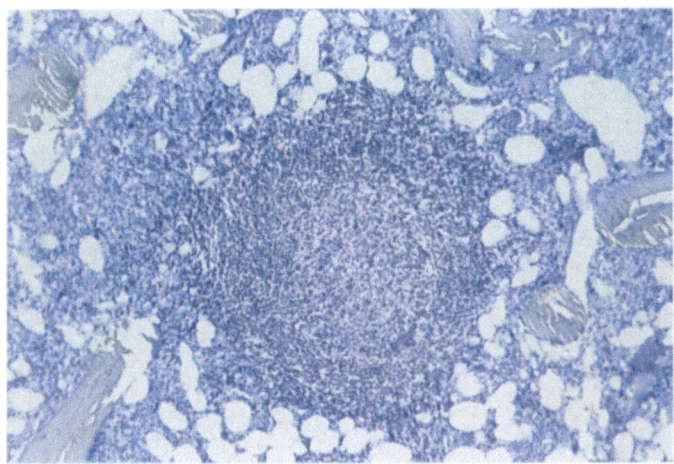

Fig. 1.71 Lymphoid follicle in normal bone marrow

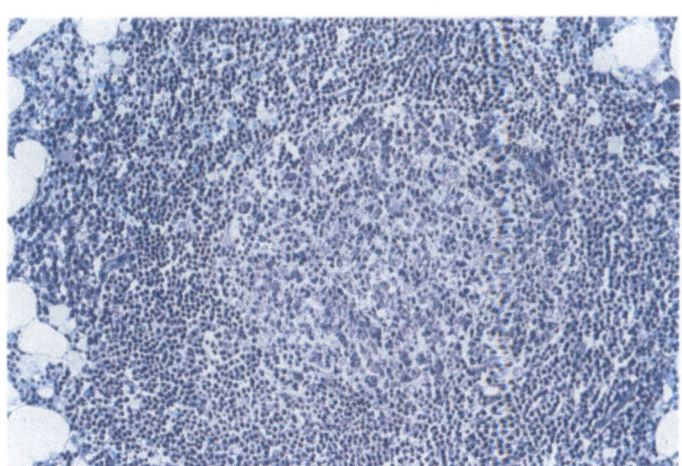

Fig. 1.72 Germinal centre of lymphoid follicle in previous figure

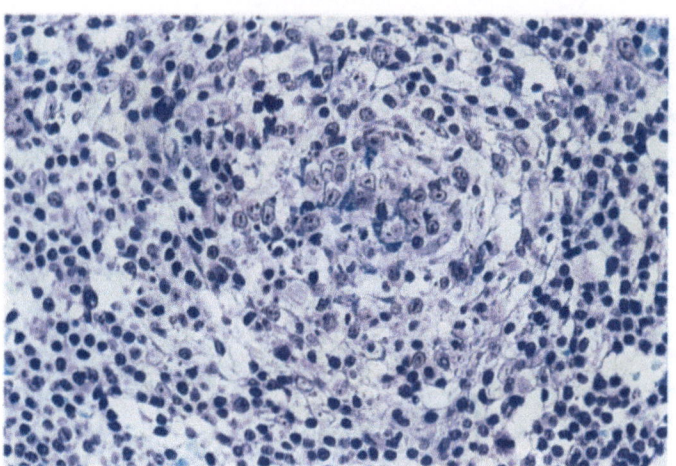

Fig. 1.73 Follicle centre cells of lymphoid follicle in normal bone marrow

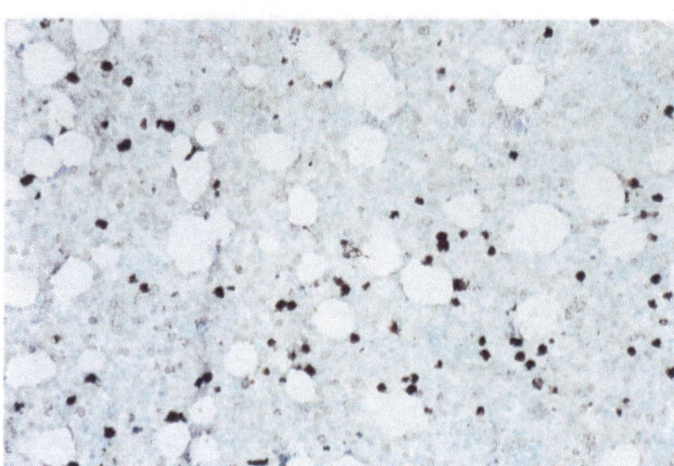

Fig. 1.74 Diffusely scattered B lymphocytes in normal bone marrow. Cryostat section, CD 19

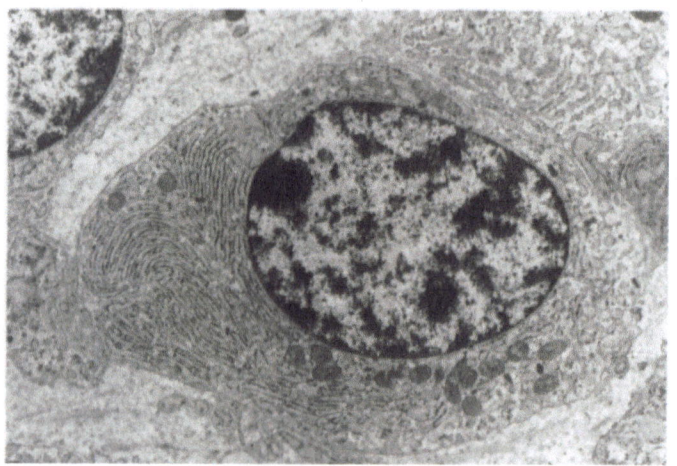

Fig. 1.75 Normal plasma cell. Note mitochondria and rough endoplasmic reticulum. EM × 20 000

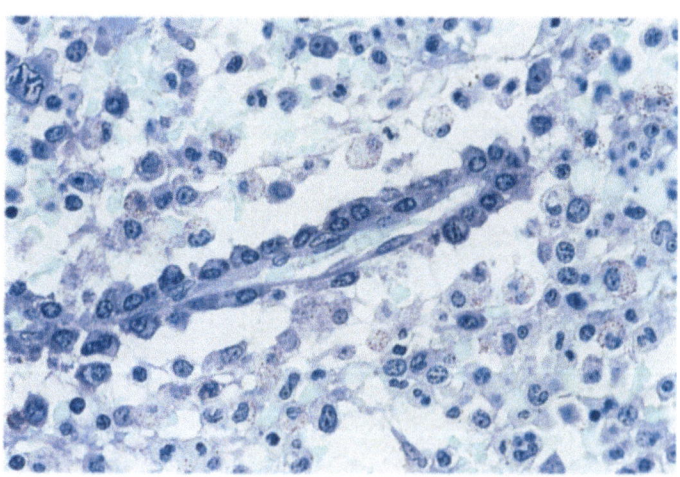

Fig. 1.76 Perivascular plasma cells in longitudinal section

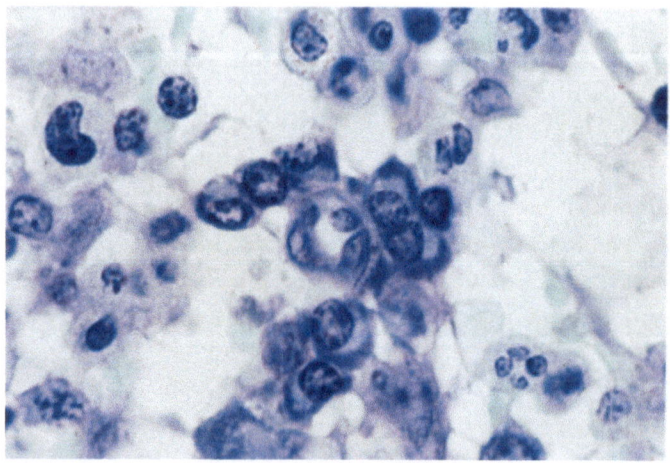

Fig. 1.77 Perivascular plasma cells in cross-section

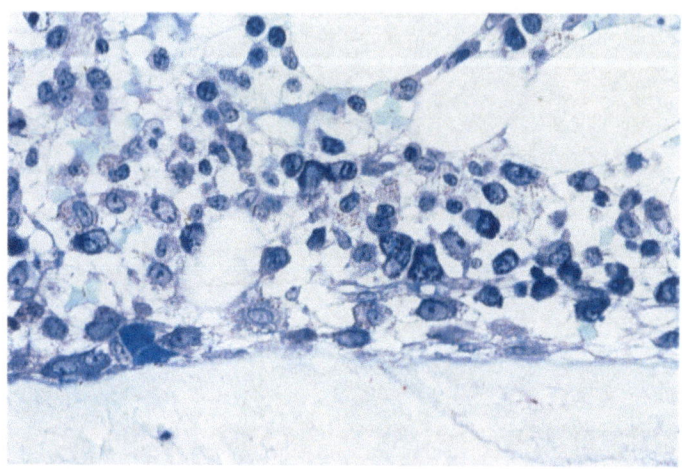

Fig. 1.78 Interstitial plasma cells in normal bone marrow

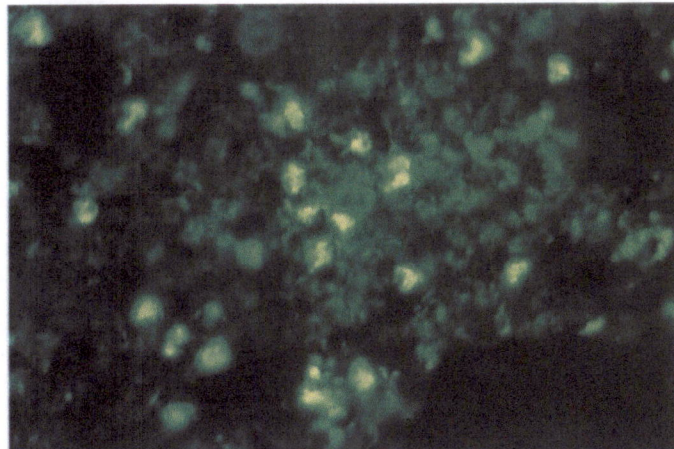

Fig. 1.79 Immunohistology on cryostat sections: FITC-labelled antibody to IgG. Plasma cells show green fluorescence

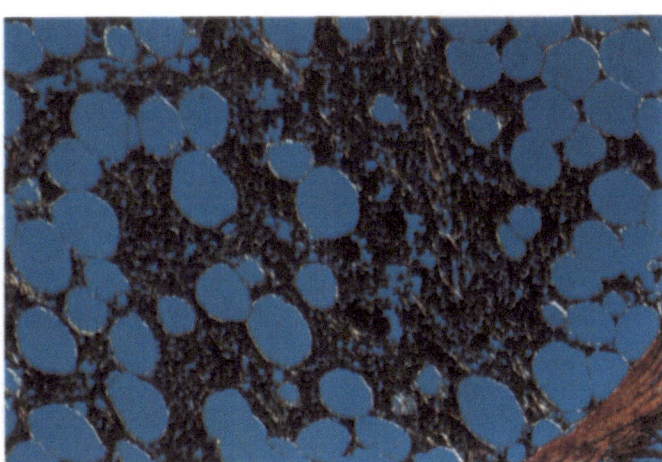

Figs 1.80–1.84 Sections of normal bone marrow stained by Gomori's stain for reticular fibres; Fig. 1.80 viewed in polarized light; very few fibres present in the marrow

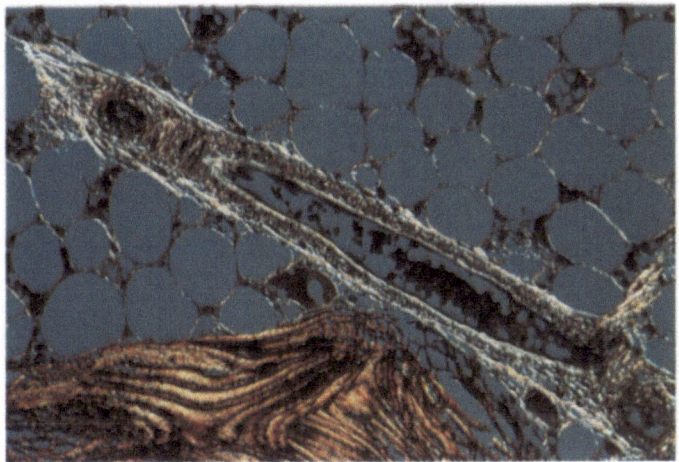

Fig. 1.81 Note association of fibres with blood vessel in fatty bone marrow. Gomori, polarized light

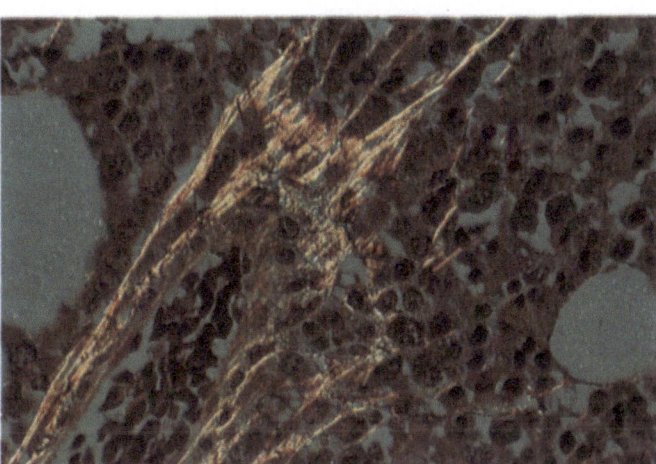

Fig. 1.82 Periarterial fibres radiating into cellular bone marrow. Gomori, polarized light

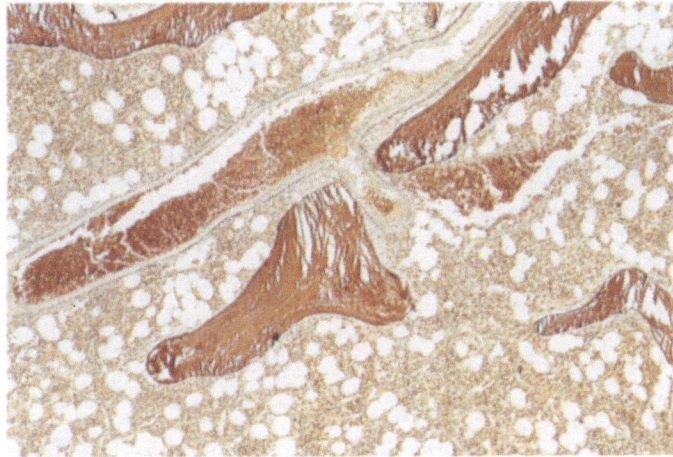

Fig. 1.83 Branching artery in close apposition to trabecular bone. Gomori

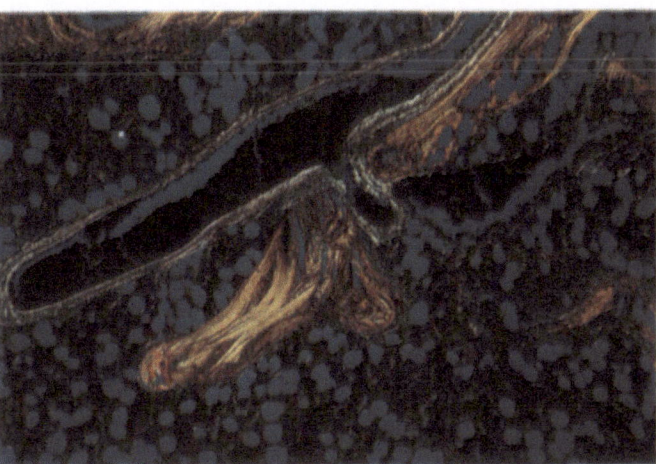

Fig. 1.84 Same as Fig. 1.83 viewed in polarized light to demonstrate perivascular fibres. Note absence of reticular fibres in normal bone marrow. Gomori

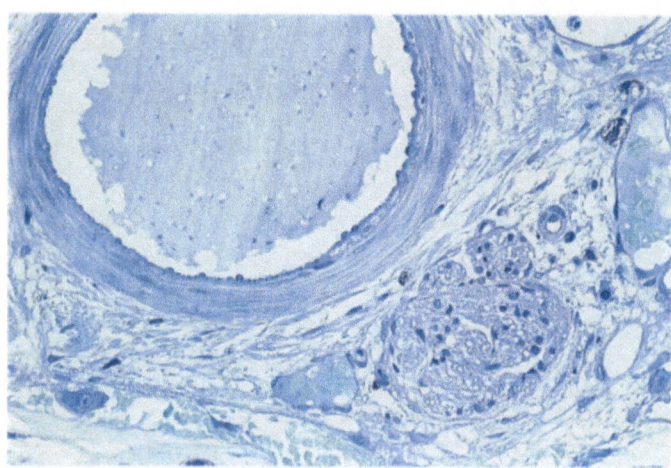

Fig. 1.85   Large artery accompanied by a nerve

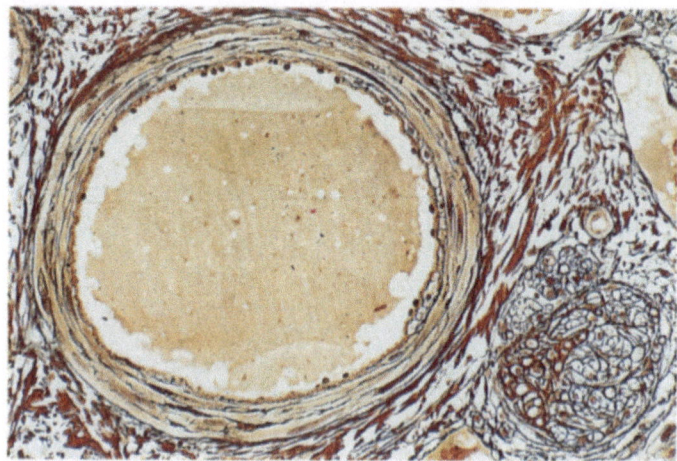

Fig. 1.86   Parallel sections stained by Gomori, wih coarse perivascular fibrosis

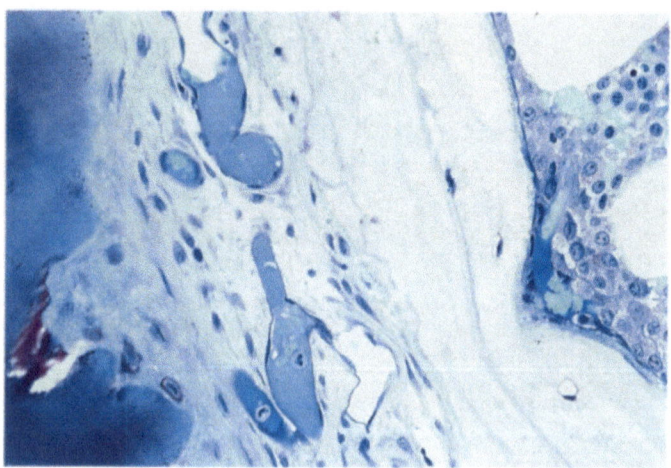

Fig. 1.87   Large blood vessels in periosteum

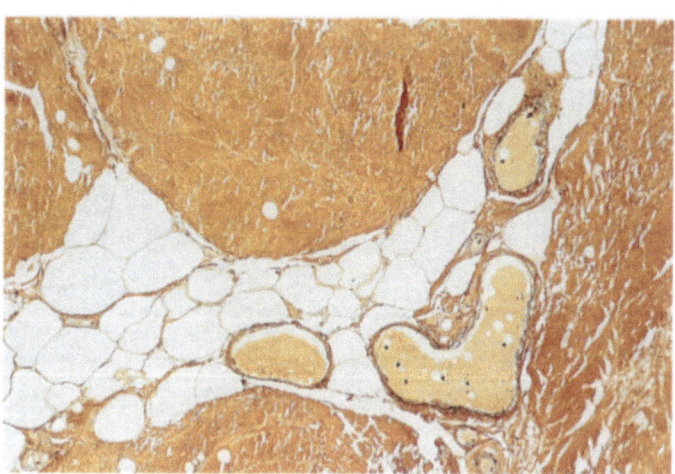

Fig. 1.88   Large blood vessels in fatty tissue between periosteum and cortical bone. Gomori

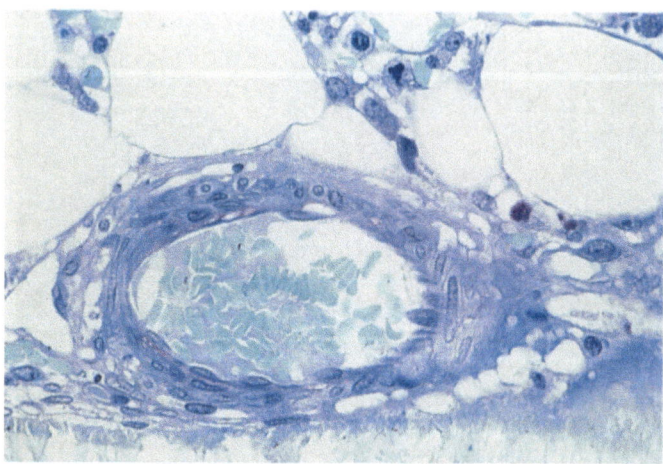

Fig. 1.89   Paratrabecular artery in cross-section

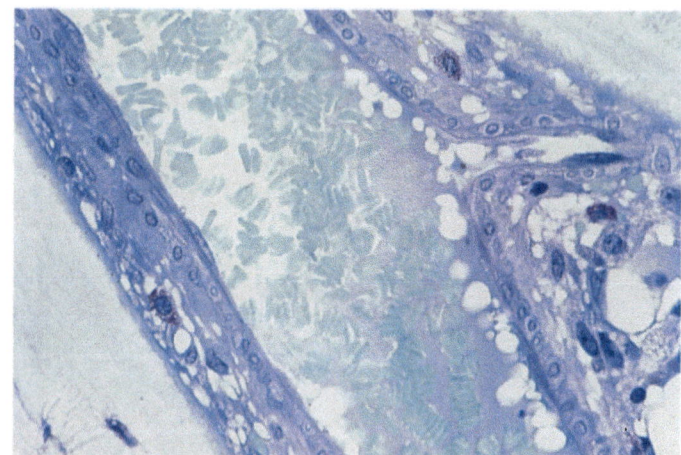

Fig. 1.90   Paratrabecular artery in longitudinal section

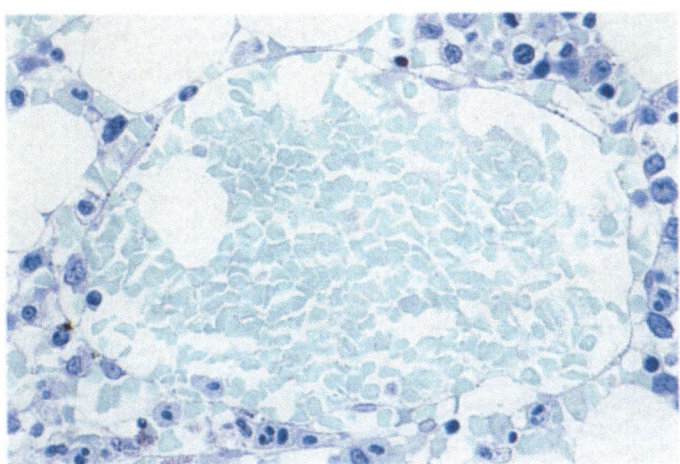

Fig. 1.91 Large sinusoid lined by single layer of endothelial cells

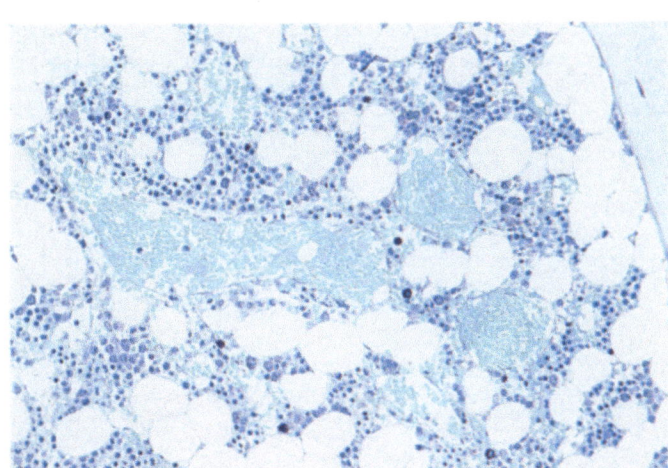

Fig. 1.92 Ectatic sinusoids filled with erythrocytes in normal bone marrow

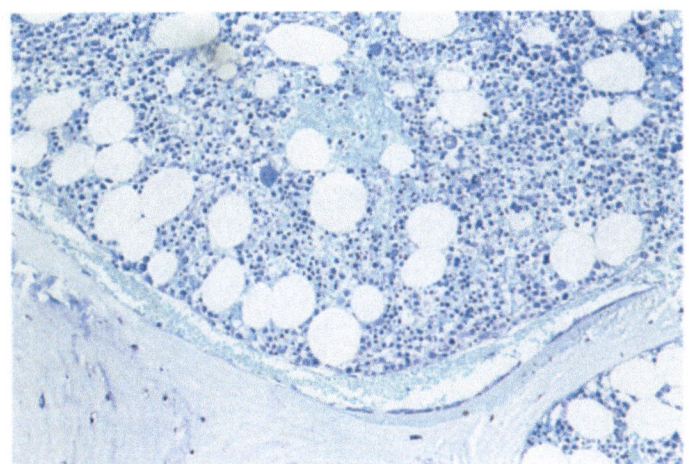

Fig. 1.93 Paratrabecular sinusoid

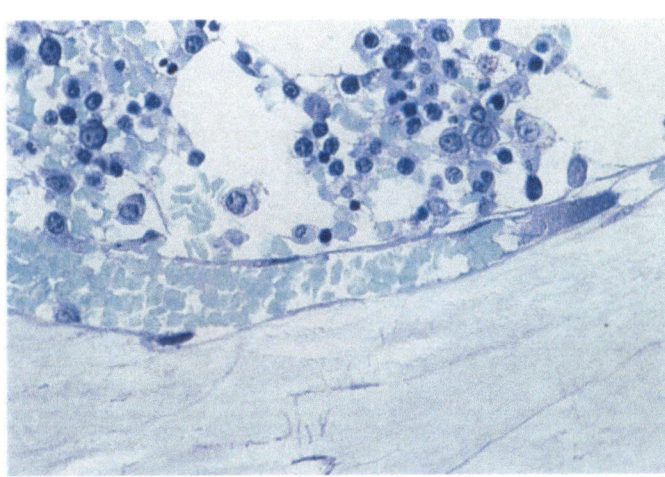

Fig. 1.94 Paratrabecular sinus with endosteum and endothelium

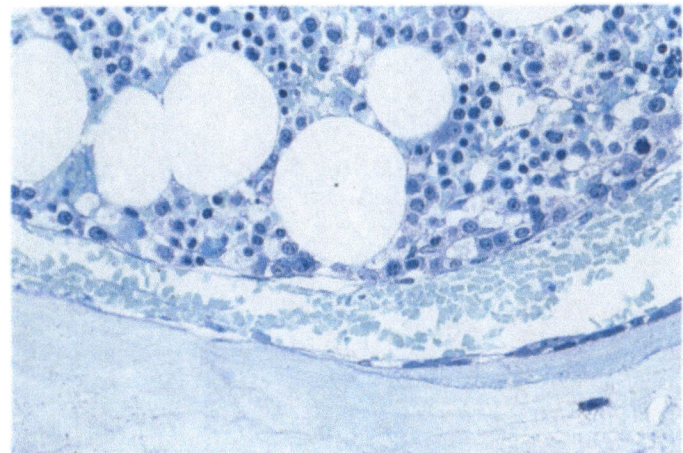

Fig. 1.95 Paratrabecular sinus with osteoblasts (right) on layer of osteoid

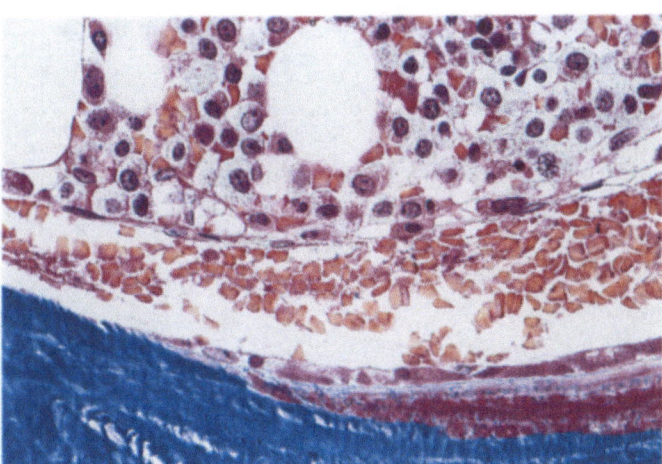

Fig. 1.96 Broad paratrabecular sinus with seam of osteoblasts and layer of osteoid. Ladewig

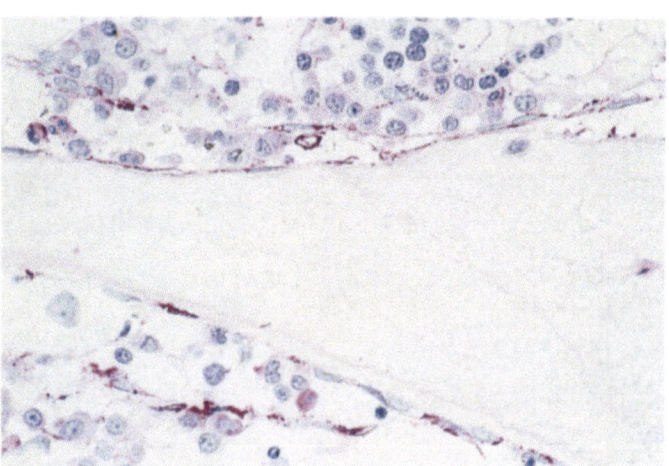

Fig. 1.97 Bone biopsy section stained by PAS: note PAS postive sinusoidal endothelium and endosteal lining cells

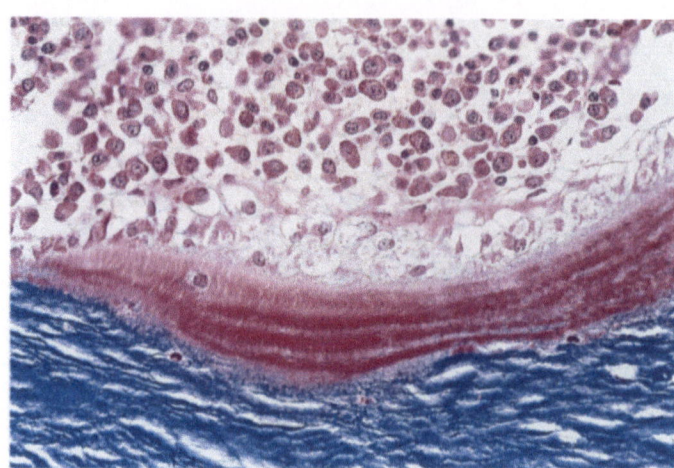

Fig. 1.98 Seam of active osteoblasts with layers of osteoid (red). Note one osteoblast enveloped by osteoid (incipient osteocyte). Ladewig

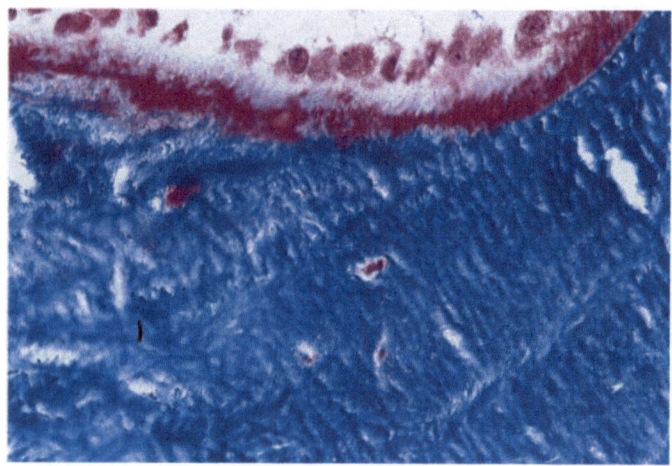

Fig. 1.99 Cuboidal osteoblasts, one layer of osteoid (red) and mineralized bone (blue) with osteocytes. Ladewig

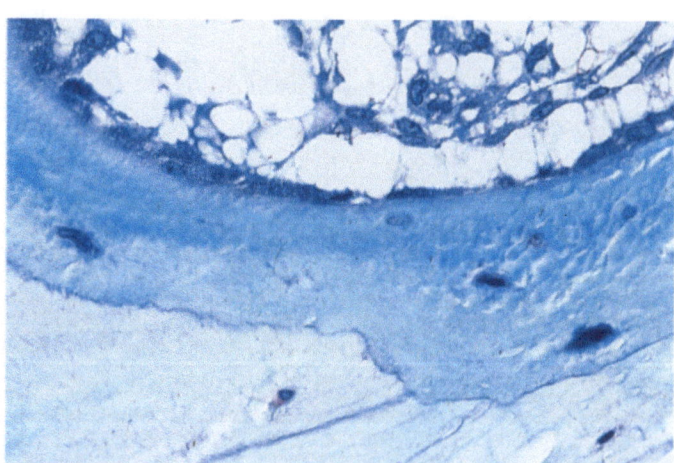

Fig. 1.100 Seam of osteoblasts and broad layer of osteoid. Note osteocytes in osteoid

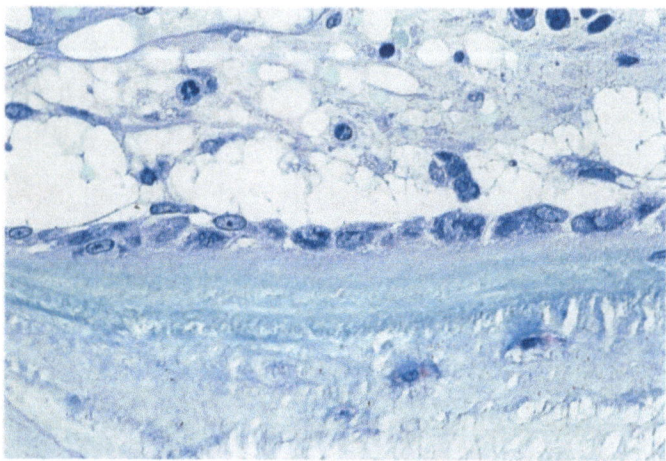

Fig. 1.101 Note osteoblast and endothelial association at trabecular surface (left and right of centre)

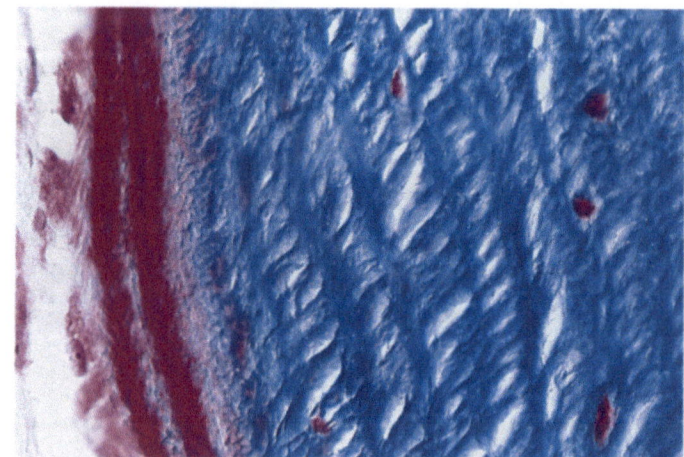

Fig. 1.102 Note lamellae of osteoid and calcified bone. Ladewig

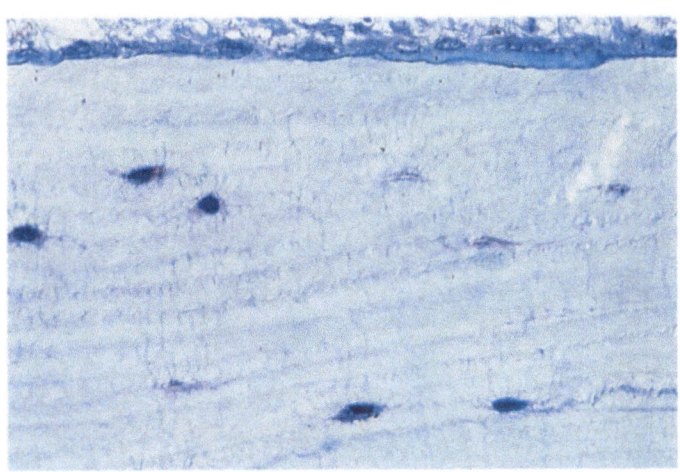

Fig. 1.103 Osteocytes between lamellae of calcified bone with canaliculi radiating out from the lacunae

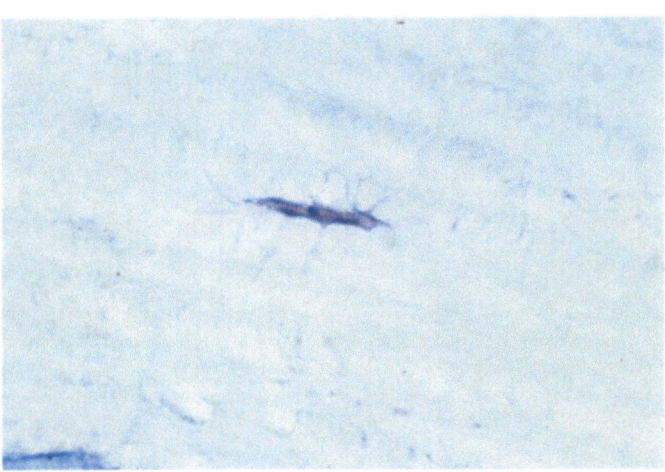

Fig. 1.104 Higher magnification of part of Fig. 1.103, osteocyte with canaliculi

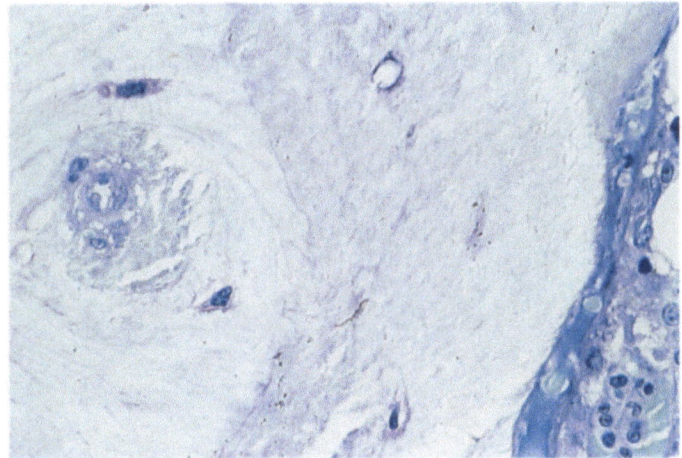

Fig. 1.105 Haversian canal in cortical bone

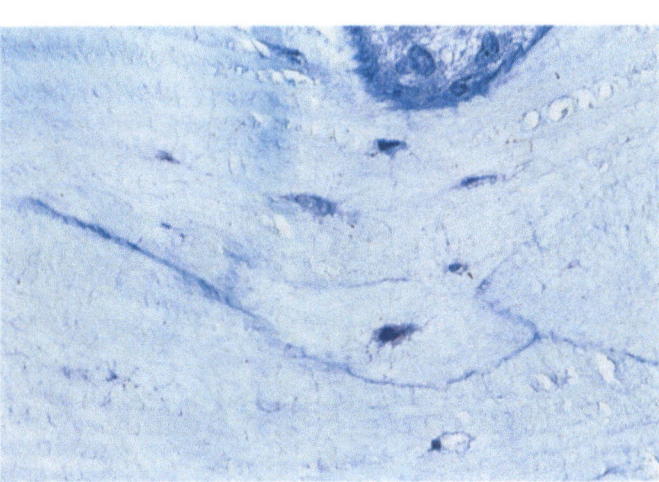

Fig. 1.106 Cement lines (evidence of previous remodelling) in lamellar bone

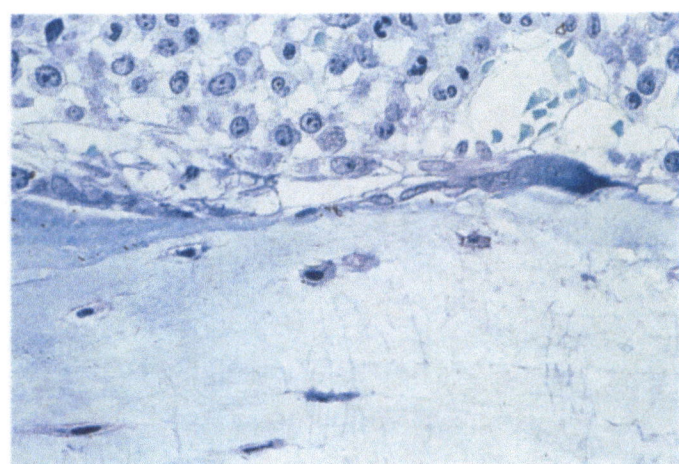

Fig. 1.107 Bone remodelling unit with osteoclast, osteoblasts, fibres and blood vessels

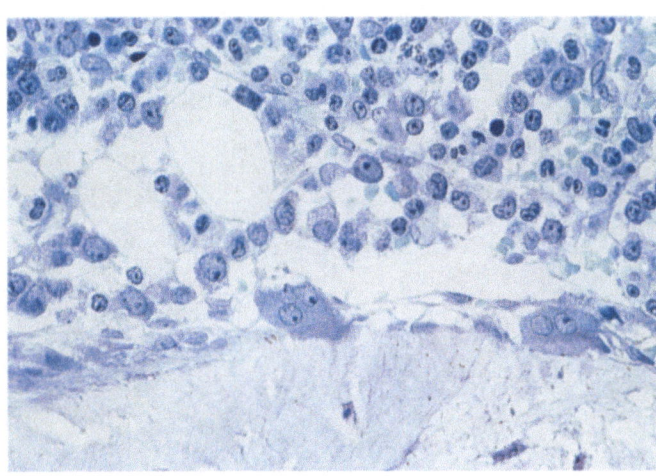

Fig. 1.108 Note binucleate osteoclasts on osseous surface between endosteal cells

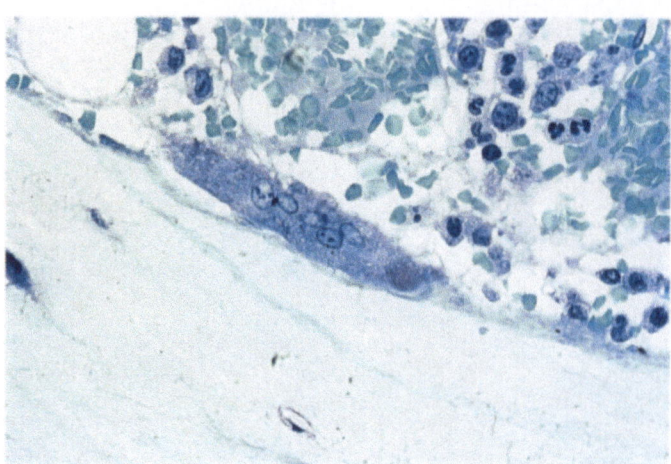

Fig. 1.109 Multinucleate osteoclast on trabecular surface

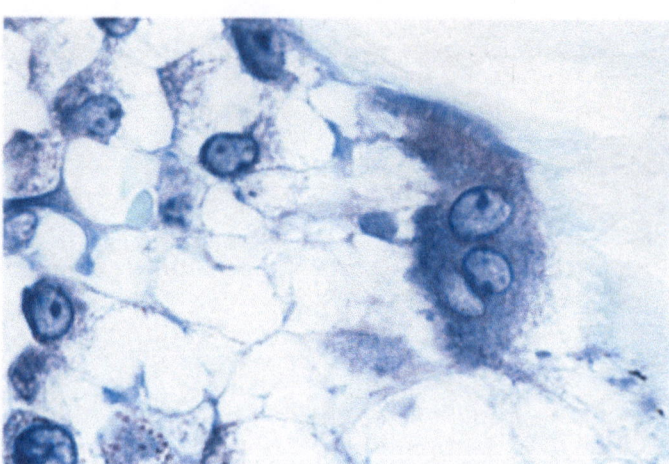

Fig. 1.110 High magnification of osteoclast on trabecular surface. Note variability in cytoplasmic staining

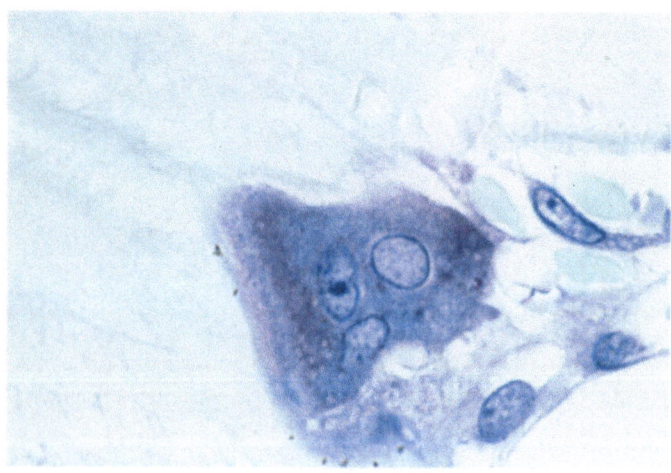

Fig. 1.111 Osteoclast in erosion cavity (Howship's lacuna)

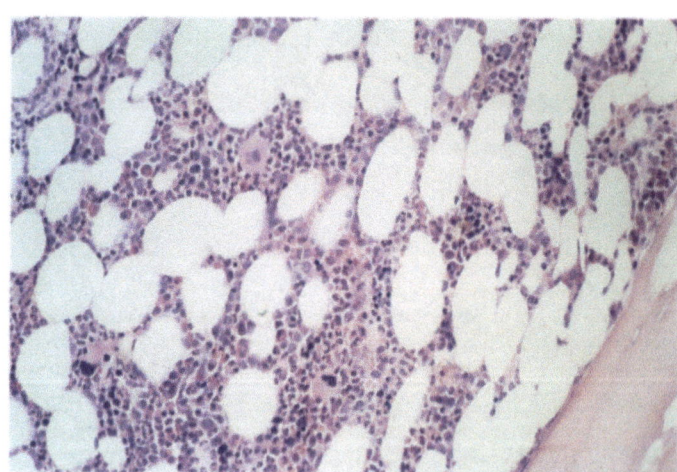

Figs 1.115–1.124 Examples of sections of decalcified paraffin-embedded biopsies.

Fig. 1.115 Low-power view of normal cellular bone marrow. H&E

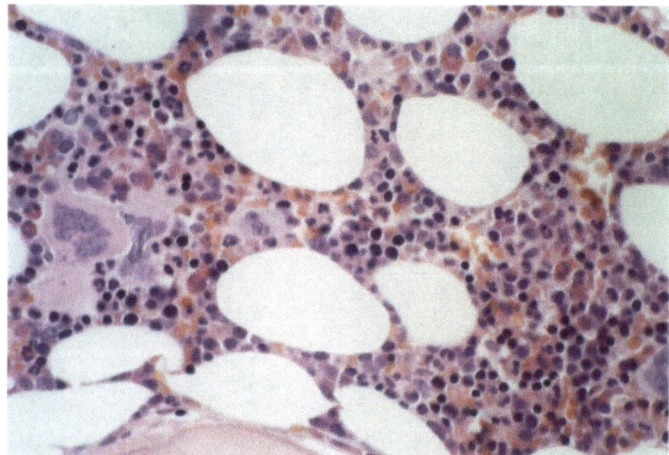

Fig. 1.116 Higher magnification of Fig. 1.115 showing haematopoiesis. H&E

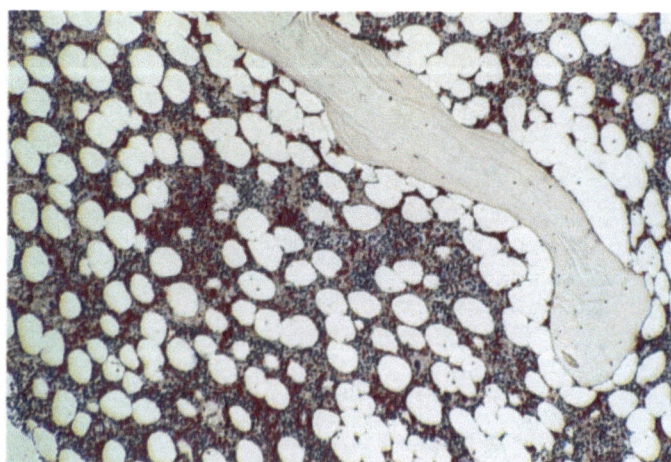

Fig. 1.117 Section stained by Leder showing reaction in myeloid tissue, none in the other cell lines

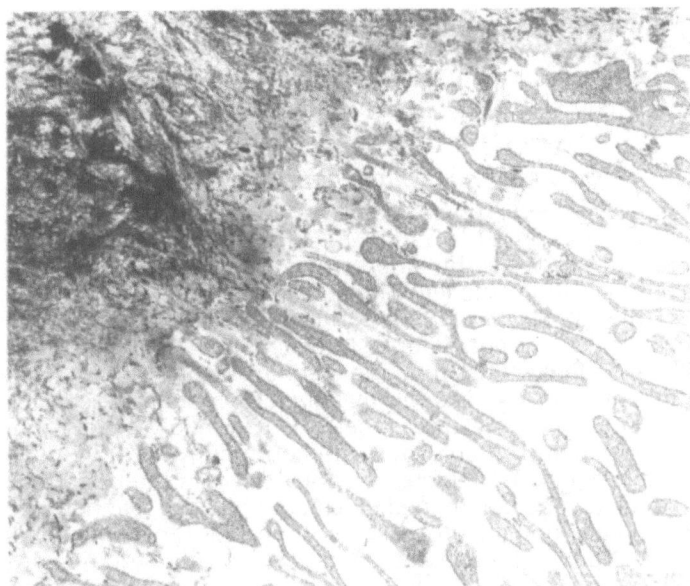

Fig. 1.113 High magnification of ruffled membrane shown in Fig. 1.112. EM × 40 000

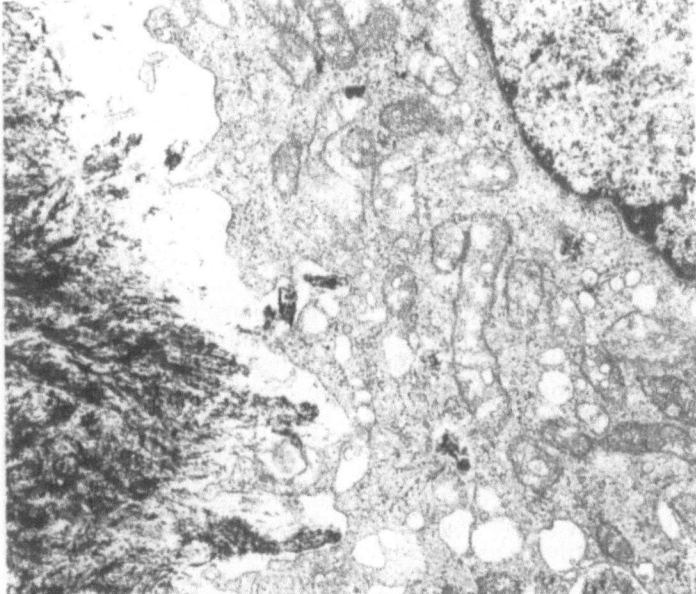

Fig. 1.114 Part of osteoclast on bone. Note smooth surface, mitochondriae and vacuoles containing electron-dense particles (fragments of bone). EM × 40 000

marrow biopsy sections[52]. Optical measurements by means of graticules or grids in the eyepiece are still used with or without computerized evaluation of the results.

References

1. Ellis, L. D., Jensen, W. N. and Westerman, M. P. (1964). Needle biopsy of bone marrow. *Arch. Intern. Med.*, **114**, 213
2. Burkhardt, R. (1971). Bone marrow and bone tissue. *Colour Atlas of Clinical Histopathology*. Berlin: Springer
3. Jamshidi, J. and Swaim, R. W. (1971). Bone marrow biopsy with unaltered architecture: a new biopsy device. *J. Lab Clin. Med.*, **77**, 335
4. Duhamel, G. (1974). *Histopathologie clinique de la moelle osseuse*. Paris: Masson
5. Block, M. (1976). *Text Atlas of Haematology*. Philadelphia: Lea and Febiger
6. Rywlin, A. M. (1976). *Histopathology of the Bone Marrow*. Boston: Little Brown
7. Krause, J. R. (1981). *Bone Marrow Biopsy*. Edinburgh: Churchill Livingstone
8. Moosavi, H., Lichtman, M. A., Donnelly, J. A. and Churukian, C. J. (1981). Plastic-embedded human marrow biopsy specimens. *Arch. Pathol. Lab. Med.*, **105**, 269
9. Westerman, M. P. (1981). Bone marrow needle biopsy: an evaluation and critique. *Sem. Haematol.*, **18**, 293
10. Rowden, G., Sacher, R. A. and More, N. S. (1982). Plastic embedded specimens for evaluation of bone marrow. In Roath, S. (ed.), *Topical Reviews in Haematology*, Vol. II Bristol: Wright
11. Islam, A. (1982). A new bone marrow biopsy needle with core securing device. *J. Clin. Pathol.*, **356**, 359
12. Frisch, B., Bartl, R. and Burkhardt, R. (1982). Bone marrow biopsy in clinical medicine. An overview. *Haematologia*, **3**, 245
13. Bartl, R., Frisch, B. and Burkhardt, R. (1982). *Bone Marrow Biopsies Revisited. A New Dimension for Haematologic Malignancies*. Basel: Karger (2nd edn 1985)
14. Burkhardt, R., Frisch, B. and Bartl, R. (1982). Bone biopsy in haematological disorders. *J. Clin. Pathol.*, **35**, 257
15. Frisch, B. and Bartl, R. (1984). *Bone Marrow Biopsies Updated*. Bibliotheca Haematologica 50. Basel: Karger
16. Wittels, B. (1985). *Surgical Pathology of Bone Marrow – Core Biopsy Diagnosis*. Philadelphia: Saunders
17. Schaefer, H. E. (1985). Beckenkammbioptische Diagnostik. Osteologie – Haematologie – Onkologie – metabolische Störungen. *Internist*, **26**, 453
18. Beckstead, J. H. (1986). The bone marrow biopsy. A diagnostic strategy. *Arch. Pathol. Lab. Med.*, **110**, 175
19. Burns, W. A. and Yook, C. R. (1988). Plastic sections and ultrastructural techniques in the evaluation of bone marrow pathology. *Hematol. Oncol. Clin. N. Am.*, **2**, 525
20. Thiele, J., Fisher, R., Zankovich, R. and Diehl, V. (198). The significance of histologic bone marrow examination for the diagnosis of haematologic diseases. *Med. Klin.*, **83**, 643
21. Islam, A. and Henderson, E. A. (1988). Value of long-core biopsy in the detection of discrete bone marrow lesions. *Histopathology*, **12**, 641
22. Bartl, R., Frisch, B. and Burkhardt, R. (1989). Bone marrow histology. In Catovsky, D. (ed.), *Methods in Haematology. The Leukemic Cell*. Edinburgh: Churchill Livingstone
23. Lips, P., Van Ginkel, F. C. and Netelenbos, J. C. (1985). Bone marrow and bone remodelling. *Bone*, **6**, 343
24. McDougall, L. G., Pettifor, J. M. and Patel, J. M. (1987). Bone growth and haemopoiesis: steroid reversible anaemia, myelofibrosis and increased bone formation in a child. *Br. J. Haematol.*, **66**, 5
25. Burgio, G. R., Arico, M., Caselli, D., Beluffi, G. and Calligaro, A. (1987). Bone and bone marrow syndromes: a causal, not only casual, connection? *Haematologia*, **72**, 363
26. Burkhalter, J. L. and Patel, B. R. (1983). Radionuclide bone scan as an aid in localizing lesion for bone biopsy. *Skeet. Radiol.*, **9**, 246
27. Prasad, R. and Olson, W. H. (1987). Bone marking for biopsy using radionuclide bone imaging. *Cancer*, **60**, 2205
28. Lalor, B., Freemont, A. and Carlile, S. (1986). An improved transilial crest bone biopsy drill for quantitative histomorphometry. *Bone*, **7**, 273
29. Hodgson, S. F., Johnson, K. A., Muhs, J. M., Lufkin, E. G. and McCarthy, J. T. (1986). Out patient percutaneous biopsy of the iliac crest: methods, morbidity and patient acceptance. *Mayo Clin. Proc.*, **61**, 28
30. Bartl, R., Frisch, B., Buchenrieder, B. *et al.* (1984). Multiparameter studies on 650 bone marrow biopsy cores. Diagnostic value of combined utilisation of imprints, cryostat and plastic sections in medical practice. *Bibl. Haematologica*, **50**, 1
31. Frisch, B., Lewis, S. M., Burkhardt, R. and Bartl, R., (1985). *Biopsy Pathology of Bone and Bone Marrow*. London: Chapman and Hall
32. Islam, A. and Frisch, B. (1985). Plastic embedding in routine histology. I: Preparation of semi-thin sections of undecalcified marrow cores. *Histopathology*, **9**, 1263
33. Trubowitz, S. and Davies, S. (eds) (1982). *The Human Bone Marrow: Anatomy, Physiology and Pathophysiology*, Vols I and II Boca Raton, Florida: CRC Press
34. Gulati, G. L., Ashton, J. K. and Hyun, B. H. (1988). Structure and function of the bone marrow and haematopoiesis. *Hematol. Oncol. Clin. N. Am.*, **2**, 495
35. Zucker-Franklin, D., Greaves, M. F., Grossin, C. E. and Marmont, A. M. (1981). *Atlas of Blood Cells: Function and Pathology*. Philadelphia: Lea and Febiger
36. Mangan, K. F. (1985). T-cell-mediated suppression of haematopoiesis. *N. Engl. J. Med.*, **312**, 306
37. Nienhuis, A. W. (1988). Haematopoietic growth factors. Biologic complexity and clinical promise. *N. Engl. J. Med.*, **318**, 916

38. Navone, R., Azzoni, L. and Valente, G. (1988). Immunohistochemical assessment of ferritin in bone marrow trephine biopsies: correlation with marrow haemosiderin. *Acta Haematol.*, **80**, 194

39. Gerwitz, A. M. (1986). Human megakaryocytopoiesis. *Sem. Hematol.*, **23**, 27

40. Smith, J. G., Kyle, B. and Rowan, R. M. (1986). T4:T8 lymphocyte ratios in human bone marrow: the effect of sampling technique. *Clin. Lab. Haematol.*, **8**, 49

41. Trentin, J. J. (1971). Determination of bone marrow stem cell differentiation of stromal haemopoietic inductive microenvironments (HIM). *Am. J. Pathol.*, **65**, 621

42. Bentley, S. A. (1982). Bone marrow connective tissue and the haemopoietic microenvironment. *Br. J. Haematol.*, **50**, 1

43. Tavassoli, M., Friedenstein, A. (1983). Haemopoietic stromal microenvironment. *Am. J. Haematol.*, **15**, 195

44. Weiss, L. and Sakai, H. (1984). The hematopoietic stroma. *Am. J. Anat.*, **170**, 447

45. Singer, J. W., Keating, A. and Wight, T. N. (1985). The human haematopoietic microenvironment. In Hoffbrand, A.V. (ed.), *Recent Advances in Haematology*. Edinburgh: Churchill Livingstone, pp. 1–24

46. Gordon, M. Y., Hibbin, J. A., Kearney, L. U., Gordon-Smith, E. C. and Goldman, J. M. (1985). Colony formation by primitive haematopoietic progenitors in cocultures of bone marrow cells and stromal cells. *Br. J. Haematol.*, **60**, 129

47. Bianco, P., Costantini, M., Dearden, L. C. and Bonucci, E. (1988). Alkaline phosphatase positive precursors of adipocytes in the human bone marrow. *Br. J. Haematol.* **68**, 401

48. Deldar, A., Lewis, H. and Weiss, L. (1985). Bone lining cells and haematopoiesis: an electron microscopic study of canine bone marrow. *Anat. Rec.*, **213**, 187

49. The bone lining cell: a distinct phenotype? Editorial (1987). *Calcif. Tissue Int.*, **41**, 1

50. Chambers, T. J. (1985). The pathobiology of the osteoclast. *J. Clin. Pathol.*, **38**, 241

51. Kerndrup, G., Pallesen, G., Melsen, F. and Mosekilde, L. (1980). Histomorphometrical determination of bone marrow cellularity in iliac crest biopsies. *Scand. J. Haematol.*, **24**, 110

52. Henning, A. (1975). Kritische Betrachtungen zur Volumen-und Oberflächenmessung in der Mikroskopie. *Zeiss Werkzeitschr.*, **30**, 78

Appendix

Methods

Though this atlas is not primarily concerned with techniques, a brief section on methodology is perhaps appropriate, especially in view of the fact that there is still some controversy as to which is the most effective way to process bone biopsies[1–5]. There are several possibilities: (1) paraffin embedding after decalcification – this enables the use of the sections for a range of antibody and enzyme reactions (Figs 1.115–1.124, 1.130–1.135); (2) embedding in a water-miscible plastic, which preserves a greater number of antigens and enzymes; (3) embedding in methyl-methacrylate which provides excellent morphology but does not preserve antigenic and enzymic reactivity; (4) cryostat sections which offer the greatest possibilities for demonstration of antigens, enzymes, and other cellular constituents (Figs 1.125–1.126). Each method has its advantages and drawbacks, and its proponents[6–11].

Probably the most effective way to obtain a maximum of information is to use a combination as indicated in Figs 1.5 and 1.6. In this way optimal histology (either paraffin or plastic) is combined with the use of immunohistology, enzyme histochemistry[12] and electron microscopy, as required. Examples of these techniques will be given in the appropriate chapters in this atlas. In addition, the investigation of bone marrow biopsy sections with monoclonal antibodies provides an alternative to cellular techniques for immunophenotyping of pathological bone marrow infiltrates (at least in some cases). Most membrane, cytoplasmic and nuclear antigens are preserved in frozen sections which can therefore be used as adjuncts

to the evaluation of routinely processed bone marrow biopsies. Moreover, the biopsies (or portions thereof) can be processed quickly, can be stored for long periods of time and studied when convenient or required.

Value of immunological phenotyping

Immunological phenotyping of bone marrow cryostat sections (Figs 1.127–1.135) offers advantages in the diagnosis and subtyping of lymphoid infiltration, lymphomas and acute leukaemias, as well as in the detection of metastatic tumour cells. This technique has also been shown to be capable of distinguishing an early relapse in various leukaemias from regenerating bone marrow. Even minimal infiltrations of malignant lymphomas can be detected, in some cases where marrow involvement is not clearly demonstrable by histomorphology. Furthermore, the residual normal haematopoiesis within the neoplastic tissue can be determined in a more objective manner than in conventionally processed sections, and this may be an important factor in assessment of prognosis. Additionally, the morphological identification of the precursors of the three cell lines, as well as of monocytes, macrophages and lymphocytes, is confirmed and supplemented. Thus, for example, the detection of different types of lymphocytes is possible; or the recognition in pathological specimens of small, lymphoid-like, immature megakaryocytes, which cannot be identified in routinely processed biopsies. Another example is provided by cases of MDS and chronic leukaemias, in which the number of macrophages and monocytes detected immunohistochemically is usually greater than that in routinely processed and stained sections. The immunohistochemical investigation of frozen sections therefore gives a more complete picture and a deeper insight into the biological processes of various diseases, and into the functional state of the neoplastic tissue. This enables more comprehensive diagnostic and prognostic assessment. The immunohistological techniques used to obtain the sections illustrated in this atlas are briefly outlined below.

Bone marrow biopsies were taken with an 11-gauge Jamshidi needle (CAT. No. VRC 4011, A. R. Horwell Ltd., UK) under local anaesthesia from the posterior iliac crest and divided into two halves. Biopsies smaller than 35 mm^2 bone marrow area were not processed for immunohistology. One half of the biopsy was embedded in methyl-methacrylate without decalcification for conventional histology. The other half was soaked for 2–28 h in Histocon® (Cat. No. 0582, Polysciences Inc., Warrington, PA, USA) either at room temperature or at 4 °C, after which the biopsy cylinder was snap-frozen in liquid nitrogen and stored at − 180 °C. The biopsies were usually cut within 1–6 days (median 2 days). For sectioning, the biopsy was placed on a small tissue holder covered with OCT (Cat. No. 4583, Raymond Lamb, London, UK) and cut at 3–5 μm in a cryostat at − 18 °C to − 33 °C (median − 22 °C), depending on the amount of adipose tissue present. The sections were mounted on albuminized glass slides and air-dried; they could be kept at 4 °C for up to 16 h. Before incubation with antibodies the slides were fixed in cold ethanol (− 4 °C) for 5 min then soaked in cold chloroform (− 4 °C) for 3 min and air-dried. In all cases frozen sections were obtained which included three to 10 (median 5) fields of intact bone marrow including paratrabecular tissue. A representative section of each bone marrow was stained with H&E prior to incubation, to ascertain that sufficient marrow was present. Sections with less than three fields of evaluable bone marrow were not incubated for immunohistology. The antibodies used; their reactivities; sources; and published references are given in Table 1.3. The method used for visualization of the end product is that of Cordell *et al.* 1984[15].

(Continued on p. 36)

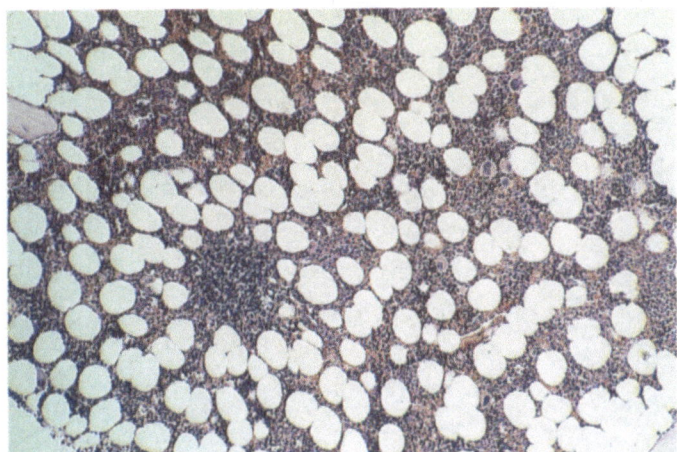

Fig. 1.118 Small lymphoid nodule in normal bone marrow. H&E × 70

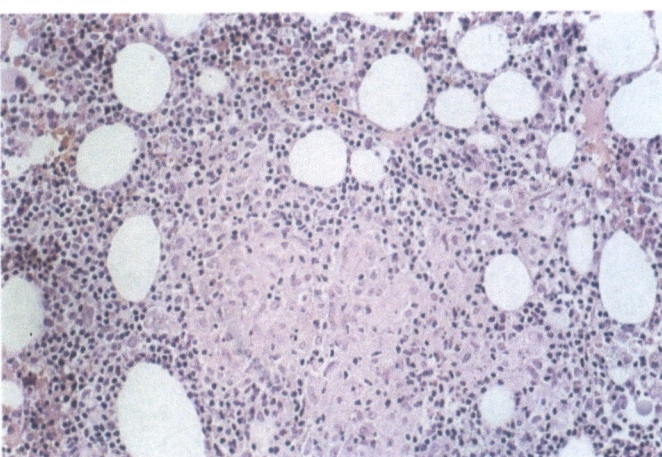

Fig. 1.119 Granuloma in bone marrow in a patient with tuberculosis. H&E

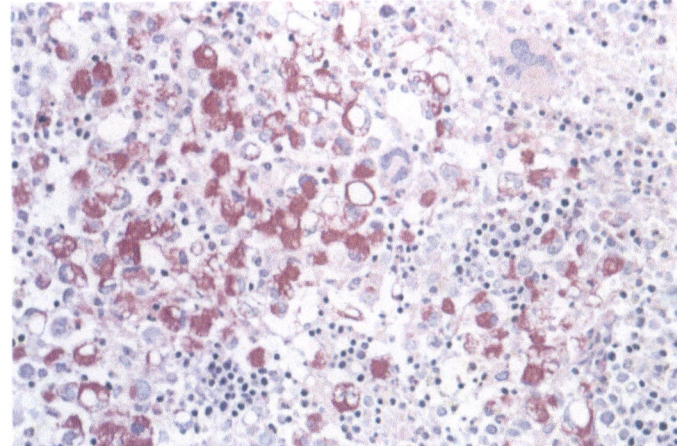

Fig. 1.120 Paraffin section. Tumour cell emboli in blood clot among haematopoietic tissue. PAS

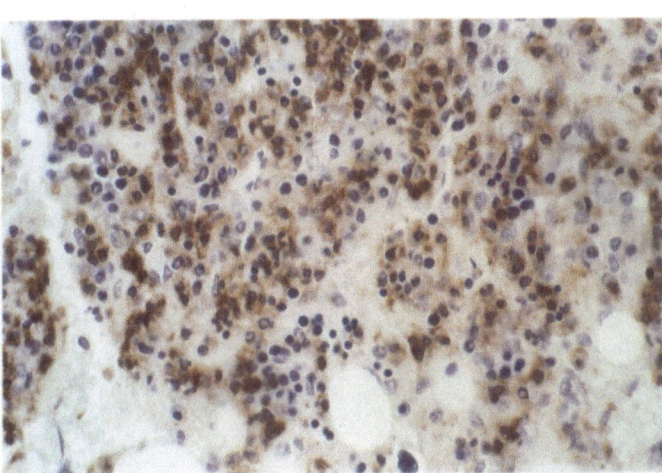

Fig. 1.121 Bone biopsy section of patient with malignant lymphoma and bone marrow involvement, stained with UCHL I (a pan T cell marker)

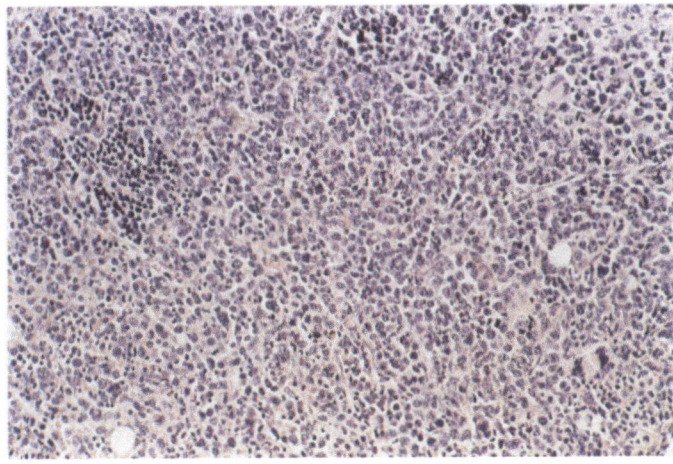

Fig. 1.122 Diffuse infiltration of bone marrow in multiple myeloma. H&E

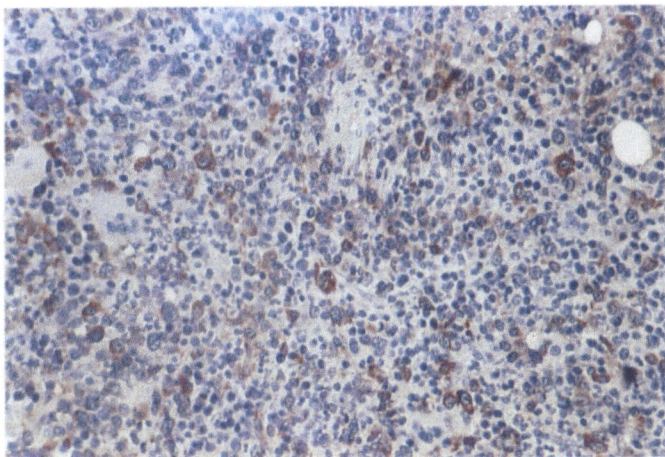

Fig. 1.123 Myeloma cells reactive with antibody to IgA

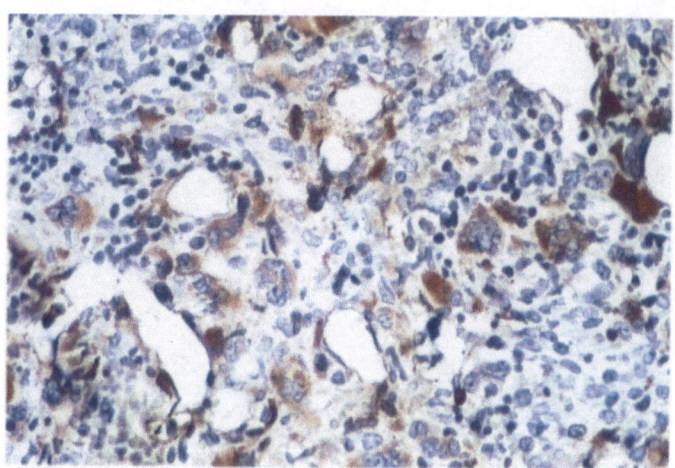

Fig. 1.124 Section of bone biopsy of patient with acute myelofibrosis (AMF), incubated with F. VIII-related antigen. Reaction expressed in megakaryocytes and endothelial cells

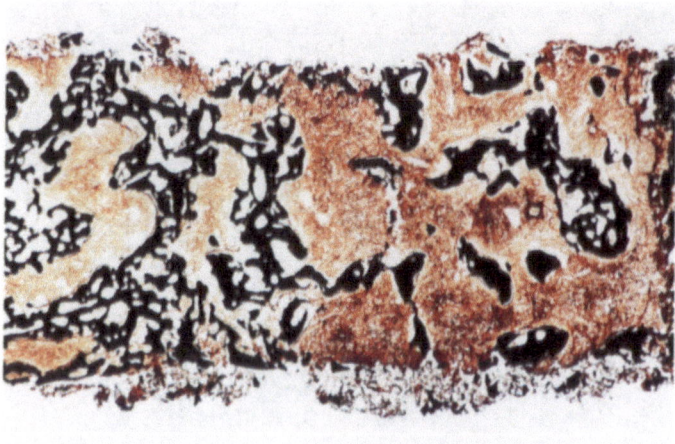

Fig. 1.125 Cryostat section of bone biopsy of patient with osteomyelosclerosis (OMS) showing altered trabecular bone structure. Gomori

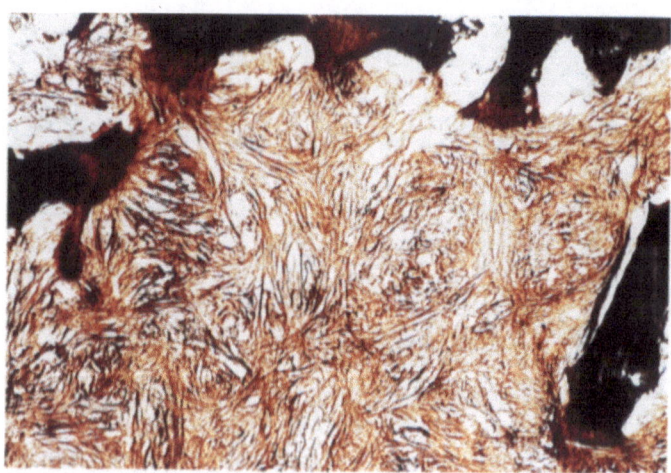

Fig. 1.126 Higher magnification of Fig. 1.125 showing extensive fibrosis of marrow cavities. Gomori

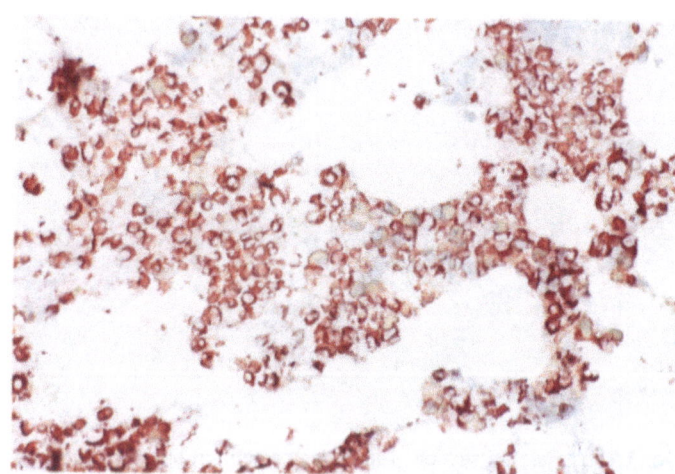

Fig. 1.127 Cryostat section of normal bone biopsy. Immuno-staining with VIM2, which reacts with myeloid and monocytic cells

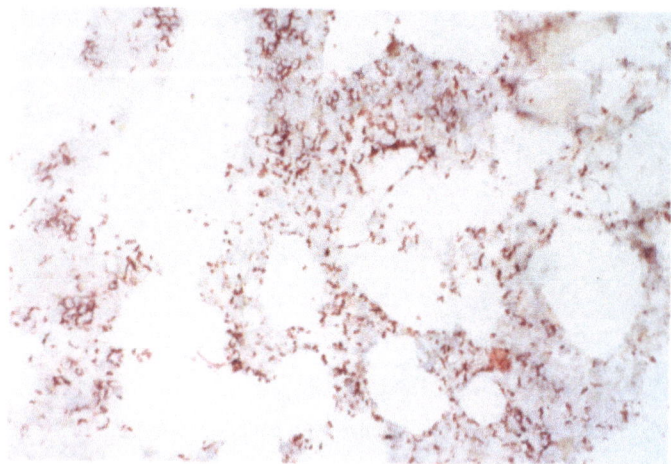

Fig. 1.128 Cryostat section of normal bone biopsy. Immuno-staining with VIEG, which reacts with erythroid cells

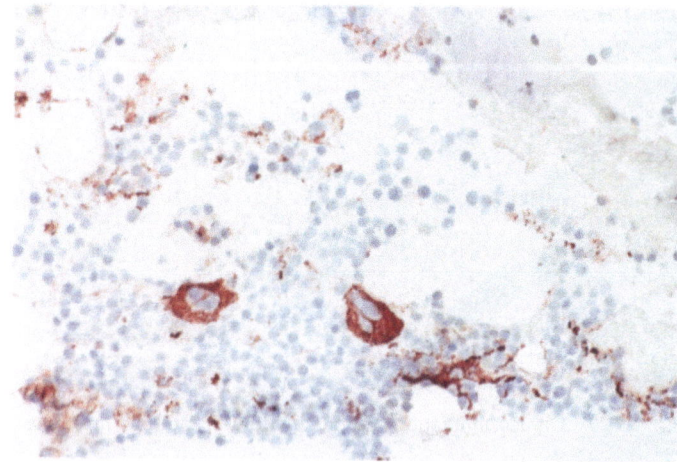

Fig. 1.129 Cryostat section of bone biopsy of patient with immunocytoma. Immunostaining with F. VIII-related antigen which reacts with megakaryocytes and endothelial cells

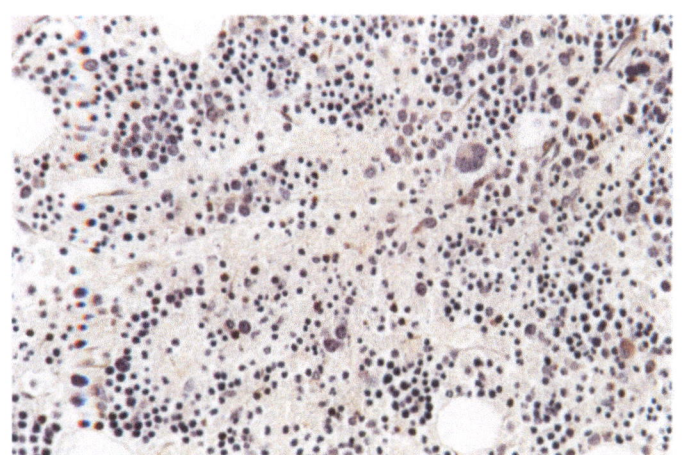

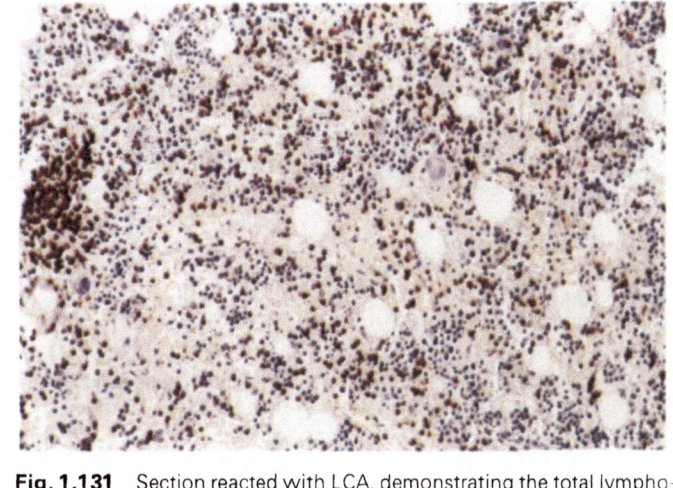

Figs 1.130–1.132 Sections of paraffin-embedded bone biopsy of 58-year-old patient after severe pancytopenia with aplastic bone marrow (cause unknown); this biopsy taken during regenerative phase.

Fig. 1.130 This section shows left-shifted, regenerating haematoporesis. Section reacted with MB2 (B-cell marker); note only isolated positive cells, upper right

Fig. 1.131 Section reacted with LCA, demonstrating the total lymphocyte population

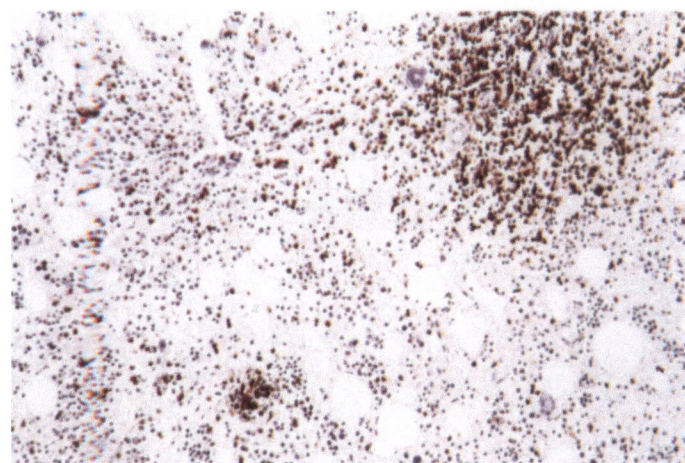

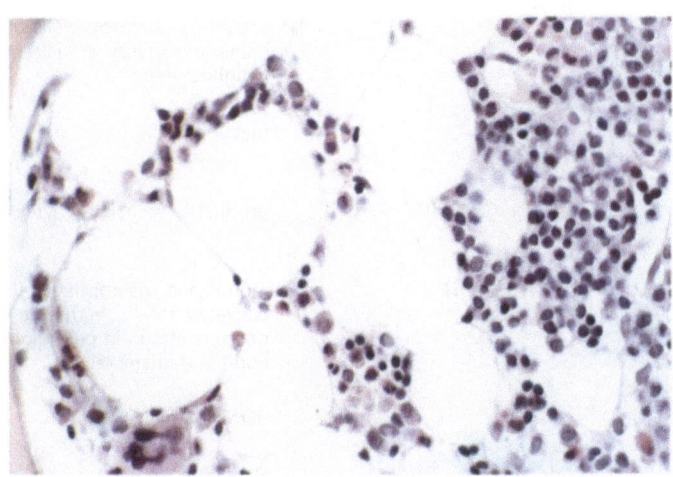

Fig. 1.132 Section reacted with VCHL1 (T-cell marker) note positive nodule and diffuse infiltration of T cells

Figs 1.133–1.135 Sections of bone biopsy of 60-year-old patient with moderate, peripheral lymphocytosis, no evidence found for lymphoma

Fig. 1.133 Section stained by B-cell marker MB2; only isolated positive cells.

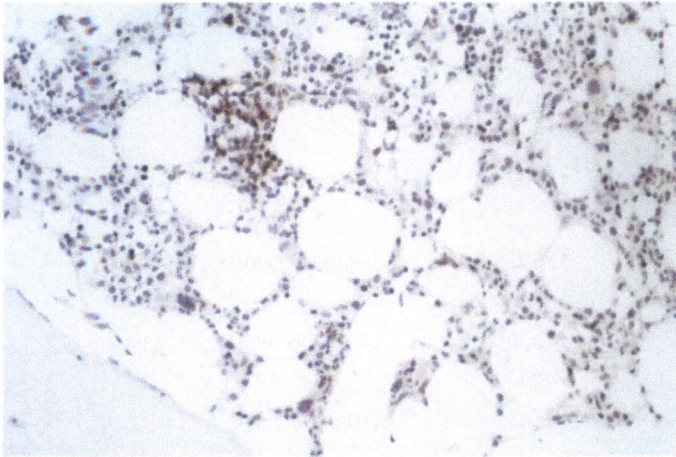

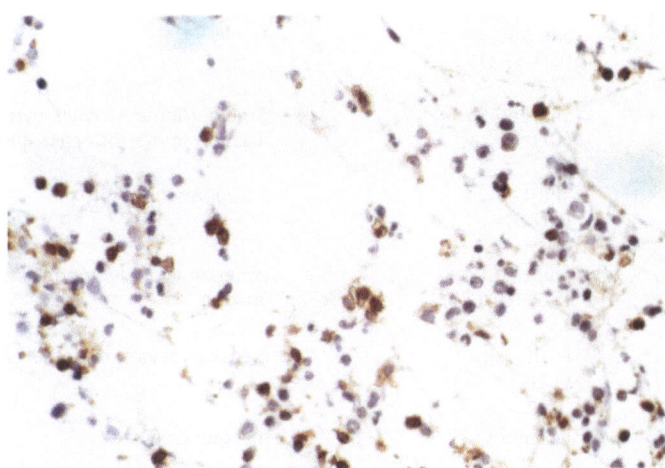

Fig. 1.134 Section reacted with VCHL; note that the nodule (Fig. 1.133, upper right) is positive for the T-cell marker

Fig. 1.135 Another part of the section in Fig. 1.134, showing interstitial T cells which have reacted with the antibody

Table 1.3 Antibodies and their cell reactivity

Antibody (Reference)	Main specificity	Dilution in PBS (pH 7.6)	Source
VIM 8 (1)	granulocytes	1 : 100	Prof. Knapp, Vienna
VIM D2 (2)	monocytes, endothelial cells	1 : 300	Prof. Knapp, Vienna
VIM D2 (3)	myelomonocytic cells (granulocytes, monocytes)	1 : 50	Prof. Knapp, Vienna
My 7 (CD 13) (4)	myelomonocytic cells, endothelial cells	1 : 20	Coulter, Krefeld, FRG
Ki-M6	blood monocytes, tissue macrophages excluding accessory cells of T- or B-cell immune response	1 : 500	Behring/Marburg, FRG
Ki-M8	blood monocytes, tissue macrophages excluding accessory cells of T- or B-cell immune response, follicle mantle lymphocytes	1 : 500	Behring/Marburg, FRG
VIEG 4 (5)	glycophorin A (erythroid cells)	1 : 300	Prof. Knapp, Vienna
VIPL 1 (CDw40) (6)	gp IIb/IIIa megakaryocytes, platelets	1 : 500	Prof. Knapp, Vienna
anti-HLA-DR (7)	monocytes, macrophages, B lymphocytes, activated T cells, immature myeloid and possibly erythroid cells, some null cells and Langerhans cells	1 : 200	Becton, Dickinson, CA, USA
to Ig G	gamma chain specific	1 : 200	Dako, Denmark
anti Leu 14 (CD 22) (8)	B cells	1 : 50	Becton Dickinson, CA, USA
anti pan B (CD 19)	B cells	1 : 100	Dako, Denmark
anti E-rec (CD 2) (9)	T cells	1 : 200	Dako, Denmark
anti Leu 4 (CD 3) (10)	T cells	1 : 100	Becton Dickinson CA, USA
anti Leu 3a (CD 4)	T-helper/inducer, weak cytoplasmic reaction in macrophages and monocytes	1 : 100	Becton Dickinson CA, USA
anti Leu 2a (CD 8)	T-suppressor/cytotoxic	1 : 100	Becton Dickinson, CA, USA
anti CALLA (CD 10) (11)	common acute lymphoblastic leukaemia antigen	1 : 50	Becton Dickinson, CA, USA
F VIII rag (12)	megakaryocytes, endothelial cells	1 : 300	Dako, Denmark
Desmin (13)	myogenic cells	1 : 10	Dako, Denmark
Transferrin-rec. (OKT 9) (14)	erythroid cells, lymphoblasts, tumour cell lines, monocytes	1 : 20	Dako, Denmark

References for Appendix

1. Gatta, K. C., Heryet, A., Brown, D. C. and Mason, D. Y. (1987). Is it necessary to embed bone marrow biopsies in plastic for haematological diagnosis? *Histopathology*, **11**, 1
2. Murray, G. I. (1988). Is wax on the wane? *J. Pathol.*, **156**, 187
3. Plastic or paraffin? Editorial (1989). *Lancet*, **1**, 139
4. Murray, G. I. and Ewen, S. W. B. (1989). Plastic or paraffin? *Lancet*, **1**, 387.
5. Bennett, K. W., Winstanley, T. G., Taylor, A. K. M. and Shorthouse, A. J. (1989). Plastic or paraffin? *Lancet*, **1**, 653.
6. Warnke, R. A. and Rouse, R. V. (1985). Limitations encountered in the application of tissue section immunodiagnosis to the study of lymphomas and related disorders. *Human Pathol.*, **16**, 326
7. Beckstead, J. H. (1985). Optimal antigen localization in human tissues using aldehyde-fixed plastic-embedded sections. *J. Histochem Cytochem.*, **33**, 954
8. Freedman, A. S. and Nadler, L. M. (1987). Cell surface markers in hematologic malignancies. *Sem. Oncol.*, **14**, 193
9. Archimbaud, E., Islam, A. and Preisler, H. (1987). Immunoperoxidase detection of myeloid antigens in glycolmethacrylate-embedded human bone marrow. *J. Histochem. Cytochem.*, **35**, 595
10. Wolf, E., Hantschieck, M. and Dominok, G. (1988). Immuno- and enzymehistochemical studies of methacrylate-embedded biopsy material, especially iliac crest biopsies. *Acta Histochem.*, Suppl. (Jena), **35**, 179
11. Casey, T. T., Cousar, J. B. and Collinson, R. D. (1988). A simplified platic embedding and immunohistologic technique for immunophenotypic analysis of human haematopoietic and lymphoid tissues. *Am. J. Pathol.*, **131**, 183
12. Leder, L. d. (1964). Ueber die selektive fermentcytochemische Darstellung von neutrophilen myeloischen Zellen und Gewebsmastzellen im Paraffinschnitt. *Klin. Wochenschr.*, **42**, 533

References for Table 1.3

1. Knapp, W., Majdic, O., Stockinger, H., Bettelheim, P., Liszka, K., Köller, U. and Peschel, Ch. (1984). Monoclonal antibodies to human myelomonocyte differentiation antigens in the diagnosis of acute myeloid leukemia. *Med. Oncol. Tumour Pharmacother.*, **4**, 257
2. Majdic, O., Bettelheim, P., Liszka, K. and Lutz, D. (1982). Leukämiediagnostik mit monoklonalen Antikörpern. *Wien Klin. Wochenschr.*, **94**, 387
3. Majdec, O., Bettelheim, P., Stockinger, H., Aberer, W., Liszka, K., Lutz, D. and Knapp, W. (1984). M 2, a novel myelomonocytic cell surface antigen and its distribution on leukemic cells. *Int. J. Cancer*, **33**, 617
4. Griffin, J. D., Ritz, J., Nadler, M. and Schlossman, S. F. (1981). Expression of myeloid differentiation antigens on normal and malignant myeloid cells. *J. Clin. Invest.*, **68**, 932
5. Knapp, W., Majdic, O., Holter, W., Stockinger, H. and Köller, U. (1985). Überlegungen zur therapeutischen Verwendung monoklonaler Antikörper. *Wien Klin. Wochenschr.*, **97**, 97
6. Vainschenker, W., Deschamps, J. F., Bastin, J. M., Guichard, J., Titeux, M., Breton-Gorius, J. and McMichael, A. (1982). Two monoclonal antiplatelet antibodies as markers of human megakaryocyte maturation. Immunofluorescent staining and platelet peroxidase detection in megakaryocyte colonies and *in vivo* cells from normal and leukemic patients. *Blood*, **59**, 514
7. Lampson, L. A. and Levy, R. (1980). Two populations of Ia-like molecules on a human B-cell line. *J. Immunol.*, **125**, 293
8. Stein, J., Gerdes, J. and Mason, D. Y. (1982). The normal and malignant germinal centre. *Clin. Haematol.*, **11**, 531
9. Thurlow, P. J., Lovering, E. K., d'Apice, A. J. F. and McKenzie, I. F. C. (1983). A monoclonal anti-pan T cell antibody: *in vitro* and *in vivo* studies. *Transplantation*, **36**, 212
10. Beverley, P. C. L. and Callard, E. (1981). Distinctive functional characteristics of human 'T' lymphocytes defined by E rosetting or a monoclonal anti-T cell antibody. *Eur. J. Immunol.*, **11**, 329
11. Ritz, J., Pesando, J. H., Sallan, S. E., Clavell, L. A., MacConarty, N., Rosenthal, P. and Schlossman, S. F. (1981). A monoclonal antibody to human lymphoblastic leukaemia antigen. *Nature*, **283**, 583
12. Mukai, K., Rosai, J. and Burgdorf, W. H. C. (1980). Localization of factor VIII rag in vascular cells using an immunoperoxidase method. *Am. J. Surg Pathol.*, **4**, 273
13. Osborn, M. and Weber, K. (1983). Biology of disease: tumor diagnosis by imtermediate filament typing: a novel tool for surgical pathology. *Lab. Invest.*, **48**, 372
14. Sutherland, R., Delia, D., Schneider, C., Newnson, R., Kemshead, J. T. and Greaves, M. (1981). Ubiquitous cell surface glycoprotein on tumor cells is proliferation-associated receptor for transferrin. *Proc. Natl. Acad. Sci. USA*, **78**, 4515
15. Cordell, J. L., Falini, B., Erber, W. N., Gosh, A. K., Abdulaziz, Z, Mac Donald, S., Pulford, K. A. F., Stein, H. and Mason, D. Y. (1984). Immunoenzymatic labeling of monoclonal antibodies using immune complexes of alkaline phosphatase and monoclonal anti-alkaline phosphatase (APAAP complexes). *J. Histochem. Cytochem.*, **32**, 219

Cytopenias

This term refers to a decrease (or decreases) in the levels of any of the formed elements of the peripheral blood. The cause(s) may be ineffective or reduced production, increased peripheral utilization and/or destruction without a balanced matching increase in production, or a combination of these mechanisms. The numerous possible causes for peripheral cytopenias are given in textbooks of haematology; here conditions will be illustrated in which a bone marrow biopsy provides diagnostically useful information.

Aplastic Anaemia

Aplastic or hypoplastic anaemia (Figs 2.1–2.14) is an 'umbrella' term for a variety of disorders characterized by reduction in the formed elements of the blood (pancytopenia, referring to red cells, granulocytes and platelets) together with hypocellularity of the bone marrow. When hypoplasia is suspected a BMB is indicated to exclude other causes that might be responsible for the peripheral cytopenia. These include myeloproliferative and lymphoproliferative disorders, metastatic carcinomas and refractory anaemias. Aplastic anaemia may also precede other haematological disorders or neoplasias; for example hairy cell leukaemia[1].

For a reliable assessment of bone marrow cellularity a cylinder of a least 2 × 20–30 mm is required. The widespread occurrence of hypocellularity can be confirmed by isotopic scanning techniques. Occassionally, a bone marrow aspirate or biopsy may yield a hypercellular or normocellular specimen. This is due to the accidental sampling of a residual focus of haematopoiesis – the so-called 'hot spots', especially when they contain large erythropoietic islands usually showing some degree of maturation arrest and dyserythropoiesis. Representative sections of the bone marrow in hypo- and aplasia are shown in Figs 2.9–2.14. There is a drastic reduction in haematopoietic tissue which is replaced by fat cells among which are scattered haemosiderin-loaded macrophages, mast and plasma cells and lymphocytes. Sinusoids may be decreased, but the residual foci of erythroid precursors are typically situated close to sinusoids, and show maturation inhibition. Some mitotic figures may be present, and histiocytes with erythrophagocytosis may be found in the vicinity. Megakaryocytes may be absent, or widely dispersed single ones or very small clusters may be found, in addition to small groups of myeloid precursors. Varying degrees of inflammatory infiltrates – lymphoid, plasma and mast cells, eosinophils and neutrophils may be present (Figs 2.5–2.8). Increases in blasts are generally not found. In early cases the bone marrow may show interstitial oedema, serous atrophy, necrotic cells and capillaries and lipomacrophages, especially in cases due to starvation, anorexia nervosa or radiation. Immunohistology on cryostat sections is required for precise characterization of residual stromal and haematopoietic and infiltrating elements; for example, the proportion of B and T cells, and of subsets of T lymphocytes (Figs 2.13 and 2.14).

A reduction in trabecular bone (osteopenia) is also seen in hypoplasias of long duration, possibly due to inadequacy of the local blood supply. No features of bone marrow histology have yet been identified which could be used as parameters of prognostic significance and reliably predict the course of disease. However, lymphocytic infiltrations and capillary necroses were rare in cases who later recovered. Also complete fatty replacement of haematopoiesis carried a less favourable prognosis than partial aplasia at the onset of disease.

There is a very heterogeneous group of possible aetiologies for aplastic anaemia, but in most cases the cause is *not* reflected in the bone marrow picture, and in many patients the aetiology remains obscure in spite of extensive investigations. The aplastic anaemia associated with pancytopenia presumably arises from a defective stem cell (or pluripotent precursor cell) as distinct from isolated reductions in red cells, in granulocytes or in platelets which result from failure of proliferation and differentiation of the committed precursors which produce these cell lines.

When classified according to aetiology aplastic anaemia could be divided into the following broad groups:

1. Idiopathic (or unknown) which includes the constitutional[2,3] (familial or congenital e.g. Fanconi's) (Figs 2.15–2.17), and the acquired, when no history of exposure to any agent known to induce bone marrow suppression can be elicited.
2. Secondary: this group includes exposure to agents known to cause bone marrow damage depending on the extent and duration of exposure; a subgroup includes exposure to substances associated with aplastic anaemia in only a small proportion of the exposed population. The agents themselves include physical (ionising radiation), drugs: cytotoxic and other chemicals; infections: viral and some bacterial[4–8]. The recognition of chemotherapy-induced myelosuppression has now assumed additional significance with the advent of therapy with colony-stimulating factors[9]. Drug-induced myelosuppression is considered in the section on secondary myelodysplastic syndromes.

Some authors have addressed the question of the prognostic and predictive value of variations in bone marrow histology and in myeloid progenitor cells in aplastic anaemia[10]; in particular, whether the degree or grade of inflammatory infiltrate might be used as an indicator of the response to immunosuppressive therapy; but this was not confirmed in a larger series of patients[11]. Inflammatory grade had no prognostic value either in the immunosuppressed patients or in the marrow transplant group. However, complete restitution takes place after aplasia caused by starvation[12,13] (e.g. anorexia nervosa) once adequate nutrition is resumed.

In addition, the extent of the hypoplasia found at initial examination – that is the percentage of the bone marrow haematopoietic tissue that is replaced by fat cells – appears to have some bearing on the subsequent course. Partial atrophy carries a lesser risk than complete replacement.

(Continued on p. 42)

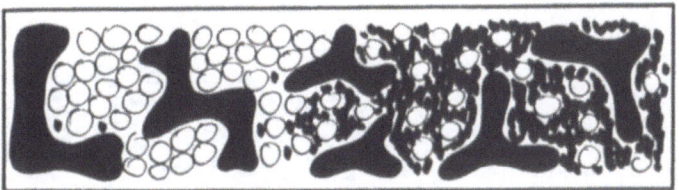

SUBCORTICAL ATROPHY

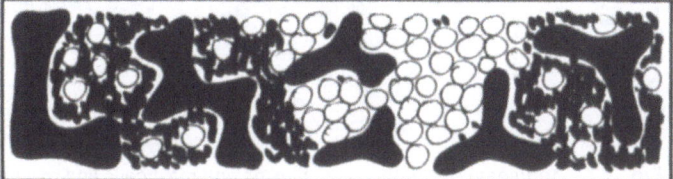

PATCHY ATROPHY

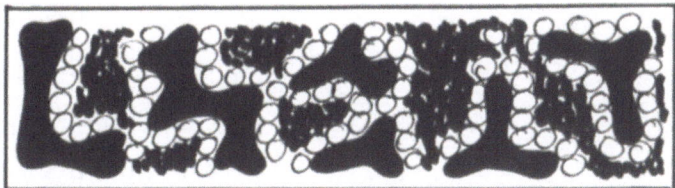

ENDOSTEAL ATROPHY (INCIPIENT OSTEOPOROSIS)

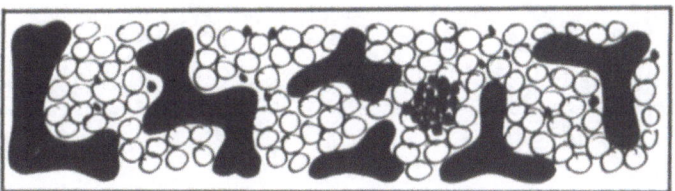

TOTAL ATROPHY (APLASTIC ANAEMIA)

Fig. 2.1 Schematic representation of types of marrow hypoplasia (atrophy)

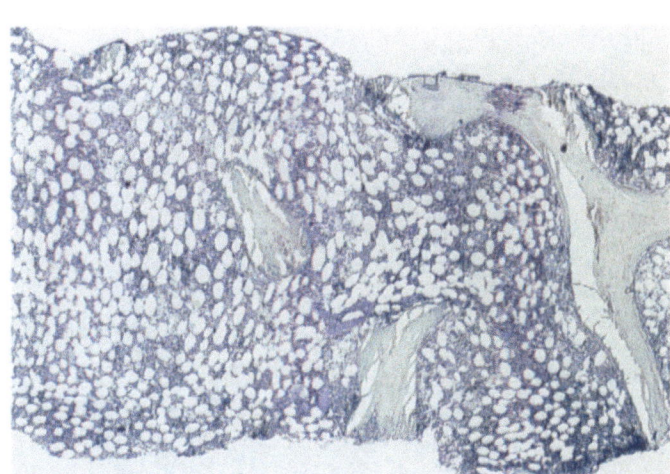

Fig. 2.2 Low magnification of bone biopsy showing hypocellular bone marrow, with fairly even distribution of fat cells and haematopoietic precursors

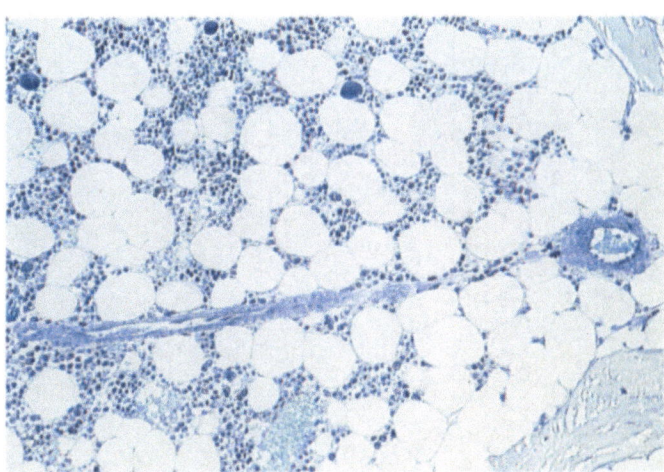

Fig. 2.3 Higher magnification of part of Fig. 2.2 showing precursors of all three cell lines

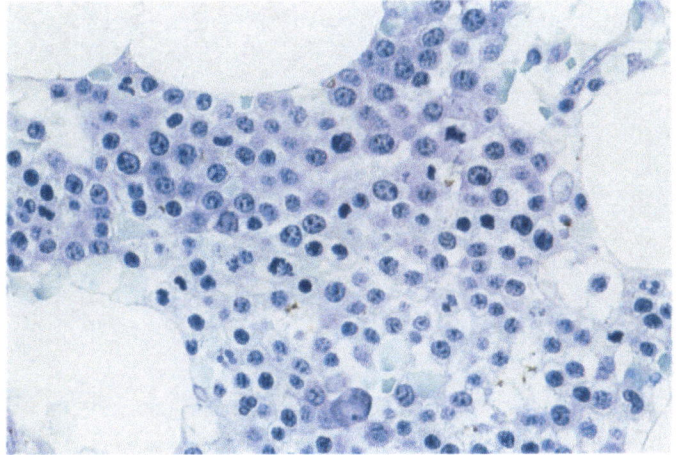

Fig. 2.4 Erythropoietic 'hot spot' in otherwise hypocellular bone marrow (not illustrated)

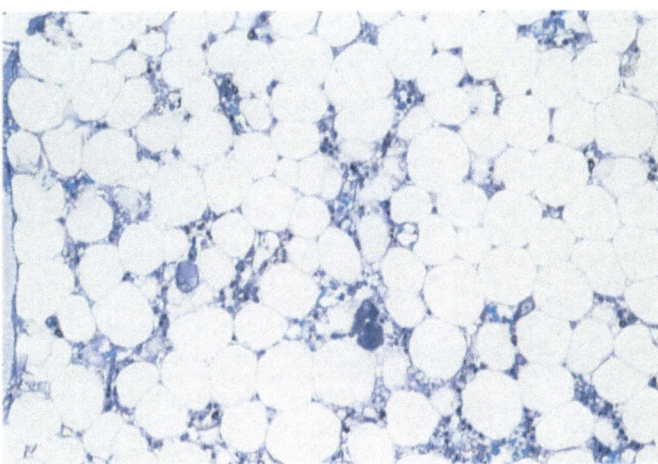

Fig. 2.5 Hypoplastic bone marrow with isolated megakaryocytes, macrophages and inflammatory cells

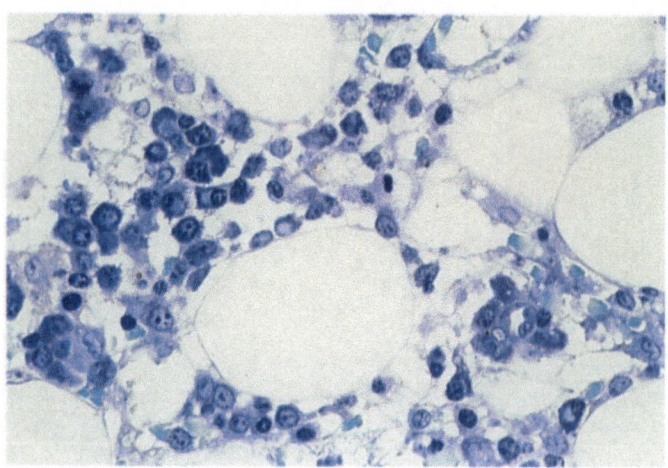

Fig. 2.6 Lymphocytic and plasmacytic infiltration in hypocellular bone marrow

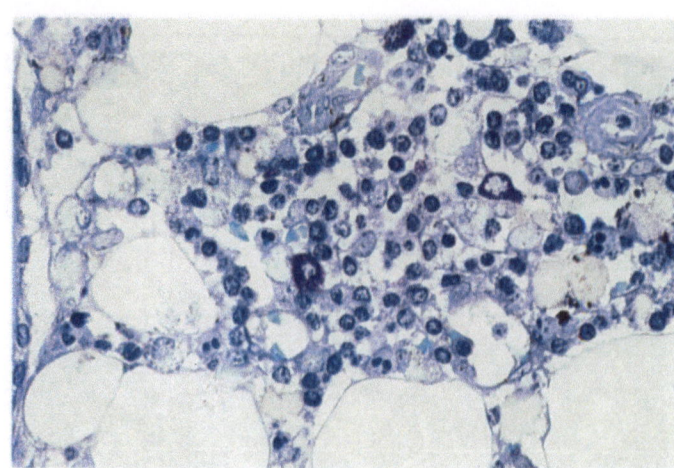

Fig. 2.7 Aggregate of lymphocytes, plasma and mast cells and macrophages

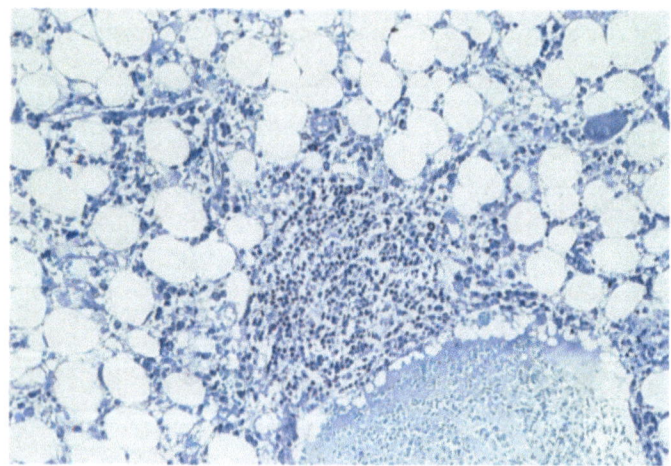

Fig. 2.8 Parasinusoidal lymphoid cell aggregate in hypocellular bone marrow. Note perivascular plasmacytosis, upper right

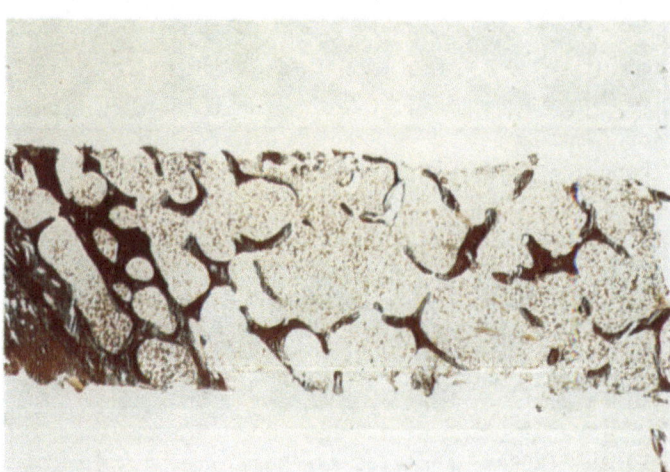

Fig. 2.9 Low magnification of bone biopsy section of patient with aplastic anaemia. Note residual haematopoiesis in subcortical region

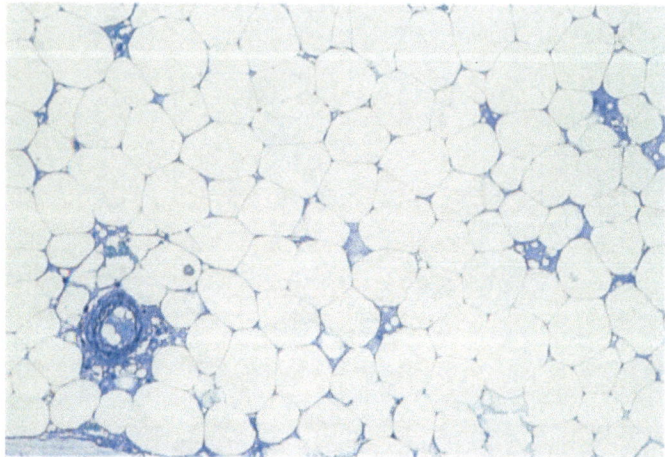

Fig. 2.10 Higher magnification of part of section shown in Fig. 2.9, fat cells, small artery, few sinusoids

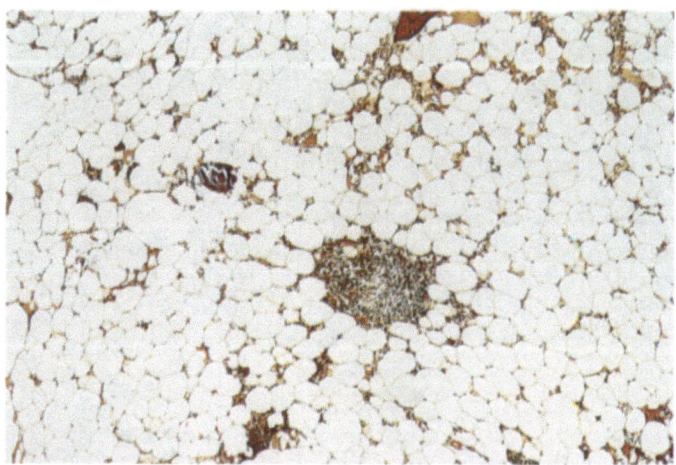

Fig. 2.11 As in Fig. 2.10, empty marrow with small lymphoid cell aggregate. Gomori

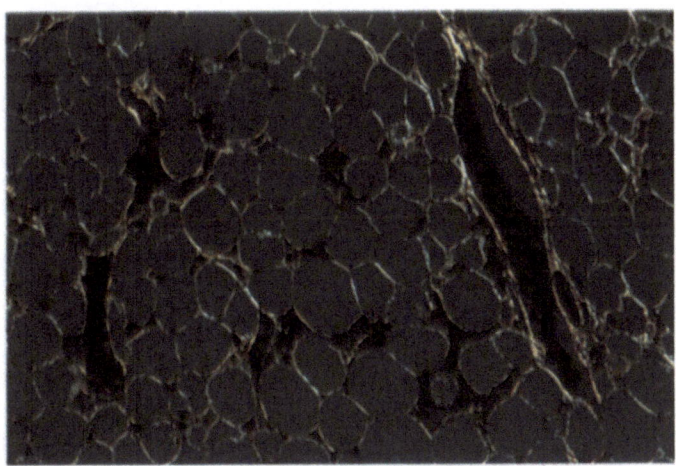

Fig. 2.12 As in Fig. 2.11, Gomori's stain viewed in polarized light. Note outlines of fat cells

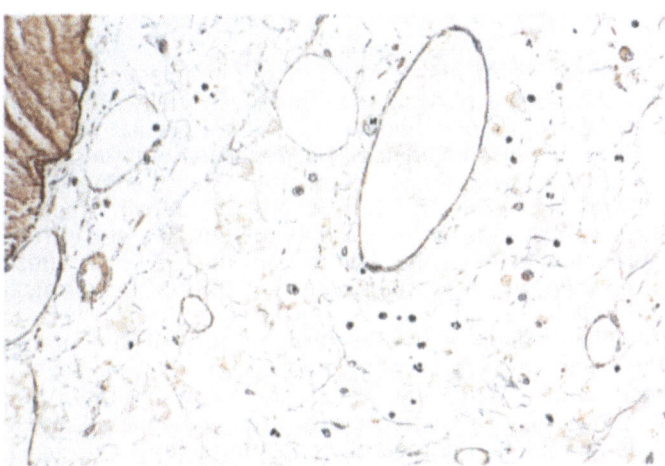

Fig. 2.13 Bone biopsy section of patient with aplastic anaemia, showing exudative myelitis. Gomori

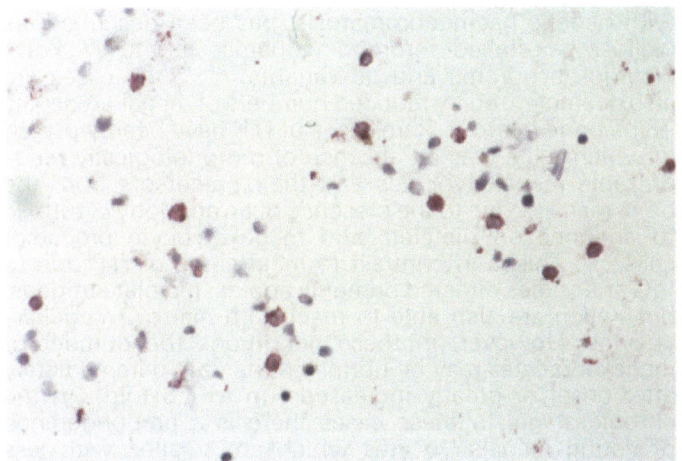

Fig. 2.14 Cryostat section from same biopsy as in Fig. 2.13. Demonstration of T lymphocytes by their reaction with CD_4 (anti Leu 3a)

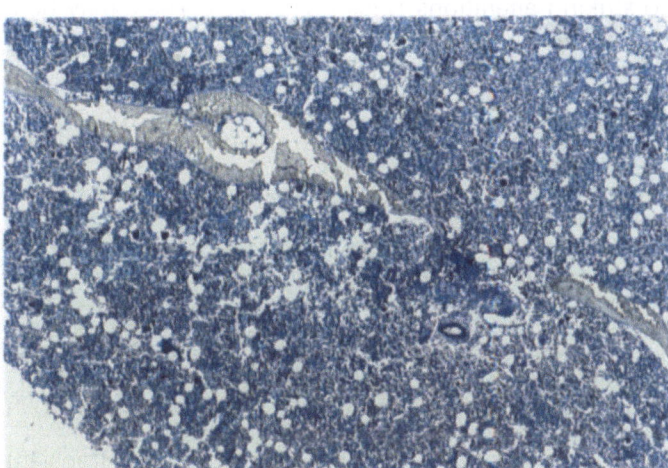

Figs 2.15–2.17 Bone biopsy section of 36-year-old male patient with dyskeratosis congenita. All these figures represent different areas from the same biopsy

Fig. 2.15 Low-power view of hypercellular area

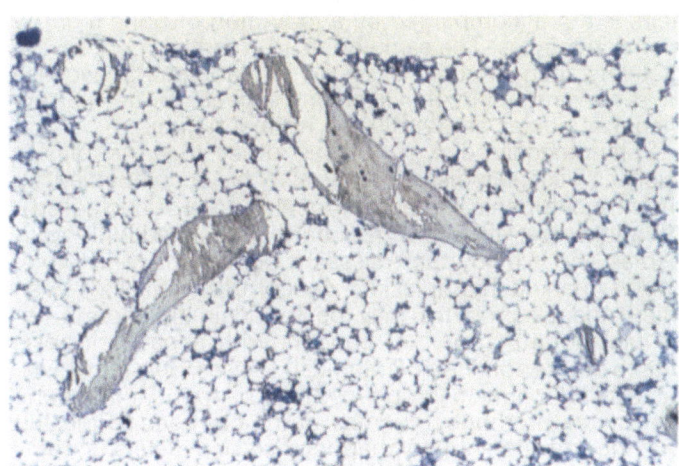

Fig. 2.16 Low-power view of hypocellular area

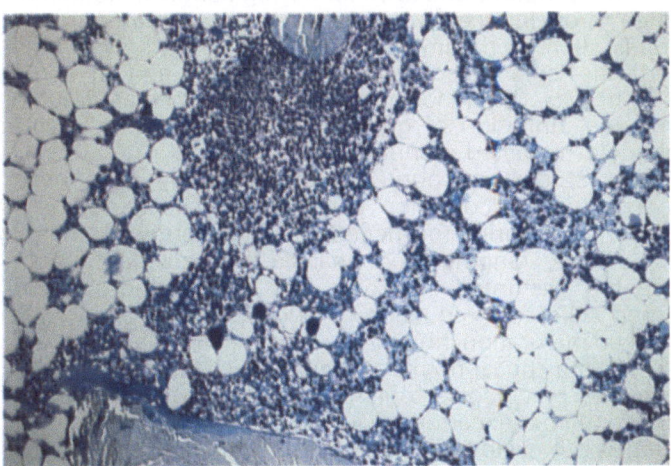

Fig. 2.17 Lymphoid cell aggregate in bone marrow with myelodysplastic features

The residual haematopoietic tissue in aplastic anaemia may show signs of dysplasia. This is especially prominent in the erythroid precursors – dyserythropoiesis.

Though aplastic anaemia is generally regarded as a disease of haematopoietic precursor cells, some cases are apparently due to failure of the microenvironment[14], and/or to defects in the microcirculation[15,16], and others to imbalances of regulatory mechanisms. However, these cases cannot be recognised by routine histological methods.

Selective depression of erythropoiesis occurs in chronic renal disorders and in patients on haemodialysis; several factors have been implicated, including inhibition by aluminium in the latter group. The anaemia in these patients may be improved by chelating agents.

Pure Red Cell Aplasia

This may be acute or chronic. The chronic type is either congenital – the Blackfan-Diamond syndrome – or acquired, with selective inhibition of erythropoiesis.

At low magnification the bone marrow histology shows no striking alterations (Figs 2.18–2.22). There may be a patchy, localized replacement by fat cells, together with areas of normal cellularity; but at high power these contain only an isolated erythroblast or two, with no erythroid islands. Megakaryocytes and granulopoietic precursors appear within normal limits. Iron-containing stromal cells are increased, as are macrophages containing cellular debris, and mast and plasma cells; aggregates of lymphoid cells may be present.

There are numerous potential causes of secondary pure red cell aplasia, including immunological, as in cold haemagglutinin disease and thymoma, or in cases associated with systemic lupus erythematosus and primary autoimmune hypothyroidism, and imbalance of T-cell subsets[17,18]. It may also occur in lymphoproliferative disorders, especially CLL and T-cell proliferations; and in myeloproliferative disorders, for example CML.

Viral infections are responsible for some of the transient erythroblastopenias of childhood, while the aplastic crisis in sickle cell disease has been associated with Parvovirus infection[19].

Granulocytopenia

This may rarely be constitutional, as in cyclic neutropenia, which is probably due to abnormal regulation, or acquired, often drug-induced[19-25]. It may occur in autoimmune states such as rheumatoid arthritis, in Felty's syndrome (arthritis, splenomegaly and leukopenia) and in some lymphomas. One mechanism is antibody-mediated autoimmune inhibition of granulopoiesis; another is T-lymphocyte-mediated granulopoietic failure.

Few studies on bone marrow histology have been reported in this condition, particularly in the acute phase (Fig. 2.23). During this period the bone marrow histology is variable, ranging from marked hypocellularity with oedema, disrupted sinusoids and extravasation of red blood cells, to a reduction in myeloid precursors and/or marked maturation inhibition, while the other cell lines and the stroma appear normal. When there is little reduction in myeloid precursors, together with marked maturation arrest, the bone marrow histological picture may resemble that of promyelocytic leukaemia, (Fig. 2.24), due to the absence of all the late maturational stages. Peripheral neutropenia, together with a cellular bone marrow, is typically seen in the autoimmune conditions mentioned above, e.g. rheumatoid arthritis and Felty's syndrome. Drug-induced agranulocytosis may be due to direct toxicity, in which case myelopoiesis may be absent, or be antibody-mediated as in ibuprofen-associated pure white

cell aplasia[26], in which a circulating complement-dependent antibody profoundly inhibited the growth of myeloid progenitors in vitro.

Extensive necrosis of the bone marrow with profound granulocytopenia may also occur after drug-induced bone marrow toxicity. The bone marrow histology showed extensive necrotic tissue occupying the intertrabecular areas and small patches of residual haematopoiesis infiltrated by lymphocytes and plasma cells.

Thrombocytopenias

Three main mechanisms are distinguished: defective production, accelerated loss, destruction or utilization and abnormal distribution. As with the other cytopenias, they may be classified into primary and secondary. The primary group includes consitutional and congenital thrombocytopenia[27-30] (e.g. Tar syndrome due to greatly reduced numbers of megakaryocytes – Fig. 2.25) and some cases of idiopathic thrombocytopenic purpura (ITP). In the former types the marrow is cellular with virtual absence of megakaryocytes. Thrombocytopenia, together with genetic haemochromatosis, has been described, as well as sex-linked thrombocytopenias in the Wiskott-Aldridge syndrome and its variants[30,31]. Such cases are also characterized by reduced numbers of megakaryocytes in the bone marrow. Rare cases of ITP have been reported in which there was an absence of morphologically recognizable megakaryocytes and their precursors from the bone marrow, due to the presence of an antibody cytotoxic to antigens on platelets and megakaryocyte precursor cells[32,33]. This is in contrast to most cases of ITP due to IgG antibodies directed primarily against platelet antigens, but which are also able to react with marrow megakaryocytes. However, in these conditions the number of megakaryocytes may be normal in the period immediately after onset or greatly increased (up to 4.8-fold), in the chronic stage. In these cases there is a preponderance of young megakaryocytes which are smaller, with less convoluted nuclei; but some larger ones are also present.

When a reduction in platelets is due to cytotoxic agents[34], and is part of an aplastic condition, the picture is that of an aplastic anaemia with reduction in megakaryocytes. Thrombocytopenia may be a presenting symptom of a pre-leukaemic condition (described in the section on myelodysplastic syndromes). The thrombocytopenia which occasionally occurs after drugs such as nalidixic acid, is not accompanied by a reduction of bone marrow megakaryocytes. The same holds true for the reduction in platelets seen in some cases of hypothermia[35], because of sequestration in the liver and spleen. Bone marrow megakaryocytes are within the normal range.

Splenomegaly due to causes other than neoplasias such as vascular disease may also be accompanied by thrombocytopenias (megakaryocytes are not decreased). Alcoholic liver disease is frequently associated with cytopenias, and in many such cases the bone marrow histology shows marked hypoplasia[36]. In contrast, small or even micro-megakaryocytes may be found in the normo- or cellular bone marrows of patients with hepatic cirrhosis due to other (non-haematological) causes. Sea-blue histiocytes and foamy macrophages may be found in the bone marrow in thrombocytopenias, and it has been suggested that they develop due to phagocytosis of platelets. Thrombocytopenia may be found in almost any type of autoimmune disease; megakaryocytes in the bone marrow are normal or increased (with the exceptions mentioned above). In thrombotic thrombocytopenic purpura[37] (TTP) the bone marrow architecture is essentially normal, megakaryocytes are within the normal range or increased and clumps of platelet may be found in small arterioles in

(Continued on p. 46)

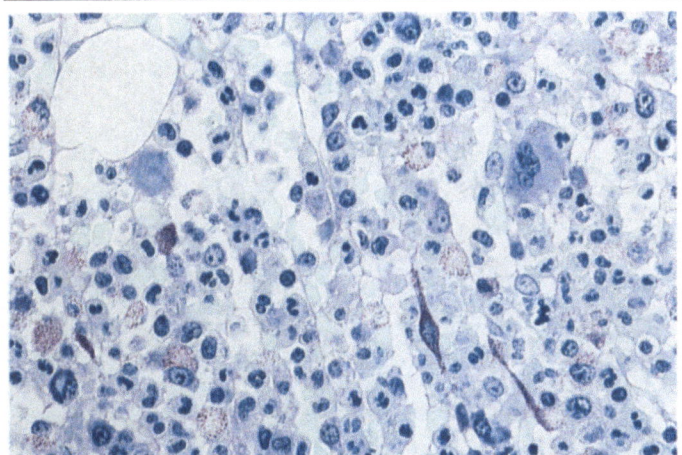

Fig. 2.18 · Section of bone biopsy of patient with pure red cell aplasia no erythroid islands present

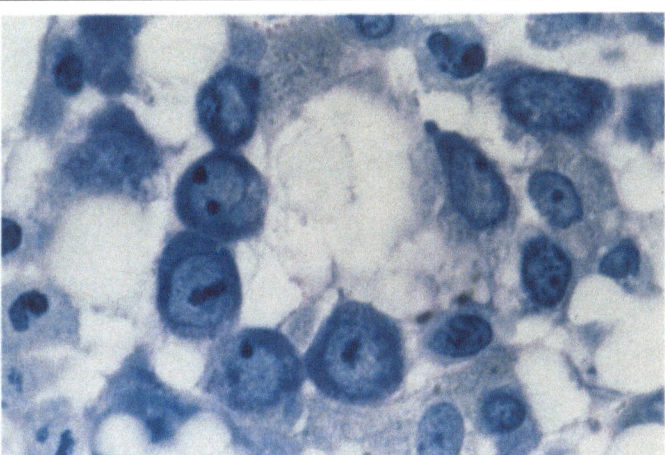

Fig. 2.19   Higher magnification of part of section shown in Fig. 2.18, showing one group of early erythroblasts

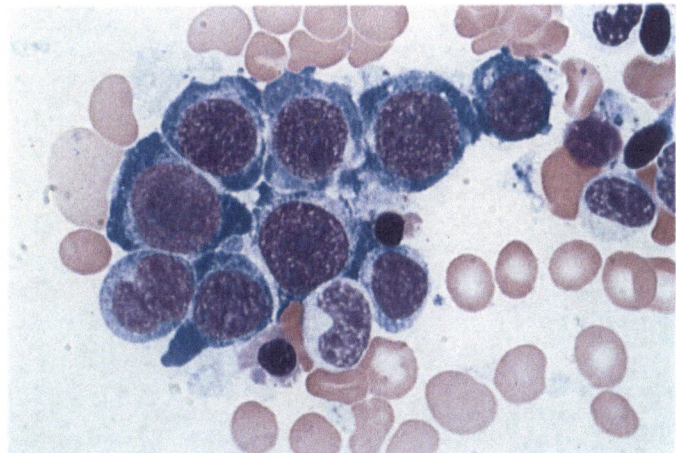

Fig. 2.20   Part of smear of aspirate of patient with pure red cell aplasia, there were no normoblasts (except for the two included here), early erythroblasts, maturation arrest; note one with two nuclei

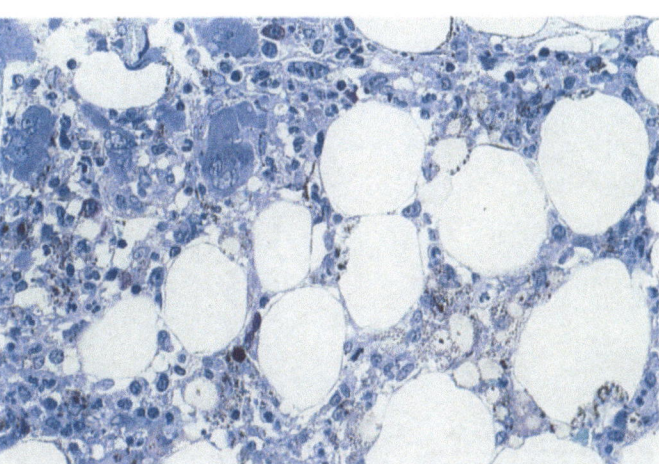

Fig. 2.21   Section of bone biopsy of patient with pure red cell aplasia; showing granulopoiesis, megakaryocytes, plasma, mast and lymphoid cells and macrophages with haemosiderosis

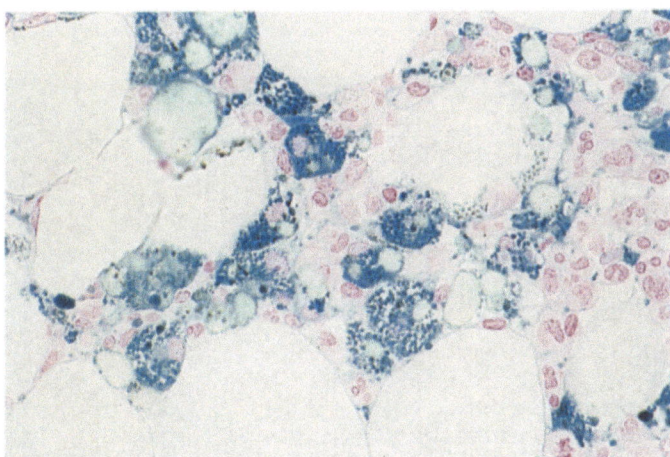

Fig. 2.22   Section parallel to Fig. 2.21, stained with Berlin blue showing iron deposition in macrophages and stromal cells

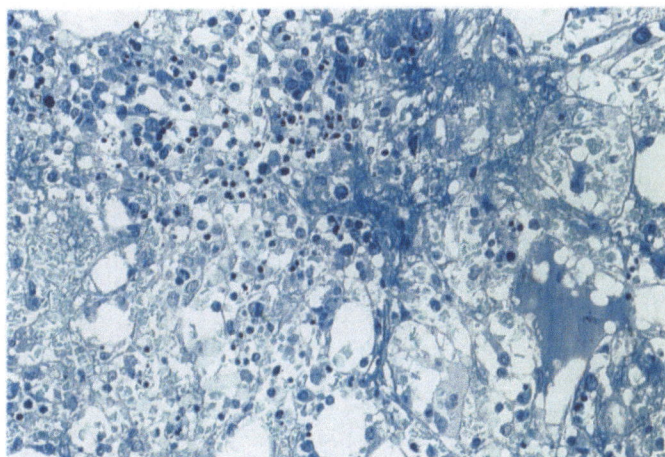

Fig. 2.23   Section of bone biopsy of patient with agranulocytosis, showing areas of necrosis, and deposition of fibrin in the bone marrow

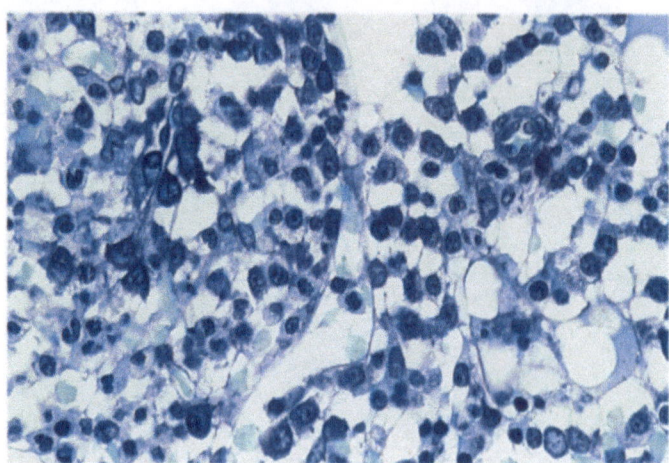

Fig. 2.24 Section of bone biopsy of patient with agranulocytosis, high magnification to show early haematopoietic precursors, with maturation arrest

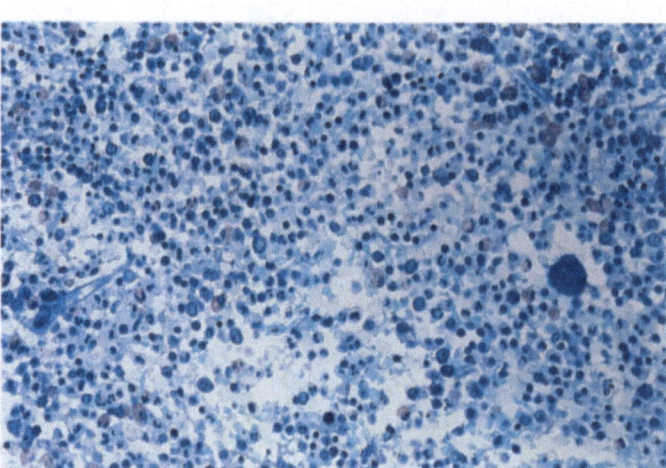

Fig. 2.25 Section of bone biopsy of patient with TAR syndrome (thrombocytopenia and absent radii); hypercellular bone marrow with one megakaryocyte

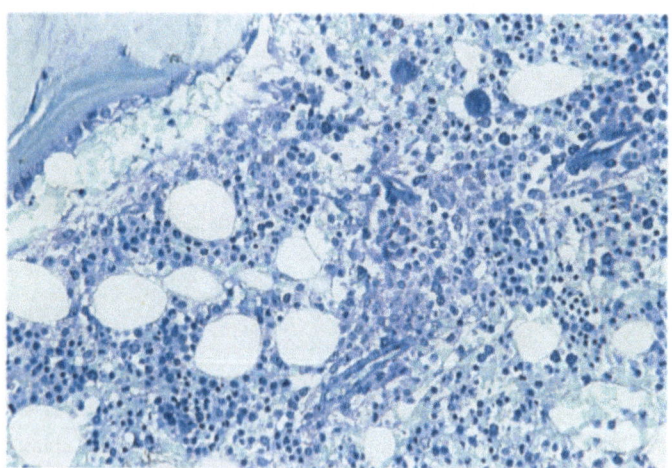

Fig. 2.26 Section of bone biopsy of patient with chronic hepatitis, showing myelodysplastic features, granulopoiesis with left shift and small megakaryocytes

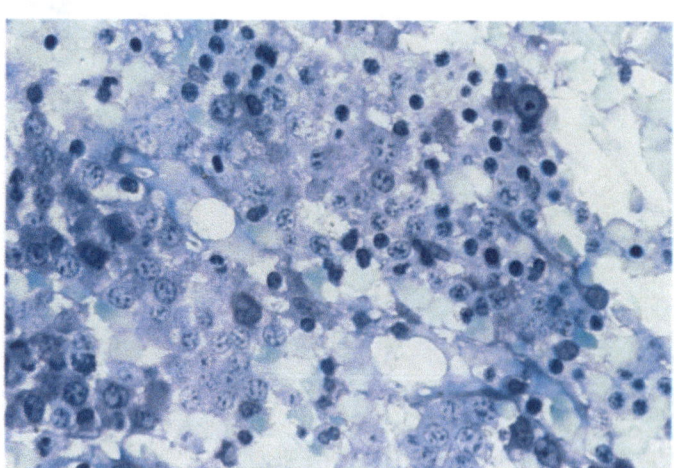

Fig. 2.27 Section of bone biopsy of patient with hepatic cirrhosis showing erythroid islands with megaloblastoid features and maturation arrest. Note lymphocytic infiltration

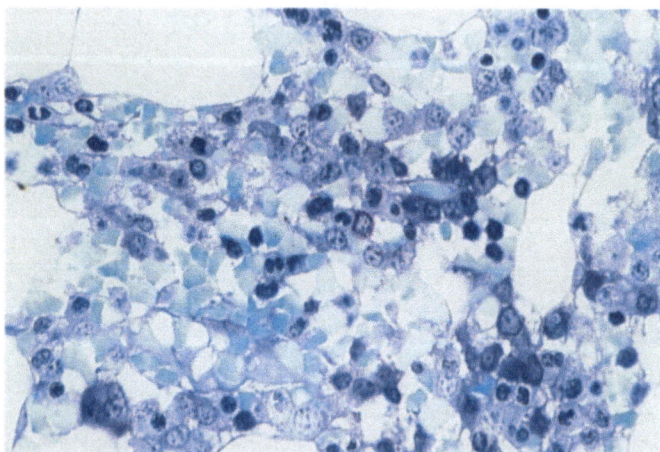

Fig. 2.28 Same case as Fig. 2.27, showing myelopoiesis with left shift, some megaloblastic erythroblasts, lymphocytes and mast cells

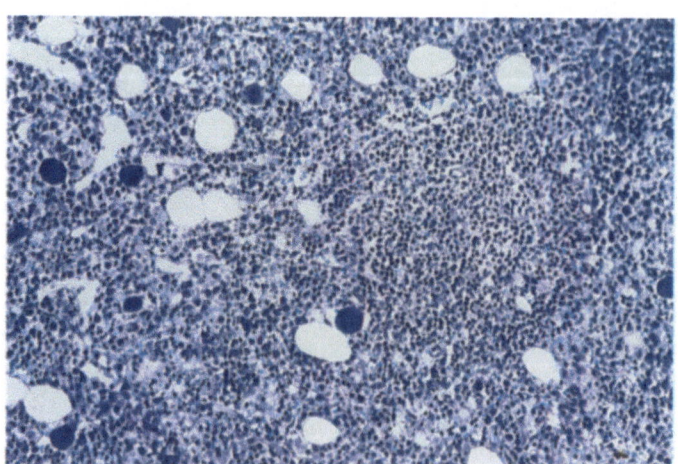

Fig. 2.29 Hypercellular bone marrow with large lymphoid nodule in bone biopsy of patient with rheumatoid arthritis

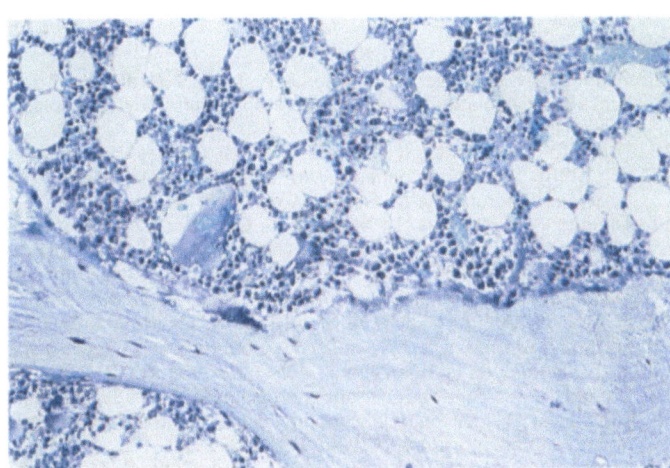

Fig. 2.30 Osteoclastic resorption in another patient with rheumatoid arthritis

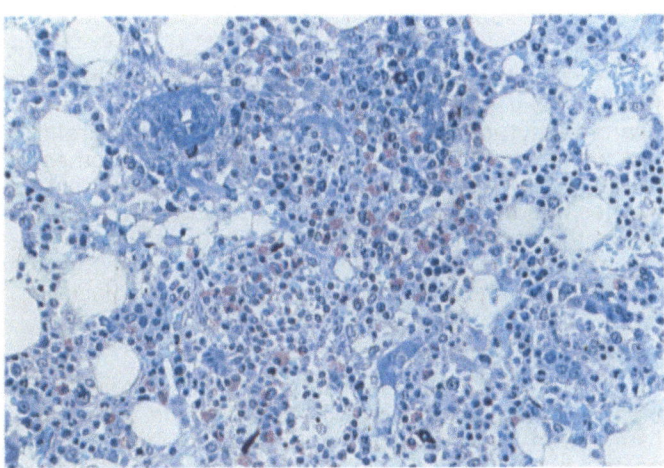

Fig. 2.31 Section of bone biopsy of patient with rheumatoid arthritis showing lymphocytosis and eosinophilia

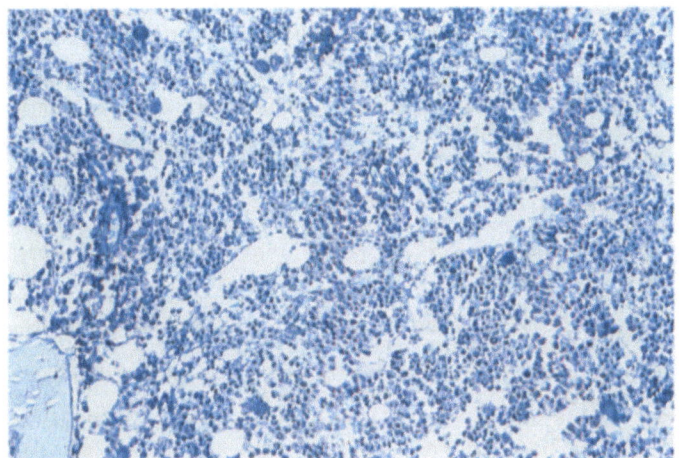

Fig. 2.32 Section of bone biopsy of patient with Felty's syndrome (arthritis, leucopenia and splenomegaly); cellular bone marrow with myeloid left shift

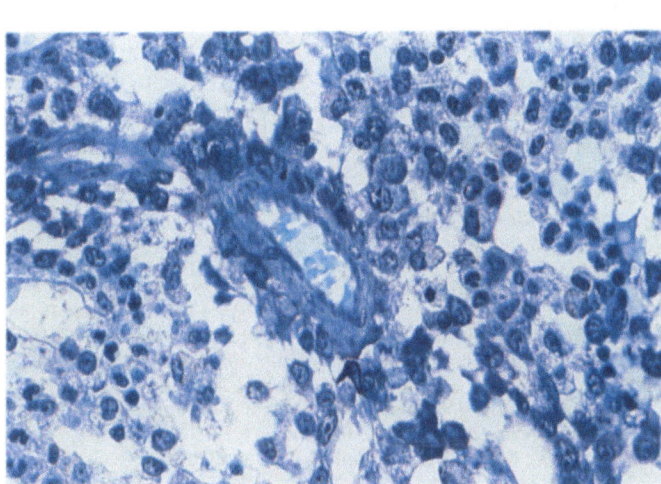

Fig. 2.33 Higher magnification of area from Fig. 2.31, showing early myeloid precursors

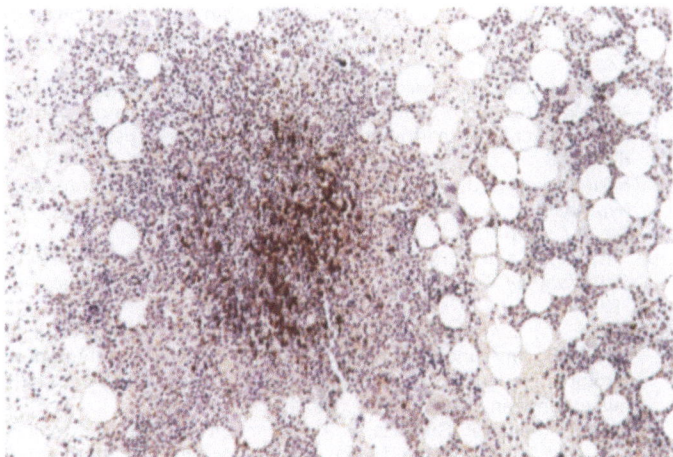

Fig. 2.34 Section of paraffin-embedded bone biopsy of patient with rheumatoid arthritis; B-lymphocytes are positive with the antibody MB2

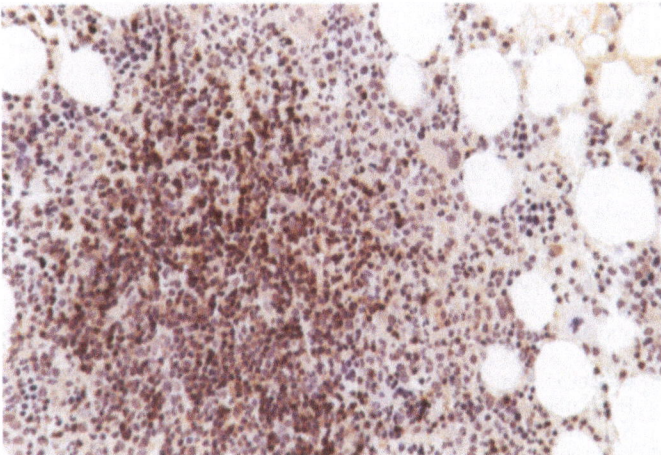

Fig. 2.35 Section parallel to that in Fig. 2.34, stained by LCA (leucocyte common antigen) indicating the mixed nature of the lymphoid nodules in rheumatoid arthritis

the bone marrow, coating the plaques of fibrinoid necrosis of the blood vessel walls.

Thrombocytopenia in the myelo- and lymphoproliferative disorders and the myelodysplastic syndromes is considered in the appropriate sections. The bone marrow changes due to chemotherapy and radiotherapy are dealt with in the section on secondary myelodysplasias.

Pancytopenias with hypercellular bone marrows are considered in the section on primary myelodysplasias.

Anaemia of Chronic Diseases

This is due to a number of factors, including impaired response by the bone marrow and defects in the metabolism of iron. Among the conditions in which this type of anaemia occurs are: chronic infections, chronic inflammatory non-infectious conditions, malignancies, chronic renal and hepatic disorders[38]. Iron-containing cells in the bone marrow are usually increased. In hepatic and rheumatic diseases the peripheral cytopenia may be accompanied by a cellular bone marrow, often showing maturation arrest (Figs 2.26–2.35). However, in cases of hepatic disease due to alcohol abuse, the bone marrow may be hypocellular.

References

1. Krause, J. R. (1984). Aplastic anemia terminating in hairy cell leukemia. A report of two cases. *Cancer*, **53**, 1533

2. Colvin, B. T., Baker, H., Hibbin, J. A., Gordon-Smith, E. C. and Gordon, M. Y. (1984). Haemopoietic progenitor cells in dyskeratosis congenita. *Br. J. Haematol.*, **56**, 513

3. Gutman, A., Frumkin, A., Adam, A., Block-Shtacher, N. and Rozenszajn, L. A. (1978). X-linked dyskeratosis congenita with pancytopenia. *Arch. Dermatol.*, **114**, 1667

4. MacDougall, L. G., Pettifor, J. M. and Patel, J. M. (1987). Bone growth and haemopoiesis: steroid reversible anaemia, mylofibrosis and increased bone formation in a child. *Br. J. Haematol.*, **66**, 5

5. Doney, K., Storb, R., Buckner, C. D. and Thomas, E. T. (1988). Treatment of gold-induced aplastic anaemia with immuno-suppressive therapy. *Br. J. Haematol.*, **68**, 469

6. Dhingra, K., Michels, S. D., Winton, E. F. and Gordon, D. S. (1988). Transient bone marrow aplasia associated with non-A, non-B hepatitis. *Am. J. Hematol.*, **29**, 168

7. Tzakis, A. G., Arditti, M., Whitington, P. F., Yanaga, K., Esquivel, C., Andrews, W. A., Markowka, I., Malatak, J. and Freese, D. K. (1988). Aplastic anemia complicating orthotopic liver transplantation for non-A, non-B hepatitis. *N. Engl. J. Med.*, **319**, 393

8. Brodsky, E., Zeidan, Z., Biger, Y. and Schneider, M. (1989). Topical application of chloramphenicol eye ointment followed by fatal bone marrow aplasia. *Isr. J. Med. Sci.*, **25**, 54

9. Antman, K. S., Griffin, J. D., Elias, A., Socinski, M. A., Ryan, L., Cannistra, S. A., Odette, D., Whitley, M., Frei III, E. and Schnipper, L. E. (1988). Effect of recombinant human granulocyte-macrophage colony-stimulating factor on chemo-therapy-induced myelosuppression. *N. Engl. J. Med.*, **319**, 593

10. Hinterberger, W., Geissler, K., Fisher, M., Lechner, K. and Kabrna, E. (1985). Aplastic anemia: assessment of myeloid progenitor cells in the bone marrow and blood provides prognostic information. *Acta Haematol.*, **73**, 1

11. Sale, G. E., Rajantie, J., Doney, K., Appelbaum, F. R., Storb, R. and Thomas, K. D. (1987). Does histologic grading of inflammation in bone marrow predict the response of aplastic anaemia patients to antithymocyte globulin therapy? *Br. J. Haematol.*, **67**, 261

12. Smith, R. R. L. and Spivak, J. L. (1985). Marrow cell necrosis in anorexia nervosa and involuntary starvation. *Br. J. Haematol.*, **60**, 525

13. Maisel, D., Lim, J. Y., Pollock, W. J., Yatani, R. and Liu, P. I. (1988). Bone marrow necrosis: an entity often overlooked. *Ann. Clin. Lab. Sci.*, **18**, 109

14. Islam, A. (1988). Do bone marrow fat cells or their precursors have a pathogenic role in idiopathic aplastic anaemia? *Med. Hypotheses*, **25**, 209

15. Zoumbos, N. C., Gascon, P., Djeu, J. Y., Trost, S. R. and Young, N. S. (1985). Circulating activated suppressor T lymphocytes in aplastic anaemia. *N. Engl. J. Med.*, **312**, 257

16. Tork-Storb, B., Doney, K., Sale, G., Donnall Thomas, E. and Storb, R. (1985). Subsets of patients with aplastic anemia identified by flow microfluorometry. *N. Engl. J. Med.*, **312**, 1015

17. Taniguchi, S., Shibuya, T., Morioka, E., Okamura, T., Okamura, S., Inaba, S. and Niho, Y. (1988). Demonstration of three distinct immunological disorders on erythropoiesis in a patient with pure red cell aplasia associated with thymoma. *Br. J. Haematol.*, **68**, 473

18. El Mouzan, M. I., Ahmad, M. A. M., Al Fadel Saleh, M., Al Sohaibani, M. O. and Al Gindan, Y. M. (1988). Myelofibrosis and pancytopenia in systemic lupus erythematosus. *Acta Haematol.*, **80**, 219

19. Conrad, M. E., Studdard, H. and Anderson, L. J. (1988). Aplastic crisis in sickle cell disorders: bone marrow necrosis and human parvovirus infection. *Am. J. Med. Sci.*, **295** 212

20. Wright, D. G., Dale, D. C., Fauci, A. S. and Wolff, S. M. (1981). Human cyclic neutropenia: clinical review and long-term follow-up of patients. *Medicine*, **60**, 1

21. Young, G. A. R. and Vincent, P. C. (1980). Drug-induced agranulocytosis. *Clin. Haematol.*, **9**, 483

22. Analgesics, agranulocytosis, and aplastic anaemia: a major case–control study (1986). *Lancet*, **2**, 899

23. Evans, D. I. K. (1988). Granulocytopenia due to fusidic acid. *Lancet*, **2**, 95

24. International Agranulocytosis and Aplastic Anaemia Study (1988). Risk of agranulocytosis and aplastic anaemia in relation to use of antithyroid drugs. *Br. Med. J.*, **297**, 262

25. Neftel, K. A., Woodtly, W., Schmid, M., Frick, P. G. and Fehr, J. (1986). Amodiaquine induced agranulocytosis and liver damage. *Br. Med. J.*, **292**, 721

26. Mamus, S. W., Burton, J. D., Groat, J. D., Schulte, D. A., Lobell, M. and Zanjani, E. D. (1986). Ibuprofen-associated pure white-cell aplasia. *N. Engl. J. Med.*, **314**, 624

27. Hall, J. G., Levin, J., Kuhn, J. P., Ottenheimer, E. J., von Berkunn, K. A. P. and McKusick, V. A. (1969). Thrombocytopenia with absent radius. *Medicine*, **48**, 411

28. Griffiths, A. D. (1983). Constitutional aplastic anemia: a family with a new X-linked variety of amegakaryocytic thrombocytopenia. *J. Med. Genet.*, **20**, 361

29. Koneti Rao, A. and Holmsen, H. (1986). Congenital disorders of platelet function. *Sem. Hematol.*, **23**, 102

30. Greaves, A., Pickering, C., Martin, J., Cartwright, I. and Preston, F. E. (1987). A new familial "giant platelet syndrome" with structural, metabolic and functional abnormalities of platelets due to a primary megakaryocyte defect. *Br. J. Haematol.*, **65**, 429

31. Mulnes, J. P., Schofield, K. P. and Low-Beer, T. S. (1986). Genetic haemochromatosis and thrombocytopenia. *Lancet*, **2**(8519), 1336

32. Hoffman, R., Zaknoen, S., Yang, H. H., Bruno, E., LoBuglio, A. F., Arrowsmith, J. B. and Prchal, J. T. (1985). An antibody cytotoxic to megakaryocyte progenitor cells in a patient with immune thrombocytopenic purpura. *N. Engl. J. Med.*, **312**, 1170

33. Smeets, R. E. and Hillen, H. F. (1988). Acquired amegakaryocytic thrombocytopenic purpura. Treatment with high-dose dexamethasone pulse therapy and review of the literature. *Neth. J. Med.*, **32**, 27

34. Rio, B., Andreau, G., Nicod, A., Arrago, J. P., Dutrillaux, F., Samama, M. and Zittoun, R. (1986). Thrombocytopenia in veno-occlusive disease after bone marrow transplantation or chemotherapy. *Blood*, **67**, 1773

35. Easterbrook, P. J. and Davis, H. P. (1985). Thrombocytopenia in hypothermia: a common but poorly recognised complication. *Br. Med. J.*, **291**, 23

36. Frisch, B., Lewis, S.M., Burkhardt, R. and Bartl, R. (1985). *Biopsy Pathology of Bone and Bone Marrow*. (London: Chapman and Hall)

37. Asada, Y., Sumiyoshi, A., Hayashi, T., Suzumiya, J. and Kaketani, K. (1985). Immunohistochemistry of vascular lesion in thrombotic thrombocytopenic purpura, with special reference to Factor VIII related antigen. *Thromb. Res.*, **38**, 469

38. De la Serna, F. J., Gilsanze, F., Ruilope, L. M., Praga, M., Rodicio, J. L. and Alcazar, J. M. (1988). Improvement in the erythropoiesis of chronic haemodialysis patients with Desferrioxamine. *Lancet*, **1**, 1009

Hyperplasias

3

Erythrocytes

A raised red cell count (secondary polycythaemia or erythrocytosis), without leukocytosis or thrombocytosis, is due to stimulation of erythropoiesis by increased levels of erythropoietin[1]. This may be congenital, as a result of abnormal haemoglobins, or acquired, as in pulmonary or vascular diseases, or residence at high altitudes, or due to various tumours such as renal carcinoma, cerebellar adenomas and uterine myomas or due to drugs[2]. In secondary erythrocytosis the bone marrow shows a normal architectural pattern and cellularity is normal to increased with numerous erythroid islands (Fig. 3.1). Iron stores are not depleted (provided there is no iron deficiency) and marrow reticulin is normal.

In 'pseudo' or stress polycythaemia due to a reduced plasma volume, the red cell mass is not increased and the bone marrow histology is normal.

Leukaemoid Reactions

These may involve neutrophilic or eosinophilic granulocytes, lymphocytes or monocytes. The peripheral blood values and pictures may mimic those seen in leukaemias, especially chronic myeloid leukaemia (CML) (Figs 3.2–3.8). Leukaemoid reactions may occur in numerous conditions including infections and inflammatory states, in allergies, in response to drugs, burns, and neoplasms[3,4]. Eosinophilia may be found especially in allergic disorders, parasitic infections, immune and collagen diseases[5].

It may not be possible to distinguish a leukaemoid reaction and CML on bone marrow histology alone (Figs 3.2, 3.3, 3.6 and 3.7). The overall marrow cellularity is increased and fat cells may be virtually absent, replaced by granulocytic precursors. In the reactive state numerous polymorphonuclear leukocytes are dispersed throughout the marrow. The hyperplastic granulopoiesis is perivascular and intertrabecular, without the broad paratrabecular seams of early myeloid precursors seen in CML. Charcot–Leyden crystal-containing cells are found in the bone marrow whenever there is also an element of eosinophilic hyperplasia. Megakaryocytes are within the normal range or somewhat increased, but show no marked atypical morphological features or clustering. In CML basophils are increased – in the bone marrow and in the peripheral blood – this is usually not seen in leukaemoid reactions.

Thrombocytosis

Transient elevations in the platelet counts may occur after splenectomy, in acute or chronic inflammations, after bleedings and after operations and after administration of some drugs[6]. Thrombocytosis may be observed in patients with Hodgkin's disease, malignant lymphomas and various carcinomas. (Figs 3.9–3.14). In these secondary conditions (providing there is no bone marrow involvement) the bone marrow architectural pattern is normal, with normal to increased cellularity and a mild to moderate increase in megakaryocytes both in size[7] and in number but without the marked polymorphism and clustering

which characterize neoplastic megakaryocytic proliferations. However, megakaryocytes in the bone marrow may not be increased in some of these reactive conditions even in the presence of high peripheral blood platelet counts.

Lymphocytosis

The differential diagnosis between reactive and neoplastic lymphoid infiltrations in the bone marrow is considered in the section on lymphoproliferative disorders (Fig. 3.15). Polyclonal peripheral blood lymphocytosis is likely to be reactive rather than neoplastic, as in some cigarette smokers[8,9]. Malignant thymoma may be accompanied by lymphocytosis[10]. Lymphocytosis may also occur in disorders of the immune system[11] (see Chapter 8).

Plasmacytosis

Reactive bone marrow plasmacytosis has been reported in numerous conditions (Figs 3.16–3.19). In reactive plasmacytosis the plasma cells are dispersed throughout the marrow, singly, or in groups of two or three, and are clustered around capillaries and small blood vessels. These bone marrow pictures may resemble those seen in early or in smouldering MM and in monoclonal gammopathy (see Chapter 8). Reactive plasmacytosis is especially common in allergic and autoimmune states, and in certain cytopenias, especially drug-induced.

Mast Cells

Increases in bone marrow mast cells have been observed in many conditions, often together with bone marrow plasma- and lymphocytosis (Figs 3.20–3.27). In most reactive conditions the mast cells are found along the walls of sinusoids and small blood vessels as well as among the marrow elements (Figs 3.20–3.22). Mast cell granulomas are not seen in most of the reactive conditions. Mast cells are also increased in areas of osseous remodelling (Figs 3.23–3.24), in osteoporosis during the active phase, and sometimes in the vicinity of metastases, especially in association with angiogenesis. Increased mast cells in the bone marrow are found in hypoplasias (Fig. 3.25) and in post-chemotherapy bone marrows. Mast cells may be especially prominent in patients with hyperglobulinaemias, and in certain lymphoproliferative disorders in the bone marrow – such as immunocytoma (Fig. 3.26). In addition, an increase in mast cells is seen in myeloproliferative disorders and in myelodysplasias – especially sideroblastic anaemias (Fig. 3.27) (see appropriate chapters).

Dyserythropoiesis

This is a broad term used to describe morphological (and functional and kinetic) abnormalities of erythropoiesis[3]. Morphologically these abnormalities are more readily recognized in smears of bone marrow aspirates (Figs 3.28 and 3.29), and by electron microscopy, than in histological

(Continued on p. 53)

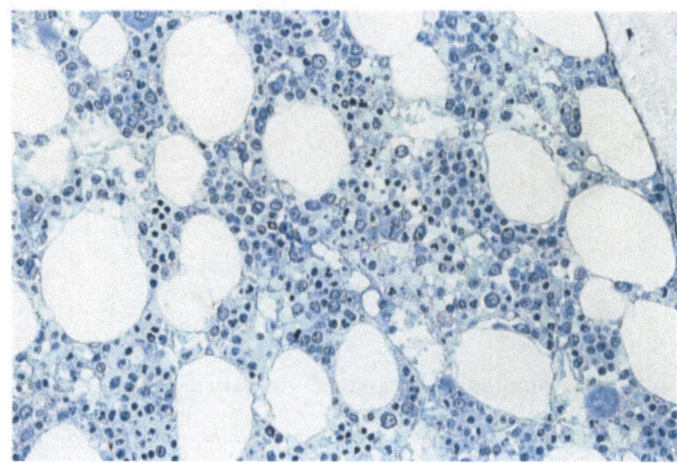

Fig. 3.1 Bone biopsy section of a 59-year-old patient with secondary erythrocytosis. Note normocellular bone marrow

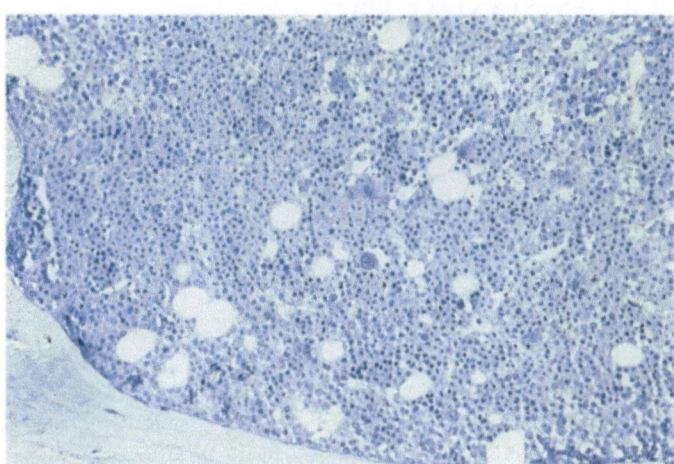

Figs 3.2–3.8 Bone biopsies of patients with leukaemoid reaction due to infections
Fig. 3.2 Low power to show increased cellularity consisting mainly of hyperplastic myelopoiesis

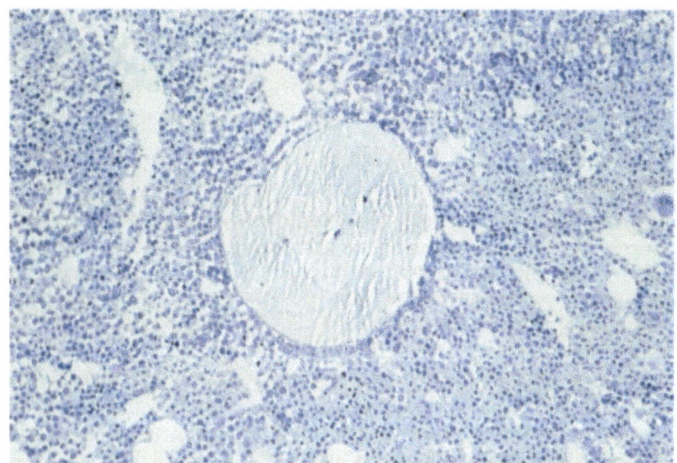

Fig. 3.3 Section of bone biopsy of patient with leukaemoid reaction, showing cuff of immature myeloid cells around an ossicle

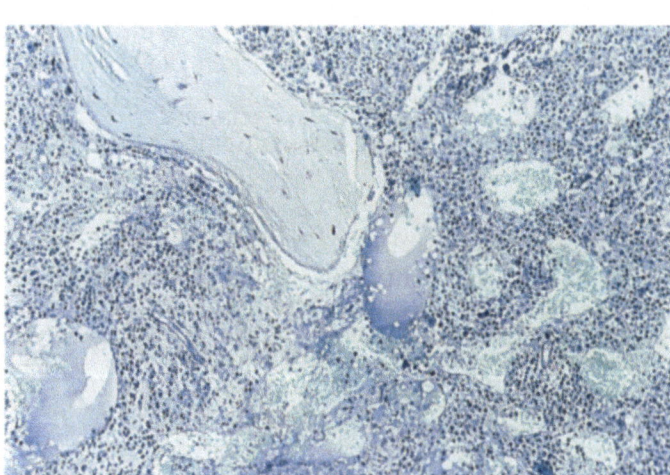

Fig. 3.4 Section showing myeloid hyperplasia, disorganization of marrow and necrosis of marrow cells

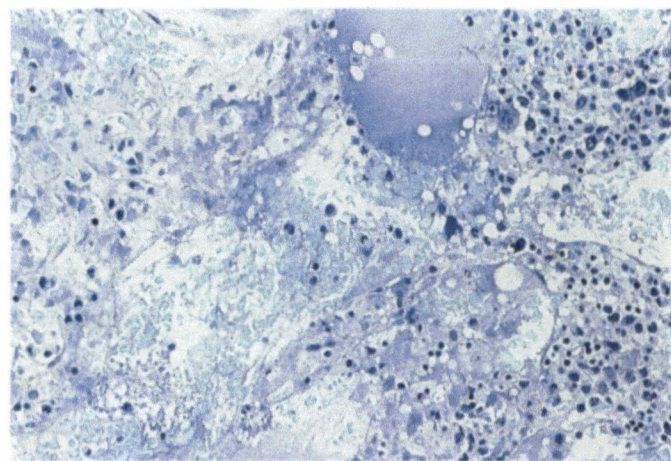

Fig. 3.5 Higher magnification (same case as Fig. 3.4) showing disruption of sinusoidal endothelium, deposition of fibrin, aggregates of red blood cells and of platelets

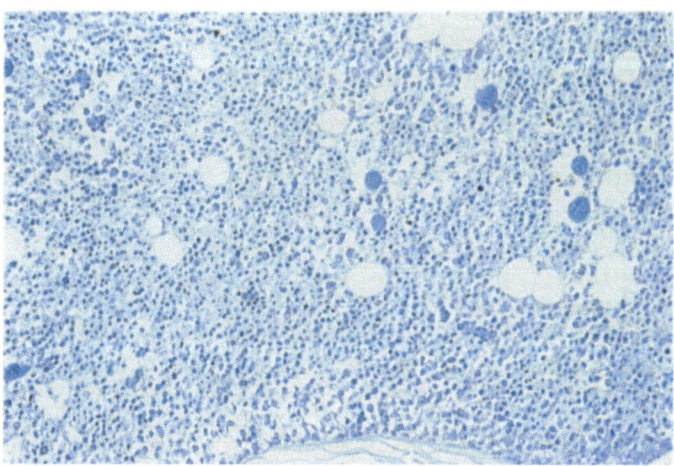

Fig. 3.6 Section of bone biopsy of patient with cancer of lung and raised white cell count. Bone marrow picture resembles that in CML

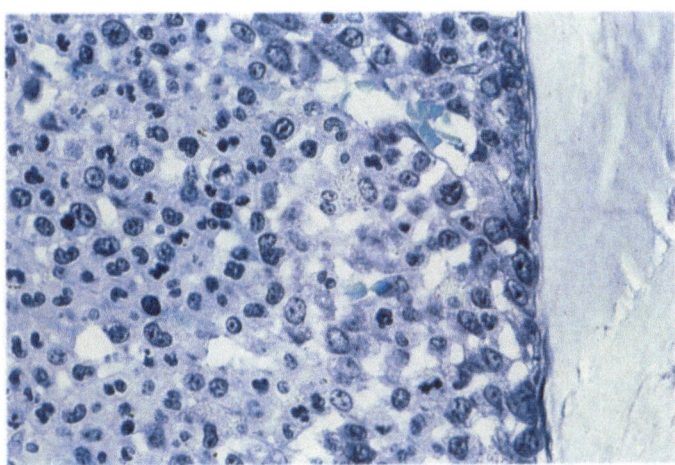

Fig. 3.7 Higher magnification of area from Fig. 3.6 showing myeloid precursors at trabecular surface

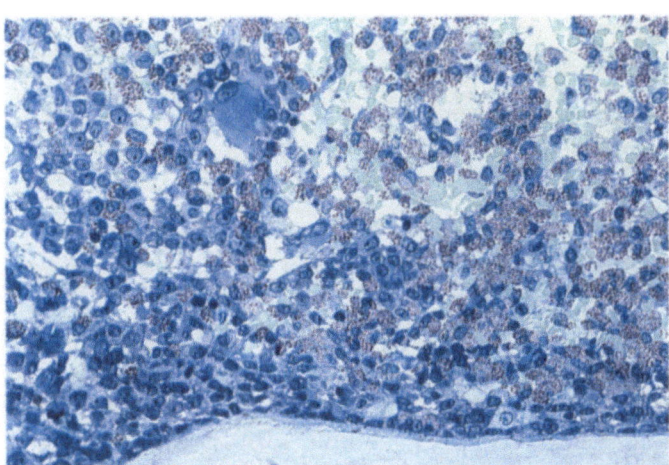

Fig. 3.8 Section of bone biopsy of patient with eosinophilia, showing hyperplasia of the eosinophilic cell line at the trabecular surface

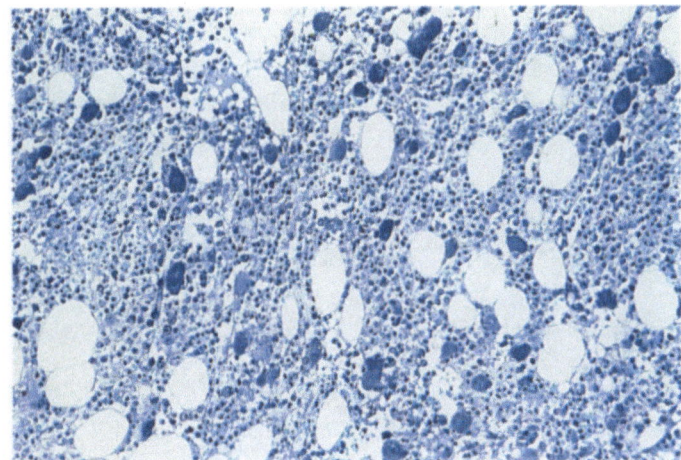

Fig. 3.9 Section of bone biopsy of patient with thrombocytosis, but no clusters of polymorphic megakaryocytes were found; lung cancer was later diagnosed

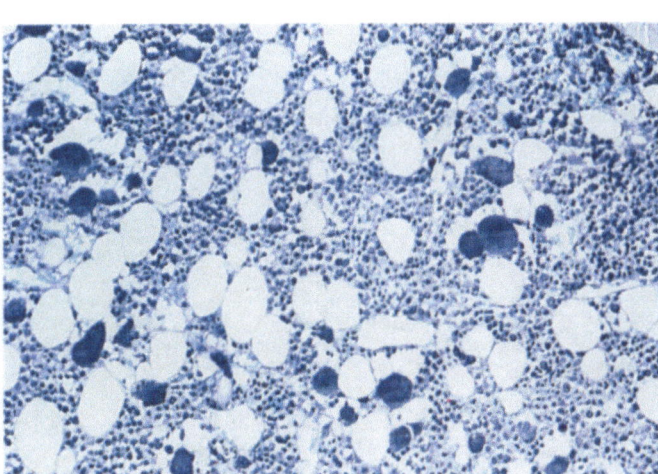

Fig. 3.10 Section of bone biopsy of patient with metastatic cancer, but no involvement in the biopsy, megakaryocytic hyperplasia

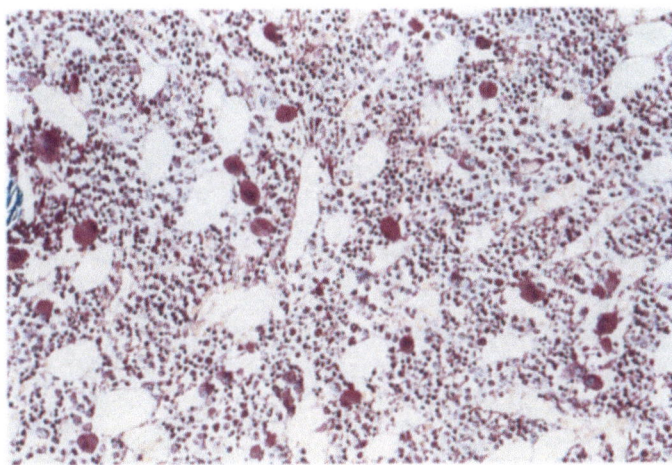

Fig. 3.11 Section of bone biopsy of patient with malignant melanoma, hyperplasia of megakaryocytes near the metastases. Ladewig

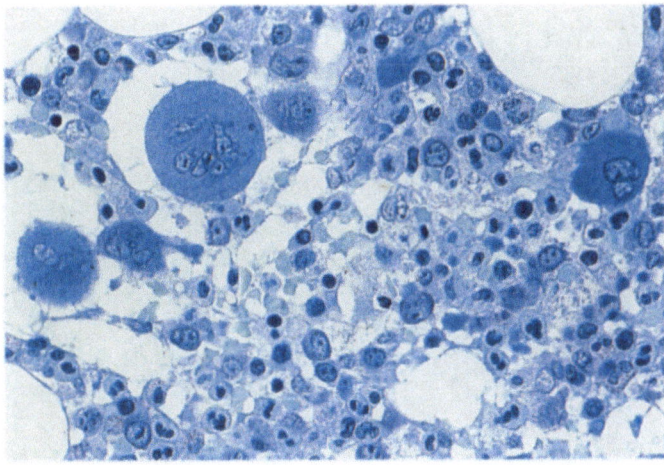

Figs 3.12–3.14 Sections of bone biopsies of patients with reactive thrombocytosis

Fig. 3.12 Megakaryocytes range in size from small to very large

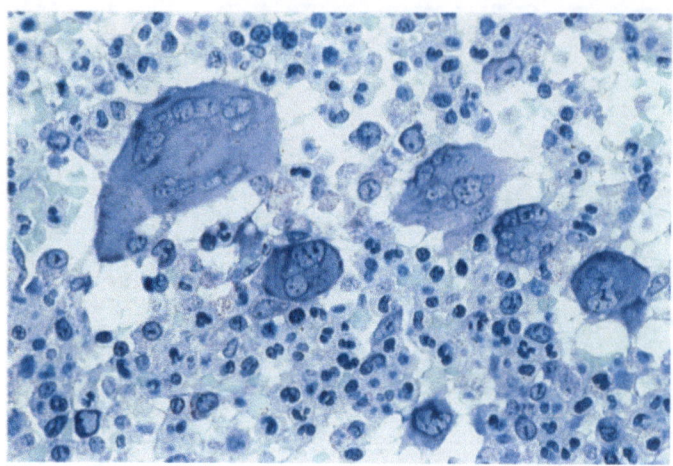

Fig. 3.13 Configuration of megakaryocyte nuclei resembles that in myeloproliferative disorders. Note also range in size and megakaryoblast

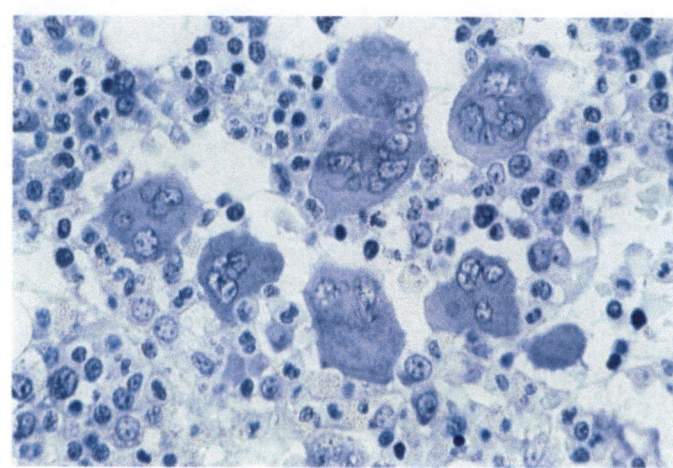

Fig. 3.14 Cluster of large megakaryocytes around a sinus, on this appearance alone, a diagnosis of a reactive condition would be difficult

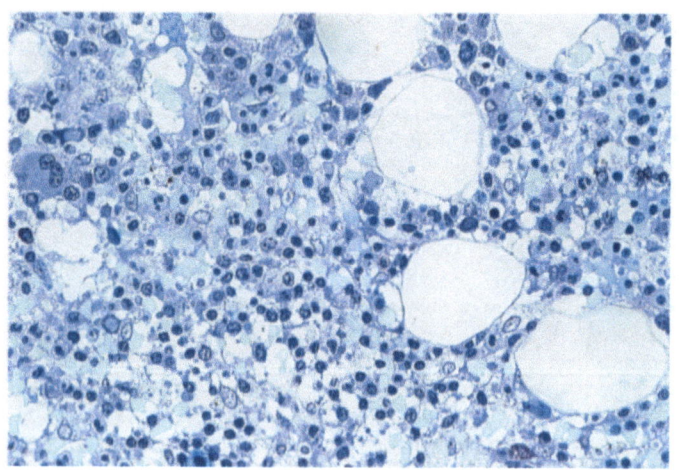

Fig. 3.15 Interstitial lymphocytosis in the bone marrow, this is possible to identify in good plastic sections

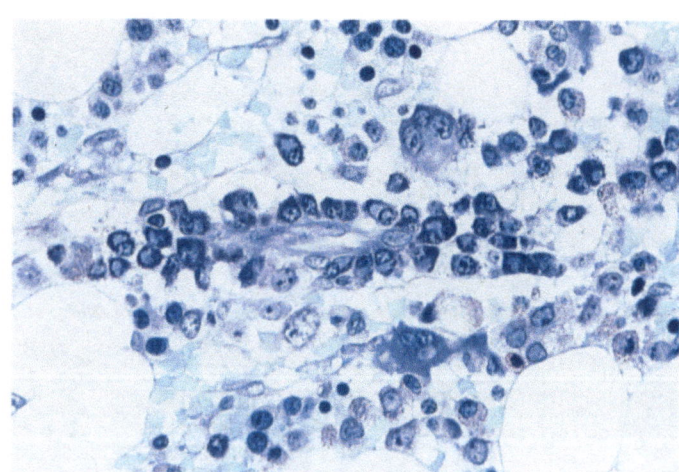

Fig. 3.16 Reactive plasmacytosis, mainly perivascular

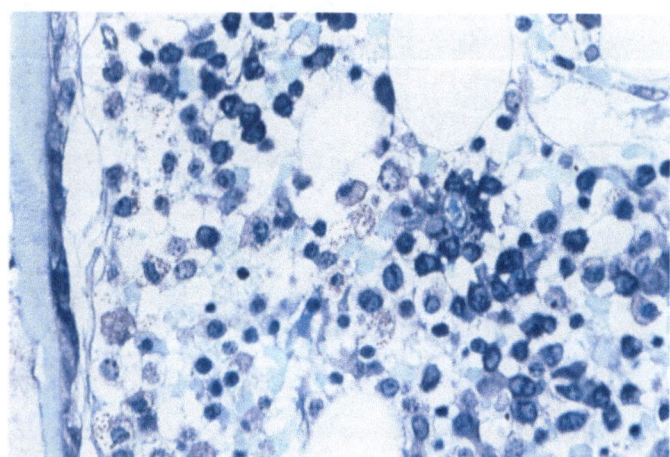

Fig. 3.17 Interstitial reactive plasmacytosis. Plasma cells in somewhat oedematous bone marrow

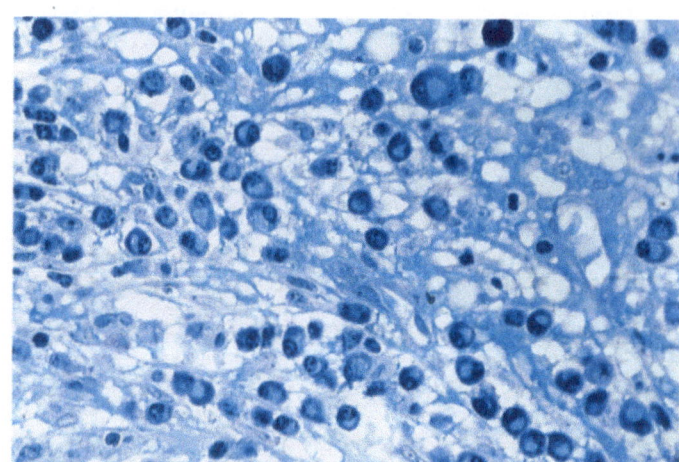

Fig. 3.18 Myelitis and plasmacytosis in bone biopsy of patient after chemotherapy for Hodgkin's disease. There had been no bone marrow involvement

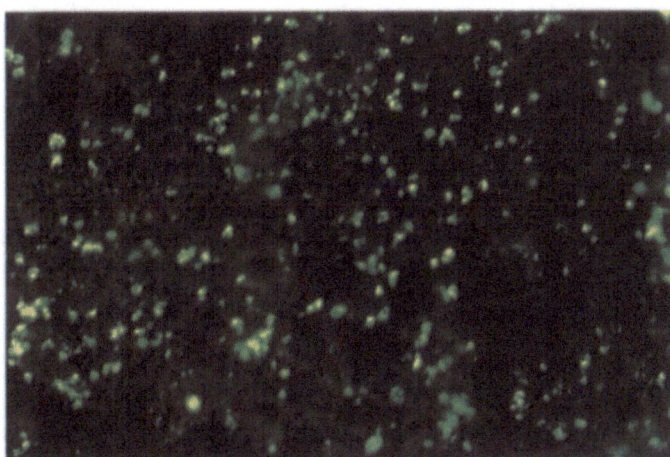

Fig. 3.19 Cryostat section incubated for demonstration of IgG with FITC-labelled antibody. Positive plasma cells identified by green fluorescence; inflammatory bone marrow reaction

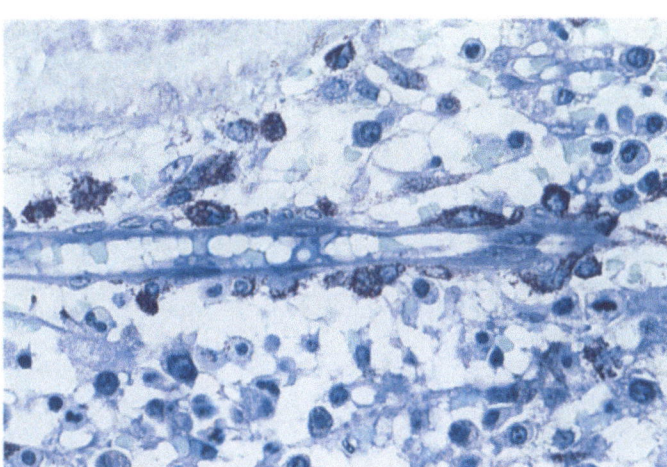

Figs 3.20-3.22 Reactive bone marrows in patients with infections showing perivascular and interstitial mast cells

Fig. 3.20 Perivascular mast cells, capillary in longitudinal section

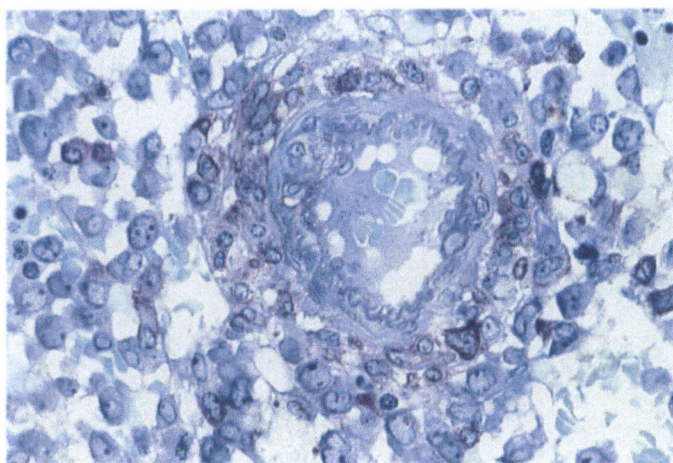

Fig. 3.21 Mast cells around an artery

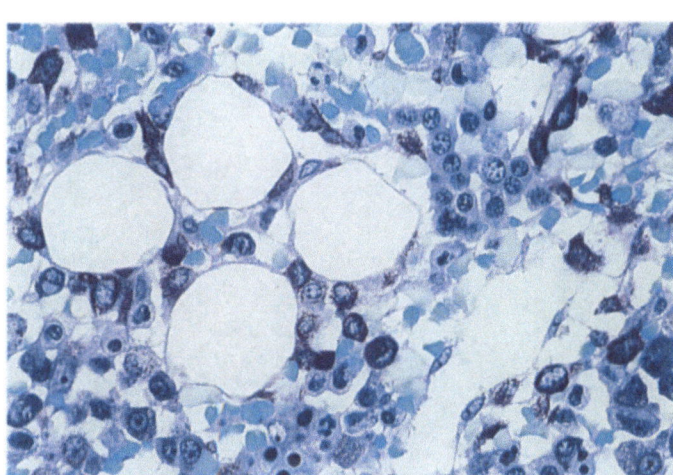

Fig. 3.22 Mast cells among haematopoietic and fat cells

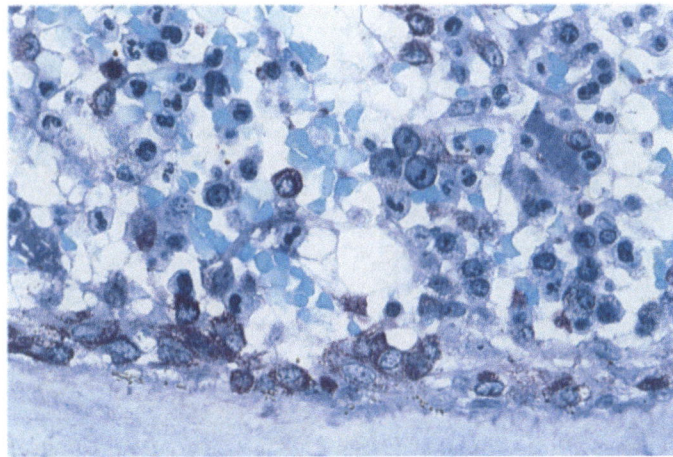

Fig. 3.23 Mast cells at trabecular surface in patient with incipient osteopenia

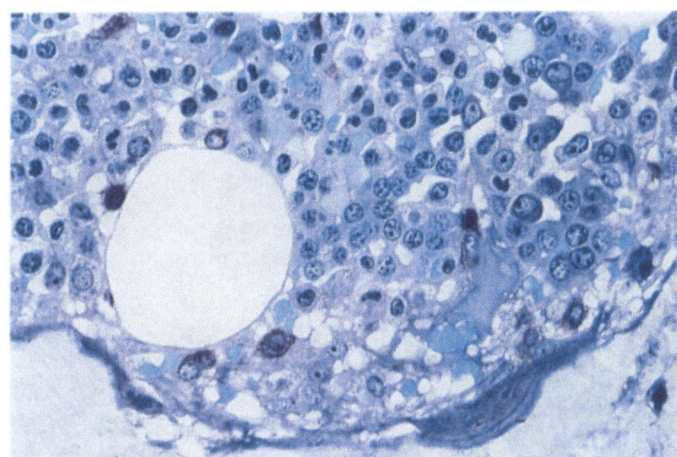

Fig. 3.24 Mast cells and osteoclast at trabecular surface

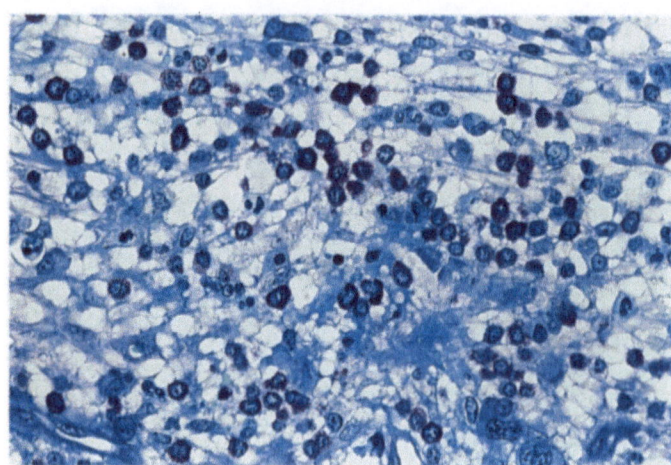

Fig. 3.25 Mast cell hyperplasia in a 74-year-old female patient with sclerosing myelitis of unkown aetiology

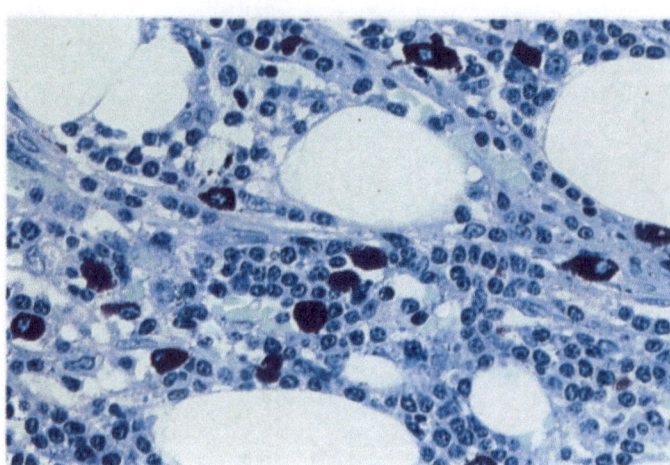

Fig. 3.26 Mast cells in areas of lymphocytic infiltration in the bone marrow in a patient with a lymphoproliferative disorder (immunocytoma)

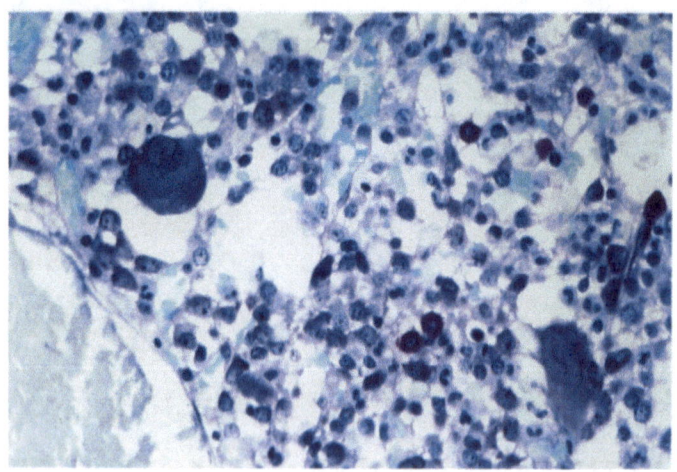

Fig. 3.27 Mast cells in bone biopsy of patient with sideroblastic anaemia

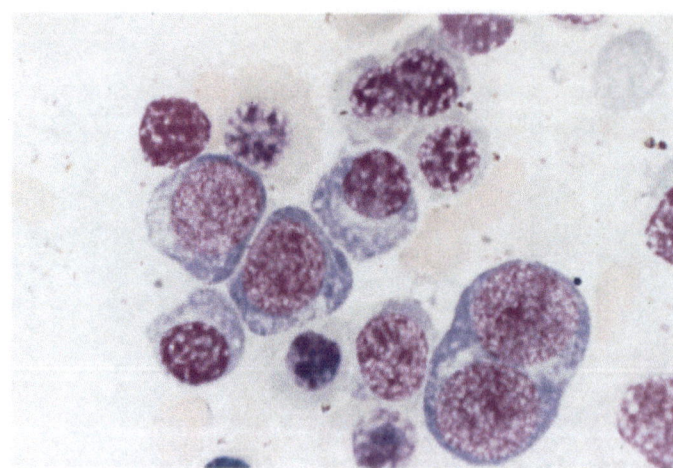

Fig. 3.28 Smear of aspirate of patient with congenital dyserythropoietic anaemia. Note megaloblastic erythropoiesis and binucleate erythroblasts

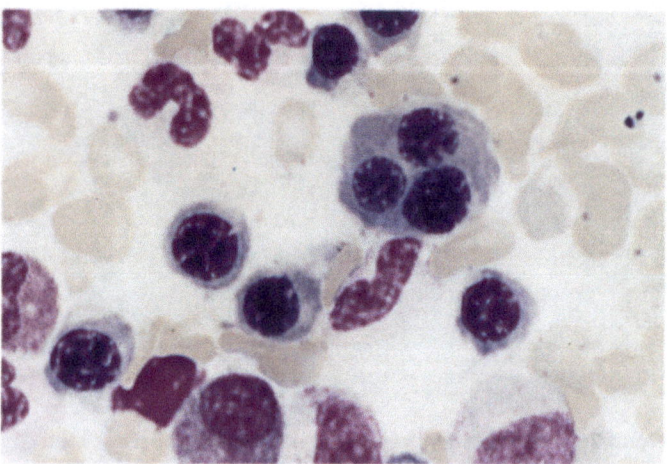

Fig. 3.29 As Fig. 3.28, showing trinucleate normoblast

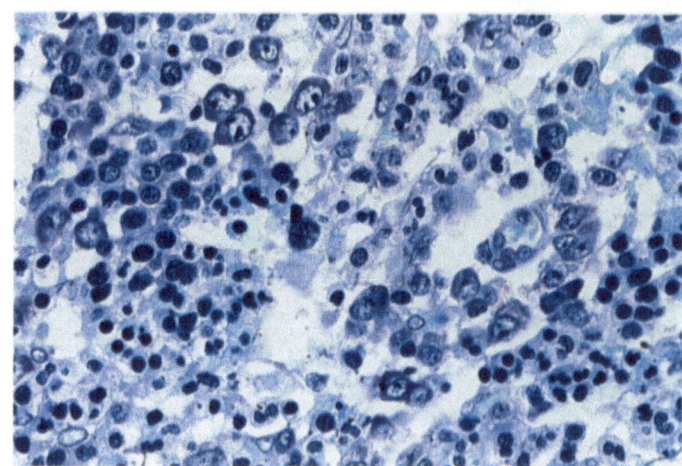

Fig. 3.32 Dyserythropoiesis in patient with polycythaemia vera (PV), note especially the late normoblasts

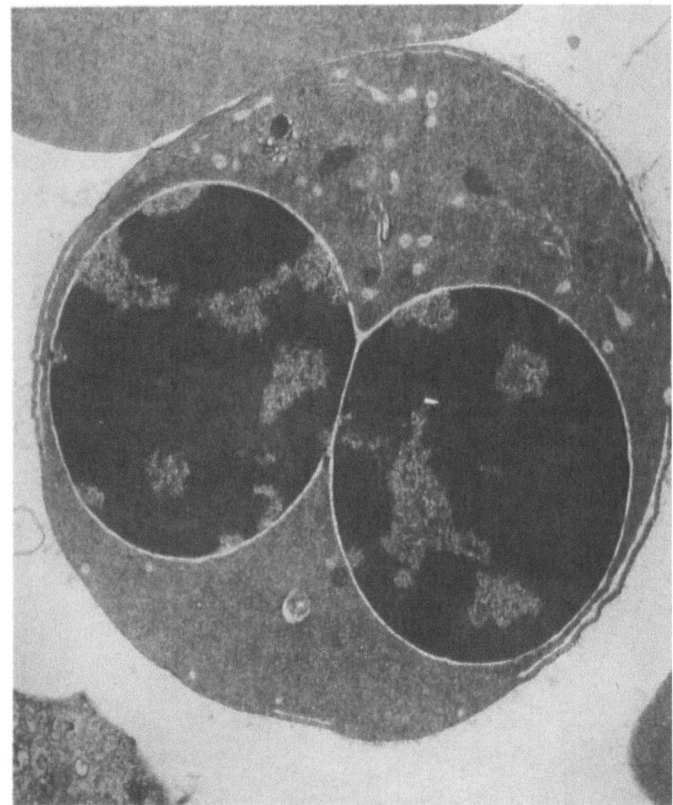

Fig. 3.30 Electron micrograph of binucleate normoblast with peripheral cisterna. × 15 000

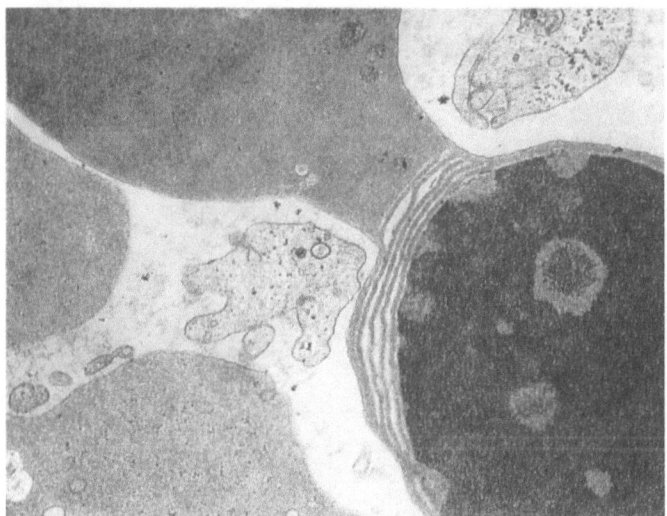

Fig. 3.31 Electron micrograph of normoblast: extrusion of nucleus together with accessory membranes. × 1500

sections of the bone marrow (Figs 3.30 and 3.31). Nevertheless, they can also be seen in the sections, especially if widespread and at high magnification.

Dyserythropoiesis is divided into congenital and acquired. The congenital group includes the congenital dyserythropoietic anaemias (CDA I, II, III) and their variants; the haemoglobinopathies; the thalassaemic syndromes; and others. Bone biopsies are not usually taken in these conditions, as the diagnosis is generally made by other biochemical and haematologic tests and if the bone marrow is examined this is done by aspirate. These congenital conditions are characterized by hyperplastic and ineffective erythropoiesis with variable degrees of haemolysis and anomalies of iron metabolism.

Acquired dyserythropoiesis occurs in numerous con-

ditions such as deficiencies – vitamin B_{12}, folate, iron – in haematologic malignancies, and in myelodysplastic syndromes (Figs 3.32–3.34).

Haemolytic Anaemias

Bone biopsies are rarely of diagnostic significance, but may help in differential diagnosis when a malignancy is thought to be a contributing factor. The bone marrow is generally cellular with reduced fat cells due to the hyperplastic erythropoiesis (Figs 3.35–3.37). But hypoplasia and even an 'aplastic crisis' may occur which is due to a temporary failure of erythropoiesis. These 'crises' may be precipitated by infections, especially viral, and by other stresses[12]. In chronic haemolytic states there may be extramedullary haematopoiesis in the liver and spleen, and extension of red marrow into the shafts of the long bones. Drug-induced haemolysis may also occur in patients on chemotherapy[13,14]. In these cases the haemolysis may contribute to a cytopenia already present due to cytoxicity and/or replacement by metastases.

Erythroid Hyperplasias

Erythroid hyperplasia is also seen in iron deficiency, but the precursors are small and poorly haemoglobinized and there is ineffective erythropoiesis. In extreme cases the marrow may be hypocellular. In contrast, the anaemias associated with chronic disorders are due to defective iron metabolism and the bone marrow cellularity is generally within the normal range or decreased without dyserythropoietic features. Iron in the stromal cell is increased. Deposition of iron in cells both of the reticuloendothelial system and in the erythroblasts – sideroblastosis – may be found in many different conditions all associated with anaemia. These include megaloblastic anaemias, haematological malignancies, myelodysplastic syndromes, inflammatory diseases, alcohol abuse, and others.

Haemosiderosis and Haemochromatosis

These are characterised by iron accumulation in cells of the reticuloendothelial system (Figs 3.38–3.40). The former is due to tranfusion overload, less frequently seen now since the advent of chelating agents. It still occurs in hereditary conditions such as the thalassaemias and others, in which children are regularly transfused to maintain their haemoglobin levels. In adults haemosiderosis may be seen in patients frequently transfused because of aplastic anaemia or malignancies. It is not possible on purely morpholigical grounds to distinguish haemochromatosis from haemosiderosis in the bone marrow. Haemochromatosis occurs as a primary familial condition; or in association with various hepatic disorders[15,16]. With increasing iron overload the number of iron-containing stromal cells is greatly increased and there is deposition in endothelial cells, in osteoblasts and endosteal cells, as well as on the osteoid seams. The cancellous bone may be outlined by a layer of iron.

Megaloblastic Erythropoiesis

Erythropoiesis with megaloblastoid or megaloblastic features is found in the presence of defective DNA synthesis as in B_{12} or folate deficiency, in accelerated haematopoiesis due to haemolysis or haemorrhage, in congenital anomalies as in the CDAs, in acquired conditions and in malignancies of the haematopoietic systems (Figs 3.41–3.44).

The erythroid precursors are larger than normal with large nuclei having a fine chromatin pattern. In the granulocytic series there are giant metamyelocytes,

(Continued on p. 56)

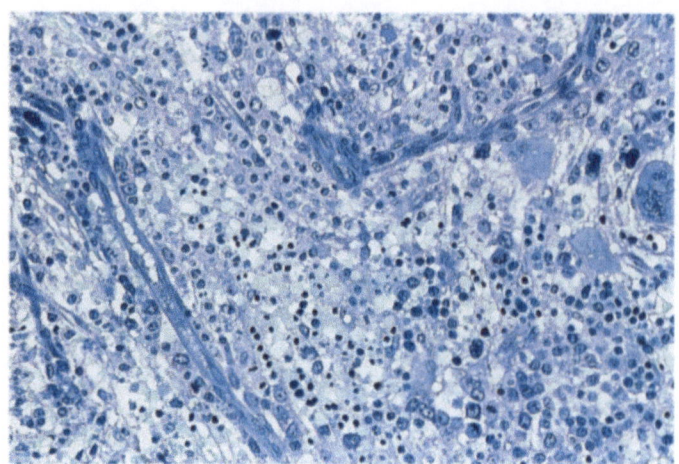

Fig. 3.33 Section of bone biopsy of patient with incipient myelofibrosis on the basis of idiopathic thrombocythaemia. Note disruption of erythroid islands, erythroblasts and late normoblasts; low-power view.

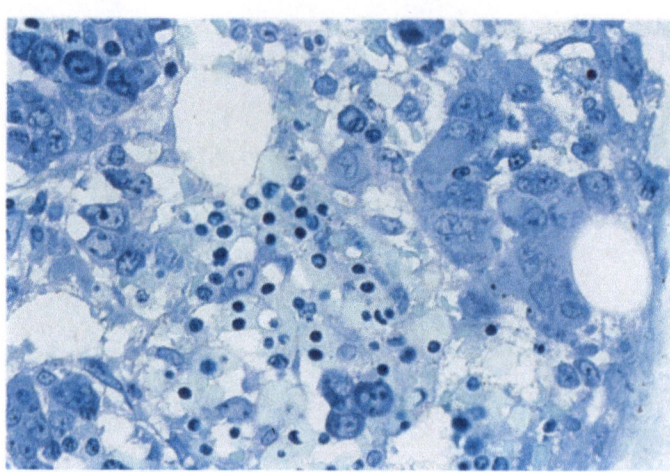

Fig. 3.34 Higher magnification of another area from Fig. 3.33, showing erythroblasts and dyserythropoietic normoblasts

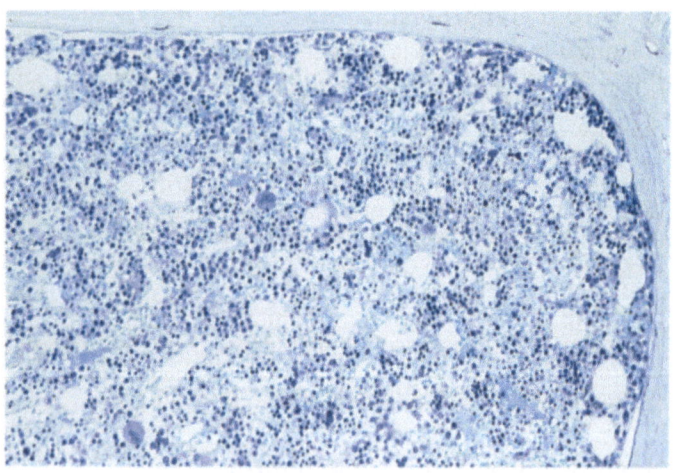

Fig. 3.35 Section of bone biopsy of patient with drug-induced haemolysis; showing hyperplastic erythropoiesis with numerous erythroid islands, low-power view

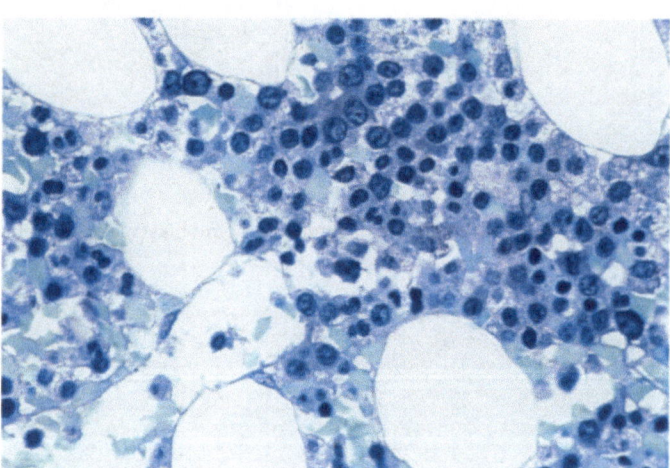

Fig. 3.36 Higher magnification of area from Fig. 3.35, showing erythroblasts at all maturational stages

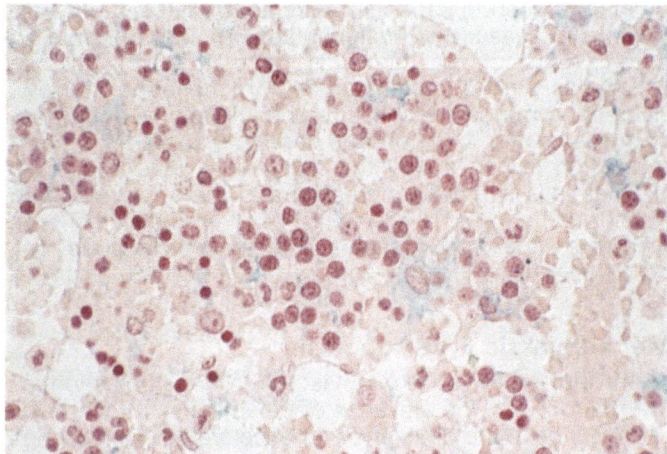

Fig. 3.37 Same case as in Fig. 3.35, section of biopsy stained by Berlin blue. There is a faint blue 'wash' in the stromal cells

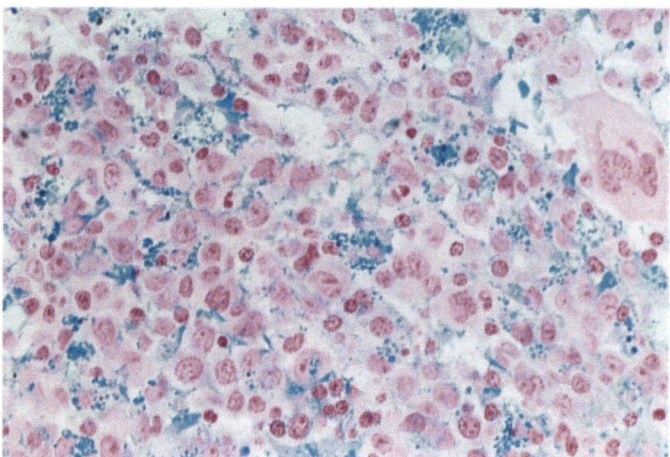

Fig. 3.38 Section of bone biopsy of patient with haemosiderosis, showing massive iron deposition in stromal cells

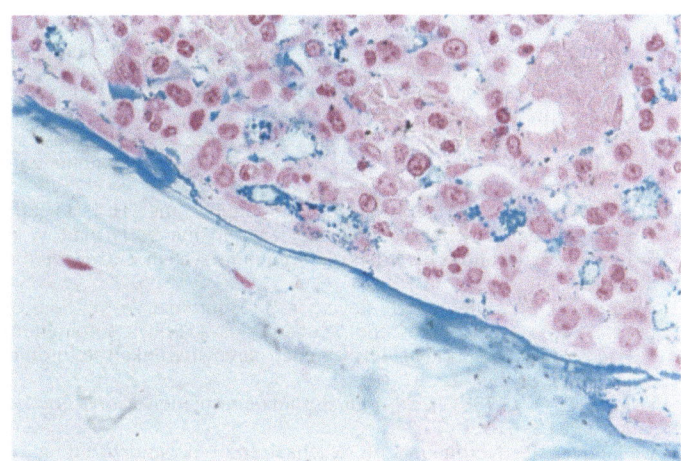

Fig. 3.39 Same as above, iron deposition on osteoid, and in osteoblasts

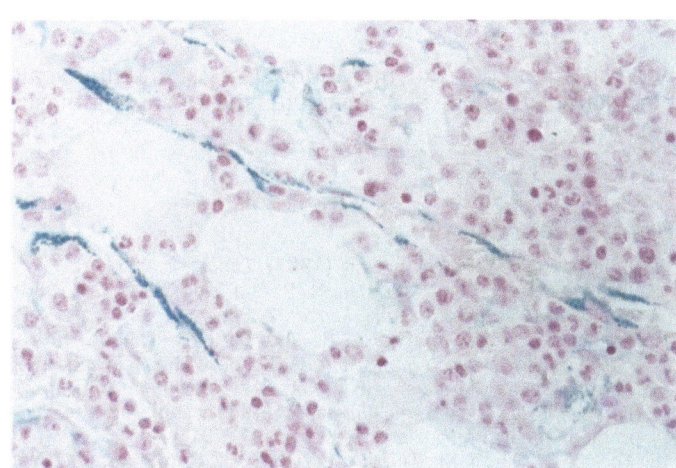

Fig. 3.40 Section of bone biopsy of patient with metastatic cancer and anaemia after blood transfusion. Deposition of iron in endothelial cells

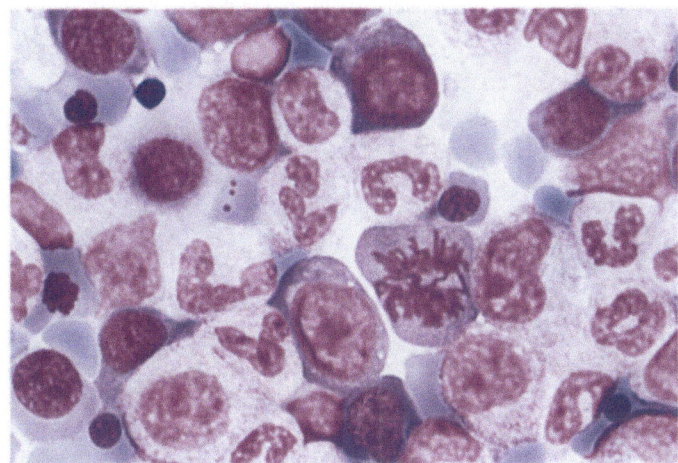

Fig. 3.41 Megaloblasts in smear of bone marrow aspirate of patient with vitamin B$_{12}$ deficiency

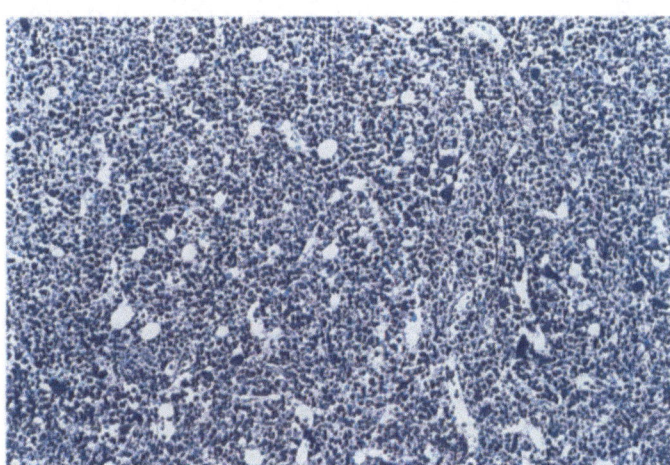

Fig. 3.42 Megaloblastic erythropoiesis in bone biopsy of patient with vitamin B$_{12}$ deficiency; low power showing densely packed marrow

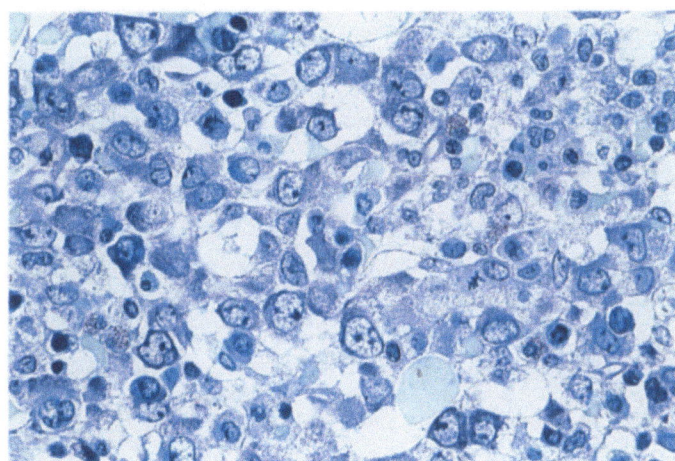

Fig. 3.43 Higher magnification, same biopsy as Fig. 3.42. Note numerous early erythroblasts with megaloblastic features

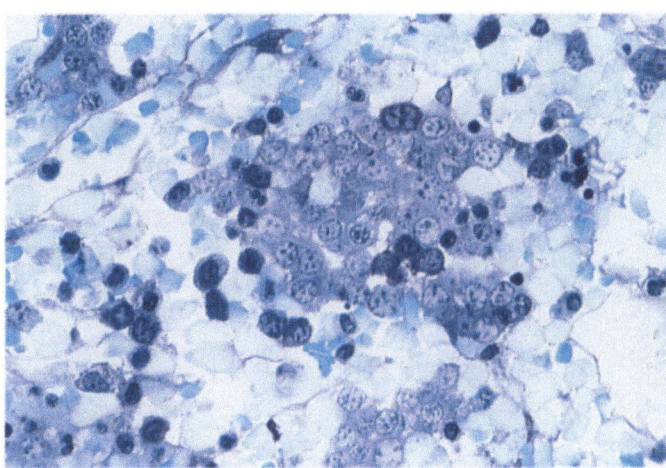

Fig. 3.44 Section of bone biopsy of patient with hepatic disease showing erythropoiesis with megaloblastoid features

hypersegmented polymorphonuclears; multinucleate megakaryocytes are also characteristic of megaloblastic anaemia.

References

1. Editorial. Pseudopolycythaemia (1987). *Lancet*, **2**, 603
2. Innes, A., Rowe, P. A., Burden, R. P. and Morgan, A. G. (1988). Cyclosporin and erythraemia. *Lancet*, **2**, 285
3. Frisch, B., Lewis, Burkhardt, R. and Bartl, R. (1985). *Biopsy Pathology of Bone and Bone Marrow.* (London: Chapman and Hall)
4. Pertusa-Pena, C., Llarena-Ibarguren, A., Zabala, J. A., Arruza-Echeverria, A. and Arregui-Erbina, P. (1988). Leukemoid reaction in bladder carcinoma. *Arch. Esp. Urol.*, **41**, 231
5. Teo, C. G., Singh, M., Ting, W. C., Ho, L. C., Ong, Y. W. and Seet, L. C. (1985). Evaluation of the common conditions associated with eosinophilia. *J. Clin. Pathol.*, **38**, 305
6. Itami, N., Akutsu, Y. and Yasoshima, K. (1988). Thrombocytosis after cyclosporin therapy in child with nephrotic syndrome. *Lancet*, **2**, 1018
7. Ebbe, S., Yee, T., Carpenter, D. and Phalen, E. (1988). Megakaryocytes increase in size within ploidy groups in response to the stimulus of thrombocytopenia. *Exp. Hematol.*, **16**, 55
8. Chanarin, I., Harrisingh, D., Tidmarsh, E. and Skacel, P. O. (1984). Significance of lymphocytosis in adults. *Lancet*, **2**, (8408), 897
9. Carstairs, K. C., Francombe, W. H., Scott, J. G. and Gelfand, E. W., (1985). Persistent polyclonal lymphocytosis of B lymphocytes, induced by cigarette smoking? *Lancet*, **1**, 1094
10. Schachor, Y., Radnay, J., Bernheim, J., Rozenszajn, A., Briuderman, I., Klajman, A. and Steiner, Z. P. (1988). Malignant thymoma with peripheral blood lymphocytosis. *Cancer*, **61**, 1222
11. Hirt, A., Morell, A., Frei, H., Imbach, P. and Wagner, H. P. (1988). Proliferation of lymphoid precursor cells in the bone marrow of patients with various disorders of the immune system. *Exp. Hematol.*, **16**, 38
12. Bertrand, Y., Lefrere, J. J., Leverger, G., Courouse, A. M., Feo, C., Clark, M., Schaison, G. and Soulier, J. P. (1985). Autoimmune haemolytic anaemia revealed by human parvovirus linked erythroblastopenia. *Lancet*, **2**, 382
13. Petz, L. D. (1985). Drug-induced immune hemolysis. *N. Engl. J. Med.*, **313**, 510
14. Sandvei, P., Nordhagen, R., Michaelsen, T. E. and Wolthius, K. (1987). Flurouracil (5-FU) induced acute immune haemolytic anaemia. *Br. J. Haematol.*, **65**, 357
15. Niederau, C., Fischer, R., Sonnenberg, A., Stremmel, W., Trampish, H. J. and Strohmeyer, G. (1985). Survival and causes of death in cirrhotic and in noncirrhotic patient with primary haemochromatosis. *N. Engl. J. Med.*, **313**, 1256
16. Edwards, C. Q., Griffin, L. M., Goldgar, D., Drummond, C., Skolnick, M. H. and Kushner, J. P. (1988). Prevalence of haemochomatosis among 11,065 presumably healthy blood donors. *N. Engl. J. Med.*, **318**, 1365

Stromal Reactions in Hypoplasias and Inflammatory Conditions (Infections)

4

Reactions involving the stromal components of the bone marrow accompany the cytopenias and occur in many clinical conditions with or without a decrease in one or more of the peripheral blood cells. These conditions include infections, diseases of collagen, hepatic disorders, Hodgkin's disease, malignant lymphomas and carcinomas – the last three without bone marrow involvement in the bone biopsy[1-3].

Components of the bone marrow stroma may be damaged by bacterial and chemical toxins and by radiation; though restitution after removal of the toxins or cessation of the radiotherapy is the rule. Especially vulnerable in the short term are the capillaries and sinusoids; these are liable to disruption so that the marrow compartments are no longer clearly separated. Radiation injury to sinusoids may eventually lead to their sclerosis. Damage to the microcirculation may also be seen in allergic and autoimmune states. In view of the role of an intact bone marrow stroma in normal haematopoiesis, damage to the stromal components of the microenvironment is likely to interfere with proliferation and maturation of precursor cells[4-7]. The presence of an eosinophilic fibrohistiocytic lesion in the bone marrow has been related to drug hypersensitivity[8].

In some infections the causative micro-organisms may be cultured from the bone marrow and/or demonstrated in smears, imprints or sections. For example tubercle bacilli in tuberculosis, Donovan bodies in kala-azar (leishmaniasis), *Coxiella burnetti* in Q fever, *Myobacterium leprae* in leprosy and *Mycobacterium avium intracellulare* in the acquired immune deficiency syndrome (AIDS).

In chronic inflammations affecting the bone marrow, haematopoiesis and fat cells are decreased, while fibroblasts, reticulum and collagen fibres, capillaries and sinusoids are increased, and interspersed with macrophages, mast and plasma cells.

Five morphological types of inflammatory reactions (Fig. 4.1) in the bone marrow have been described[9]:

1. Acute 'exudative' or 'necrotic' type: necrosis of haematopoietic cells and small blood vessels with oedema, but there is residual haematopoiesis and frequently neutrophilia (Figs 4.2 and 4.3).
2. Chronic atrophic type: also referred to a gelatinous transformation, serous atrophy, or exudative myelitis (Fig. 4.4)[10]. Both haematopoietic tissue and fat cells are reduced – but there is an uneven distribution of the atrophic areas which may alternate with cellular ones. The affected regions are infiltrated with lymphocytes, plasma and mast cells (Fig. 4.5). This type of reaction is found in chronic infections, in malignancies (especially gastric carcinoma) in the absence of metastases in the bone marrow biopsy, and in poor nutrition.
3. Chronic fibrotic type, also called sclerosing myelitis (Figs 4.6–4.9). In addition to the reduction in the normal haematopoietic and fat tissues, and an exudative and inflammatory reaction as described above, there is a marked fibrotic component. This consists of both reticulum and collagen fibres and sometimes osteoblastic new bone formation.
4. Chronic 'proliferative' or 'leukaemoid' type, characterized by a normo- to hypercellular bone marrow infiltrated by plasma, mast and lymphoid cells with neutrophilia, eosinophilia or megakaryocytosis (Figs 4.10 and 4.11).
5. Chronic, granulomatous type[11,12]: the main types of granulomas encountered in the bone marrow are: the so-called giant cell granulomas, lipid and epithelioid cell (with or without lymphocytes); and mast cell granulomas, but the latter are seen exclusively in systemic mastocytosis (Figs 4.12–4.27). Other cells such as macrophages (the precursors of the epithelioid and giant cells), fibroblasts, mast, plasma and lymphoid cells and granulocytes may be found in and around a granuloma. Granulomas may be found in hypo-, normo- and hypercellular bone marrows. Granulomas may be large or small, single or multiple, inter- or paratrabecular, and consist of a heterogeneous cell population together with capillaries, fibroblasts and fibres. In some cases confluence may occur, so that the borders are blurred and large areas of marrow are occupied. Lipid granulomas consist of lipo-macrophages together with a variable mixture of the accompanying cells described above. Occasionally isolated giant cells may be found both in normal marrows and when there is involvement by a myelo- or lymphoproliferative or other disorders.

In sarcoidosis, the characteristic granulomas may be found in the BMB; there may be multiple bone lesions on X-ray or scan (Fig. 4.19)[13,14]. The granulomas are composed of epithelioid and giant cells cuffed by blood vessels, fibres and lymphocytes. Schauman or asteroid bodies are rarely found in the granulomas in the bone marrow. Vitamin D may be metabolized by the granulomatous tissue and cause hypercalcaemia through stimulation of osteoclastic bone resorption. Morphologically, granulomas due to sarcoidosis or to tuberculosis are not distinguishable in the bone marrow (Figs 4.20–4.22). This is because, unlike in other tissues, necrosis is not usually seen in bone marrow granulomas due to tuberculosis. Numerous agents have the ability to evoke granuloma formation. These include mycobacteria, fungi, toxoplasma, histoplasma, some viruses and various foreign bodies or materials (Figs 4.23 and 4.24)[15]. Granulomas in the bone marrow may also be found in various haematological malignancies such as multiple myeloma, malignant lymphomas and Hodgkin's disease, as well as in patients with non-haematological malignancies; and as a reaction to some drugs (Figs 4.25–4.27). Haemophagocytosis by macrophages may be increased in bone marrows with granulomas (Fig. 4.28).

Osteomyelitis

In the acute phase there is a maximal infiltration of polymorphonuclear cells and necrosis of both marrow and bone, sometimes referred as to suppurative destructive necrosis (Figs 4.29–4.33). Osteolytic lesions may ensue[16],

(Continued on p. 63)

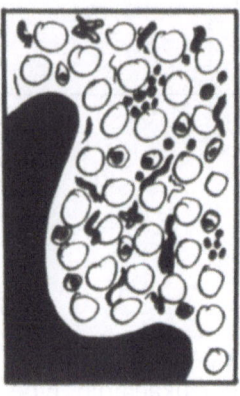 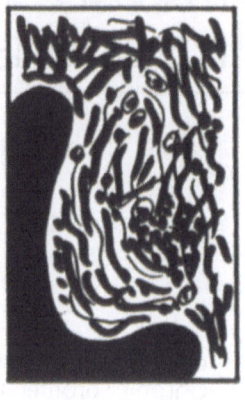 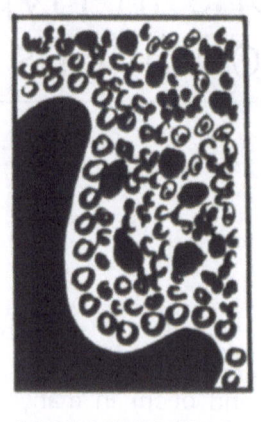 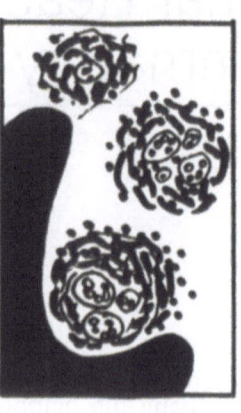

ATROPHIC   FIBROTIC   PROLIFERATIVE   GRANULOMATOUS

Fig. 4.1   Schematic representation of bone marrow in chronic inflammations

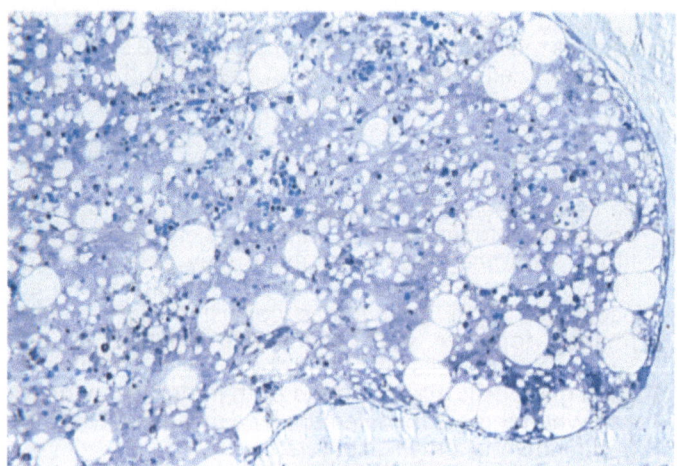

Fig. 4.2   Acute exudative type with disorganization of the marrow architecture, degeneration of haematopoietic elements and oedema

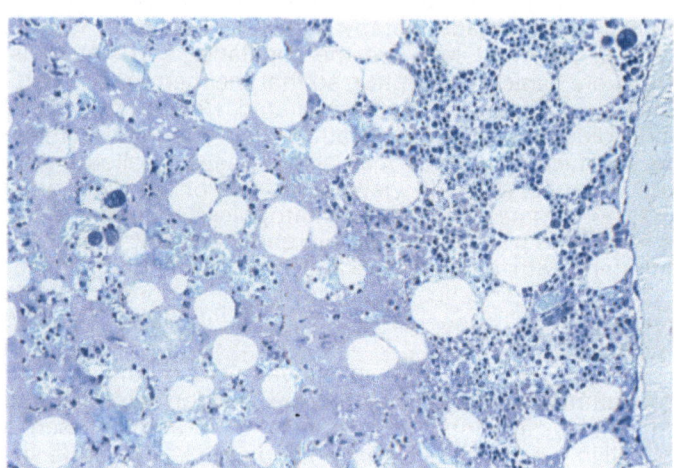

Fig. 4.3   Another area from same section as in Fig. 4.2, showing residual precursor cells and megakaryocytes

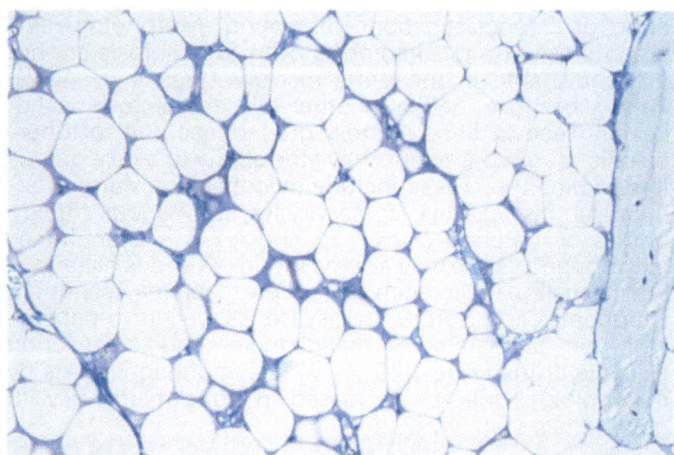

Fig. 4.4   Example of gelatinous transformation of bone marrow as occurs in patients with inadequate nutrition, or with gastric carcinoma

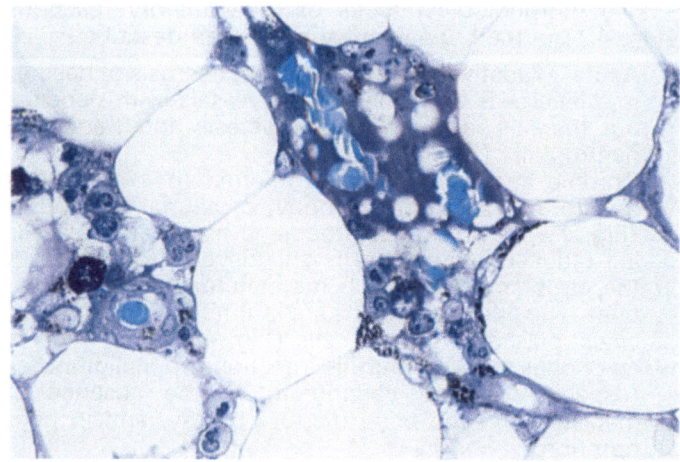

Fig. 4.5   Higher magnification of part of Fig. 4.4, showing mast cells, neutrophils and plasma cells

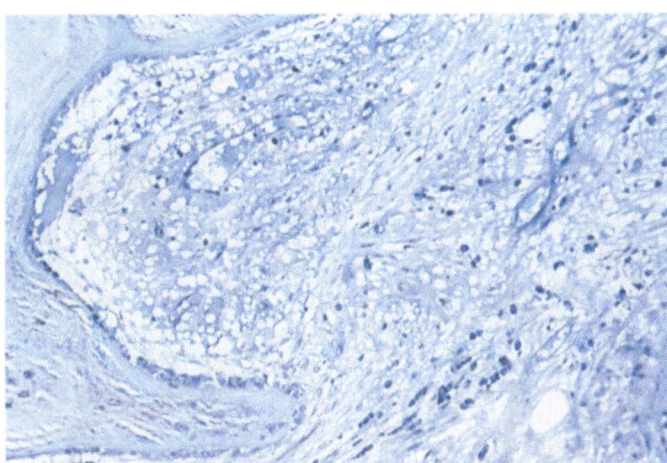

Fig. 4.6 Section of bone biopsy with sclerosing myelitis, i.e. chronic inflammation, fibrotic type. Note absence of haematopoiesis, fibrosis, and osteoblasts on osteoid seams

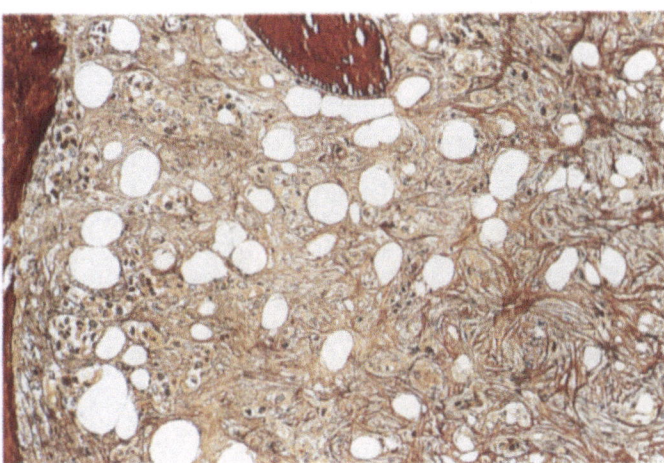

Fig. 4.7 Section of bone biopsy with sclerosing myelitis, and residual haematopoietic cells between the fibers. Gomori

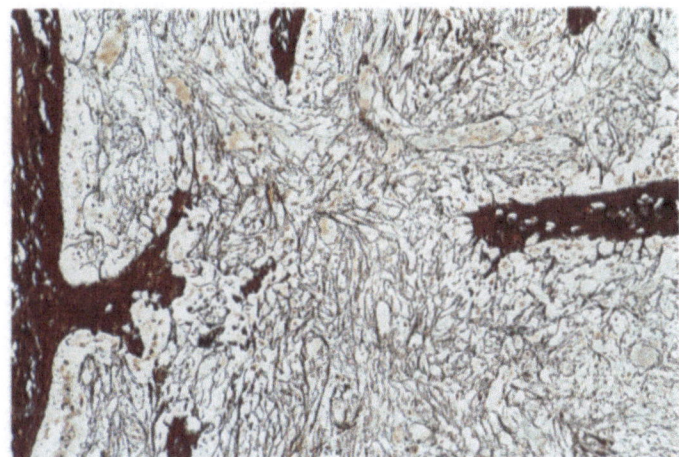

Fig. 4.8 Section of bone biopsy with sclerosing myelitis, with no residual haematopoiesis. Note sprouts of bone to which the fibres are attached. Gomori's reticulin stain

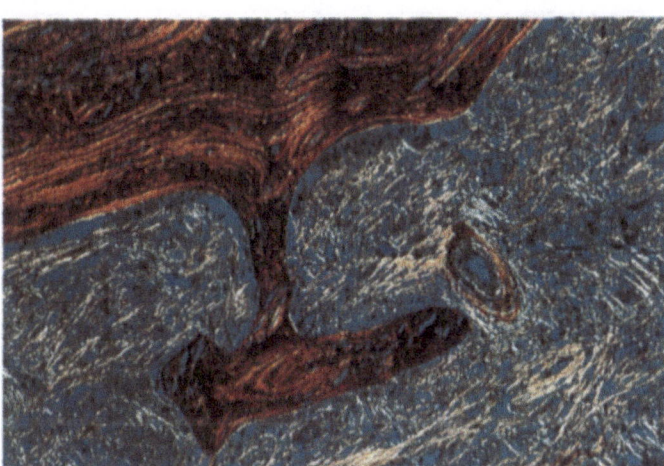

Fig. 4.9 Section from same biopsy as in Fig. 4.8, stained by Gomori, viewed in polarized light, development of osteomyelosclerosis. These bone marrows show reduction or absence of haematopoietic tissue and varying degrees of fibrosis, and of osteoblastic new bone formation. It is of interest that in these conditions there is fibrosis in the absence of megakaryocytes, in contrast to the myeloproliferative disorders

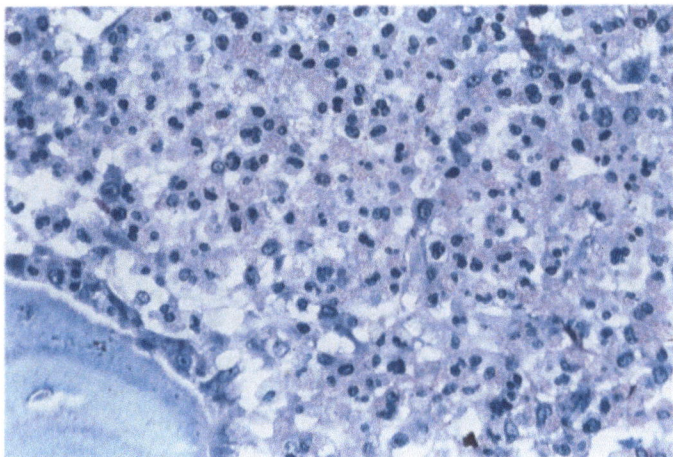

Fig. 4.10 Chronic proliferative type of inflammatory reaction in the bone marrow, bone biopsy section showing hypercellular bone marrow with eosinophilia

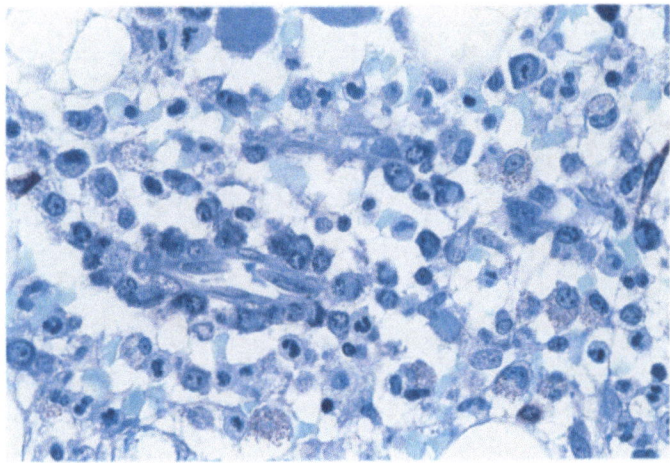

Fig. 4.11 As in Fig. 4.10, section showing eosinophilia, lymphocytosis and plasmacytosis

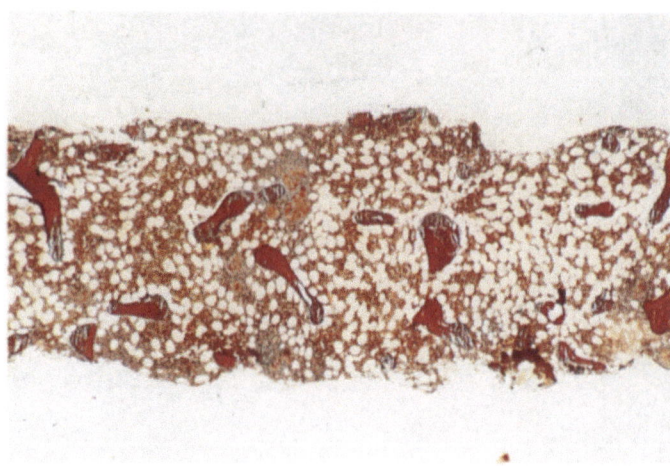

Fig. 4.12 Low-power view of bone biopsy section with several granulomas. Gomori

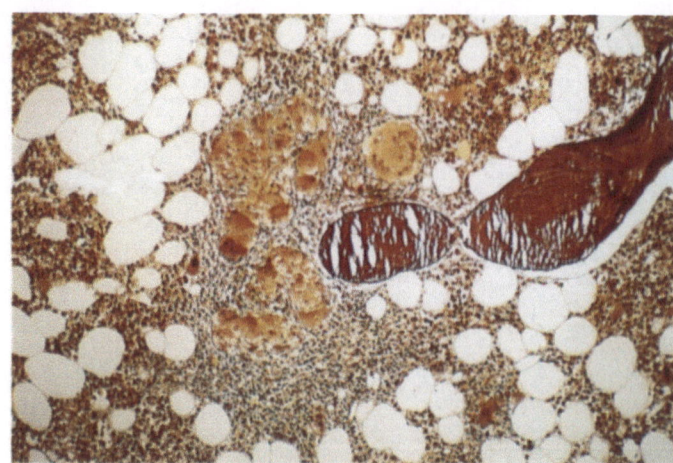

Fig. 4.13 Higher magnification of area from Fig. 4.12, showing details of the granuloma: composed of multiple giant cells, and lymphocytes. Gomori

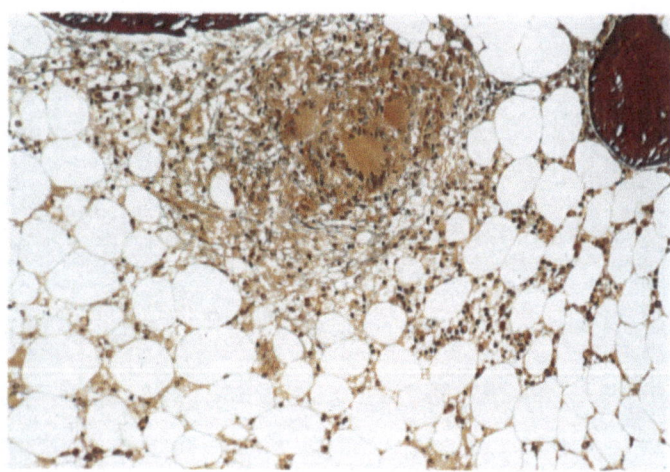

Fig. 4.14 Small granuloma in hypocellular bone marrow, composed mainly of giant cells, epithelioid cells and reticular fibres. Gomori

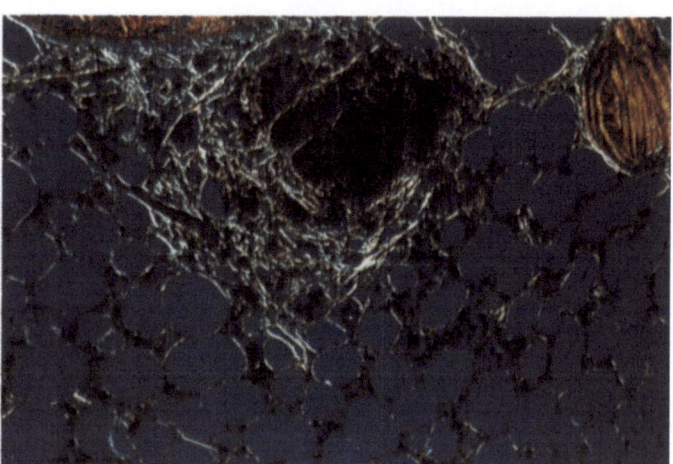

Fig. 4.15 Same area as in Fig. 4.14, viewed in polarized light: granuloma surrounded by reticular fibre network

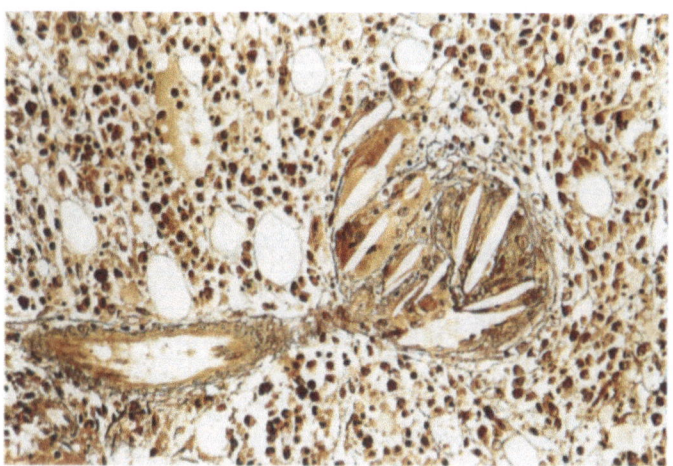

Fig. 4.16 Lipid granuloma; the inclusions have been dissolved out during processing. Gomori

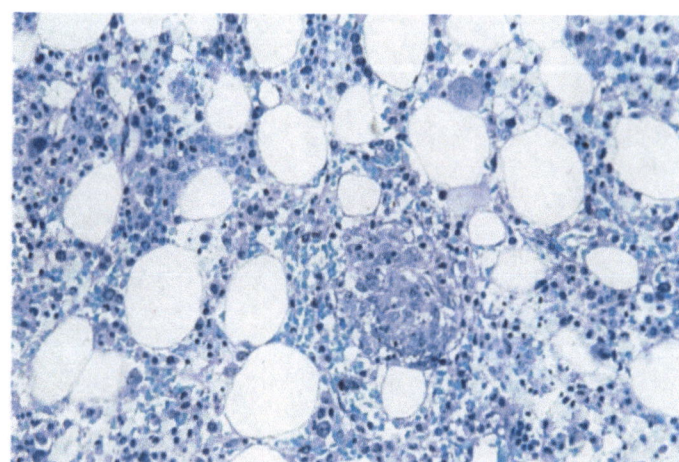

Fig. 4.17 Section of bone biopsy of patient with prostatic cancer, but no metastases in biopsy. Section showing small epithelioid cell granuloma

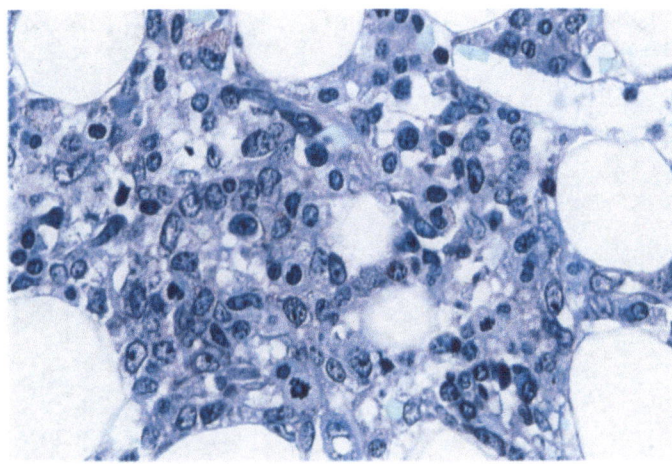

Fig. 4.18 Poorly defined epithelioid cell granuloma in section of bone biopsy of patient with breast cancer

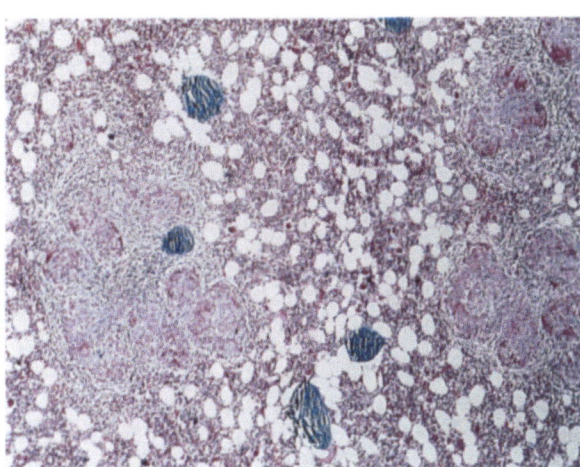

Fig. 4.19 Multiple giant cell granulomas in bone biopsy of patient with sarcoidosis. Ladewig

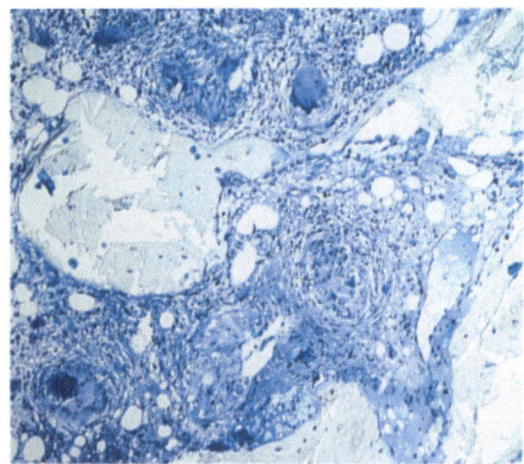

Fig. 4.20 Low-power view of section of bone biopsy of patient with TB, showing confluent giant cell granulomas

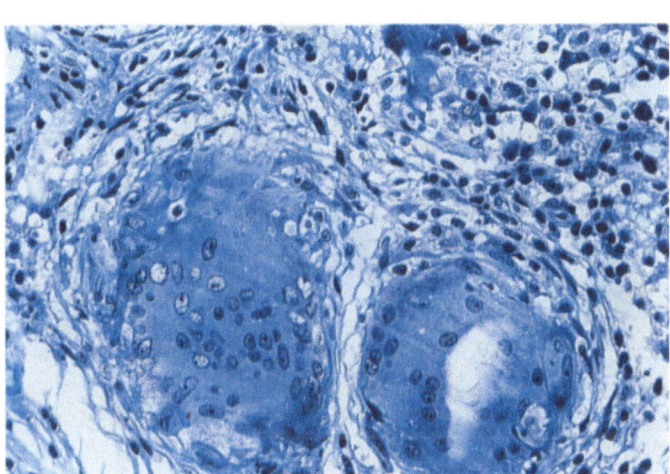

Fig. 4.21 Higher magnification of area in Fig. 4.20 showing multinucleated giant cells

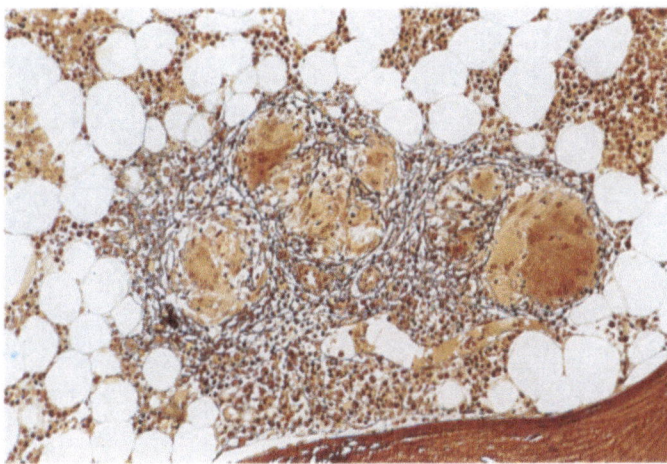

Fig. 4.22 Section of bone biopsy of patient with myelodysplastic syndrome who was found to have TB. Gomori

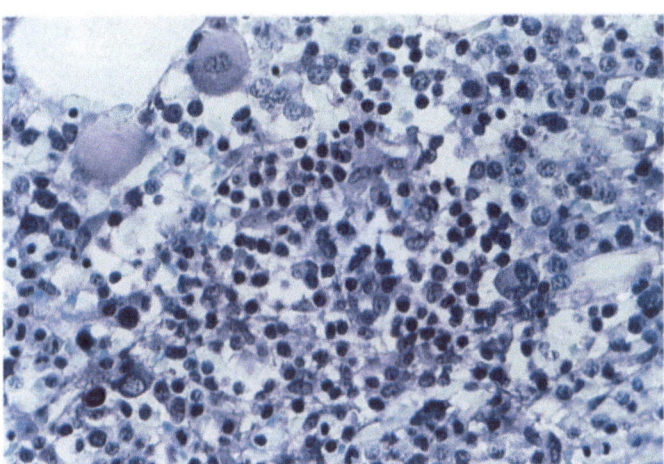

Fig. 4.23 Sections of bone biopsy of a 38-year-old patient with subfebrile temperature, massive splenomegaly and pancytopenia. The marrow contained numerous small granulomas consisting of epithelioid and lymphoid cells. The patient underwent splenectomy, and Donovan bodies were found in imprints of the spleen

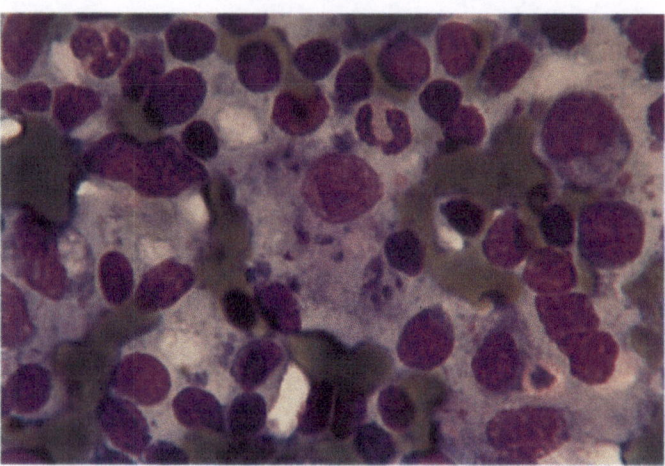

Fig. 4.24 Imprint of spleen at splenectomy (see Fig. 4.23): macrophage containing Donovan bodies; these were not found in the bone marrow in spite of intensive investigation

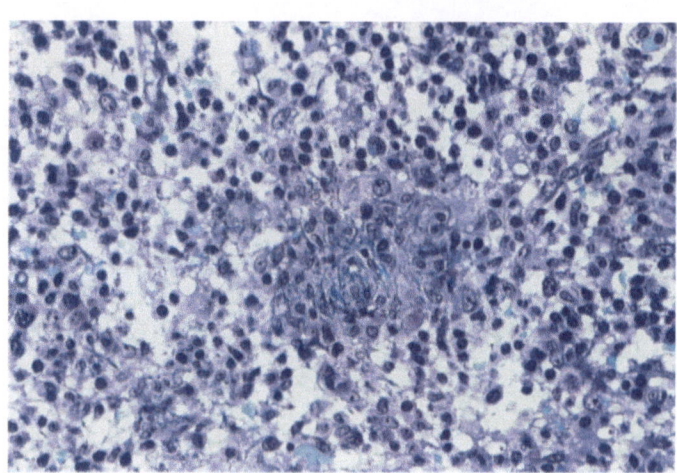

Fig. 4.25 Epithelioid granuloma in bone marrow of patient with malignant lymphoma

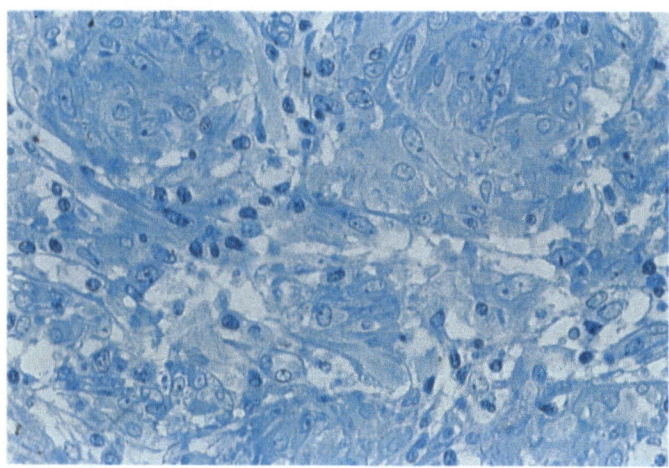

Fig. 4.26 Epithelioid cell granulomas in patient with Hodgkin's disease

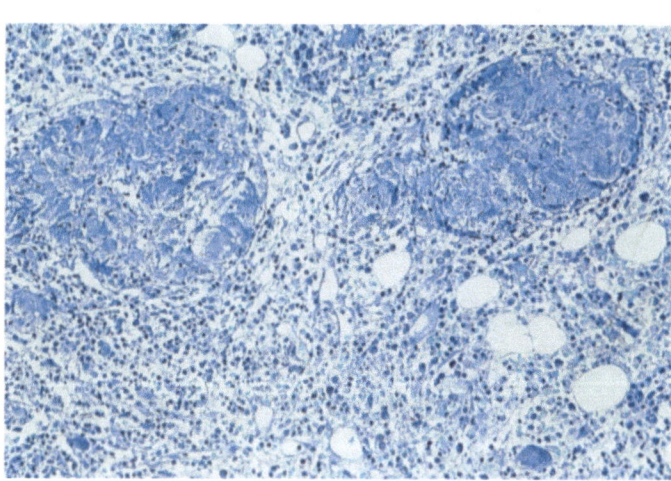

Fig. 4.27 Granulomas in bone biopsy of patient with haemolytic anaemia

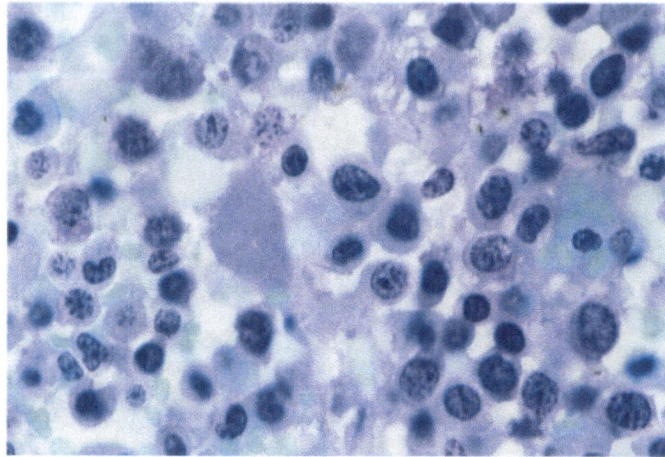

Fig. 4.28 Haemophagocytosis in bone biopsy with granulomas

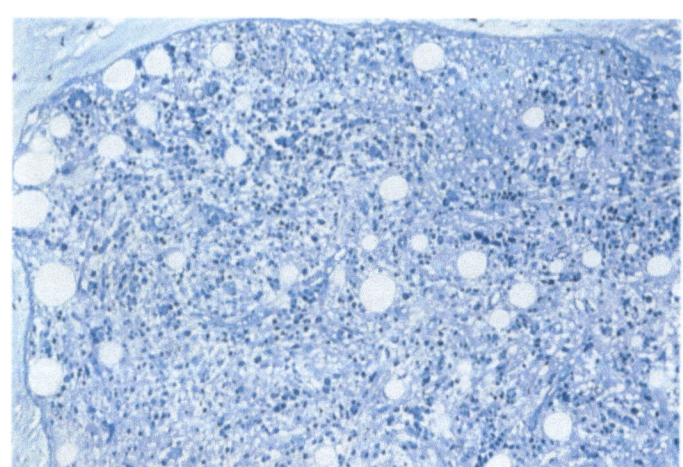

Fig. 4.29 Bone biopsy of child with osteomyelitis. Degeneration of haematopoietic tissue, disorganization, inflammatory reaction, lipid macrophages and developing sclerosis

visible on X-ray before the phase of reactive repair including osteoblastic new bone formation, which may result in a dense sclerosis (Garré's sclerosing osteomyelitis). The source and the site of entry of the causative organisms may not always be apparent; fractures, operations and superficial injuries are among the possibilities which can lead to haematogenous spread of organisms to the bone marrow. Osteolytic lesions in the elderly may be mistaken for malignant metastases[17].

Bone Marrow Necrosis

This may result not only from bacterial osteomyelitis but also from many other infections, toxins and inflammatory states. Bone marrow necrosis may be found in rapidly growing malignancies – leukaemias, lymphomas and metastases[18]. Necrosis in the bone marrow in sickle cell disease is due to vascular obstruction. Thrombosis of a blood vessel also results in ischaemia and degeneration in the surrounding tissue. In anorexia nervosa the gelatinous transformation of the bone marrow is preceded and accompanied by necrosis of haematopoietic cells (Fig. 4.34).

Blood Vessels

Alterations in blood vessels – such as arteriosclerosis (especially in diabetic patients), thrombosis and vasculitis – may affect vessels in the bone marrow as in any other organ (Figs 4.35–4.41). Haematopoiesis in the areas surrounding the affected vessels is eventually replaced by fat cells. The trabecular bone is also reduced – localized osteopenia. Vascular changes are one of the factors contributing to localized patchy marrow atrophy, especially in the older age groups (Fig. 4.42).

Primary and Secondary Amyloidosis

Amyloid may be deposited in the walls of sinusoids, as well as of small blood vessels, occasionally even larger ones (Figs 4.43 and 4.44). It may also be found as an amorphous substance deposited interstitially between the haematopoietic and fat cells (Figs 4.45 and 4.46). Interstitial and vascular amyloidosis may occasionally be seen in the same biopsy section. However, vascular is more common than interstitial amyloidosis in the bone marrow: both lead to loss of haematopoietic tissue in the affected areas. In Giemsa-stained sections amyloid appears as an amorphous deposit stained blue (Fig. 4.45). It is generally advisable to stain a parallel section with Congo red and to check for green fluorescence in polarized light as a control (Figs 4.44 and 4.47).

Secondary amyloidosis may develop in some chronic inflammatory states, in rheumatoid arthritis[19], and in familial Mediterranean fever; it has been seen in patients with cancer, and in patients on haemodialysis. In the last group, B_2 microglobulin is the major constituent of the amyloid fibres[20]. Amyloidosis of immunoglobulin origin (so called because it develops from light chains of immunoglobulins), is found in a small percentage of patients with plasma cell dyscrasias including multiple myeloma. Two other types are also recognized – primary amyloidosis in which no predisposing cause is apparent and some rare forms of hereditary amyloidosis. The different types of amyloid may be characterized by immunological techniques[21]. The clinical and laboratory features of primary amyloidosis have been reviewed recently[22].

References

1. Krech, R. and Thiele, J. (1985). Histopathology of the bone marrow in toxic myelopathy. A study of drug-induced lesions in 57 patients. *Virchows arch. (Pathol. Anat).*, **405**, 225
2. Sprigley, J. R., Vellend, H., Palmer, N., Phillips, M. J., Geddie, W. R., Van Nostrand, A. W. and Edwards, V. D. (1985). Q-fever, the liver and bone marrow pathology. *Am. J. Surg. Pathol.*, **9**, 752
3. Tavassoli, M. (1987). Structural alterations of marrow during inflammation. *Blood Cells*, **13**, 251
4. Bentley, S. A. (1982). Bone marrow connective tissue and the haemopoietic microenvironment. *Br. J. Haematol.*, **50**, 1
5. Tavassoli, M. and Friedenstein, A. (1983). Hemopoietic stromal microenvironment. *Am. J. Hematol.*, **15**, 195
6. Weiss, L. and Sakai, H. (1984). The hematopoietic stroma. *Am. J. Anat.*, **170**, 447
7. Gordon, M. Y., Hibbin, J. A., Kearney, L. U., Gordon-Smith, E. C. and Goldman, J. M. (1985). Colony formation by primitive haemopoietic progenitors in cocultures of bone marrow cells and stromal cells. *Br. J. Haematol.*, **60**, 129
8. Rywlin, A. M., Hoffman, E. P. and Ortega, R. S. (1972). Eosinophilic fibrohistiocytic lesion of bone marrow: A distinctive new morphologic finding, probably related to drug hypersensitivity. *Blood*, **40**, 464
9. Frisch, B., Lewis, S.M., Burkhardt, R. and Bartl, R. (1985). *Biopsy Pathology of Bone and Bone Marrow*. London: Chapman and Hall
10. Woessner, S., Lafuente, R., Martin, E., Florensa, L. and Marill, M. R. (1988). Gelatinous transformation of the bone marrow. Cytohistologic, histochemical and ultrastructural study of a case. *Sangre-(Barc.)*, **33**, 147
11. Vilalta-Castel, E., Valdes-Sanchez, M. D., Guerra-Vales, J. M., Teno-Esteban, G., Garzon, A., Lopez, J. I., Ricard, M. P., Abarca, M. and Garcia-Diaz, J. D. (1988). Significance of granulomas in bone marrow: a study of 40 cases. *Eur. J. Haematol.*, **41**, 12
12. Bhargava, B. A. and Farhi, D. C. (1988). Bone marrow granulomas: clinicopathologic findings in 72 cases and review of the literature. *Hematol. Pathol.*, **2**, 43
13. Mankin, H. J. and Rosenberg, A. E. (1988). A 25-year-old man with multiple bone lesions, hilar lymphadenopathy, and a pericardial effusion. *N. Engl. J. Med.*, **319**, 1209
14. Muthuswamy, P. P., Lopez-Majano, V., Raginwala, M. and Trainor, W. E. (1987). Serum angiotensin-converting enzyme (SACE) activity as an indicator of total body granuloma load and prognosis in sarcoidosis. *Sarcoidosis*, **4**, 142
15. Pelstring, R. J., Kim, C. K., Lower, E. E. and Swerdlov, S. H. (1988). Marrow granulomas in coal workers' pneumoconiosis. A histologic study with elemental analysis. *Am. J. Clin. Pathol.*, **89**, 553
16. Thompson, D., Bannister, P. and Murphy, P. (1988). Vertebral osteomyelitis in the elderly. *Br. Med. J.*, **296**, 1309
17. Foss, A. and Markus, H. (1988). Osteolytic lesions in elderly diabetic woman. *Br. Med. J.*, **296**, 280
18. Bevilacqua, G., Abadessa, A., Consolini, R., Frijia, M., Nardi, M. and Macchia, P. (1985). Bone marrow necrosis foreshadowing acute lymphoid leukemia. *Am. J. Pediatr. Hematol. Oncol.*, **7**, 228
19. Maury, C. P. J. and Teppo, A. M. (1985). Rheumatoid factors and amyloidosis in rheumatoid arthritis. *Br. Med. J.*, **291**, 1015
20. Brancaccio, D., Gallieni, M., Padovese, P., Anelli, A., Coggi, G. and Ulsenghi, C. (1988). Dialysis amyloidosis with massive popliteal deposition of B_2-microglobulin amyloid. *Lancet*, **2**, 802
21. Chastonay, P. and Hurlimann, J. (1986). Characterization of different amyloids with immunological techniques. *Pathol. Res. Pract.*, **181**, 657
22. Kyle, R. A. and Greipp, P. R. (1983). Amyloidosis (AL). Clinical and laboratory features in 229 cases. *Mayo Clin. Proc.*, **58**, 665

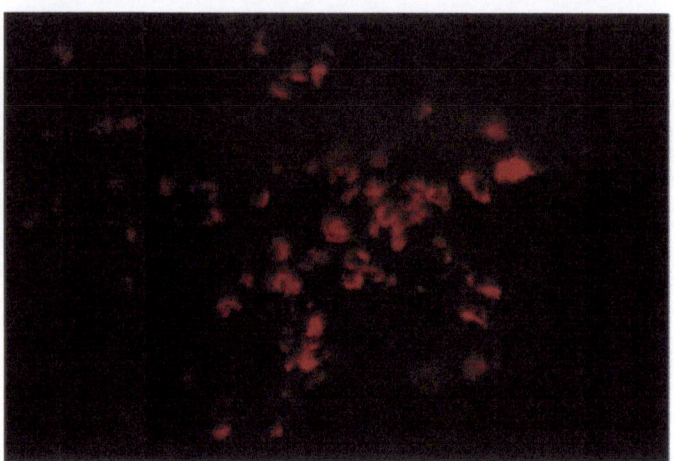

Fig. 4.30 Cryostat section of same case as in Fig. 4.29, antibody to IgG, plasma cells stained red with rhodamine

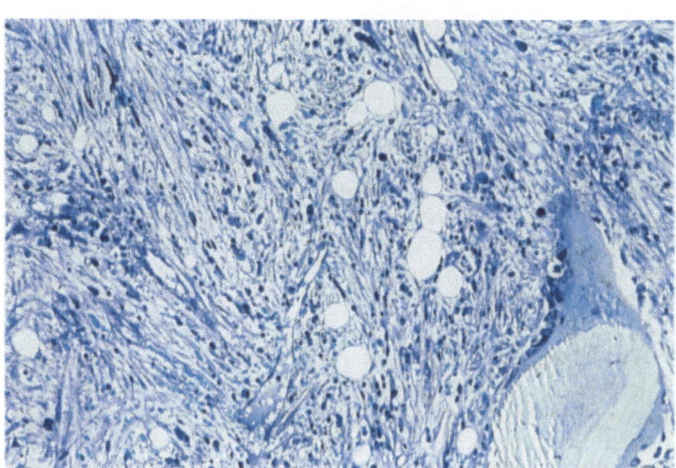

Fig. 4.31 Sclerosis of bone marrow developing in case of osteomyelitis. Note osteoblastic new bone formation

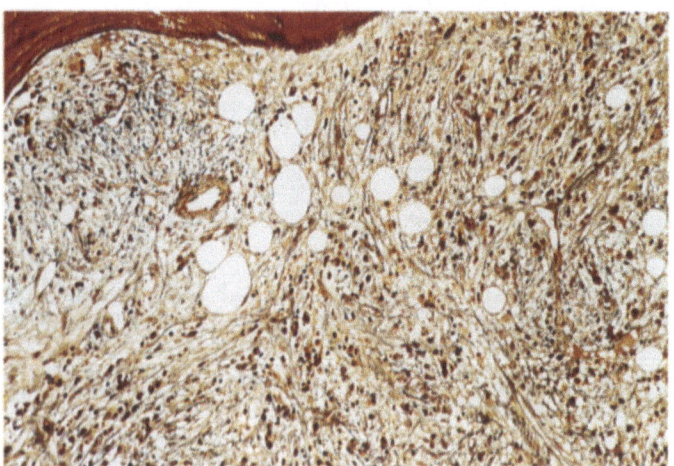

Fig. 4.32 Part of same biopsy as in Fig. 4.31, section stained by Gomori showing extensive fibrosis

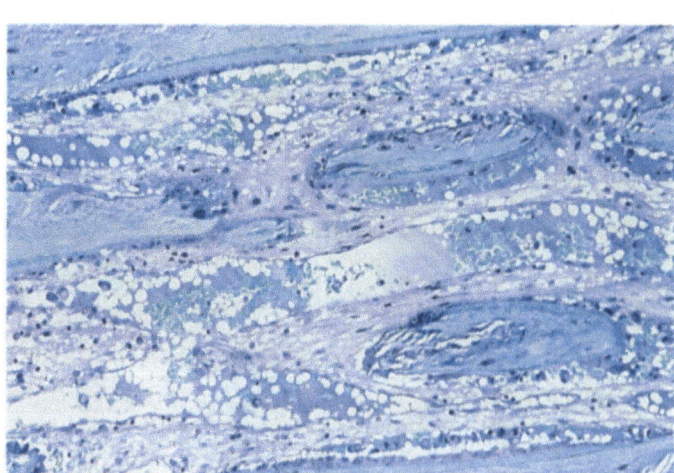

Fig. 4.33 Section of bone biopsy of patient with previous osteomyelitis, now illustrating development of osteomyelosclerosis. Note absence of haematopoietic tissue

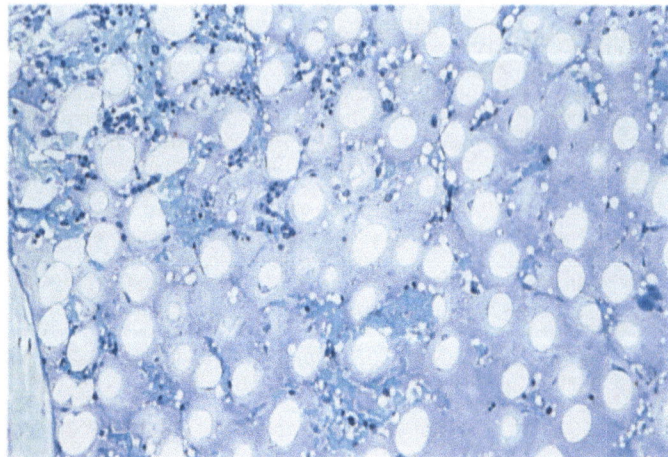

Fig. 4.34 Section of bone biopsy of patient with anorexia nervosa and excessive weight loss. Section showing gelatinous transformation of bone marrow

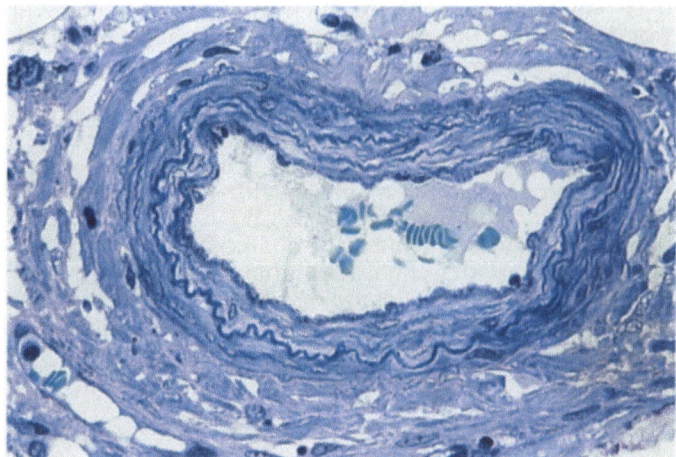

Figs 4.35–4.39 Bone biopsies of patients with diabetes illustrating sclerosis of blood vessel walls (arteries, arterioles and sinusoids)

Fig. 4.35 Sclerosis of wall of artery in bone biopsy of patient with diabetes

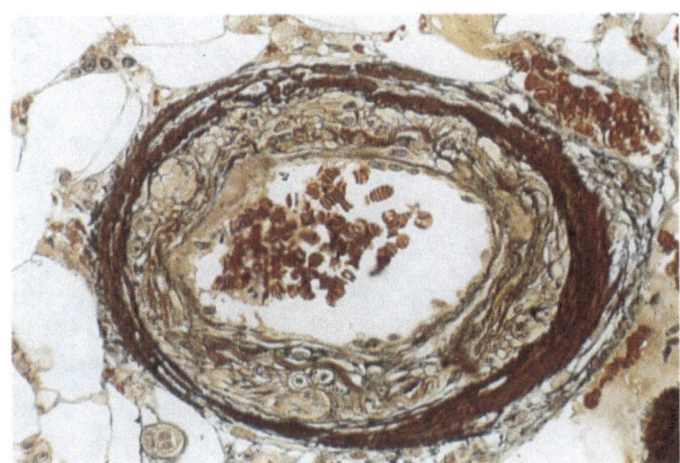

Fig. 4.36 Cross-section of artery, ossified fibres. Gomori

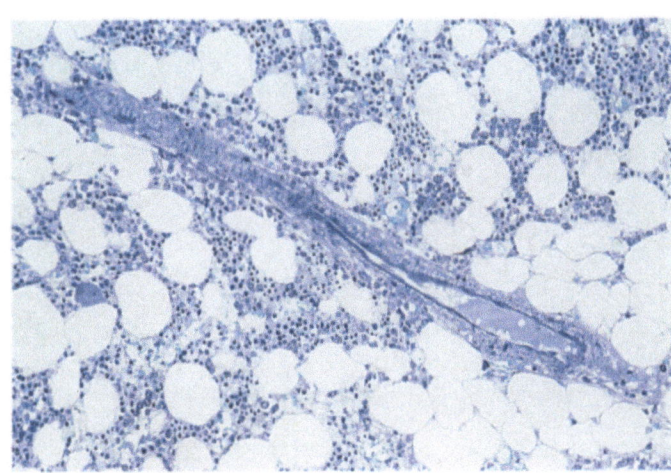

Fig. 4.37 Small artery, longitudinal cut

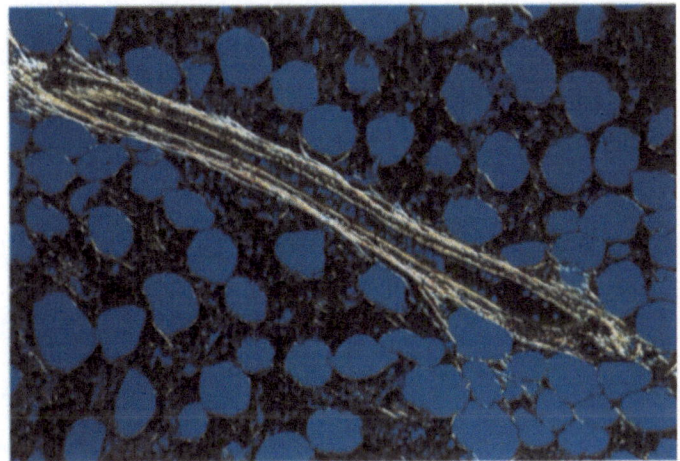

Fig. 4.38 Parallel section to that in Fig. 4.37. Gomori's stain viewed in polarized light, fibres surrounding wall of artery

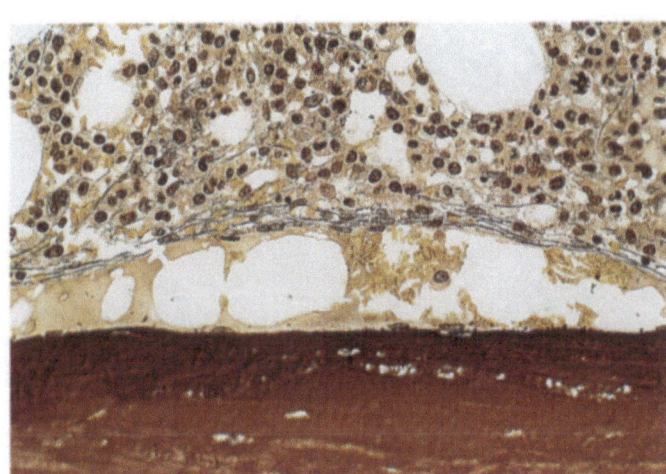

Fig. 4.39 Section showing sclerosis of wall of paratrabecular sinus. Gomori

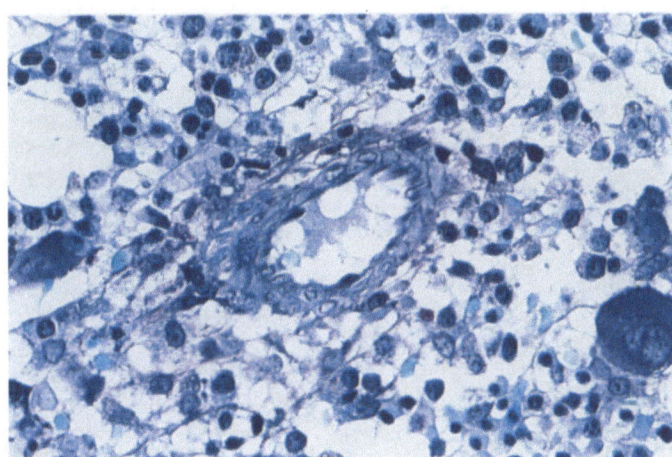

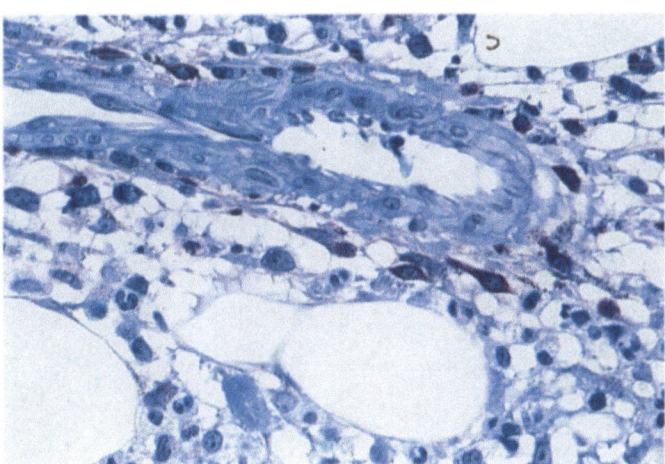

Fig. 4.41 Blood vessel cut in longitudinal section illustrating the mast cells

Figs 4.40 and 4.41 Bone biopsy sections illustrating blood vessels with varying degrees of inflammatory reactions, including perivascular plasma cells and mastocytosis

Fig. 4.40 Blood vessel cut in cross-section, oedema and fibres in surrounding marrow

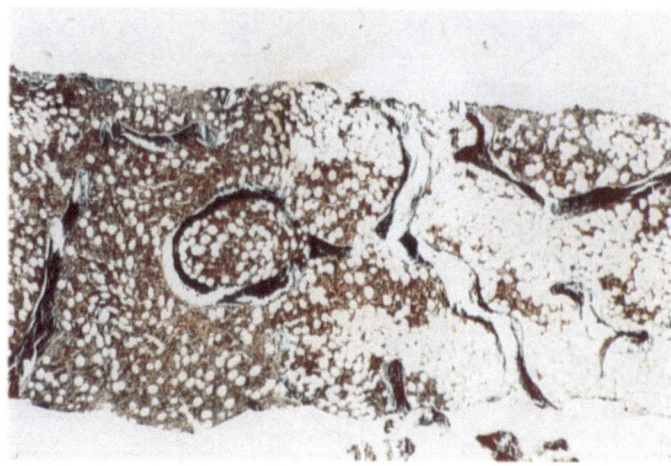

Fig. 4.42 Low-power view of bone biopsy illustrating hypocellular area in part of bone biopsy with inadequate blood supply due to vascular disease. Gomori

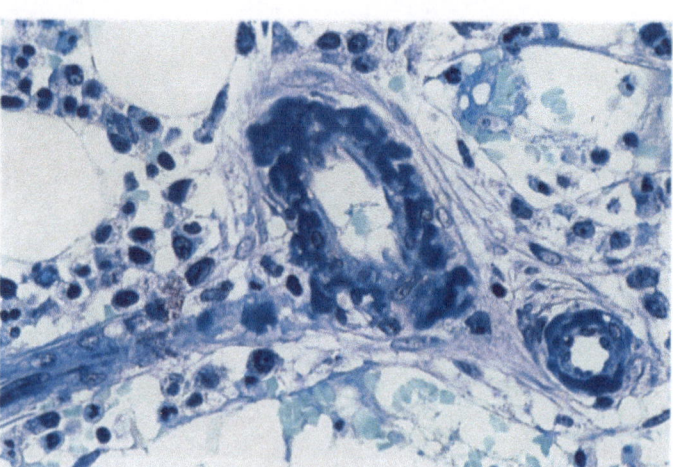

Fig. 4.43 Deposition of amyloid in wall of blood vessels. Note deposits in walls of large and small arteries

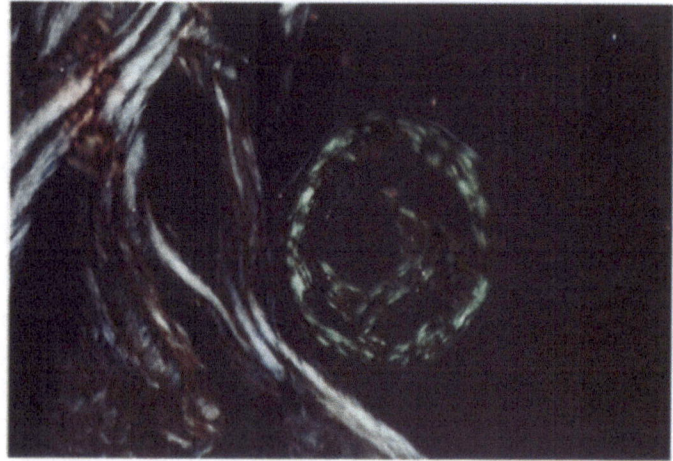

Fig. 4.44 Section from same biopsy as in Fig. 4.42 stained by Congo red, viewed in polarized light and showing green fluorescence

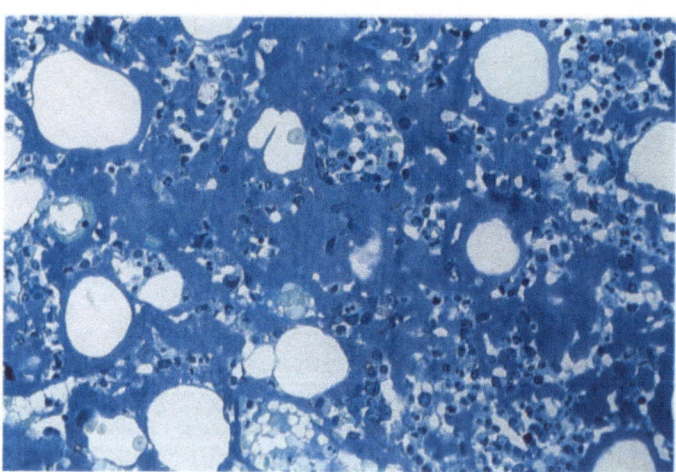

Fig. 4.45 Interstitial amyloidosis stained blue in the Giemsa-stained section

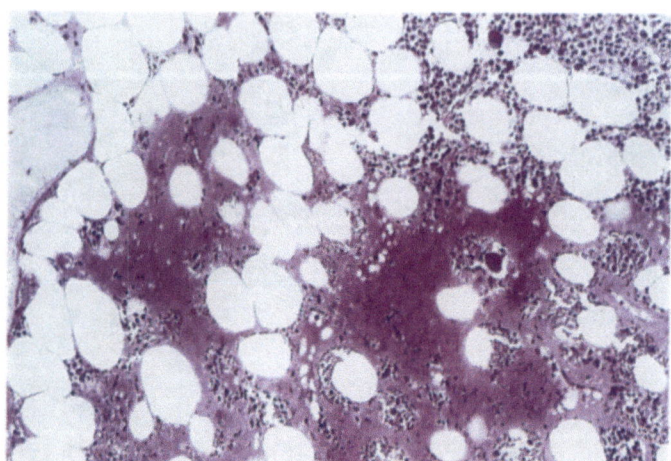

Fig. 4.46 Same case as in Fig. 4.44; bone biopsy section stained with methyl violet. The deposits of amyloid are stained red

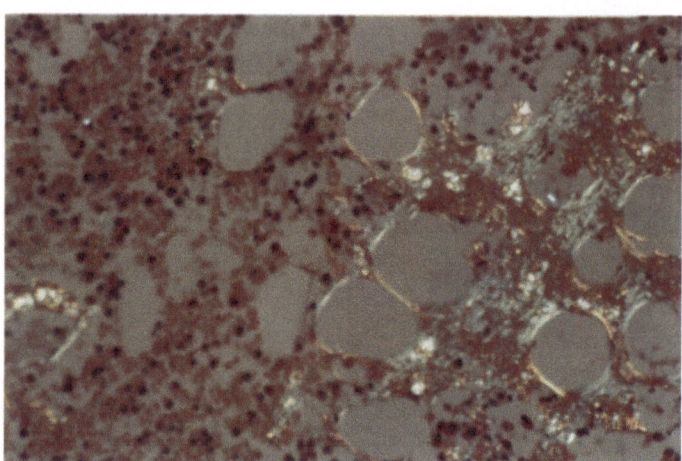

Fig. 4.47 Section of paraffin-embedded bone biopsy of patient with primary amyloidosis, stained with Congo red and viewed in polarized light showing interstitial deposits of amyloid

Primary and Secondary Myelodysplastic Syndromes

5

The designation 'myelodysplastic syndromes' (MDS) refers to a group of disorders having in common progressive (often fatal) cytopenia(s) together with ineffective haematopoiesis in the bone marrow. The MDS are considered to be pre-leukaemic conditions[1]. The MDS include the idiopathic acquired (primary) syndromes and the secondary conditions. In both types of MDS there are alterations in proliferation, development and structure of both haematopoietic and stromal elements in the bone marrow. Recent evidence suggests that the MDS result from neoplastic transformation at the level of a pluripotent stem cell, which is capable of differentiation for variable periods of time[2,3]. But the inherent defect results in some degree of morphological and functional abnormality in the erythroid, granulocytic or megakaryocytic cell lines, generally in all three. Eventually the ability to differentiate is lost and acute leukaemia ensues.

The primary MDS (i.e. the idiopathic acquired MDS) (Fig. 5.1) represent early phases of stem cell aberrations, that may precede acute or chronic myeloproliferative disorders, while the secondary MDS constitute the haematopoietic consequences of exogenous agents[4–6]. Recommendations for a morphological, immunological and cytogenetic working classification of the primary and therapy-related myelodysplastic disorders have recently been published[7].

Primary MDS

These occur mainly in people over 50–60 years of age, but have also been observed in children, though rarely[8].

The French, American, British (FAB) cooperative study group classified the MDS into five subtypes[9], which have prognostic significance[10–12]. One of the main criteria for these subdivisions was the percentage of blasts in the peripheral blood and in smears of the bone marrow aspirate. The FAB classification has also been applied to bone marrow histology[13]. The FAB subtypes of the MDS are: refractory anaemia (RA)[14], acquired idiopathic

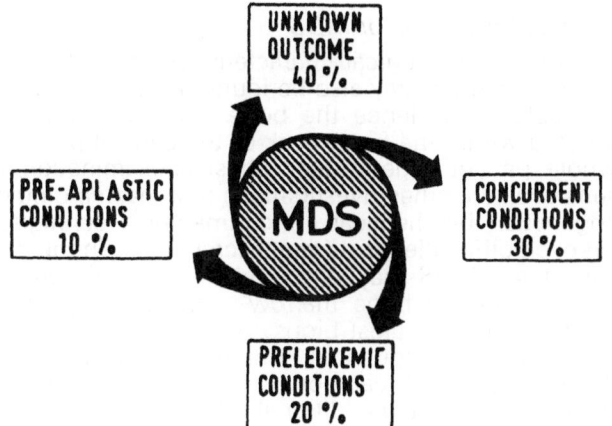

Fig. 5.1 Possible associations and aetiologies in primary acquired myelodysplastic syndromes. Other conditions may contribute or be responsible in 30% of cases, while no cause is discovered and the eventual outcome remains unclarified in about 40% of cases

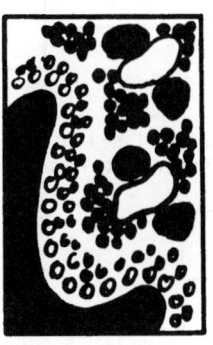 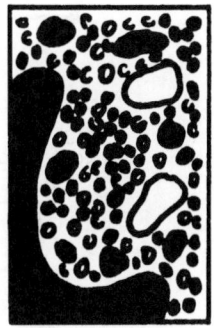

NORMAL   MYELODYSPLASIA

Fig. 5.2 Sketch of normal marrow architecture: paratrabecular granulopoiesis, intertrabecular and perisinusoidal erythroid islands and megakaryocytes. In myelodysplasia there is topographic disorganization with the precursors of the three cell lines found in all marrow regions

sideroblastic anaemia (AISA), or refractory anaemia with sideroblasts (RAS), refractory anaemia with excess of blasts (RAEB)[15], refractory anaemia with excess of blasts in transformation (RAEBT) and chronic myelomonocytic leukaemia (CMML)[16]. The boundaries between these subtypes are not sharp; there is considerable overlap between them, and many unanswered questions remain concerning the biological and pathological relationships between the groups. Moreover, there is some overlap between MDS, aplastic anaemia, some forms of acute leukaemia and other myeloproliferative disorders (see Figs 5.44–5.46)[17,18]. One drawback of the FAB classification is that it cannot take into account the stromal changes which may alter the microenvironment required for normal haematopoiesis. Moreover, the proportion of the different cell lines morphologically affected or increased is reflected more accurately in bone biopsy sections than in smears of aspirates, especially when there is an increase in reticular fibres. One important example is provided by megakaryocytes in sideroblastic anaemia: there is frequently no correlation between the platelet count in peripheral blood and the number of megakaryocytes in the bone marrow[19].

From the point of view of bone marrow histology, one must take into account the histopathologic definition of dysplasia:'dysplasia comprises a loss in the regularity of the individual cells as well as a loss in their architectural orientation'. Thus myelodysplasia (Fig. 5.2) (i.e. dysplasia in the bone marrow) is characterized by alterations in the growth, maturation, organization and structure of the haematopoietic tissue including the stromal compartment[20,21]. The bone marrow may be hypercellular (the majority), normocellular or hypocellular (Figs 5.3–5.6)[22,23]. Some bone marrow sections may present alternating fatty and cellular areas. One of the most important histological parameters is the architectual disorganization: myeloid precursors in the central intertrabecular areas (abnormal localization of immature precursors – ALIP)[24], erythrons and megakaryocytes at the trabecular surface (Figs 5.7–5.12). In addition, there are alterations in the

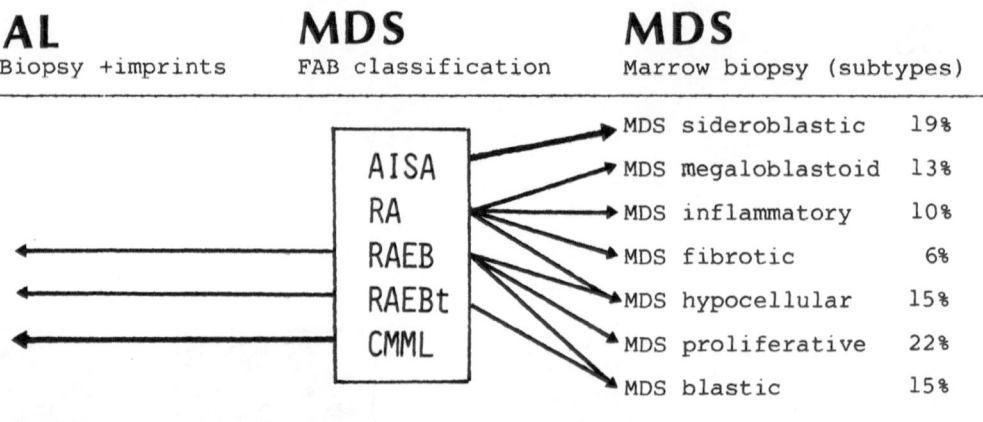

AL
Biopsy +imprints

MDS
FAB classification

MDS
Marrow biopsy (subtypes)

MDS sideroblastic	19%
MDS megaloblastoid	13%
MDS inflammatory	10%
MDS fibrotic	6%
MDS hypocellular	15%
MDS proliferative	22%
MDS blastic	15%

AISA
RA
RAEB
RAEBt
CMML

Fig. 5.37 Correlation of the FAB classification with the histological subtypes, indicated by arrows on the right-hand side. Propensity to develop acute leukaemia shown by arrows on the left side

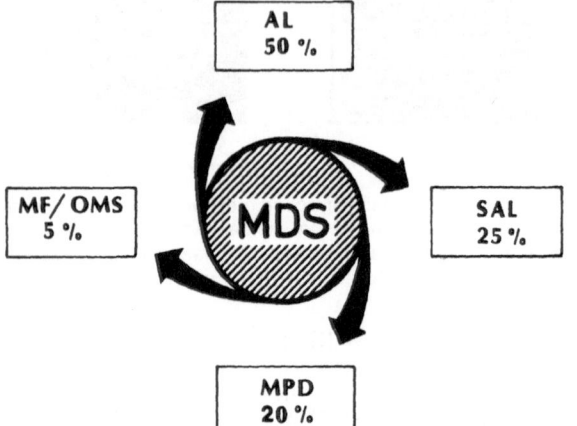

Fig. 5.39 Schematic representation of the evolution of primary myelodysplastic syndromes: about half of the cases eventually develop acute leukaemia, while the rest show a slowly progressive course developing into sub-acute or chronic myeloproliferative disorders

stromal compartment: areas of oedema, ectatic sinusoids, perivascular and interstitial fibrosis, inflammatory reactions, plasmacytosis, increased mast cells, macrophages often containing haemosiderin, lymphocytosis; one or more lymphoid aggregates may be present (Figs 5.13–5.20). In this context it is of interest that various immunological changes have been documented in MDS[25,26]. The histological criteria in MDS may be summarized as follows: (1) cellularity of the bone marrow; (2) architectural disorganization; (3) stromal reactions; (4) predominant cell line(s); (5) cellular abnormalities[27,28]; (6) ineffective haematopoiesis. On the basis of the histological criteria listed above, biopsies could be divided into seven categories: (1) MDS sideroblastic, (2) MDS megaloblastoid, (3) MDS inflammatory, (4) MDS fibrotic, (5) MDS hypocellular, (6) MDS proliferative, and (7) MDS blastic (Figs 5.21–5.36). Chronic myelomonocytic leukaemia – CMML – being by definition a leukaemia, does not, strictly speaking, belong in the group of myelodysplastic syndromes regarded as pre-leukaemic conditions (at least, not overtly leukaemic). Chronic myelomoncytic leukaemia may also follow a myelodysplastic syndrome such as refractory anaemia. Correlation of the histological types of MDS with the FAB classification is given in Fig. 5.37. The presence of ALIP in the bone biopsy sections constitutes both a diagnostic and prognostic factor. Moreover, sometimes larger aggregates of blasts may be found, and these are a warning signal for the imminent transformation to an acute leukaemia (Fig. 5.38)[19]. Haemophagocytosis has also been observed in the terminal stages of MDS[29], as in some lymphoproliferative disorders.

Evolution of disease

Many patients die as a consequence of the complications of the cytopenias (Fig. 5.39): in others, concurrent disorders such as cardiovascular diseases may be present at diagnosis, or be detected subsequently, for example metastatic carcinoma or immunologic disorders (Figs 5.40 and 5.41). Some patients develop aplastic anaemia, in others the MDS evolve into acute or smouldering leukaemias, myelofibrosis, or other chronic myeloproliferative disorders (Figs 5.42–5.46). Many retrospective and prospective studies have shown that the subgroups of the MDS have different rates of conversion to overt leukaemia[19,24,30–34]. When MDS occurs in a patient known to have a malignant solid tumour, or a second malignancy is subsequently discovered in a patient with MDS, the question arises as to whether it is a simultaneous (metachronous) condition or a paraneoplastic syndrome? One study which addressed this question has shown that a second malignancy occurred at 2.9 times the expected rate in a group of 138 patients with MDS[35].

Table 5.1 Differential diagnosis in MDS

Congenital hypoplasias	Cytotoxic dysplasias
Vitamin deficiencies	Acquired hypoplasias
Neoplasias elsewhere	Leukaemoid reactions
Rheumatic conditions	Malignant lymphomas
Haemolytic conditions	Hodgkin's disease
Chronic disorders	Myeloproliferative disorders
ARC and AIDS	

Differential diagnosis of MDS

Many of the histological characteristics of MDS, singly or in combination, may also be found in other conditions (see Table 5.1). Hence the bone marrow histology is evaluated within the framework of the clinical picture as a whole: patient's age, history, physical examination and results of all the other investigations (e.g. haematological, cytogenetic, biochemical, and imaging techniques). Moreover, difficulties and even discrepancies in the diagnosis of the MDS may occur due to: (1) discordance between different bone marrow regions – e.g. sternal aspiration and iliac crest biopsy; (2) temporal variability when comparing sequential bone marrow examinations; (3) overlapping of categories of the MDS; and (4) previously undetected additional conditions (e.g. metastases in the bone marrow) which may induce myelodysplasia.

It should be stressed that classifications based on purely morphological criteria will undoubtedly be modified in the near future. This applies to the FAB classification,

(Continued on p. 76)

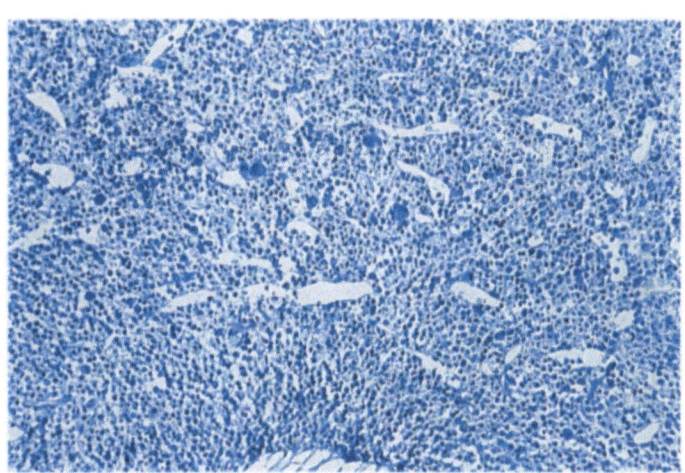

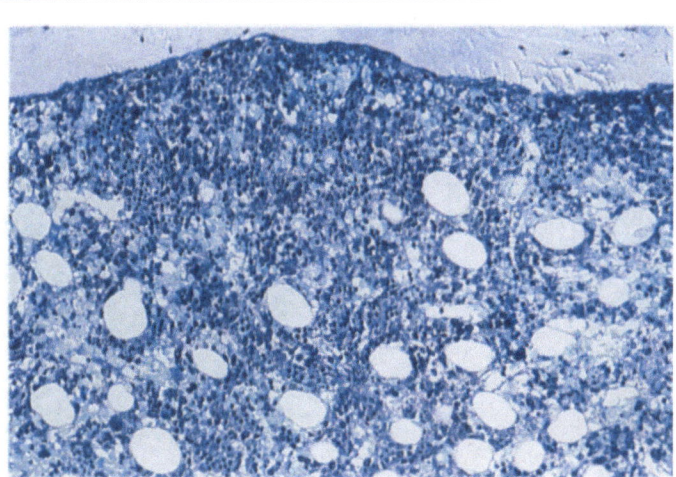

Figs 5.3–5.5 Bone biopsy sections of patients with myelodysplastic syndromes illustrating bone marrow cellularity which ranges from a densely cellular to a hypocellular bone marrow

Fig. 5.3 Hypercellular bone marrow

Fig. 5.4 Normocellular bone marrow

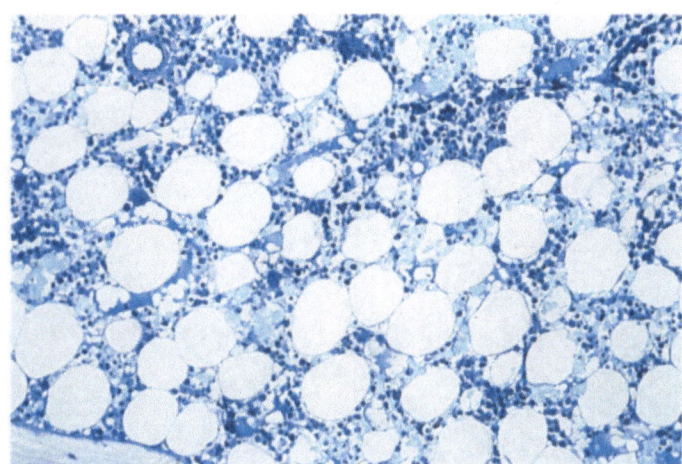

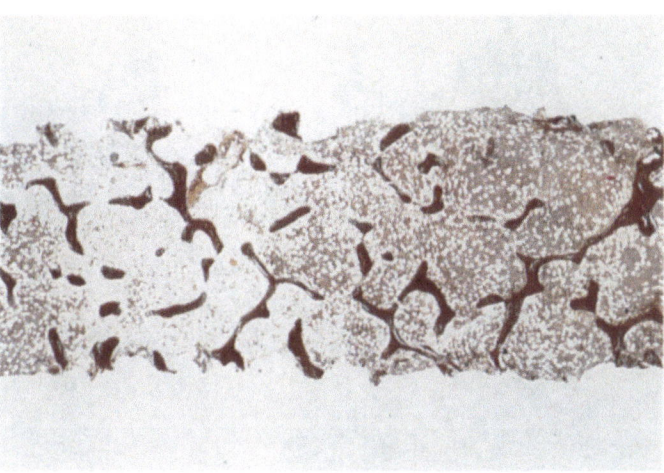

Fig. 5.5 Hypocellular bone marrow

Fig. 5.6 Low-power view of section of bone biopsy showing variable cellularity within one biopsy; stained by Gomori's stain

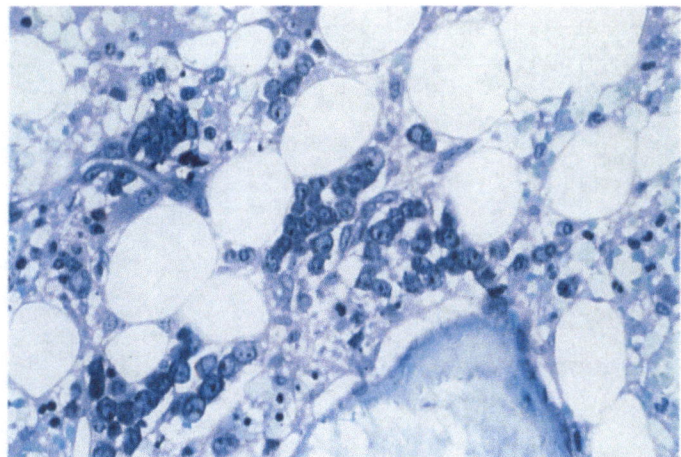

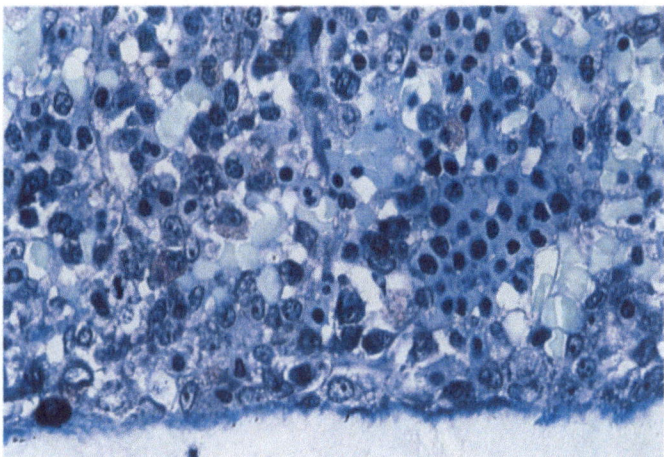

Figs 5.7–5.12 The architectural and topographic disorganization of the three cell lines in MDS

Fig. 5.7 Immature erythroblasts at trabecular surface

Fig. 5.8 High magnification of haematopoiesis at trabecular surface, note myeloid precursors, plasma cells, and erythroid island

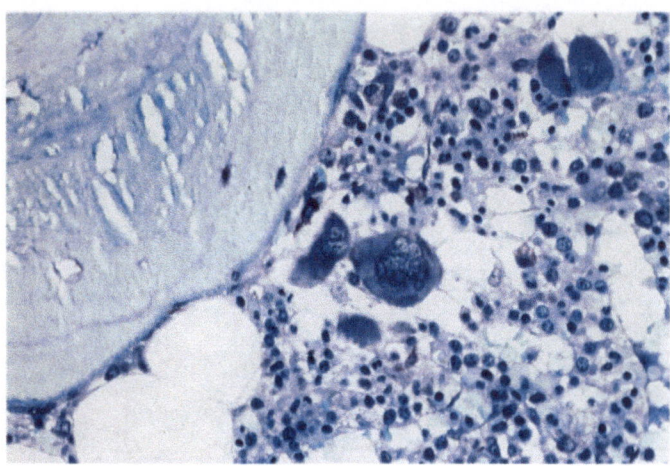

Fig. 5.9 Megakaryocytes and erythroblasts at trabecular surface

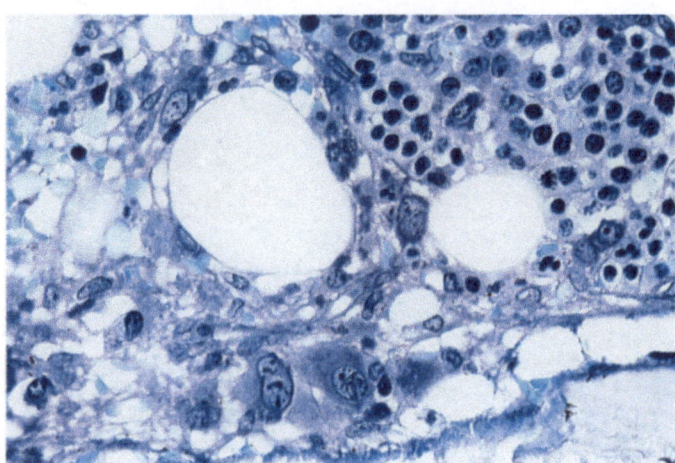

Fig. 5.10 Fibrosis and megakaryocytes at trabecular surface

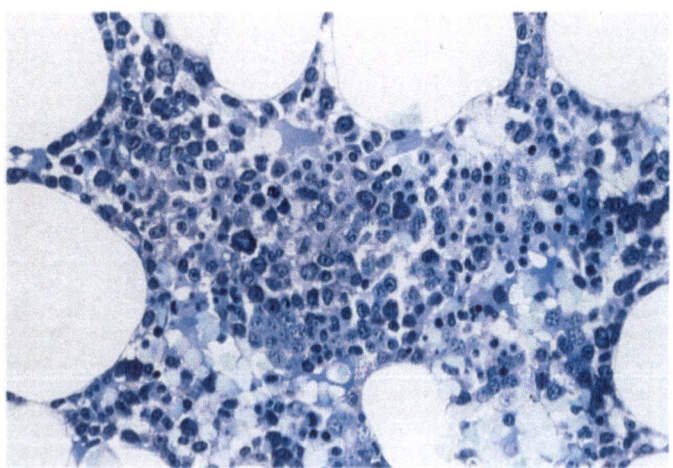

Fig. 5.11 Clusters of early myeloid precursors in central marrow area

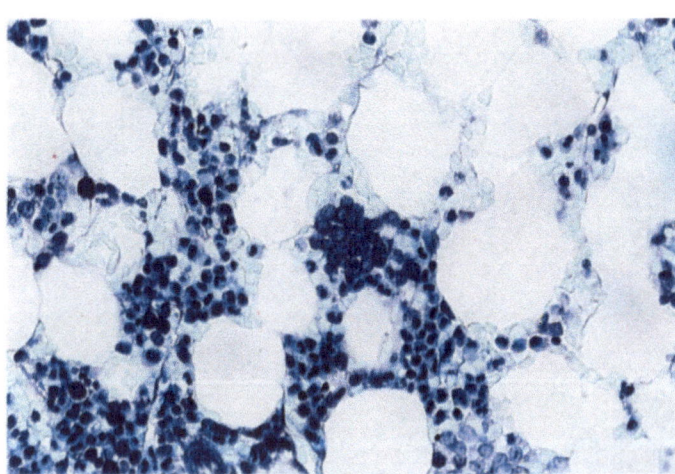

Fig. 5.12 Section of bone biopsy of patient with MDS and hypocellular bone marrow: example of abnormal localization of immature precursors – ALIP. Note central cluster of myeloblasts

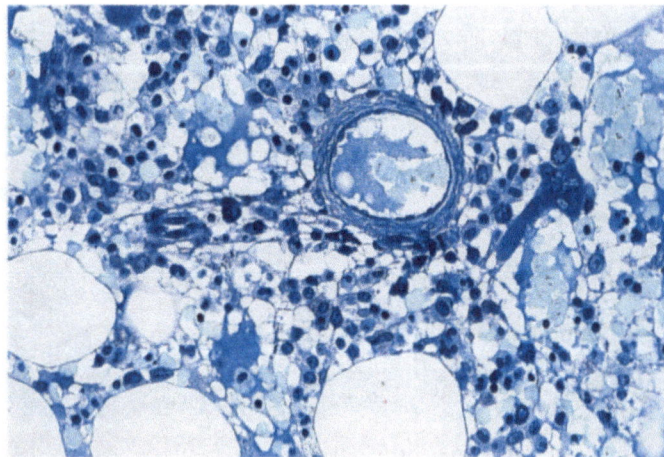

Figs 5.13–5.20 Sections of bone biopsies of patients with MDS, illustrating the stromal changes in MDS: vasculitis, increased plasma and mast cells, and fibres in the bone marrow and the dysmyelopoiesis affecting erythroid, granulolytic and megakaryocytic cell lines

Fig. 5.13 Blood vessel in loose, oedematous stroma, with plasma and lymphoid cells

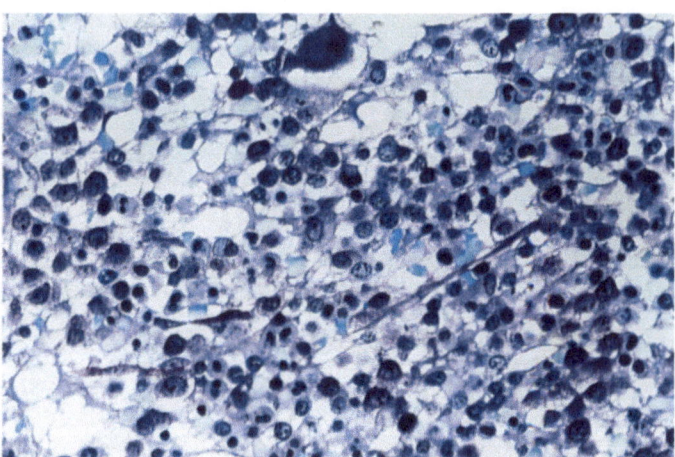

Fig. 5.14 Disorganization of marrow architecture, fibroblasts, fibers, and mast cells

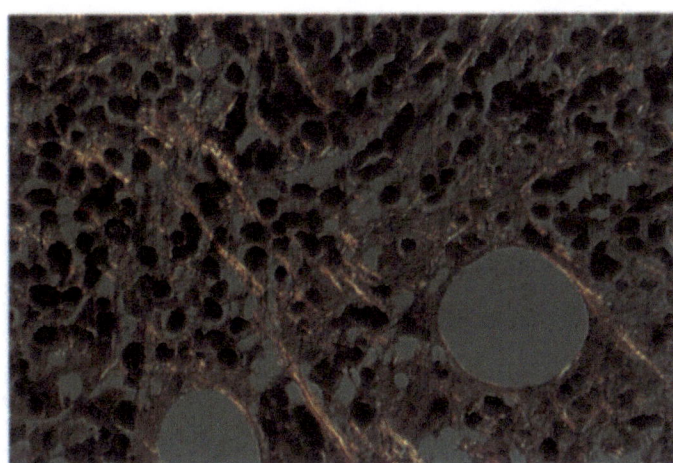

Fig. 5.15 Section of biopsy shown in Fig. 5.14, Gomori's stain, viewed in polarized light to highlight the reticular fibres

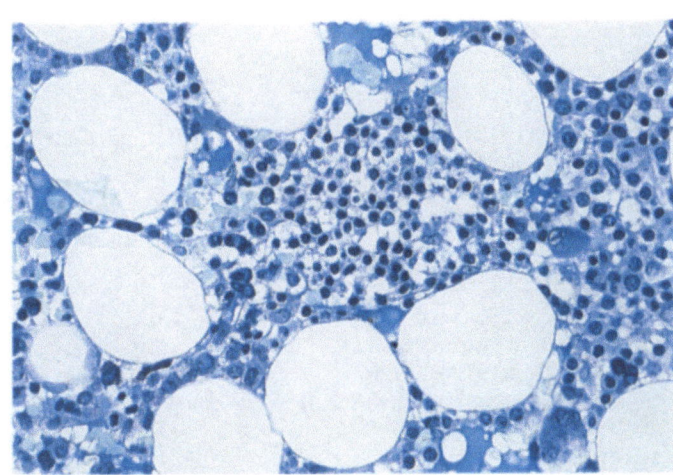

Fig. 5.16 Small lymphoid cell aggregate and micromegakaryocytes. Note also plasma cells and early myeloid precursors

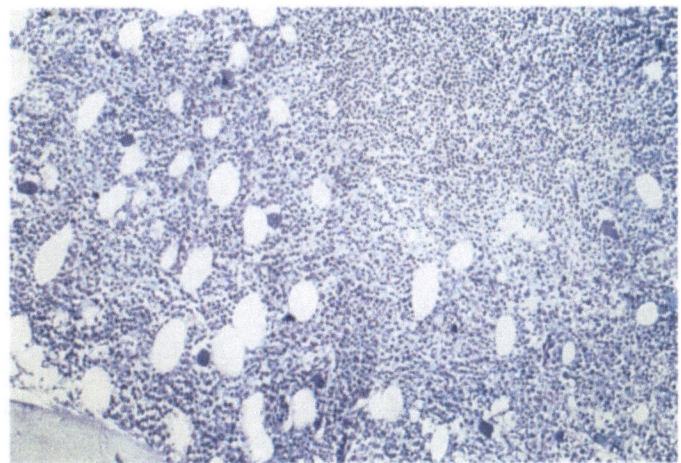

Fig. 5.17 Large lymphoid nodule in MDS

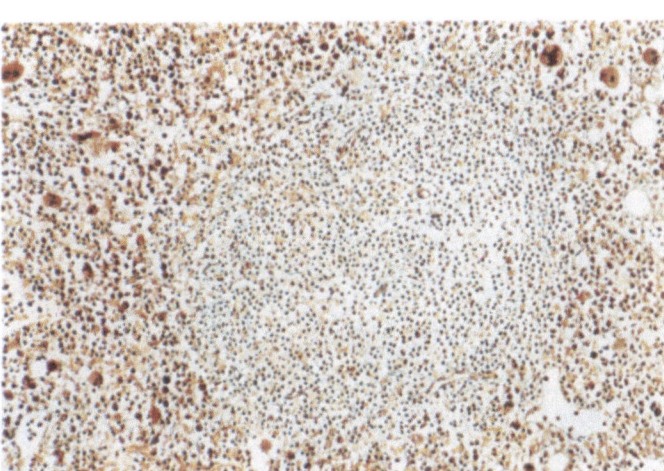

Fig. 5.18 Large lymphoid nodule in sideroblastic MDS; note hyperplasia of megakaryocytes

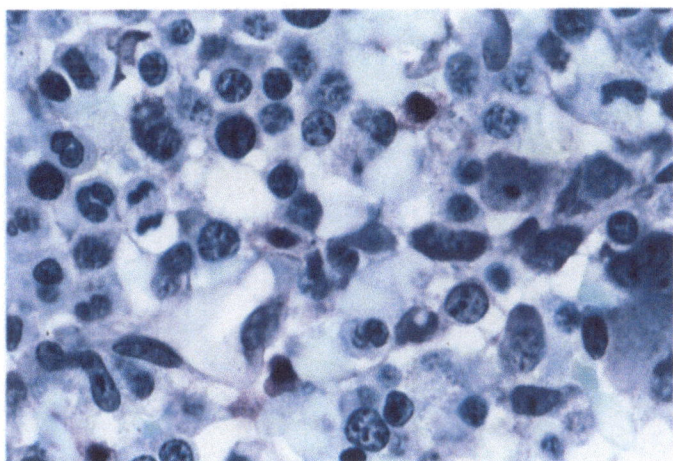

Fig. 5.19 Megaloblastoid erythroblasts and basophils

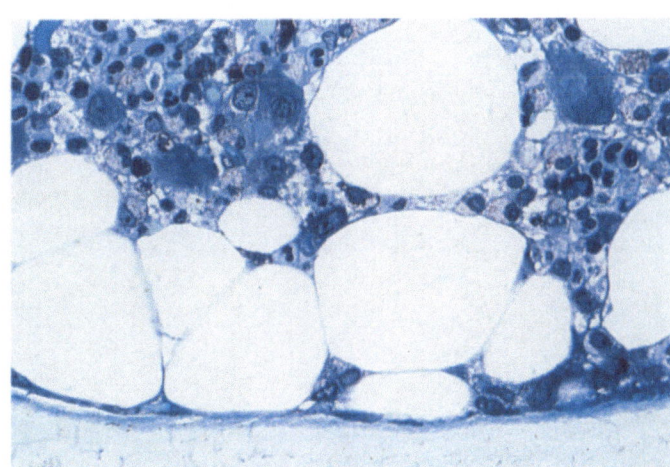

Fig. 5.20 Mononuclear megakaryocytes

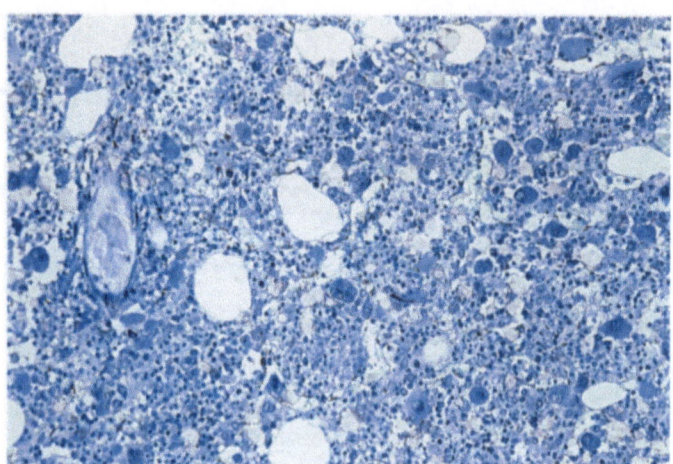

Figs 5.21–5.36 Sections of bone biopsies of patients with MDS, illustrating the histological subtypes

Fig. 5.21 MDS sideroblastic: cellular bone marrow with hyperplastic erythropoiesis and megakaryopoiesis

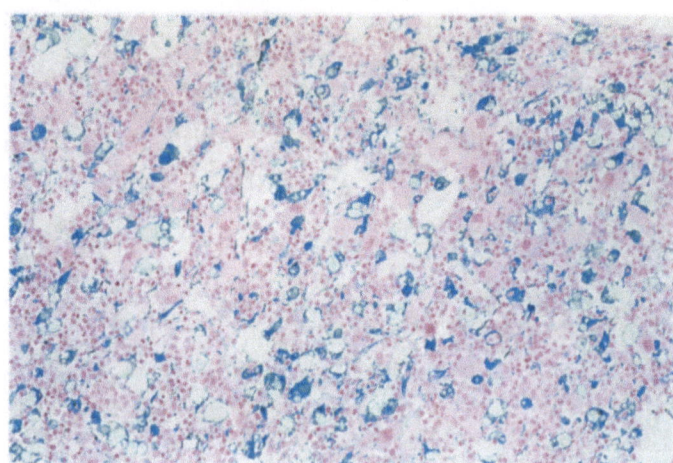

Figs 5.22 and 5.23 Stained by Prussian blue for demonstration of haemosiderin

Fig. 5.22 Overview to show great increase in iron-containing stromal cells

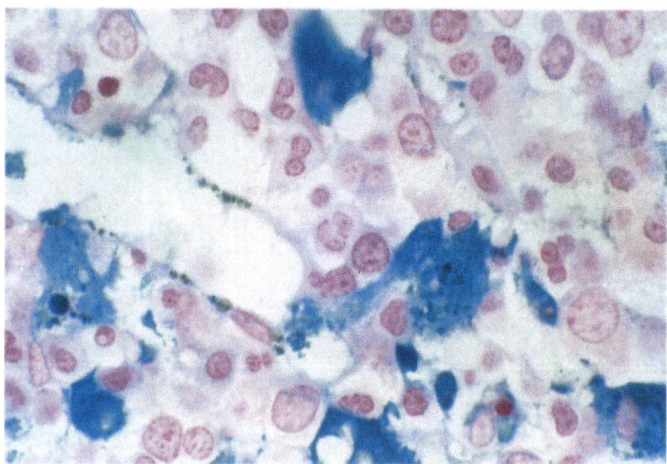

Fig. 5.23 Iron in sinus endothelium and macrophages

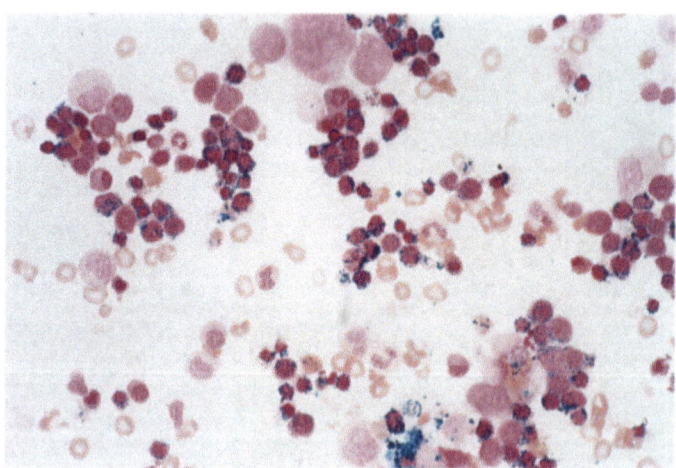

Fig. 5.24 Smear of aspirate of patient with sideroblastic MDS, illustrating ringed sideroblasts

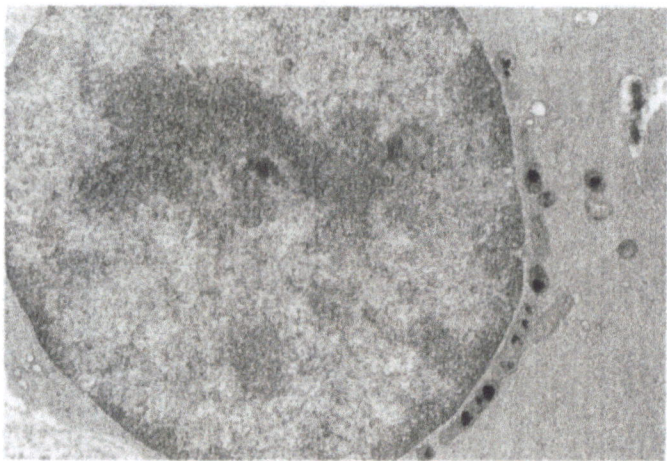

Fig. 5.25 Electron micrograph of early erythroblast with perinuclear mitochondria containing iron. × 15 000

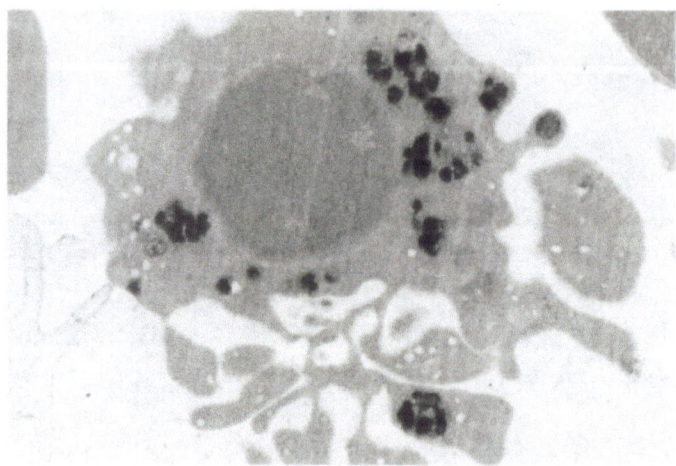

Fig. 5.26 Electron micrograph of normoblast in sideroblastic anaemia, accumulation of iron in mitochondria and siderosomes. × 20 000

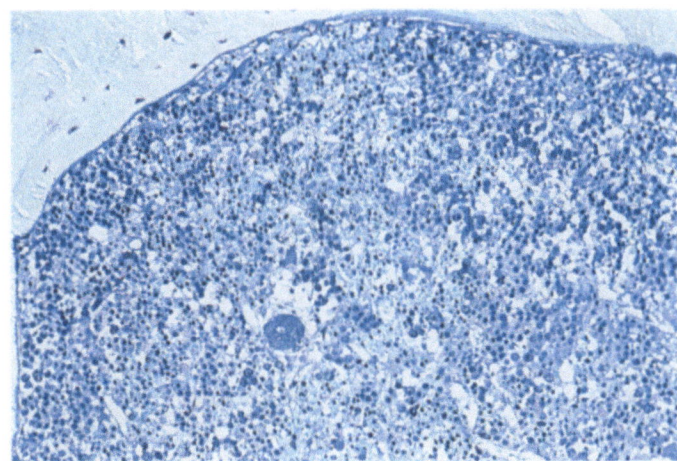

Fig. 5.27 MDS megaloblastoid: cellular bone marrow containing hyperplastic megaloblastoid erythropoiesis

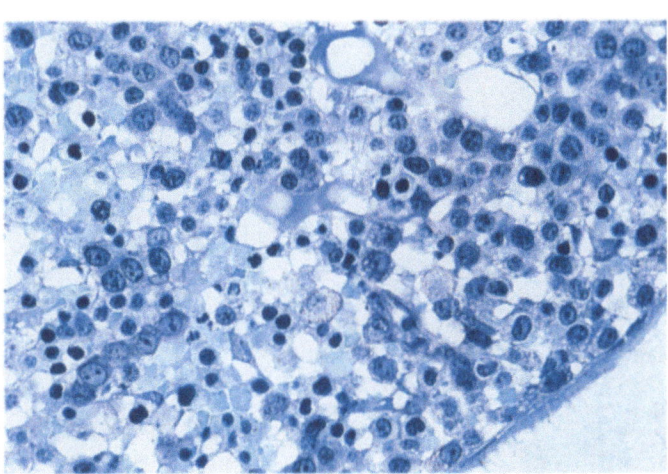

Fig. 5.28 Higher magnification of Fig. 5.27, paratrabecular area, disorganization of marrow and megaloblastoid erythropoiesis

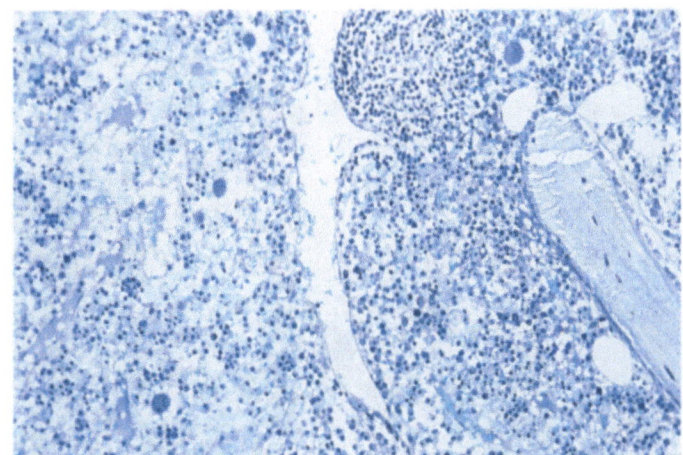

Fig. 5.29 MDS inflammatory with a looser, somewhat oedematous, marrow containing haematopoietic elements and inflammatory cells

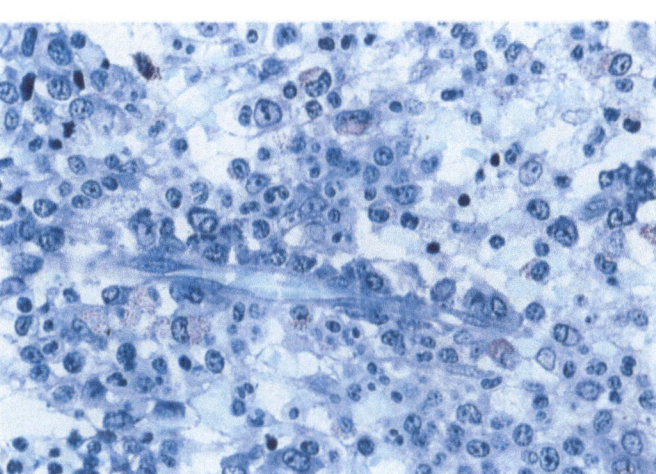

Fig. 5.30 Higher magnification of Fig. 5.29, as above, with perivascular plasymacytosis

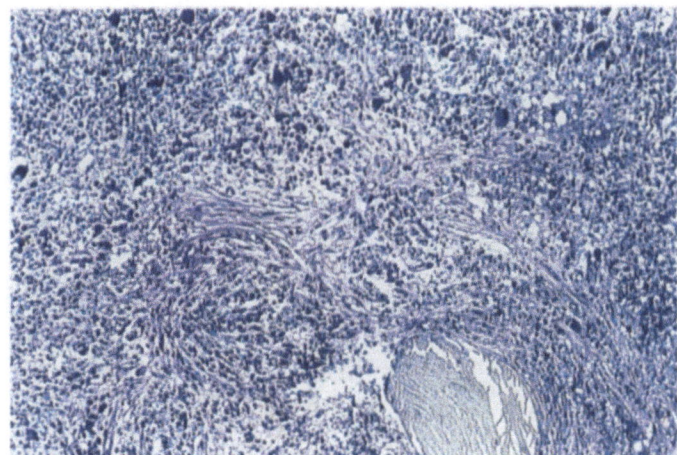

Fig. 5.31 MDS fibrotic: in this histological subtype the fibrosis may be patchy, with cellular areas in between

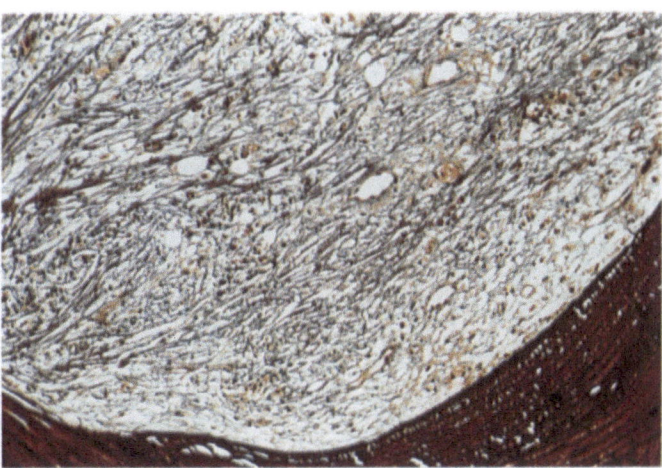

Fig. 5.32 Section of bone biopsy as in Fig. 5.31. Gomori's stain, showing fibrosis in part of the biopsy section

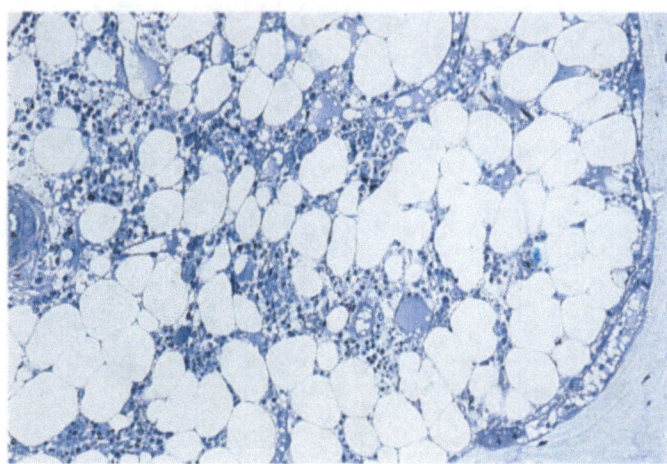

Fig. 5.33 MDS hypocellular: illustrates a case of a 73-year-old patient with refractory anaemia and a hypocellular bone with myelodysplastic features

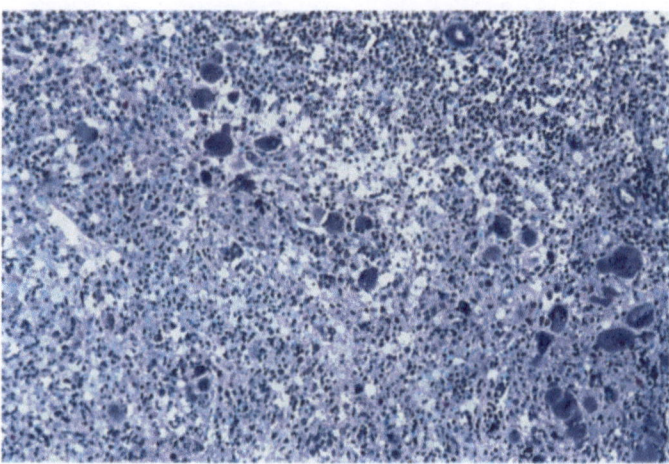

Figs 5.34 and 5.35 MDS proliferative: these sections of patients with a myelodysplastic syndrome show a hypercellular bone marrow with proliferation of all three cell lines; such cases are transitional variants between MDS and MPD

Fig. 5.34 Hypercellular marrow with replacement of fat cells and polymorphic megakaryocytes

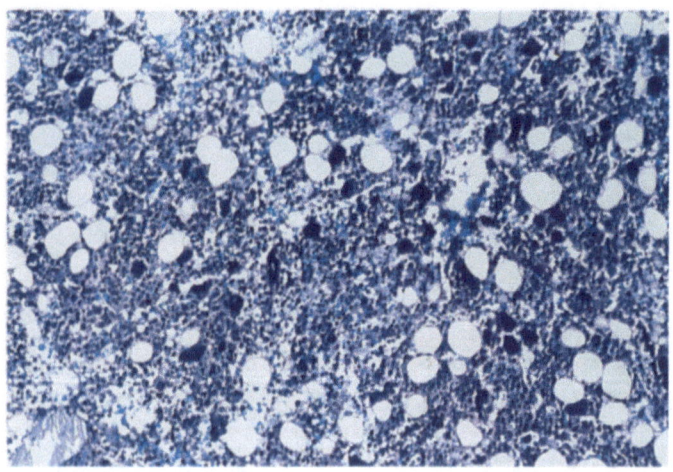

Fig. 5.35 Less densely packed marrow, megakaryocytic hyperplasia and architectural disorganization

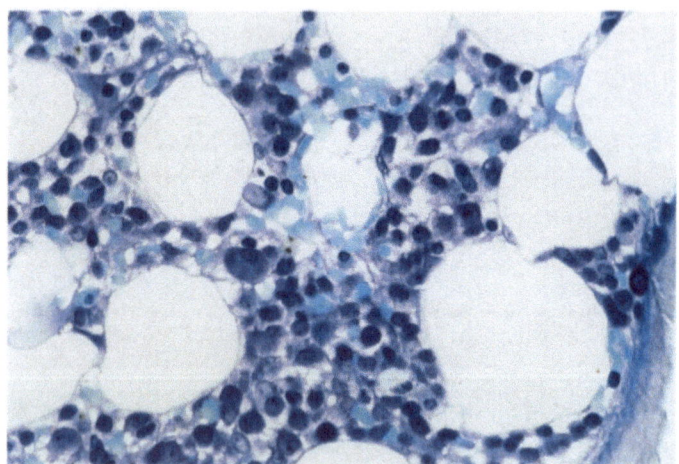

Fig. 5.36 MDS blastic, with increased blasts and early precursors in the bone marrow. This is a section of a bone biopsy of 46-year-old patient with pancytopenia, hypocellular bone marrow, increased blasts and megaloblastic erythropoiesis in the absence of any vitamin or mineral deficiency; no blasts in the peripheral blood. Over the next 2 years his peripheral blood values and bone marrow (three biopsies) remained the same. During this time he received supportive therapy, but died of sepsis

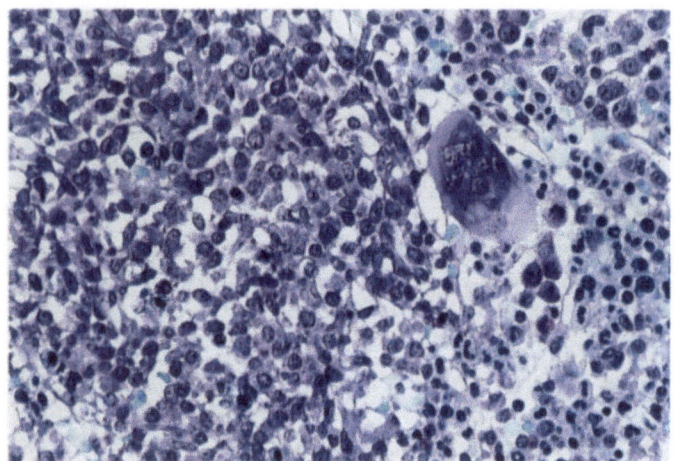

Fig. 5.38 Clone of blasts in bone marrow of a patient with MDS who developed acute leukaemia and died within a few months of this biopsy

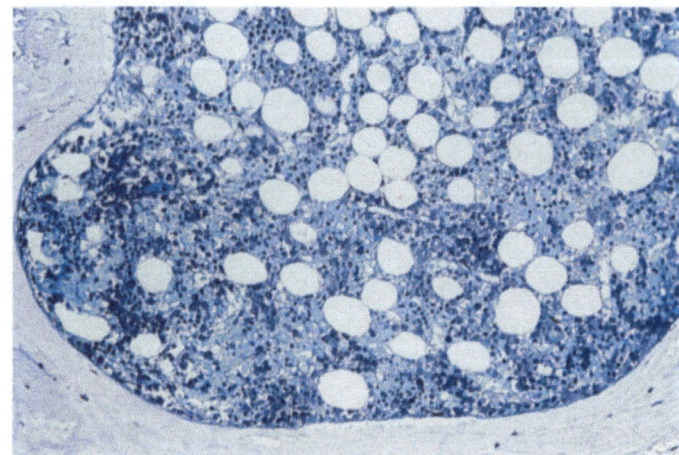

Fig. 5.40 Bone biopsy section of patient with MDS; the first indication of malignancy was the presence of the tumour cells in this biopsy. Low power showing myelodysplastic bone marrow

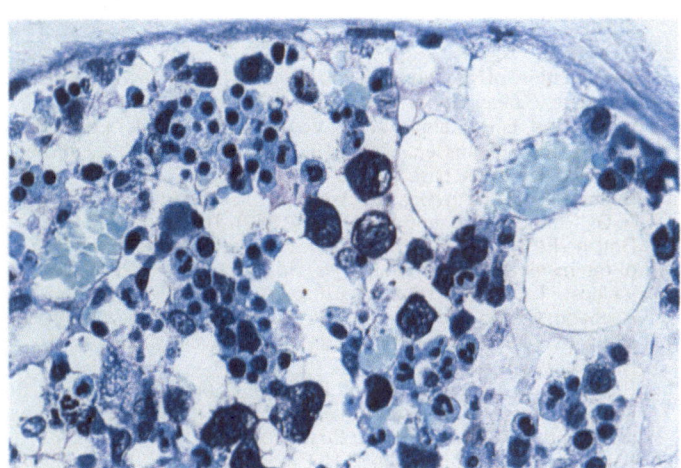

Fig. 5.41 As in Fig. 5.40, showing the tumour cells dispersed among the haematopoietic elements

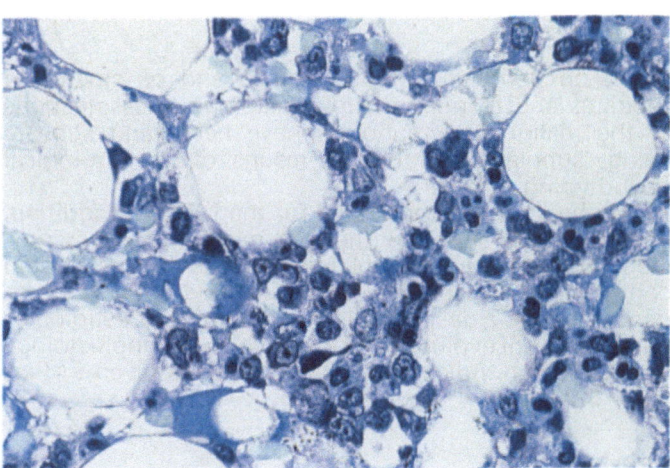

Fig. 5.42 Section of bone biopsy of patient with MDS who developed acute leukaemia; high power showing ALIP, first biopsy

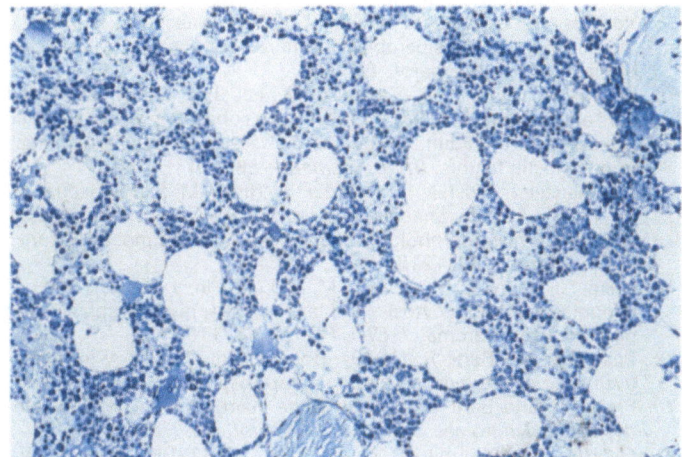

Fig. 5.43 Section of second biopsy; note infiltration of marrow with blasts, and megakaryocyte at trabecular surface (upper right)

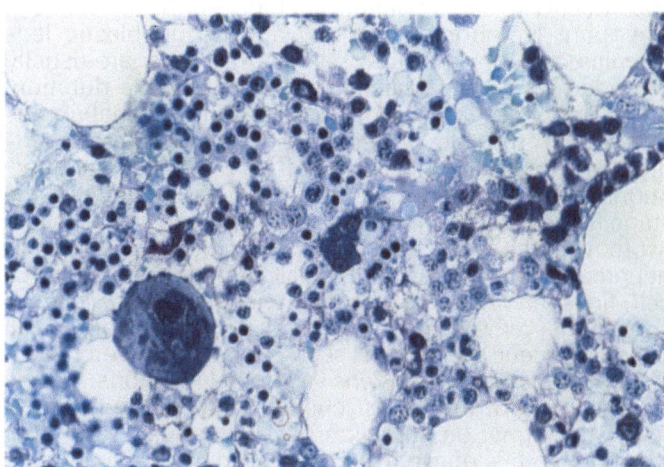

Fig. 5.44 Section of bone biopsy of 70-year-old woman who developed pancytopenia with an aplastic bone marrow which evolved to refractory anaemia, with a cellular marrow, at which time this biopsy was taken. The patient was treated with supportive therapy and a year later died of a myocardial infarction; still cytopenic but the third biopsy shortly before her death showed a cellular bone marrow with excess of blasts (RAEB)

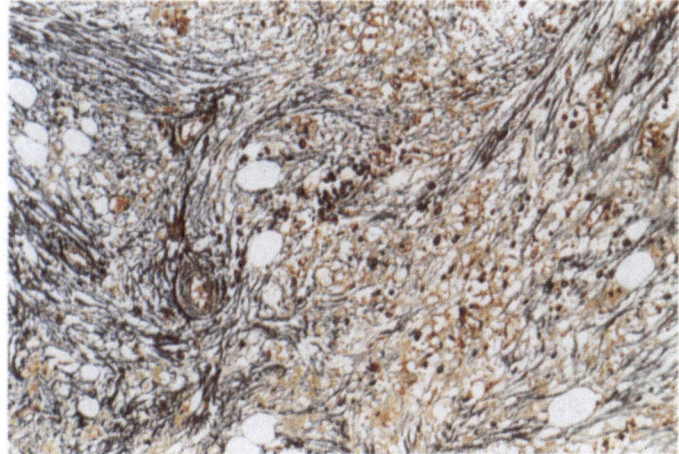

Fig. 5.45 Section of bone biopsy of patient with MDS who subsequently developed myelofibrosis, when this biopsy was taken. Gomori's stain showing fibrosis of bone marrow

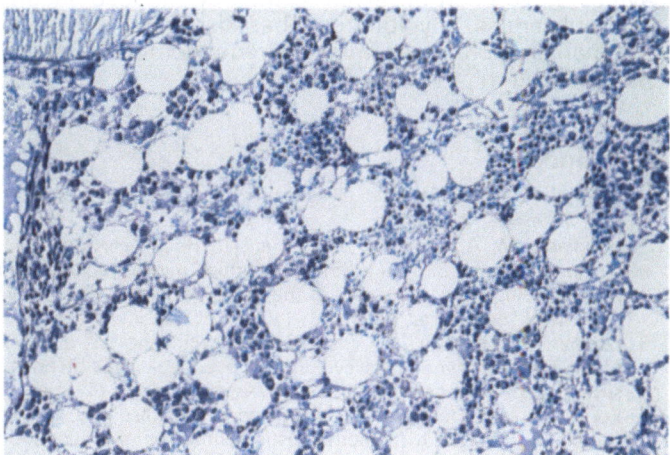

Fig. 5.46 Section of bone biopsy of patient with pancytopenia (suspected aplastic anaemia on the basis of peripheral blood findings) and myelodysplastic bone marrow; this patient later developed acute leukaemia

based on peripheral blood findings and on smears of aspirates and to bone marrow histology. Classifications of the malignant lymphomas have been, and still are being, supplemented by the results of immunological phenotyping.

This has not yet been done for the MDS. In addition, immunological studies of the bone marrow microenvironment, and of the local regulatory cells and factors, should contribute to a more precise classification of these disorders as well as a deeper understanding of their aetiologies and patterns of evolution. An example of immunohistology in MDS as an indication of its potential is given in Figs 5.47–5.50.

Secondary Myelodysplastic Syndromes

These are also known as therapy-induced myelodysplasias and secondary leukaemias which have developed (in most cases after years) in patients previously treated with cytotoxic therapy for a wide range of primary neoplasms[36]. Secondary malignancies also develop due to exposure to other toxic agents[37]. The secondary malignancies that may occur in such patients include epithelial cancers, malignant lymphomas, myeloid and lymphoblastic leukaemias; and/or pan-myeloses[38–41]. The latter are usually preceded by a pre-leukaemic phase of variable duration, often associated with cytopenia(s) and functional abnormalities of the blood cells (i.e. myelodysplastic syndromes)[42,43]. In most cases there are chromosomal alterations. The bone marrow in these syndromes reflects the stage in their development at which the biopsy was taken. Moreover, the bone marrow may be hypo-, normo- or hypercellular with morphological alterations in all three cell lines and marked stromal changes[44]. However, it should be remembered that transient depletion of all haematopoietic elements is seen after aggressive chemotherapy, together with extensive stromal reactions. Nevertheless, most of these post-chemotherapy bone marrows revert to normal on cessation of the treatment, and after the regenerative phase. Thus, a detailed history is required for the correct interpretation of the biopsy sections, as some of them may not be distinguishable from secondary MDS in its pre-leukaemic phase. The bone marrows in secondary MDS are not usually classifiable according to the FAB criteria for the primary MDS. Both an interstitial form in a hypo- or normocellular marrow, and a hypercellular form, with almost complete occupation of the marrow cavities, have been observed in therapy-induced secondary leukaemias. Myelofibrosis has also been observed; and marker techniques may be required for blast cell characterization[45] (Figs 5.51–5.64).

References

1. Koeffler, H. P. (1986). Myelodysplastic syndromes (preleukaemia). Sem. Hematol., **23**, 284
2. Baumann, M. A., Libnoch, J. A., Hansen, R. M., Heckman, M. G. and Hanson, G. A. (1985). Concurrent myelodysplasia and lymphoproliferation: a disorder of the true pluripotential stem cell? Q. J. Med., new series, **55**, 199
3. Dormer, P., Hershko, C., Voss, R. and Wilmanns, W. (1987). Myelodysplastic syndromes: evolution of overt leukaemia by one or several steps of transformation. Br. J. Haematol., **67**, 141
4. Foucar, K., Langdon II, R. M., Armitage, J. O., Olson, D. B. and Carroll, T. J. (1985). Myelodysplastic syndromes: a clinical and pathologic analysis of 109 cases. Cancer, **56**, 553
5. Verwilghen, R. L. (1986). Primary myelodysplastic syndromes. Labmedica, April-May, pp. 14–19
6. Geary, C. G. (1987). Myelodysplasia: morphology, clinical presentation and treatment. In Whittaker, J. A. and Delamore, J. W. (eds), Leukaemia. Oxford: Blackwell Scientific Publications, pp. 420–443
7. Third MIC Cooperative Study Group (1988). Recommendations for a morphologic, immunologic, and cytogenetic (MIC) working classification of the primary and therapy-related myelodysplastic disorders. Cancer Genet. Cytogenet., **32**, 1
8. van Wering, E. R., Kamps, W. A., Vossen, J. M., van der List-Nuver, C. J. A. and Theunissen, M. V. (1985). Myelodysplastic syndromes in childhood: three case reports. Br. J. Haematol., **60**, 137
9. Bennett, J. M., Catovsky, D., Daniel, M. T., Flandrin, G., Galton, D. A. G., Gralnick, H. R. and Sultan, C. (1982). The French–American–British (FAB) Co-operative Group. Proposals for the classification of the myelodysplastic syndromes. Br. J. Haematol., **51**, 189
10. Vallepsi, T., Torrabadella, M., Julia, A., Irriguibile, D., Jaen, A., Acebedo, G. and Triginer, J. (1985). Myelodysplastic syndromes: a study of 101 cases according to the FAB classification. Br. J. Haematol., **61**, 83
11. Ribera, J. M., Cervantes, F. and Rozman, C. (1987). A multivariate analysis of prognostic factors in chronic myelomonocytic leukaemia according to the FAB criteria. Br. J. Haematol., **65**, 307
12. Kerkhofs, H., Herman, J., Haak, H. L. and Leeksma, C. H. W. (1987). Utility of the FAB classification for myelodysplastic syndromes: investigation of prognostic factors in 237 cases. Br. J. Haematol., **65**, 73
13. Delacretaz, F., Schmidt, P. M., Piguet, D., Bachmann, F. and Costa, J. (1987). Histopathology of myelodysplastic syndromes. The FAB classification (proposals) applied to bone marrow biopsy. Am. J. Clin. Pathol., **87**, 180
14. Hast, R. (1986). Sideroblasts in myelodysplasia: Their nature and clinical significance. Scand. J. Haematol., **36**, (Suppl. 45). 53
15. Yoshida, Y., Oguma, S., Uchino, H. and Maekawa, T. (1987). Significance of ring sideroblasts in refractory anaemia with excess of blasts. Br. J. Haematol., **65**, 119
16. Fenaux, P., Jouet, J. P., Zandecki, M., Lai, J. L., Simon, M., Pollet J. P. and Bauters, F. (1987). Chronic and subacute myelomonocytic leukaemia in the adult: a report of 60 cases with special reference to prognostic factors. Br. J. Haematol., **65**, 101
17. Fohlmeister, I., Fischer, R., Modder, B., Rister, M. and Schaeffer, H. E. (1985). Aplastic anaemia and the hypocellular myelodysplastic syndromes: histomorphological, diagnostic and prognostic features. J. Clin. Pathol., **38**, 1218
18. Craig, A., Geary, C. G., Love, E. M. and Liu-Yin, J. (1988). Red cell hypoplasia, thrombocytosis, and leucocytosis: myelodysplastic and proliferative syndrome. J. Clin. Pathol., **41**, 1168
19. Frisch, B. and Bartl, R. (1989). Bone marrow histology in myelodysplastic syndromes: an update. (In press)
20. Frisch, B. and Bartl, R. (1986). Bone marrow histology in myelodysplastic syndromes. Scand. J. Haematol., **36**, (Suppl. 45), 21
21. Georgii, A., Vykoupil, K. F. and Buhr, T. (1988). Preleukemia: bone marrow histopathology in myelodysplasia and preleukemic syndrome. Recent Results Cancer Res., **106**, 159
22. Yoshida, Y., Oguma, S., Uchino, H. and Maekawa, T. (1988). Refractory myelodysplastic anaemias with hypocellular bone marrow. J. Clin. Pathol., **41**, 763
23. Nand, S. and Godwin, J. E. (1988). Hypoplastic myelodysplastic syndromes. Cancer, **62**, 958
24. Tricot, G., Vlietinck, R. and Verwilghen, R. L. (1986). Prognostic factors in the myelodysplastic syndromes. a review. Scand. J. Haematol., **36**(Suppl. 45), 107
25. Copplestone, J. A., Mufti, G. J., Hamblin, T. J. and Oscier, D. C. (1986). Immunological abnormalities in myelodysplastic syndromes. II. Coexistent lymphoid or plasma cell neoplasms: a report of 20 cases unrelated to chemotherapy. Br. J. Haematol., **63**, 149
26. Colombat, P. H., Renoux, M., Lamagnere, J. P. and Renoux, G. (1986). Immunologic indices in myelodysplastic syndromes. Cancer, **61**, 1075
27. Clarck, R. E., Hoy, T. G. and Jacobs, A. (1985). Granulocyte and monocyte surface membrane markers in the myelodysplastic syndromes. J. Clin. Pathol., **38**, 301
28. Kuriyama, K., Tomonaga, M., Matsuo, T., Ginnai, I. and Ichimaru, M. (1986). Diagnostic significance of detecting pseudo-Pelger-Huet anomalies and micro-megakaryocytes in myelodysplastic syndrome. Br. J. Haematol., **63**, 665
29. Prokocimer, M., Inbal, A., Gelber, M., Shohat, B., Ben-Basat, M. and Shaklai, M. (1985). Hemophagocytosis simulating malignant histiocytosis: a terminal event of the myelodysplastic syndrome. Acta. Haematol., **74**, 164
30. Tricot, G., Boogaerts, M. A., de Wolf-Peeters, C., Van den Berghe, H. and Verwilghen, R. L. (1985). The myelodysplastic syndromes: different evolution patterns based on sequential morphological and cytogenetic investigations. Br. J. Haematol., **59**, 659
31. Layton, D. M. and Mufti, G. J. (1986). Myelodysplastic syndromes: their history, evolution and relation to acute leukaemia. Blut, **53**, 432

(Continued on p. 80)

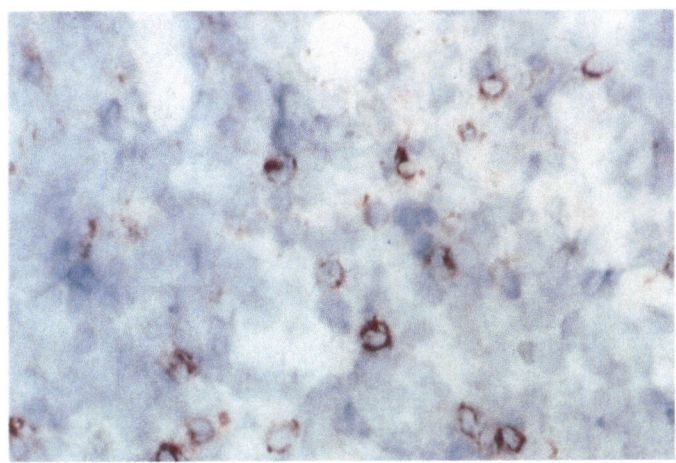

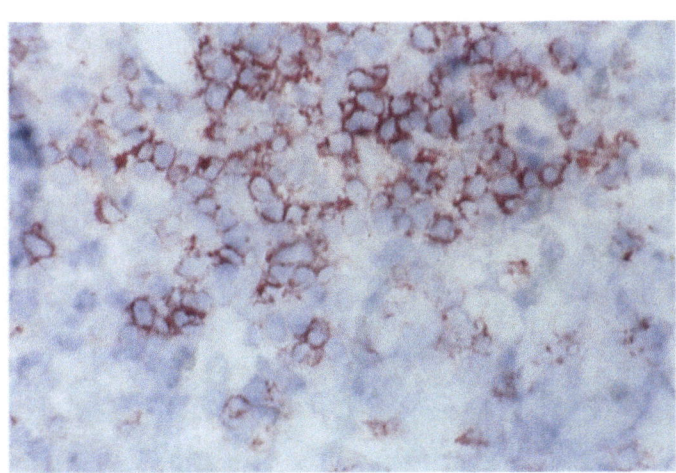

Figs 5.47–5.50 Cryostat sections of bone biopsy of 75-year-old patient with MDS (RAEB according to the FAB classification).

Fig. 5.47 Helper T-lymphocytes (CD4 positive) dispersed in the bone marrow

Fig. 5.48 Aggregate of suppressor T lymphocytes CD8 positive, as well as some single T lymphocytes among the marrow cells

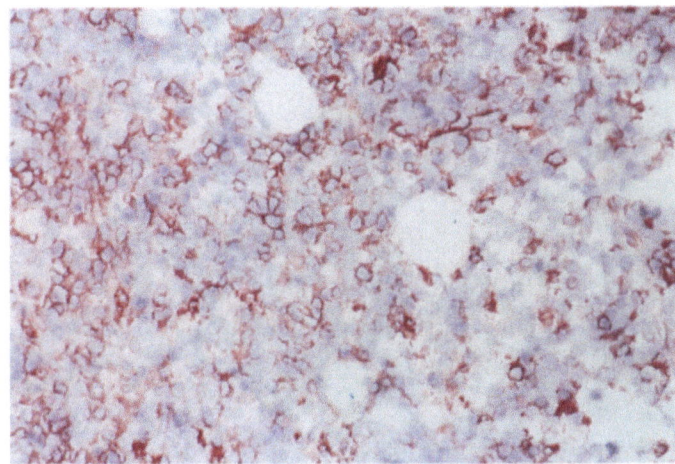

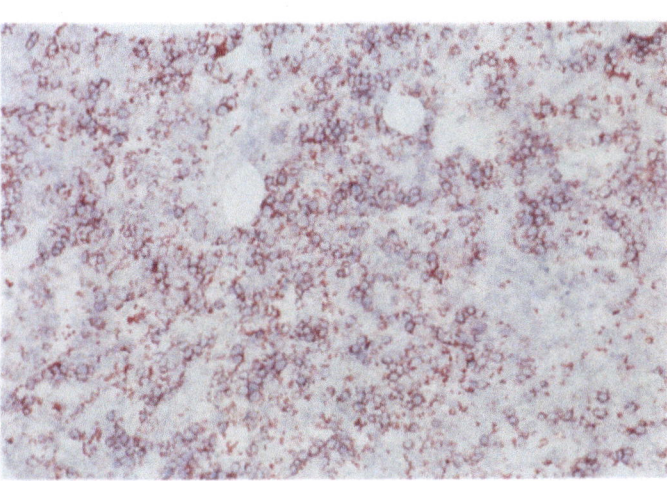

Fig. 5.49 Granulocytes and monocytes identified by their reaction with the antibody VIM 2

Fig. 5.50 Demonstration of erythropoiesis by means of the antibody VIEG 4

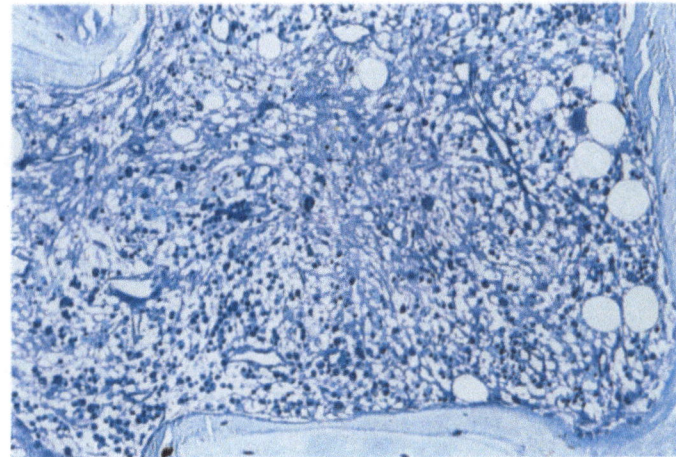

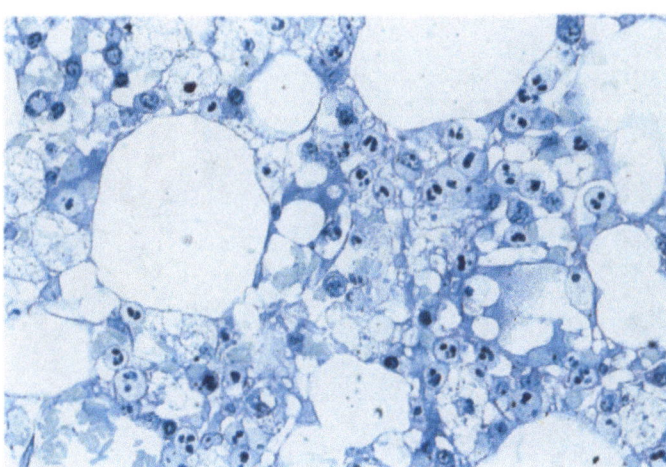

Figs 5.51–5.53 Sections of bone biopsies of patients after chemotherapy and/or radiotherapy for non-haematological malignancies.

Fig. 5.51 Low power to show widespread degeneration of bone marrow

Fig. 5.52 Higher magnification showing necrosis of marrow cells

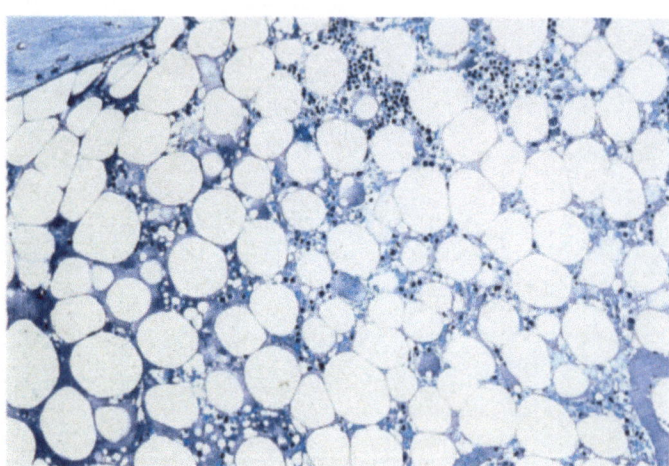

Fig. 5.53 Large areas of serous atrophy

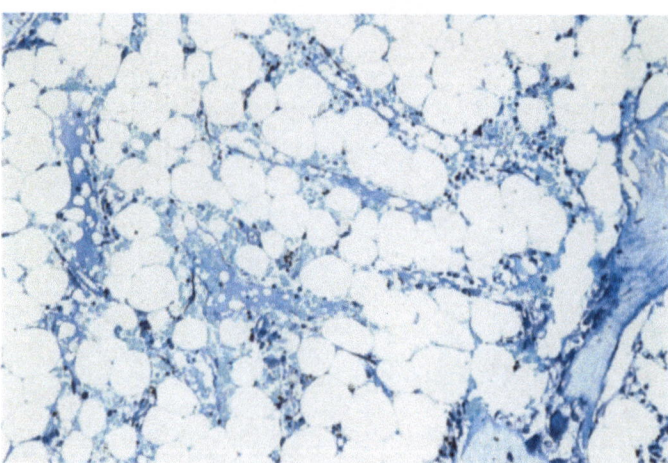

Fig. 5.54 Bone biopsy of child with toxic aplasia, note disrupted sinusoids and lymphoid infiltration

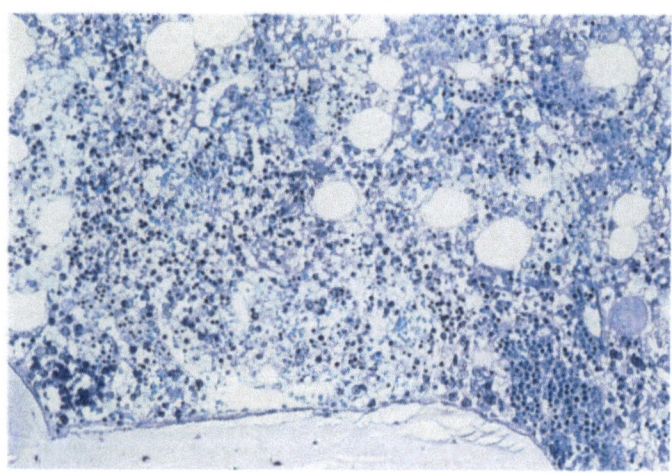

Figs 5.55–5.58 Regeneration of haematopoiesis with left shift, dysplastic features and megaloblastic erythropoiesis, in bone marrows of patients after chemotherapy

Fig. 5.55 Low power showing complete disorganization of marrow structure and markedly immature haematopoiesis

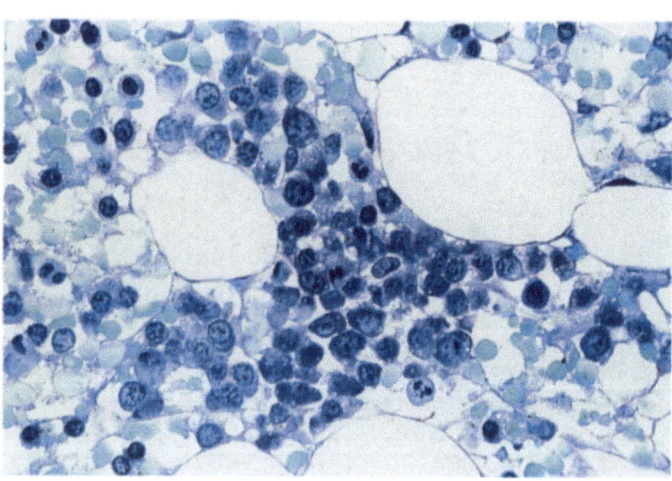

Fig. 5.56 Immature myeloid precursors in intertrabecular region – ALIP in the regenerating marrow

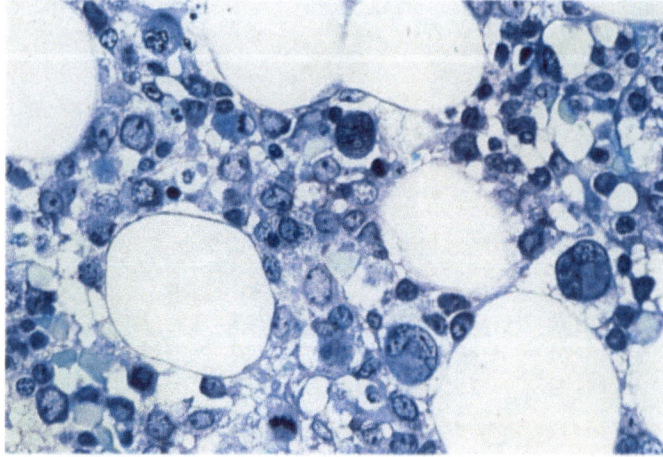

Fig. 5.57 Small megakaryocytes and immature myeloid precursors in the central marrow region

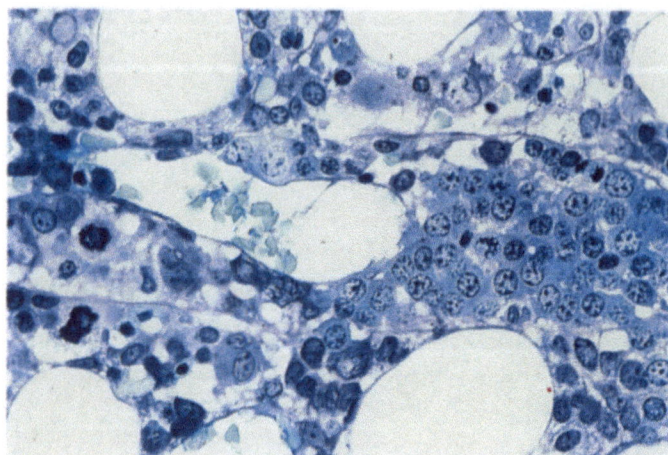

Fig. 5.58 Large cluster of erythroblasts with maturation arrest and megaloblastic features in regenerating bone marrow. Note mitotic figures

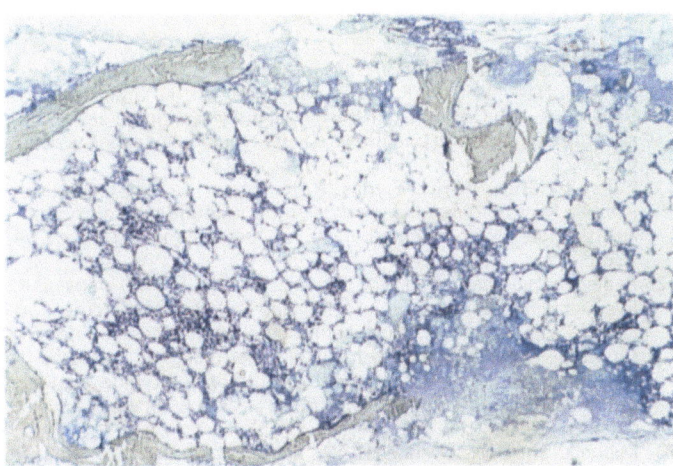

Fig. 5.59 Bone biopsy of 60-year-old patient 6 years after unilateral mastectomy for breast cancer, no radiation or chemotherapy; profound pancytopenia, presumably due to administration of methotrexate for psoriasis. Metastases had been suspected, but there were no indications on skeletal X-rays or bone scan. Information on the treatment with methotrexate was elicited only after prolonged questioning

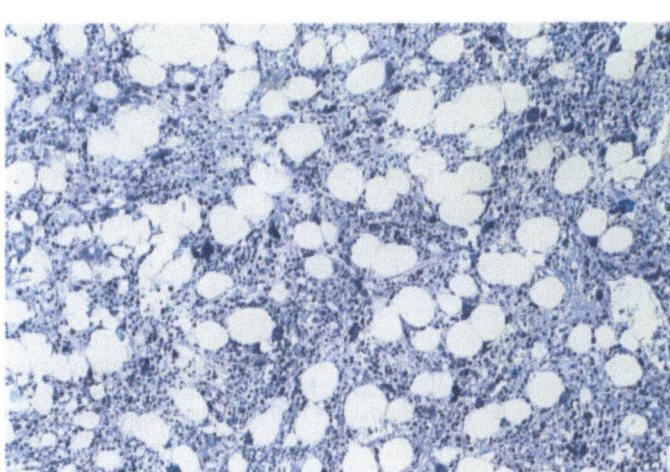

Fig. 5.60 Section of bone biopsy of patient with pancytopenia several years after cessation of therapy for multiple myeloma: secondary MDS with fibrosis

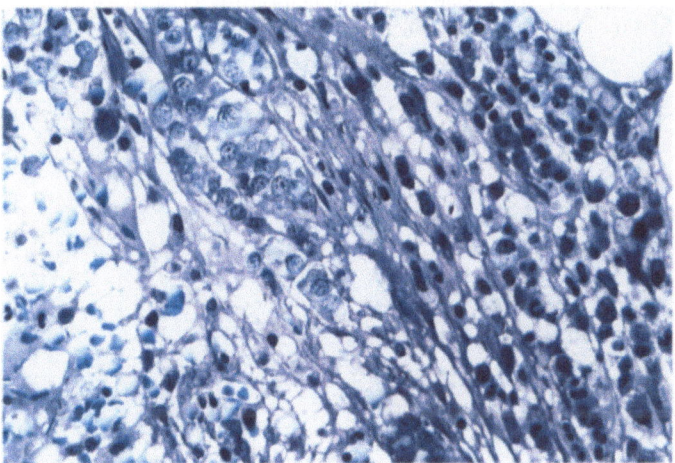

Fig. 5.61 Section of bone biopsy of patient with anaemia 2 years after operation for colon cancer; no chemotherapy or radiotherapy. Patient found to have sideroblastic anaemia. Erythroid hyperplasia and fibrosis in the bone marrow. This case possibly represents an example of a metachronous MDS

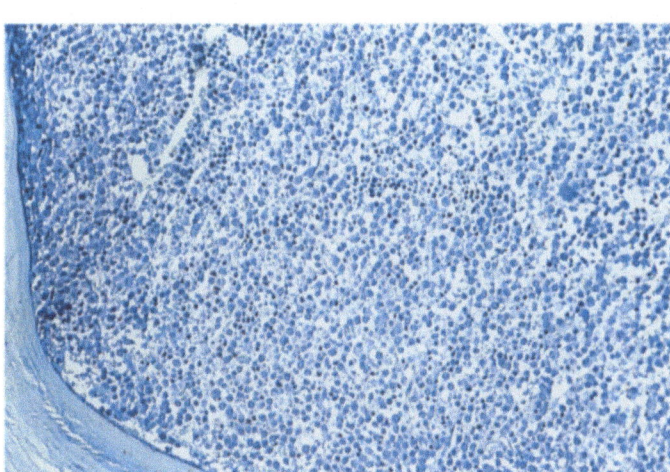

Fig. 5.62 Section of bone biopsy of patient previously treated for Hodgkin's disease who subsequently developed promyelocytic leukaemia: virtual replacement of marrow by immature granulopoiesis. Low power, illustrating the extent of the infiltration

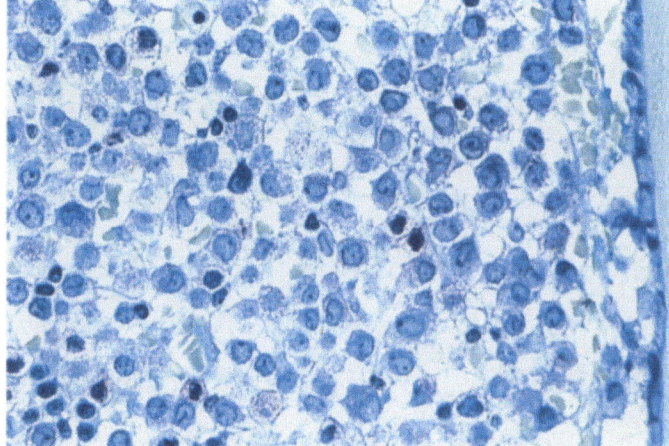

Fig. 5.63 Higher magnification showing broad paratrabecular seam of myeloblasts and promyelocytes

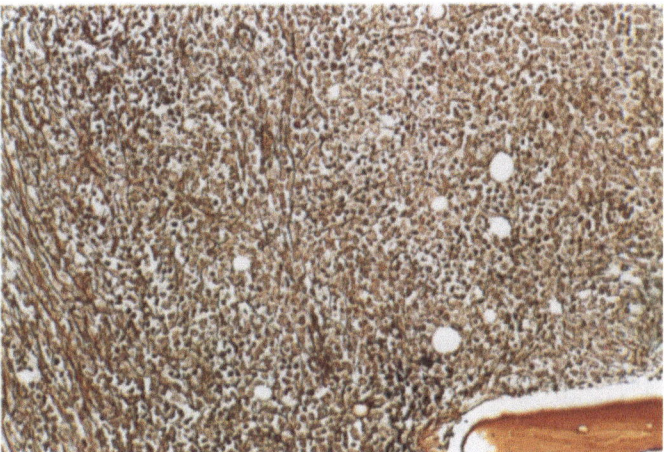

Fig. 5.64 Section of paraffin-embedded bone biopsy of patient who developed acute leukaemia, preceded by MDS with fibrosis after chemotherapy for a solid tumour

32. Bursztyn, B., Doder, D. and Ramot, B. (1987). Chronic myelomon-
    ocytic leukaemia following refractory anaemia with sideroblasts:
    Report of two cases. *Eur. J. Haematol.*, **38**, 197
33. Vandermolen, L., Rice, L., Rose, M. A. and Lynch, E. C. (1988).
    Ringed sideroblasts in primary myelodysplasia. Leukemic propensity
    and prognostic factors. *Arch. Intern. Med.*, **148**, 653
34. Bartl, R., Frisch, B. and Schmid, Ch. (1989). Evolution of myelodys-
    plastic syndromes (In press)
35. Clarck, R. E., Payne, H. E., Jacobs, A. and West, R. R. (1987).
    Primary myelodysplastic syndrome and cancer. *Br. Med. J.*, **294**,
    937
36. Cusick, J., Erskine, S., Edelman, D. and Galton, D. A. (1987). A
    comparison of the incidence of the myelodysplastic syndrome and
    acute myeloid leukaemia following Melphalan and cyclophospham-
    ide treatment for myelomatosis. A report to the medical research
    council's working party on Leukaemia in adults. *Br. J. Cancer*, **55**,
    523
37. Askow, M. (1987). Chronic lymphoid leukaemia and hairy cell
    leukaemia due to chronic exposure to benzene: report of three cases.
    Br. J. Haematol., **66**, 209
38. Tucker, M. A., d'Angio, G. J., Boice, J. D., Strong, L. G., Li, F. P.,
    Stovall, M., Stone, B. J., Green, D. M., Lombardi, F., Newton, W.,
    Hoover, R. N. and Fraumeni, J. F. (1987). Bone sarcomas linked to
    radiotherapy and chemotherapy in children. *N. Engl. J. Med.*, **317**,
    588
39. Tucker, M. A., Coleman, C. N., Cox, R. S., Varghese, A. and
    Rosenberg, S. A. (1988). Risk of second cancers after treatment for

Hodgkin's disease. *N. Engl. J. Med.*, **318**, 76
40. Janjans, N. A., Wilson, F., Gillin, M., Anderson, T., Greenberg, M.,
    Schewe, K. and Cox, J. D. (1988). Mammary carcinoma developing
    after radiotherapy and chemotherapy for Hodgkin's disease. *Cancer*,
    61, 252
41. Sofer, T., Chan, W. C., Brynes, R. K., Vogler, R. and O'Neal, Sh.
    (1984). Myeloproliferative disorder with profound hypereosinophi-
    lia associated with chemotherapy for breast cancer. *Cancer*, **54**,
    2356
42. Pedersen-Bjergaard, J., Philip, P., Pedersen, N. T., Hou-Jensen, K.,
    Svejgaard, A., Jensen, G. and Nissen, N. I. (1984). Acute non-
    lymphocytic leukemia, preleukemia, and acute myeloproliferative
    syndrome secondary to treatment of other malignant diseases. II.
    Bone marrow cytology, cytogenetics, results of HLA typing, response
    to antileukemic chemotherapy, and survival in a total series of 55
    patients. *Cancer*, **54**, 452
43. Michels, Sh. D., McKenna, R. W., Arthur, D. C. and Brunning, R.
    D. (1985). Therapy-related acute myeloid leukaemia and myelo-
    dysplastic syndrome: a clinical and morphologic study of 65 cases.
    Blood, **65**, 1364
44. Frisch, B., Bartl, R. and Chaichik, S. (1986). Therapy-induced
    myelodysplasia and secondary leukaemia. *Scand. J. Haematol.*,
    36(Suppl. 45), 38
45. Tabilio, A., Herrera, A., d'Agay, M. F., Vainchenker, W., Allard,
    C., Clauvel, J. P. and Breton-Goirus, J. (1984). Therapy-related
    leukaemia associated with myelofibrosis. Blast cell characterization
    in six cases. *Cancer*, **54**, 1382

Acute Leukaemias

6

Traditionally, the diagnosis of acute leukaemia has been, and still is, based on peripheral blood counts and on routinely stained smears of blood and bone marrow aspirates[1] (except in cases of a dry tap). Electron microscopy, cytogenetics, cytochemistry, presence of Auer rods, immunological (monoclonal antibodies) and enzyme markers are required for categorization and phenotyping[2-8]. In some cases, especially those with some degree of differentiation, the type of leukaemia may be recognized in sections of the biopsies; for example erythroblastic, megakaryoblastic and monoblastic cell lines[9].

There are two main types of bone marrow infiltration in the acute leukaemias: the hypercellular and hypocellular (Figs 6.1–6.6)[10-12]. A few early cases may show a diffuse interstitial infiltration of blasts, with partial disappearance of haematopoiesis and fat which are replaced by exudative or serous atrophy (Fig. 6.4).

Hypercellular Type

The bone marrow is hypercellular with sheets of immature cells (mainly blasts) occupying the intertrabecular spaces (Figs 6.2 and 6.3). Few normal precursors or fat cells remain. The residual haematopoiesis may show dysplastic features; disrupted sinusoids and some macrophages with cellular debris complete the picture. When the cells are very densely packed, attempts at aspiration may result in a dry tap. Other cases may have a looser infiltration so that connective tissue elements, reticulin fibres, macrophages, erythrocytes and other cells are dispersed among the blasts[13]. When rapid multiplication outstrips the blood supply, areas of necrotic cells may be found. The degree of fibrosis which accompanies these acute and subacute leukaemias varies widely from mild to marked as in acute myelofibrosis (AMF) (see below). Osteopenia, i.e. attenuation of the trabeculae with or without the presence of osteoclasts, is frequently seen. Occasionally increased osseous remodelling may be associated with hypercalcaemia and osteolytic lesions[14]; osteomalacia may develop during the course of therapy. Accelerated bone formation has also been reported[15]. Dysplastic features may occur

in cell lines other than the one directly involved in the acute leukaemia, for example dysmegakaryopoiesis in acute myelomonocytic leukaemia[16-18]. Also, proliferations affecting one myeloid cell line may predispose to acute leukaemia in another – for example, myeloblastic leukaemia in urticaria pigmentosa[19].

Hypocellular Type

There is a decrease in haematopoiesis, and an increase in fat cells between which the blasts are dispersed (Figs 6.5 and 6.6). The residual haematopoiesis may show dysplastic features. When progression is slow, this corresponds to 'smouldering leukaemia'.

Recently, a comparative study was made of bone marrow aspirates and bone marrow biopsy findings at initial diagnosis in 51 patients with acute myeloid leukaemia[20]. Differences were observed in: (1) estimated overall marrow cellularity; (2) extent of blast cell infiltration, quantity and distribution of the different cell lines in the bone marrow; (3) bone marrow infiltration with inflammatory cells. The results suggest that bone marrow biopsies complement the findings of bone marrow aspiration in the acute leukaemias and also provide additional information not otherwise obtained[21].

Acute Myelofibrosis (AMF)

Most cases of acute (or malignant) myelosclerosis[22] have now been shown to be acute or subacute leukaemias with a dominant fibrotic reaction (Figs 6.7–6.9). In many cases there is a panmyelosis – i.e. involvement of myelo-, erythro-, and megakaryocytic cell lines, or a megakaryoblastic or myeloblastic myelosis[23-26].

Promyelocytic Leukaemia

The bone marrow is hypercellular with broad paratrabecular seams of promyelocytes and myelocytes whose cytoplasm contains variable amounts of granules (Figs 6.10 and 6.11). Relatively few metamyelocytes, bands or segmented granulocytes are seen, and there is a marked decrease in erythroid precursors and megakaryocytes. Proerythro- and promegakaryocytic subtypes are also recognized (Figs 6.12–6.14).

Smouldering Leukaemia

1. A cell line similar to that in acute myeloblastic leukaemia may be present in the bone marrow for months or years together with suppression, to a variable extent, of normal haematopoiesis (Figs 6.15 and 6.16). Clearly, there is a certain amount of overlap between these cases and hypoplastic acute leukaemia and some forms of myelodysplastic syndrome, or even aplastic anaemia.
2. Smouldering (or subacute or chronic) myelomonocytic leukaemia (Figs 6.17–6.21). Though included in the classification of the myelodysplastic syndromes, which are considered to be pre-leukaemic conditions by the FAB group, it would be more logical to classify this

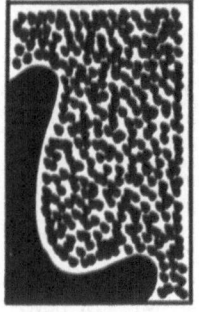
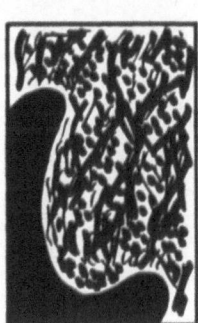

HYPERCELLULAR   HYPOCELLULAR (SMOULDERING)   ACUTE MYELOFIBROSIS

Fig. 6.1 Schematic representation of hyper- and hypocellular acute leukaemia, and acute myelosclerosis (or acute myelofibrosis)

(Continued on p. 84)

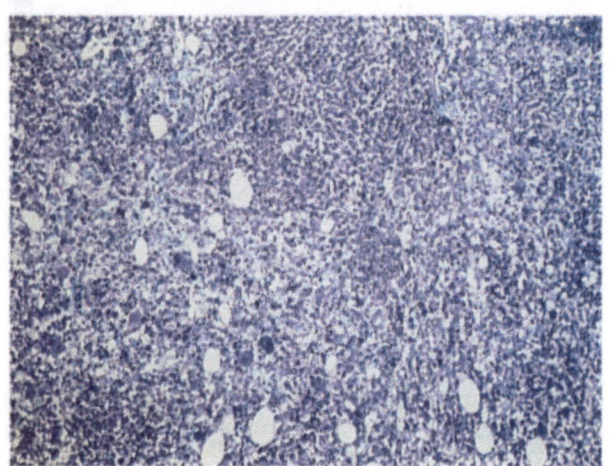

Fig. 6.2 Sections of bone biopsy of patient with the hypercellular type of acute leukaemia: densely cellular bone marrow with few remaining fat cells

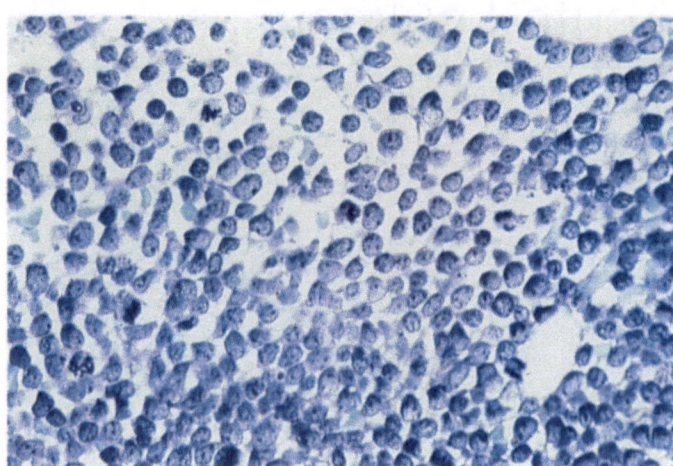

Fig. 6.3 Higher magnification of Fig. 6.2, to show the sheets of blasts

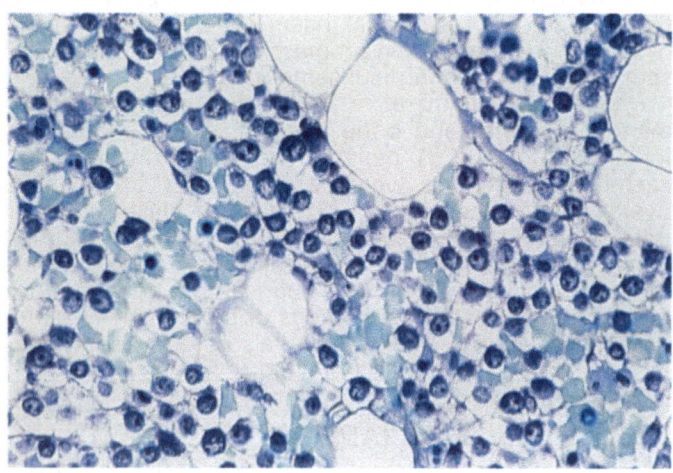

Fig. 6.4 Section of bone biopsy showing the diffuse type of infiltration

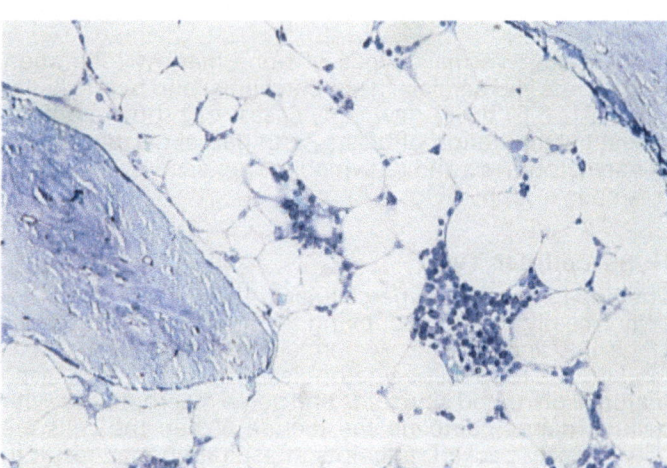

Fig. 6.5 A case of hypocellular acute leukaemia: low-power view showing fatty marrow

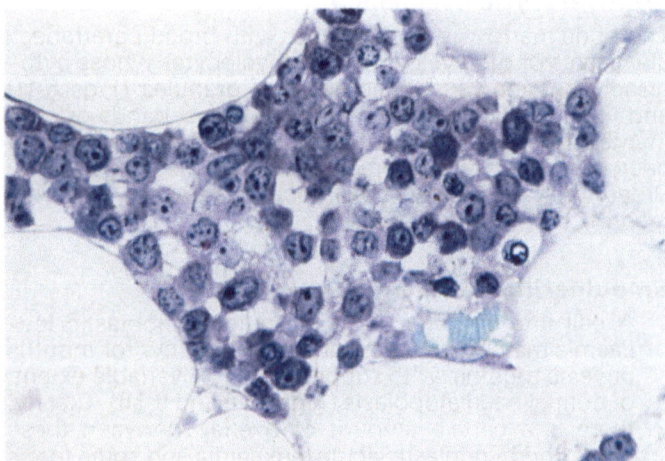

Fig. 6.6 High-power view of the cluster of immature cells (off-centre, right in Fig. 6.5)

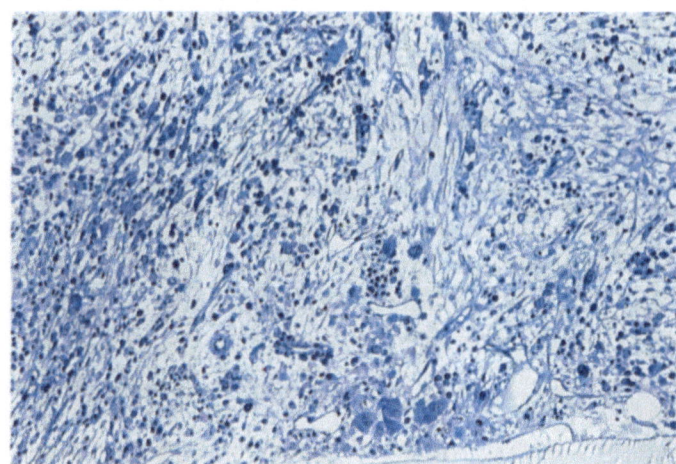

Fig. 6.7 Section of bone biopsy of patient with AMF, low power, showing haematopoietic elements between the fibres. Note cluster of megakaryocytes at trabecular surface right of centre

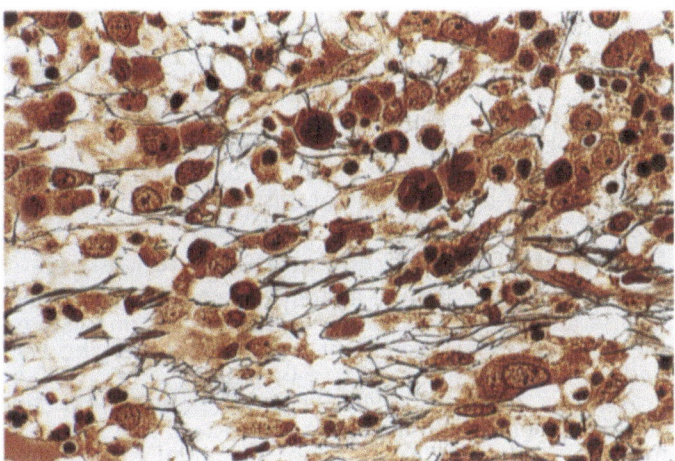

Fig. 6.8 Higher magnification of section of bone biopsy of patient with AMF, Gomori's stain. Immature haematopoietic precursors separated by the fibres

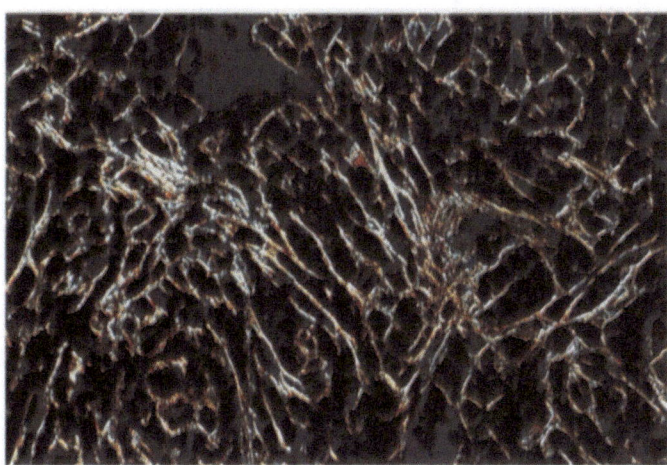

Fig. 6.9 Same as Fig. 6.8, viewed in polarized light

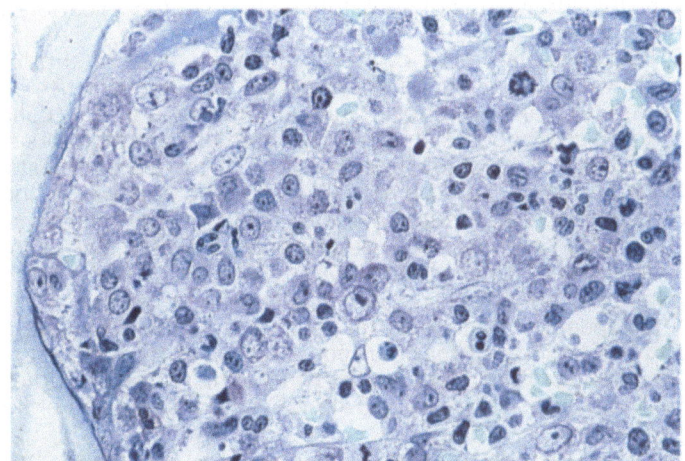

Fig. 6.10 Section of bone biopsy of patient with promyelocytic leukaemia. The myeloid cells show some degree of differentiation so that both promyelocytes and myelocytes are present with variable amounts of cytoplasm and cytoplasmic granules. High-power view of paratrabecular region

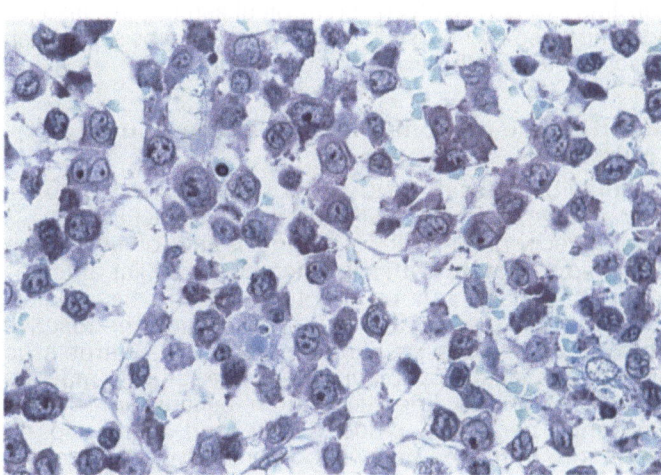

Fig. 6.11 As Fig. 6.10, from central marrow space, showing extension of the sheet of immature cells into the marrow

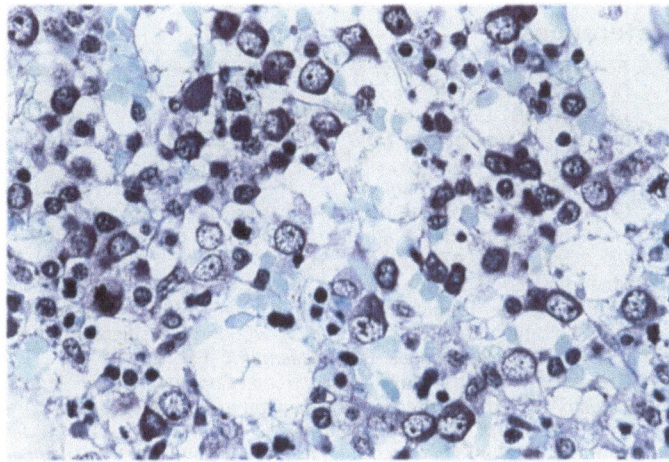

Figs 6.12–6.14 A disorder similar to promyelocytic leukaemia may affect the erythroid and the megakaryocytic cell lines so that they undergo some differentiation

Fig. 6.12 Involvement mainly of the erythroid cell line

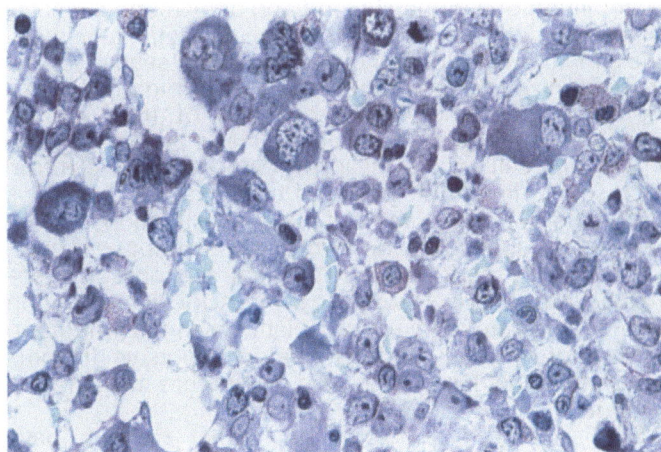

Fig. 6.13 Both erythroid and megakaryocytic lines are affected. Note promegakaryocytes

condition with the subacute leukaemias as it is already an overt leukaemia and can be recognized as such on bone marrow histology. The marrow is hypo-, normo-, or hypercellular with preservation of the overall architecture and an interstitial infiltration of monocytoid cells which may constitute 20–40% of the nucleated cell population present. These cells have round to oval or kidney-shaped nuclei, resembling those of hairy cells. A T-cell lymphoma has been associated with myelomonocytic leukaemia[27].

3. Chronic monocytic leukaemia is presumed to be a separate entity as it affects primarily the monocytic cell line (Figs 6.22–6.25). The infiltration consists of a pleomorphic cell population of monocytic cells with fairly abundant cytoplasm. These monocytic cells are larger than hairy cells.

Subacute erythroid disorders, also called di Guglielmo syndrome, or early erythroleukaemias, are characterized by a hypercellular bone marrow consisting mainly of erythroid precursors, which are pleomorphic with dyserythropoietic features (Figs 6.27–6.36). Myeloid elements are reduced while in some cases the megakaryocytic cell line is also involved. Erythroleukaemia may also be accompanied by fibrosis[28]. Erythraemic myelosis has been observed in lymphoproliferative disorders[29].

Significance of Bone Biopsies in the Acute Leukaemias

It should be noted that the value of bone marrow biopsies in the acute, and especially the subacute, leukaemias is gaining recognition both for diagnosis and for monitoring of therapy. In cases with some degree of cellular differentiation the cells can be identified in the histological sections, and the amount of infiltration and the reactive fibrosis can be assessed. Furthermore, in the erythroblastic and promegakaryocytic types a bone biopsy may be necessary for cell line recognition because of a subleukaemic peripheral blood picture and a dry tap on aspiration. In treated patients bone marrow regeneration, as well as residual nests of blasts, are more easily recognized in sections than in smears of aspirates.

Cell Lines and Phenotypic Determination in the Acute and Subacute Leukaemias

As mentioned earlier, the diagnosis of these disorders has traditionally been based on peripheral blood counts and examination of peripheral blood and bone marrow smears which constitute the basis of the internationally recognized FAB classification of the acute leukaemias. Blasts are recognized by their morphology, their high nucleocytoplasmic ratio and the finer details of their nuclear structure and nucleoli. Leukaemic blasts are assigned to a particular cell line by means of cytochemistry, electron microscopy, immunological and enzymatic studies (Figs 6.32–6.38). However, most of these investigations cannot be directly applied to bone marrow histology, though some may be performed on cryostat sections of fresh-frozen unfixed bone biopsies. Studies for determination of phenotype are required, especially when the infiltration consists of very early undifferentiated precursors. In some cases malignant lymphomas and carcinomas must also be excluded.

Studies with monoclonal and other markers have already demonstrated that morphology alone is insufficient for cell lineage determination in the acute leukaemias (Figs. 6.39–6.42). Moreover, such investigations have shown that more than one line may be involved, or that cells may possess characteristics of more than one line. When a 'dry tap' occurs on attempts at aspiration in the acute leukaemias the tests normally carried out on

smears of aspirate can be made on imprints of the biopsy; thus the FAB criteria can still be used for classification. Interdisciplinary criteria for the lymphoblastic, myeloblastic, monoblastic, erythroblastic and megakaryoblastic – as well as the mixed forms – have been established, but these are beyond the scope of this text (Figs 6.43–6.45).

Effects of Chemotherapy on the Bone Marrow

The bone marrow picture after cytotoxic therapy depends to a large degree on the amount of drugs administered, the duration of the treatment and how long or short the interval after which the biopsy was taken[30-35].

There is great variability in both parenchymal and stromal reactions of the bone marrow to the cytotoxic treatment, ranging from necrosis to almost complete aplasia with replacement by fat cells, to disruption and disorganization of the architecture of the bone marrow with reduction in haematopoietic precursors (Figs 6.46–6.53). In some cases there is extreme depletion of haematopoiesis with infiltrations of lymphoid, plasma and mast cells, macrophages with cellular debris and with haemosiderin, decrease in sinusoids or ectatic sinusoids with groups and islands of immature early precursors scattered throughout.

With less intensive cytotoxic therapy – and of shorter duration – the changes observed are also less drastic.

Some marrows show only an increase in fat cells and macrophages with otherwise normal haematopoiesis, except for a megaloblastoid aspect of the erythroblasts. In others there may be marked dysplastic changes in the haematopoietic tissue, similar to those of the myelodysplastic syndromes. Still others may resemble the bone marrow in aplastic anaemia with typical 'hot spots' – large islands of erythroblasts showing maturation arrest.

A special influence of fat cells, and of the endosteum on the process of marrow regeneration, has been postulated by some workers, on the basis of histological studies of bone biopsies before and after therapy for acute myeloid leukaemia[36].

Bone marrow pathology in transplant recipients has recently been reviewed (Figs 6.54 and 6.55)[37]. Relapse of acute myeloid leukaemia may be accompanied by myelodysplasia in all three cell lines[38].

Severe bone marrow fibrosis present before cytotoxic therapy and bone marrow transplantation may have an adverse effect on subsequent haematopoietic recovery[39].

References

1. Bennett, J. M., Catavosky, D., Daniel, M. T., Flandrin, G., Galton, D. A. G., Gralnick, H. R. and Sultan, C. (1976). (French–American–British (FAB) Co-operative Group). Proposal for the classification of the acute leukaemias. *Br. J. Haematol.*, **33**, 451

2. Bennett, J. M., Catovsky, D., Daniel, M. T., Flandrin, G., Galton, D. A. G., Gralnick, H. R. and Sultan, C. (1981). (FAB Co-operative Group). The morphological classification of acute lymphoblastic leukaemia. Concordance among observers and clinical correlations. *Br. J. Haematol.*, **47**, 553

3. Meeting Report of the Second MIC Cooperative Study Group (1988). Leuven Belgium, 15–17 September 1986 on morphologic, immunologic and cytogenetic (MIC) working classification of the acute myeloid leukaemias. *Br. J. Haematol.*, **68**, 487

4. Groupe Français de Morphologie Hématologique (1987). French Registry of Acute Leukaemia and Myelodysplastic Syndromes. Age distribution and hemogram analysis of the 4496 cases recorded during 1982–1983 and classified according to FAB criteria. *Cancer*, **60**, 1385

5. Koike, T. (1984). Megakaryoblastic leukaemia: the characterization and identification of megakaryoblasts. *Blood*, **64**, 683

6. Ming-jer Huang, Chin-Yang Li, Nichols, W. L., Ji-Hsiung Young and Katzmann, J. A. (1984). Acute leukaemia with megakaryocytic differentiaiton: a study of 12 cases identified immunocytochemically. *Blood*, **64**, 427

(Continued on p. 92)

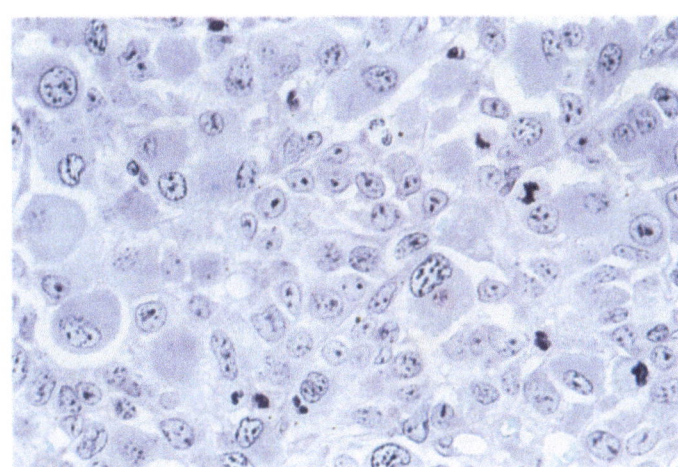

Fig. 6.14 This figure shows involvement mainly of the megakaryocytic cell line

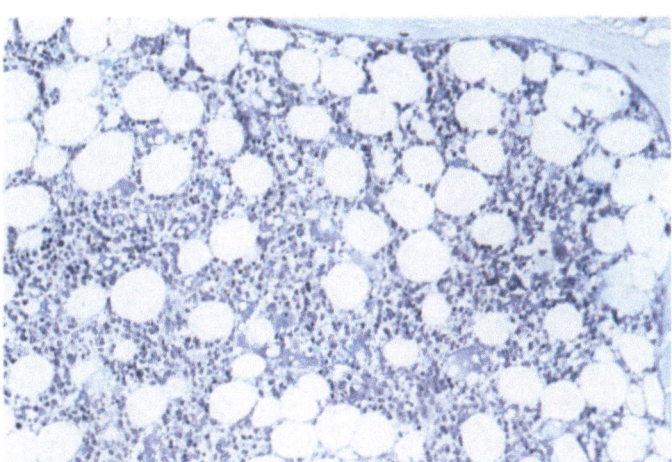

Figs 6.15 and 6.16 These sections illustrate smouldering leukaemia: the blast cell population progresses slowly with only partial suppression of normal haematopoiesis

Fig. 6.15 Low-power view showing normocellular bone marrow with interstitial infiltration

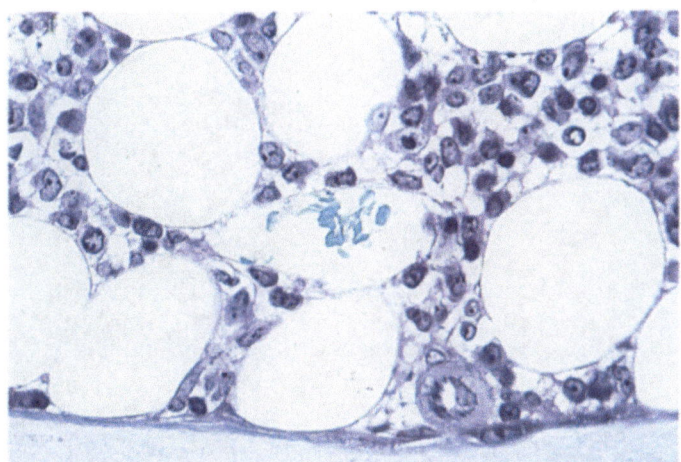

Fig. 6.16 Higher magnification illustrating oval to kidney-shaped nuclei of the monocytes

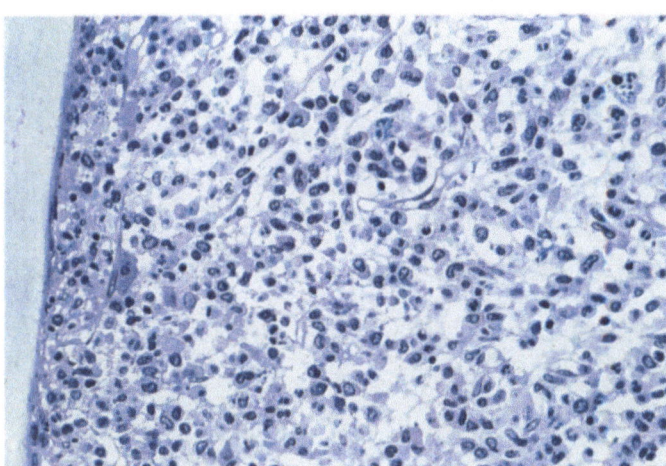

Figs 6.17–6.19 Examples of bone marrow biopsies of patients with chronic myelomonocytic leukaemia. In these cases also, some degree of haematopoietic function is maintained for variable periods of time, but eventually the normal marrow is replaced by the leukaemic cell population

Fig. 6.17 Almost complete replacement of the normal bone marrow, few residual marrow elements remain

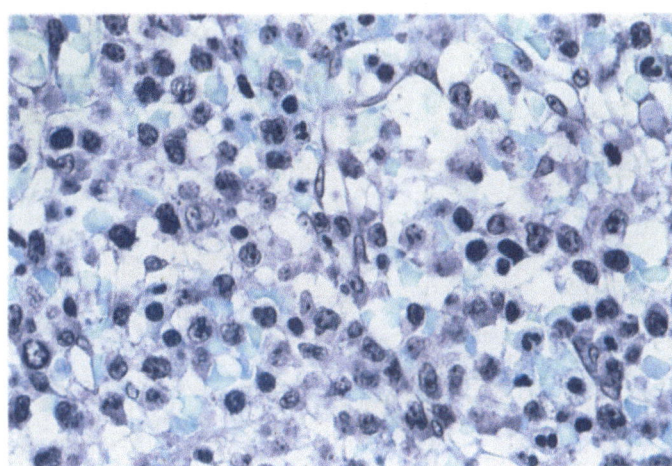

Fig. 6.18 Higher magnification of Fig. 6.17 to show the resemblance of the monocytes to hairy cells

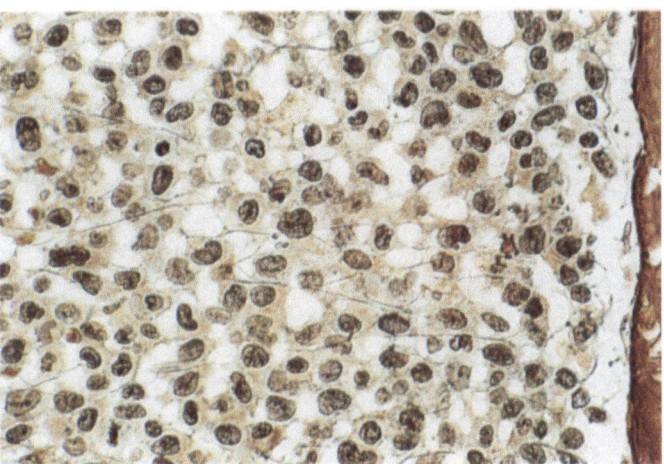

Fig. 6.19 As Fig. 6.18, stained by Gomori's stain; there is only a very delicate network of reticular fibres

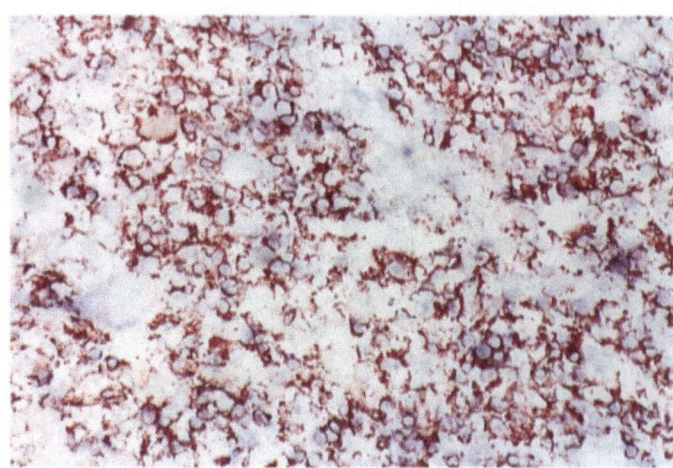

Fig. 6.20 Cryostat section of bone biopsy of patient with CMML incubated with the antibody Ki M8 which reacts with monocytes and macrophages, to show proportion of these cells present

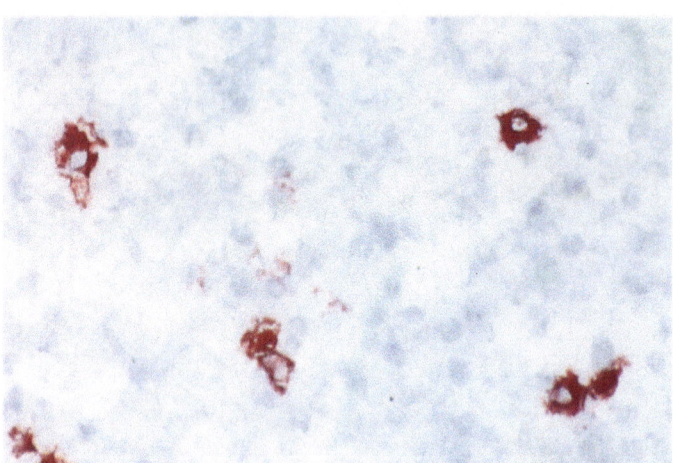

Fig. 6.21 Case of CMML, cryostat section incubated with VIPL which reacts with megakaryocytes; only a few are present

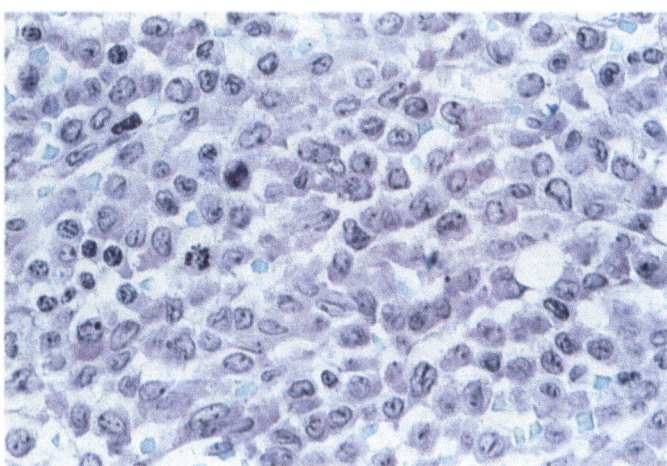

Fig. 6.22 Section of bone biopsy of patient with chronic monocytic leukaemia. High power view showing the characteristic nuclei

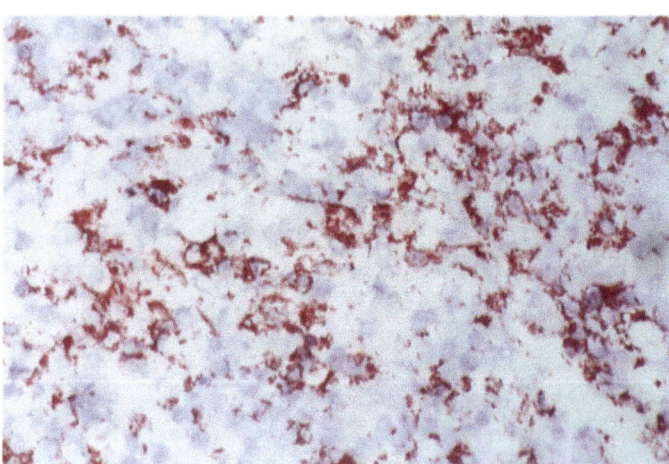

Fig. 6.23 Cryostat section of bone biopsy of patient with monocytic leukaemia incubated with the antibody Ki M8. Monocytes, macrophages and their cytoplasmic processes are stained

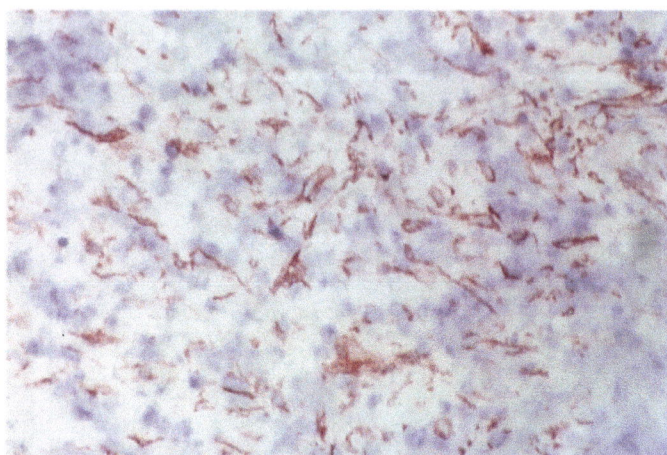

Fig. 6.24 As Fig. 6.23, cryostat section incubated with the antibody My7. Myelomonocytes and endothelial cells are stained. Note cytoplasmic processes

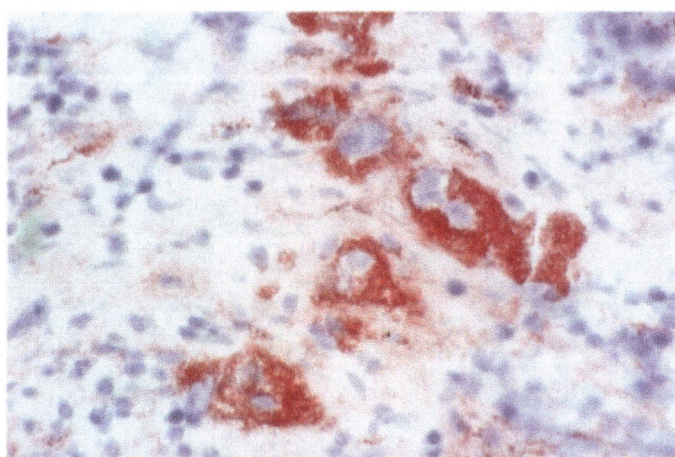

Fig. 6.25 As Fig. 6.24, demonstration of megakaryocytes by their reaction with FVIII reg

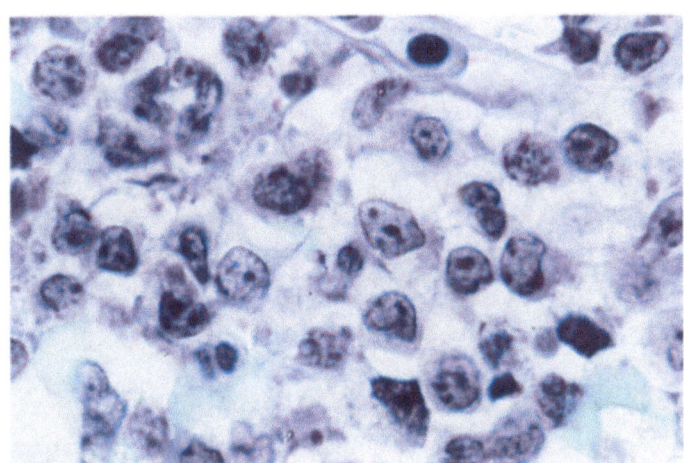

Fig. 6.26 High-power view of another case of chronic monocytic leukaemia, with less characteristic nuclei

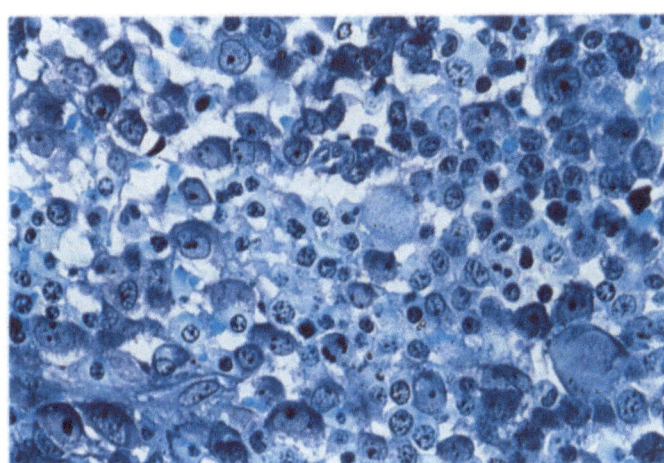

Fig. 6.27 Case of di Guglielmo syndrome, showing hypercellular bone marrow, mainly erythroid precursors, with some maturation.

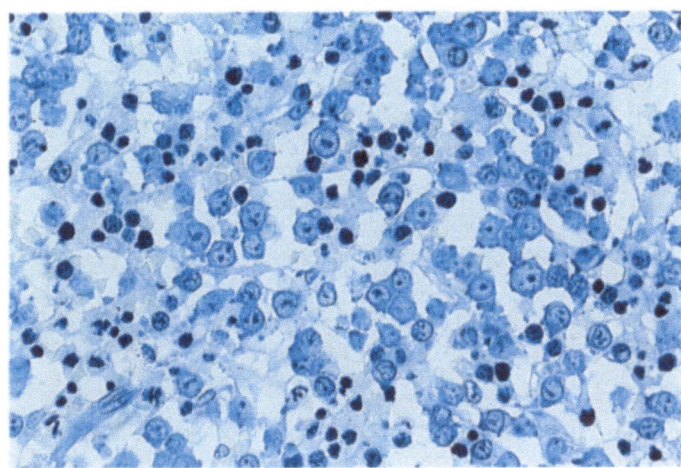

Fig. 6.28 Another case of di Guglielmo syndrome, with a greater proportion of erythroblasts

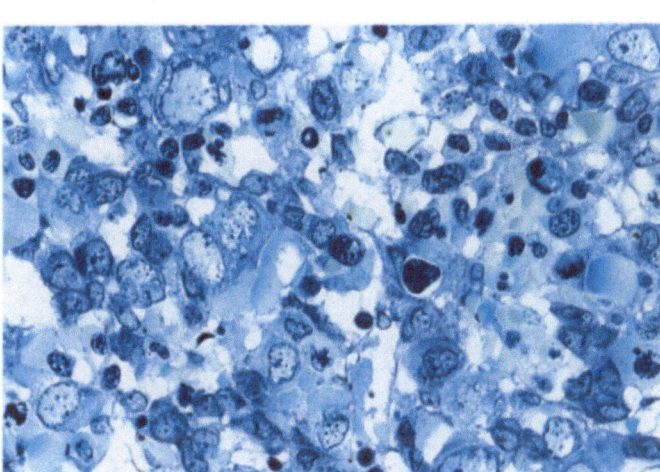

Fig. 6.29 Case of erythroleukaemia with marked dyserythropoietic features, though haemoglobulinization of the cytoplasm has occurred in some of the cells

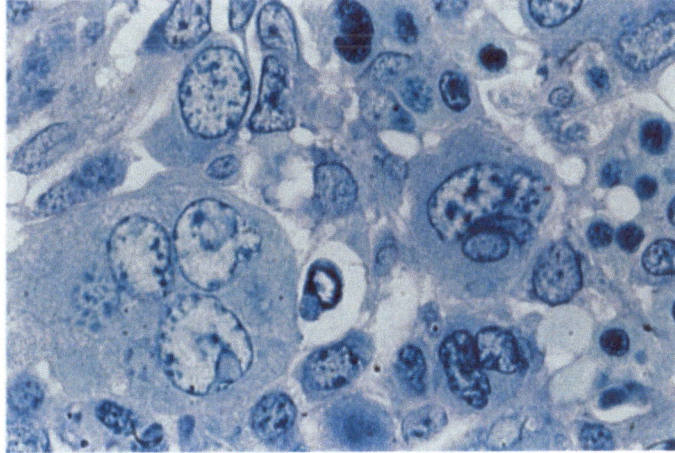

Fig. 6.30 Erythroleukaemia characterized by multinucleated erythroblasts

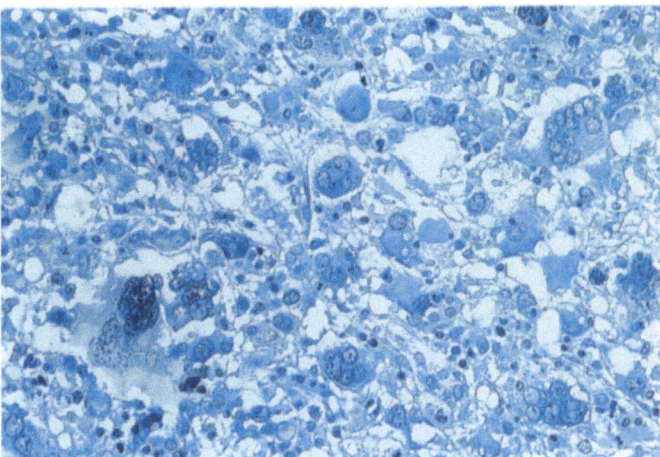

Fig. 6.31 Involvement of both the erythroid and the megakaryocytic cell lines. Note bizarre and highly pleomorphic cells

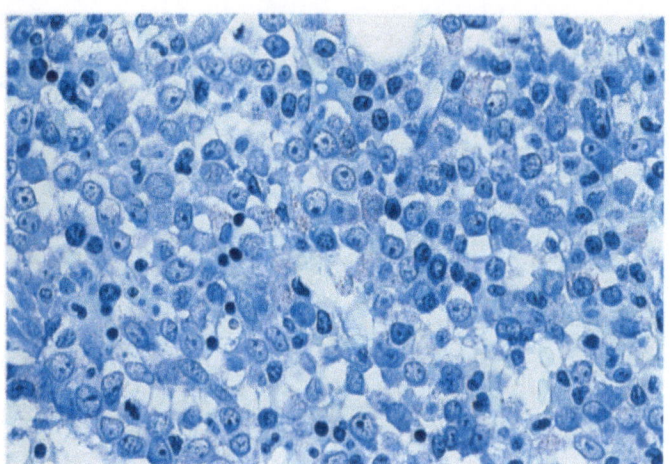

Fig. 6.32 Bone biopsy section of patient with lymphoblastic leukaemia. Note residual erythroid and myeloid precursors between the lymphoblasts

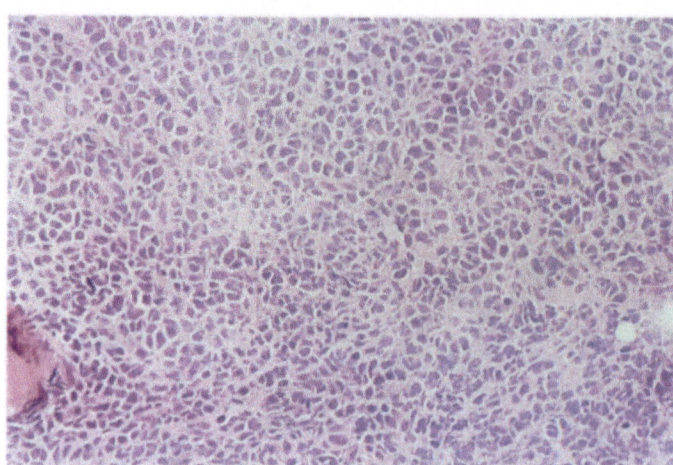

Fig. 6.33 Cryostat section of bone biopsy of patient with pre-B ALL. Residual haematopoiesis cannot be identified

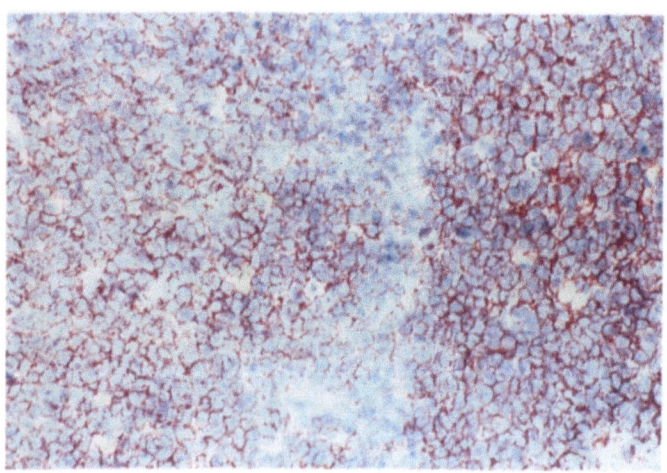

Fig. 6.34 As above, cryostat section stained by Leu 14 (CD22)

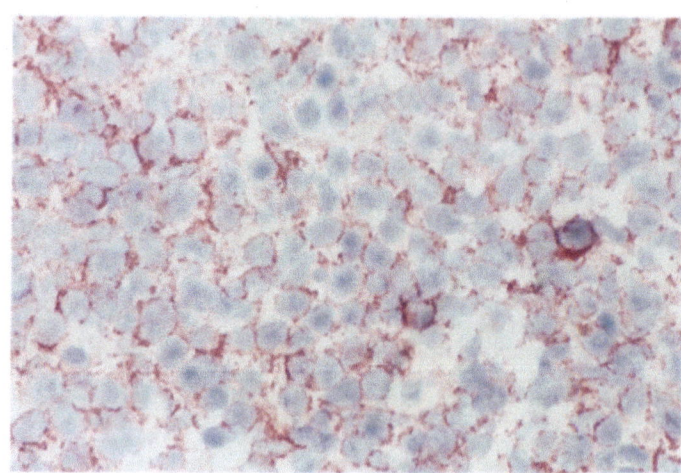

Fig. 6.35 As Fig. 6.34, cryostat section stained by the antibody to IgG heavy chain

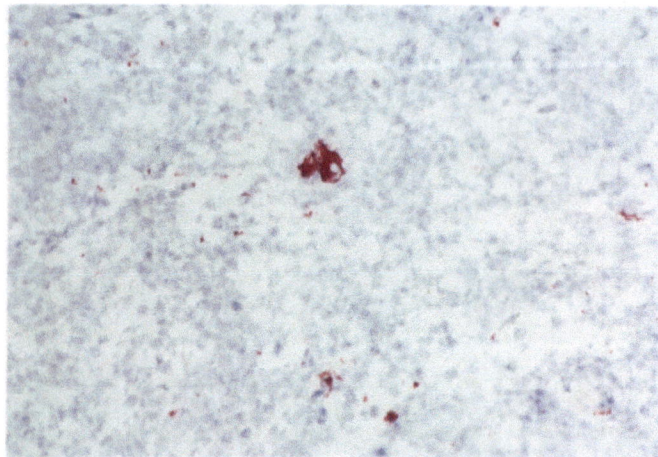

Fig. 6.36 As Fig. 6.35, residual megakaryocytes stained by the antibody VIPL1

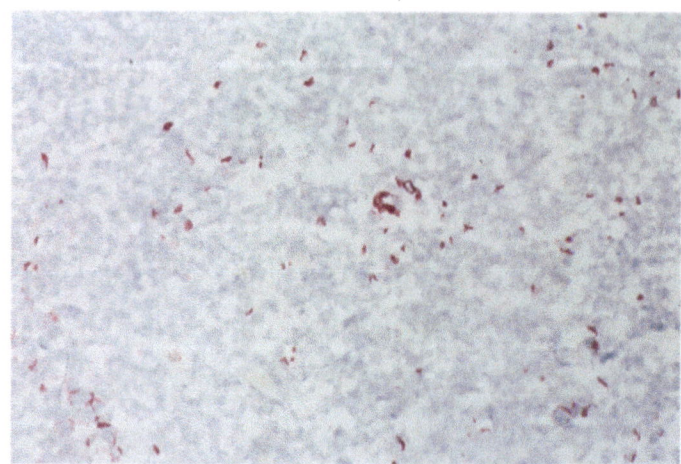

Fig. 6.37 As Fig. 6.36, isolated erythroid precursors demonstrated by their reactivity with VIEG-4

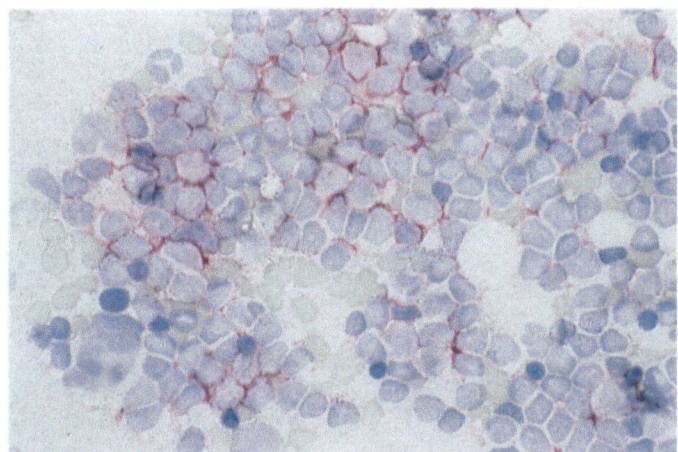

Fig. 6.38 Case of acute leukaemia, showing reactivity with the CALLA antigen

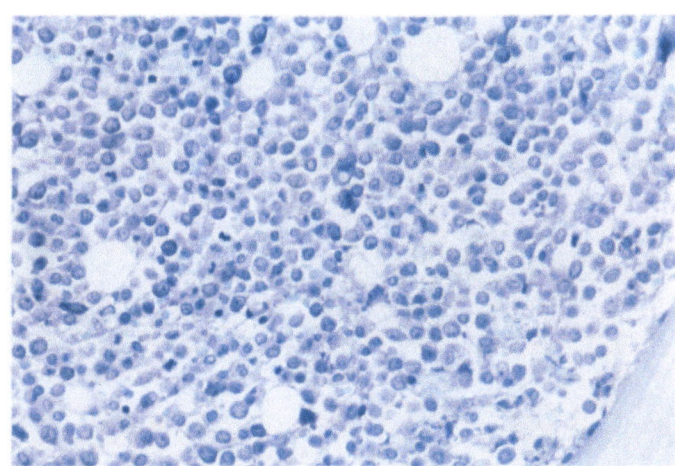

Fig. 6.39 Case of AML (FAB M2) pre-treatment bone marrow showing dense infiltration with myeloblasts

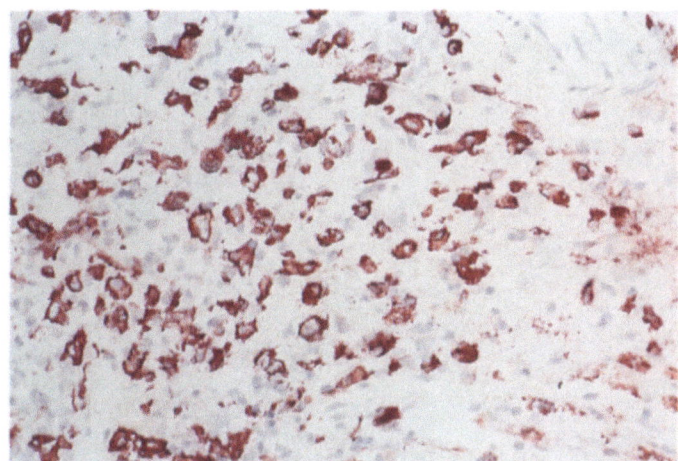

Fig. 6.40 As Fig. 6.39, cryostat section incubated with the antibody VIM2, myelomonocytic cells are stained

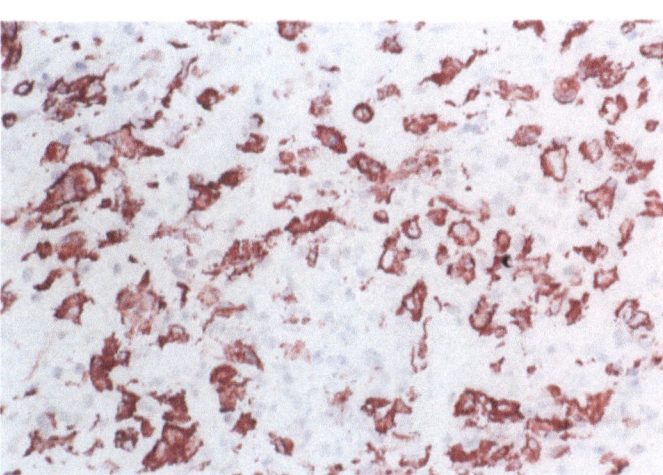

Fig. 6.41 As Fig. 6.40, cryostat section incubated with the antibody MY 7 (CD13) which reacts with myelomonocytic and endothelial cells

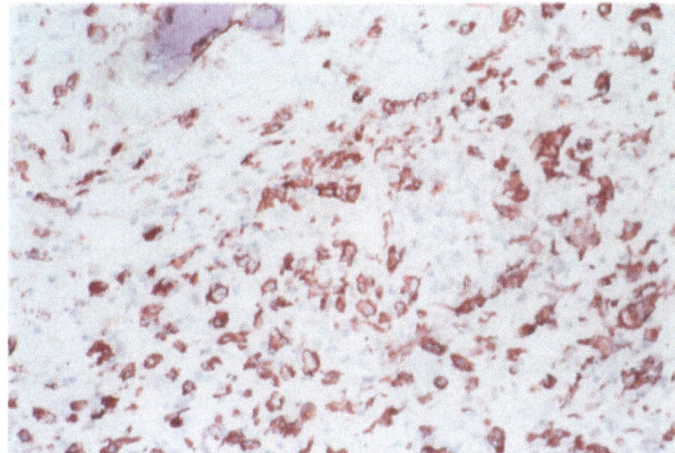

Fig. 6.42 As Fig. 6.41, cryostat section incubated with the antibody VIM 8 which stains granulocytes

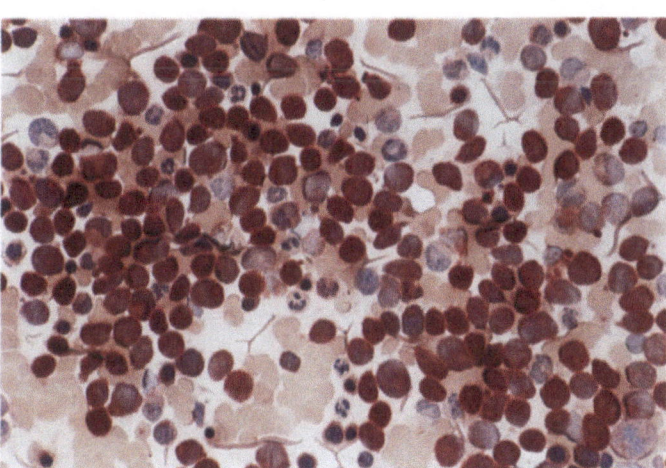

Fig. 6.43 Aspirate smear of patient with monocytic leukaemia; monocytes show α-naphthyl esterase activity

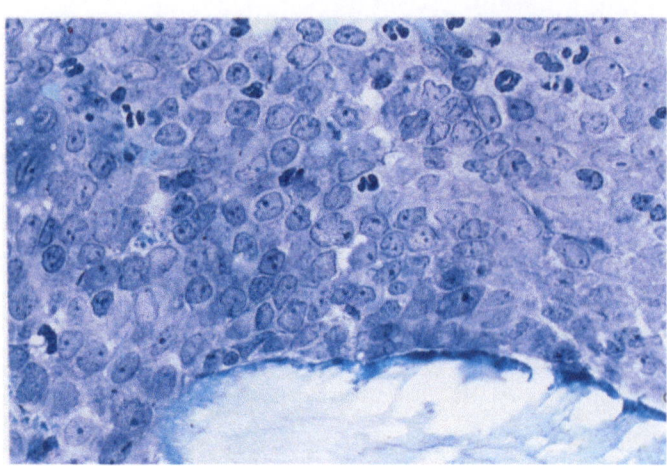

Fig. 6.44 Section of bone biopsy of patient with monoblastic leukaemia, showing fairly monomorphic sheets of blasts

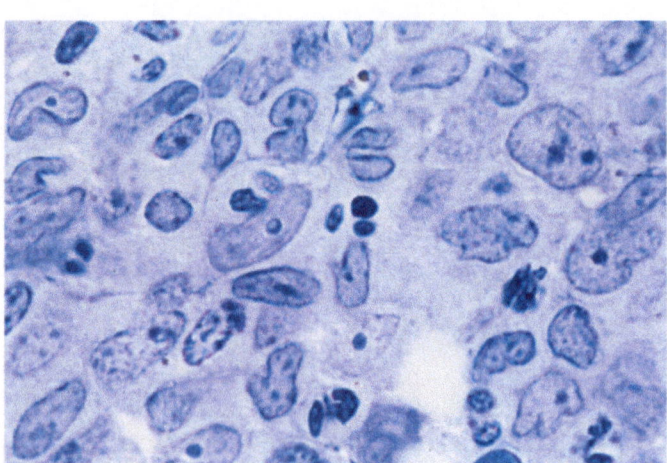

Fig. 6.45 Section of bone biopsy of another patient with monoblastic leukaemia, showing monoblasts with pleomorphic nuclei

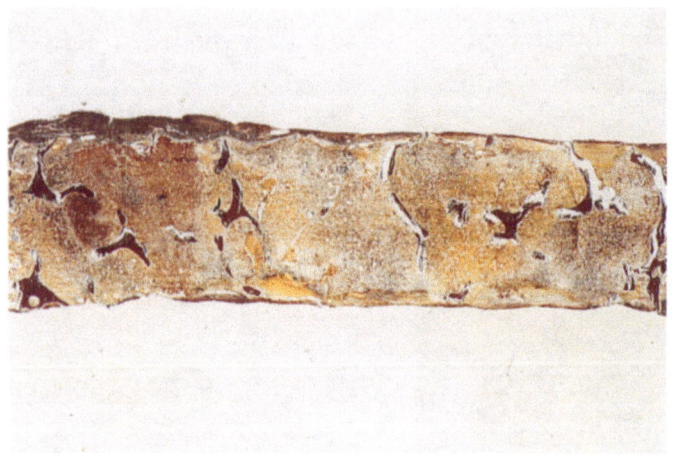

Fig. 6.46 Low-power section of bone biopsy of patient with AML after intensive chemotherapy. There is extensive degeneration and haemorrhage. Gomori

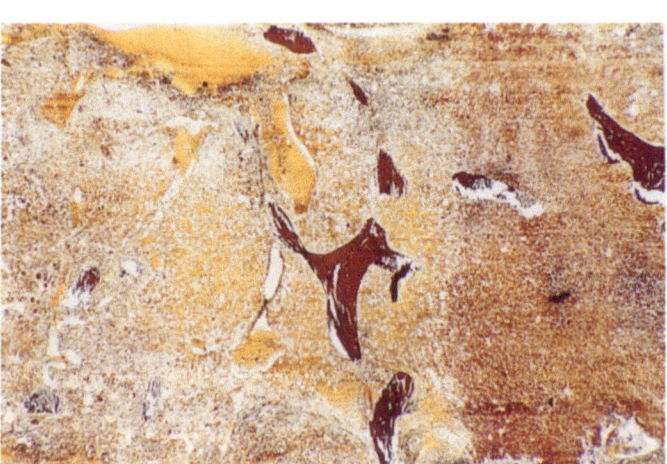

Fig. 6.47 Higher power of part of Fig. 6.46. Virtually no marrow cells left. Gomori

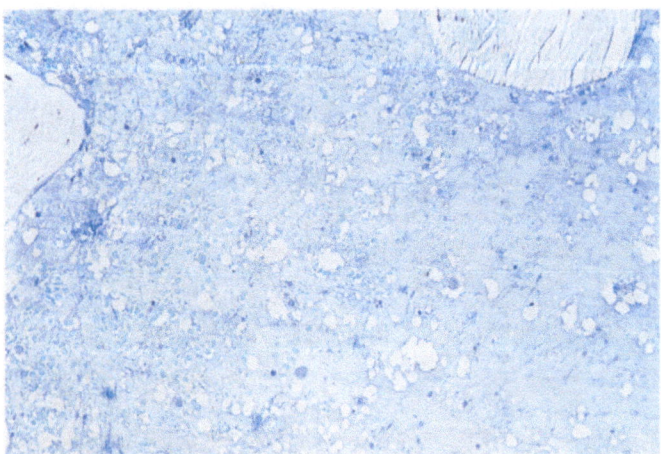

Fig. 6.48 Higher magnification of Fig. 6.46 showing complete atrophy of bone marrow

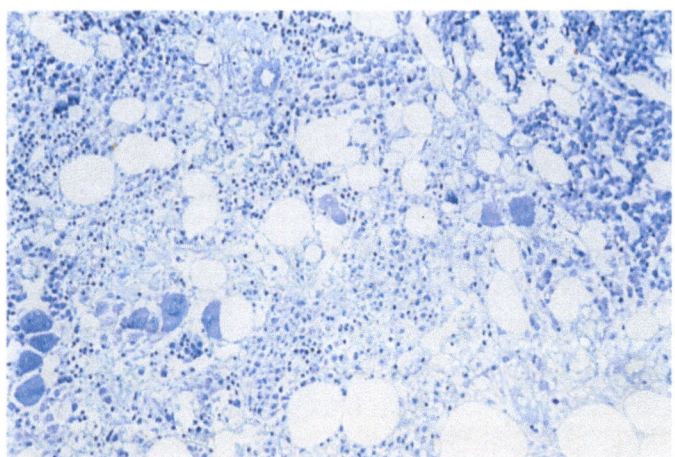

Fig. 6.49 Bone biopsy section showing partial remission after chemotherapy in patient with AML

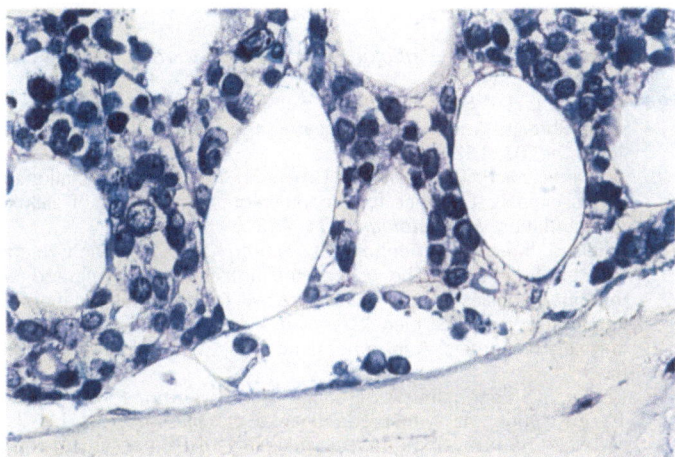

Fig. 6.50 Higher magnification of part of bone biopsy section in Fig. 6.49, showing blasts at the trabecular surface

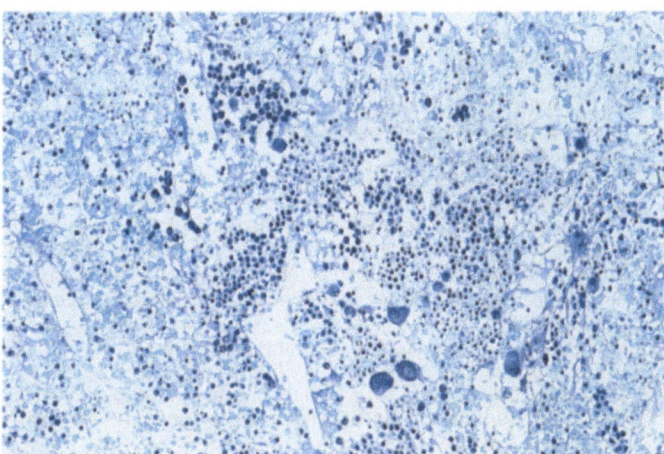

Figs 6.51–6.53 These figures illustrate progressive restitution of haematopoiesis and normal bone marrow structure

Fig. 6.51 Many early precursors but large islands of erythropoiesis showing maturation

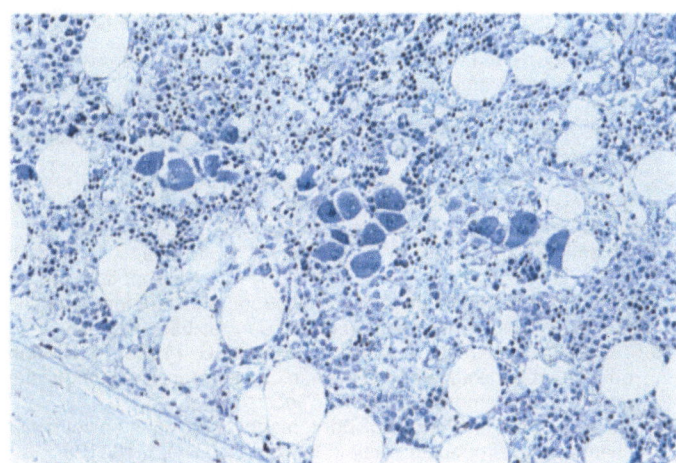

Fig. 6.52 Regenerating bone marrow with clusters of megakaryocytes

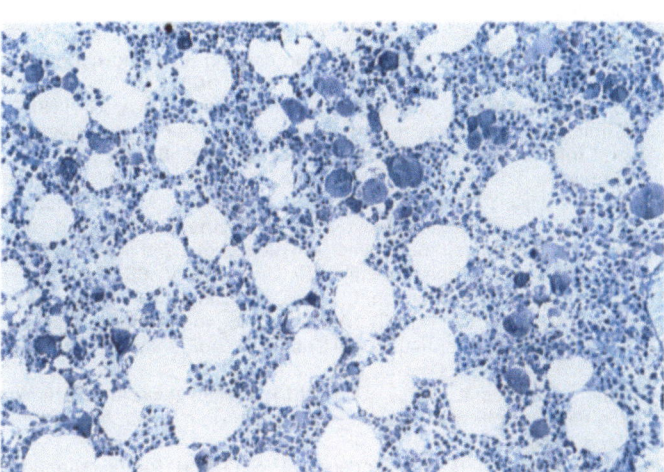

Fig. 6.53 Incipient restoration of the normal bone marrow structure, though there is still a preponderance of early precursors

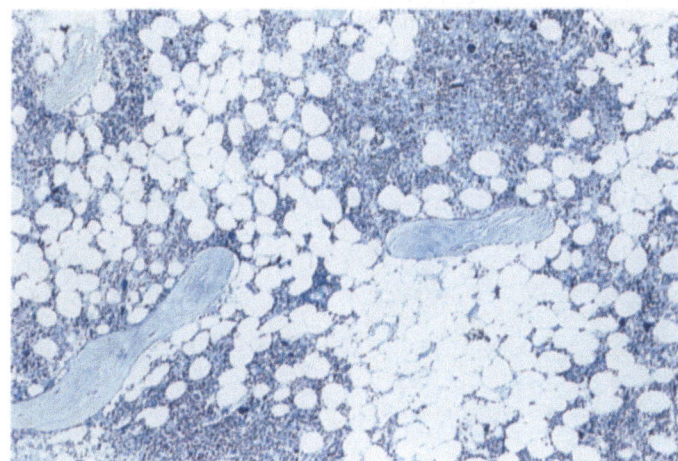

Fig. 6.54 Section of bone biopsy of patient after bone marrow transplantation for acute leukaemia; low power, showing repopulation of the bone marrow

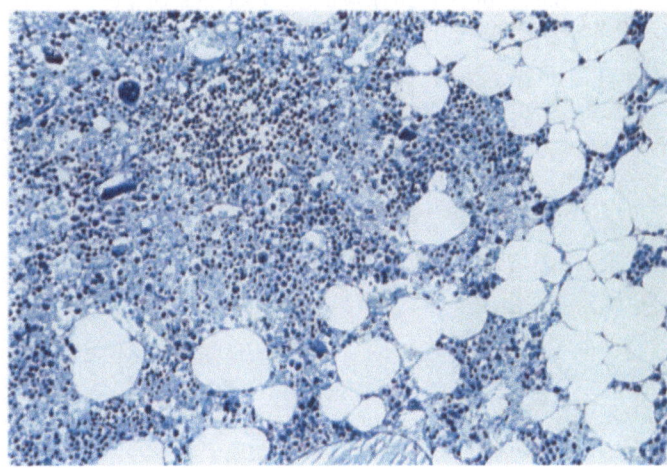

Fig. 6.55 As Fig. 6.54, higher magnification showing normal bone marrow cells and lymphoid cell aggregate

7. Eriber, W. N., Breton-Gorius, J., Villeval, J. L., Oscier, D. G., Bai, Y. and Mason, Y. (1987). Detection of cells of megakaryocyte lineage in haematological malignancies by immunoalkaline phosphatase labelling cell smears with a panel of monoclonal antibodies. *Br. J. Haematol.*, **65**, 87

8. Fialkow, P. J., Singer, J. W., Raskind, W. H., Adamson, Jacobson, R. J., Bernstein, I. D., Dow, L. W., Najfeld, V. and Veith, R. (1987). Clonal development, stem-cell differentiation, and clinical remissions in acute nonlymphoblastic leukaemia. *N. Engl. J. Med.*, **317**, 466

9. Janvier, M., Tobelem, G., Daniel, M. T., Bernheim, A., Marty, M. and Boiron, M. (1984). Acute monoblastic leukaemia. *Scand. J. Haematol.*, **32**, 385

10. Howe, R. B., Bloomfield, C. D. and McKenna, R. W. (1982). Hypocellular acute leukaemia. *Am. J. Med.*, **72**, 391

11. Maddox, A. M., Keating, M. J., Smith, T. L. *et al.* (1986). Prognostic factors for survival of 194 patients with low infiltrate leukaemia. *Leukaemia Res.*, **10**, 995

12. Berdeaux, D. H., Glasser, I., Serokmann, R., Moon, T. and Durie, B. G. (1986). Hypoplastic acute leukaemia: review of 70 cases with multivariate regression analysis. *Haematol. Oncol.*, **4**, 291

13. Manoharan, A., Horsley, R. and Pitney, W. R. (1979). The reticulin content of bone marrow in acute leukaemia in adults. *Br. J. Haematol.*, **43**, 185

14. Oscier, D. G. and Stenvenson, J. C. (1988). Ectopic production of calcitonin and hypocalcemia in acute leukemia. *Br. J. Haematol.*, **68**, 265

15. Schenkein, D. P., O'Neil, W. C., Shapiro, J. and Miller, K. B. (1986). Accelerated bone formation causing profound hypocalcemia in acute leukaemia. *Ann. Intern. Med.*, **105**, 375

16. Brito-Babapulle, F., Catovsky, D. and Galton, D. A. G. (1987). Clinical and laboratory features of de novo acute myeloid leukaemia and trilineage myelodysplasia. *Br. J. Haematol.*, **66**, 445

17. Jinnai, I., Tomonaga, M., Kuriyama, K., Matsuo, T., Nonaka, H., Amenormori, Y., Yoshida, Y., Kusano, M., Tagawa, M. and Ichimaru, M. (1987). Dysmegakaryocytopoiesis in acute leukaemias: its predominance in myelomonocytic (M4) leukaemia and implication for poor response to chemotherapy. *Br. J. Haematol.*, **66**, 467

18. Harrington, D. S., Peterson, C., Ness, M., Sanger, W., Smith, D. M. and Vaughan, W. (1988). Acute myelogenous leukaemia with eosinophilic differentiation and Trisomy-I. *Am. J. Clin. Pathol.*, **90**, 464

19. Vilter, R. W. and Wiltse, D. (1985). Preleukaemia and urticaria pigmentosa followed by acute myeloblastic leukaemia. *Arch. Intern. Med.*, **145**, 349

20. Islam, A., Frisch, B. and Henderson, E. S. (1989). Plastic embedded core biopsy – A complementary approach to bone marrow aspiration in the diagnosis of acute myeloid leukaemia. *J. Clin. Pathol.*, (In Press)

21. Islam, A. and Henderson, E. S. (1988). Bone marrow biopsy in acute myeloid leukaemia. *Hematol. Rev.*, **2**, 187

22. Lewis, S. M. and Szur, L. (1963). Malignant myelodysplastic myelosclerosis. *Br. Med. J.*, **II**, 472

23. Mahl, G., Frisch, B., Bartl, R., Kager, K., Pappenberger, R., Schlag, R. and Burkhardt, R. (1984). Acute myelofibrosis: Only one extreme in the spectrum of 'idiopathic' myelofibrosis. In Lennert, K. and Hubbner, K. (eds), *Pathology of the Bone Marrow*. Stuttgart: G. Fischler

24. Truong, L. D., Saleem, A. and Schwartz, M. R. (1984). Acute myelofibrosis. A report of four cases and review of the literature. *Medicine*, **63**, 182

25. Bernardeschi, P., Bonechi, I and Urbano, U. (1986). Acute malignant myelosclerosis. Evidence for a panmyelotic disturbance of cellular differentiation. *Haematologica*, **71**, 493

26. Thiele, J., Krech, R., Wienhold, St., Simon, K. G., Zankovich, R. and Fischer, R. (1987). The use of the anti-factor VIII method on trephine biopsies of the bone marrow for the identification of immature and atypical megakaryocytes in myeloproliferative diseases and allied disorders. A morphometric study. *Virchows Arch. B*, **54**, 89

27. Beiske, K., Langholm, R., Godal, T. and Marton, P. F. (1986). T-zone lymphoma with predominance of "plasmacytoid T-cells" associated with myelomonocytic leukaemia – a distinct clinicopathological entity. *J. Pathol.*, **150**, 247

28. Mayumi, M., Tsutsui, T., Shirane, H., Mizue, H. and Mikawa, H. (1985). Erythroleukemia with myelofibrosis – Pediatric case report and discussion of possible stem cell origin of the disorder. *Acta. Haematol. Jpn.*, **48**, 1414

29. Zanke, B. W., Johnston, J. B. and Israels, L. G. (1988). Erythemic myelosis in chronic lymphocytic leukaemia. *Cancer*, **62**, 954

30. Frisch, J., Bartl, R. and Chaichik, S. (1986). Therapy-induced myelodysplasia and secondary leukaemia. *Scand. J. Haematol.*, **36**(Suppl. 45), 38

31. Lohrmann, H. P. (1984). The problem of permanent marrow damage after cytotoxic drug treatment. *Oncology*, **41**, 180

32. Islam, A., Catovsky, D., Goldman, J. M. and Galton, D. A. G. (1984). Bone marrow fibre content in acute myeloid leukaemia before and after treatment. *J. Clin. Pathol.*, **37**, 1259

33. Brody, J. P., Krause, J. R. and Penchansky, L. (1985). Bone marrow response to chemotherapy in acute lymphocytic leukaemia and acute non-lymphocytic leukaemia. *Scand. J. Haematol.*, **35**, 240

34. Abrams, R. A., Lichter, A. S., Bromer, R. H., Minna, J. D., Cohen, M. H, and Deisseroth, A. B. (1985). The haematopoietic toxicity of regional radiation therapy. Correlations for combined modality therapy with systemic chemotherapy. *Cancer*, **55**, 1429

35. Testa, N. G., Hendry, J. H. and Molineux, G. (1985). Long-term bone marrow damage in experimental systems and in patients after radiation or chemotherapy. *Anti-Cancer Res.*, **5**, 101

36. Islam, A. (1987). Pattern of bone marrow regeneration following chemotherapy for acute myeloid leukemia. *J. Med.*, **18**, 108

37. Sale, G. E. and Buckner, C. (1988). Pathology of bone marrow in transplant recipients. *Hematol/Oncol. Clin. N. Am.*, **2**, 735

38. Brito-Babapulle, F., Catovsky, D. and Galton, D. A. G. (1988). Myelodysplastic relapse of de novo acute myeloid leukaemia with trilineage myelodysplasia: a previously unrecognized correlation. *Br. J. Haematol.*, **68**, 411

39. Rajantie, J., Sale, G. E., Deeg, H. J., Amos, D., Applebaum, F., Storb, R., Clift, R. A. and Buckner, C. D. (1986). Adverse effect of severe marrow fibrosis on hematologic recovery after chemoradiotherapy and allogenic bone marrow transplantation. *Blood*, **67**, 1693

These comprise polycythaemia vera (PV); idiopathic thrombocythaemia (IT); chronic myeloid leukaemia (CML) or chronic granulocytic leukaemia (CGL); myelofibrosis/osteomyelosclerosis (MF/OMS), as well as the variant, intermediate or transitional forms. It has now been established that they are clonal disorders of the bone marrow representing evolution from a single neoplastic cell but capable nevertheless of producing differentiated progeny for variable periods of time. Hence they comprise a spectrum of the more or less well-defined clinical entities listed above. But there are no unequivocal cytological characteristics which distinguish the cells in the CMPD for their normal counterparts in the bone marrow, at least not initially. The megakaryocytes constitute an exception: the giant forms, nuclear configurations, and clustering typical for the CMPD are not features of the reactive conditions[1-7].

Three major criteria are used for histological recognition and classification[3,7]: (1) identification of the predominant proliferative cell line(s); (2) the degree of differentiation; and (3) the connective tissue reaction – reticulin and collagenous fibres, new bone formation and the accompanying vascular proliferation and frequently inflammatory infiltrations and lymphoid nodules. However, it should be emphasized that the above groups of the CMPD are not sharply divided; they overlap – for example CML with concomitant megakaryocytic proliferation: the so-called mixed granulocytic–megakaryocytic myelosis. Moreover, a classification of the MPD should incorporate the possibility of indicating the subsequent evolution of the proliferative process[2,3,5]. Such histological transformations have been documented by serial biopsies[7]. Exceptionally, bone marrow histology is not typical. Though mostly observed in adults, myeloproliferative disorders also occur in children[8].

Polycythaemia Vera (PV)

Bone marrow histology provides a valuable additional parameter for the diagnosis of PV which is made on the basis of clinical and haematological investigations. Particularly useful is the demonstration of erythropoietin-independent growth of erythroid colonies *in vitro*[9].

The value of a bone biopsy in PV is still questioned by some authors, but in some cases the recognition of secondary polycythaemia may not be possible on clinical parameters alone. In addition, about 20% of cases of PV have a normal leucocyte and platelet count – while the number of leucocytes is often increased in secondary erythrocytosis.

In some cases all the criteria for PV of the PV Study Group cannot be met, but the bone biopsy presents the classic picture of a tri-linear hyperplasia – as may happen in patients with the Budd–Chiari syndrome. In such patients demonstration of erythropoietin-independent colony growth in culture may be particularly helpful as an additional criterion of a myeloproliferative disorder.

Certain histological features are useful in differentiating PV from secondary erythrocytosis: in the latter only the erythroid precursors are increased, megakaryocytes are quantitatively and morphologically within normal limits, iron stores are not depleted (if there is no iron deficiency) and reticulin fibres are not increased.

Bone marrow histology in PV can be subdivided into four sub-types (Figs 7.1–7.18): (1) The classic tri-linear type in which there is hyperplasia of erythroid, megakaryocytic and granulocytic cell lines; (2) the bi-linear type involving the erythroid and megakaryocytic cell lines; (3) the bi-linear type involving the erythrocytic and the granulocytic lines; and (4) the uni-linear type in which there is only erythroid hyperplasia. This is histologically similar to the picture seen in haemolysis – additional studies are of course required for diagnosis. The first – the classic tri-linear - is the most frequent. The other three types must be distinguished from the other entities in the CMPD by means of the investigations appropriate to each entity, bearing in mind the overlap and transitions that may occur between them (see above).

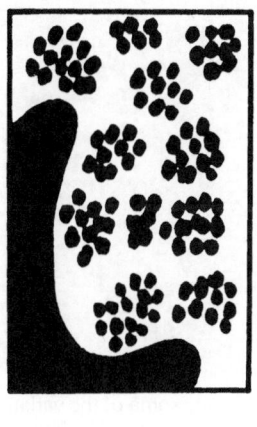
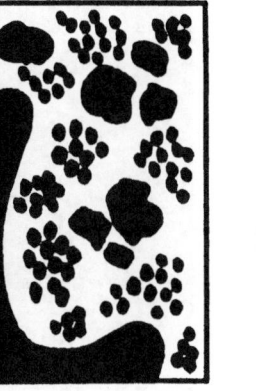
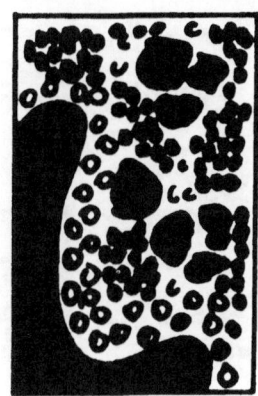

ERY	ERY	ERY	ERY
- - -	MEG	- - -	MEG
- - -	- - -	GRA	GRA

Fig. 7.1 Sketch illustrating the four histological types of PV

(Continued on p. 97)

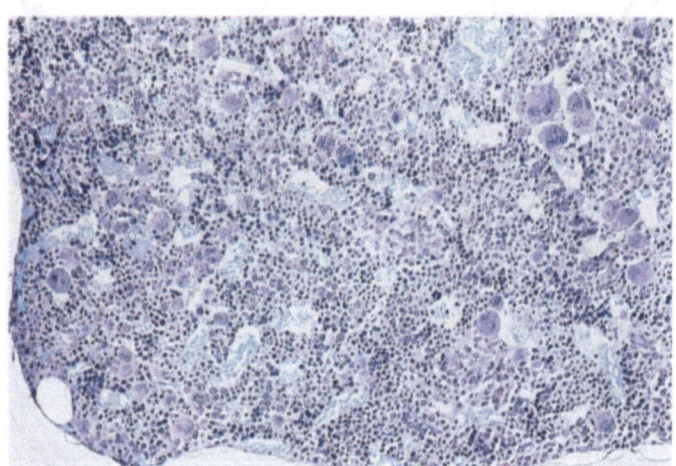

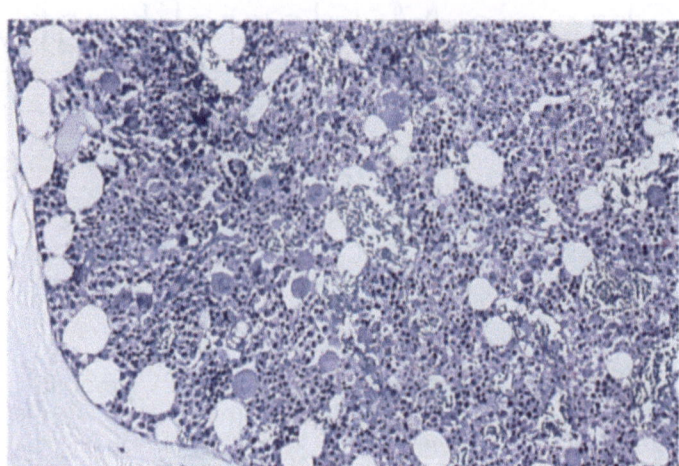

Figs 7.2–7.5   These figures illustrate the four subtypes of PV

Fig. 7.2   The classic subtype, involving the erythrocytic, megakaryocytic and granulocytic cell lines

Fig. 7.3   The erythrocytic and megakaryocytic subtype

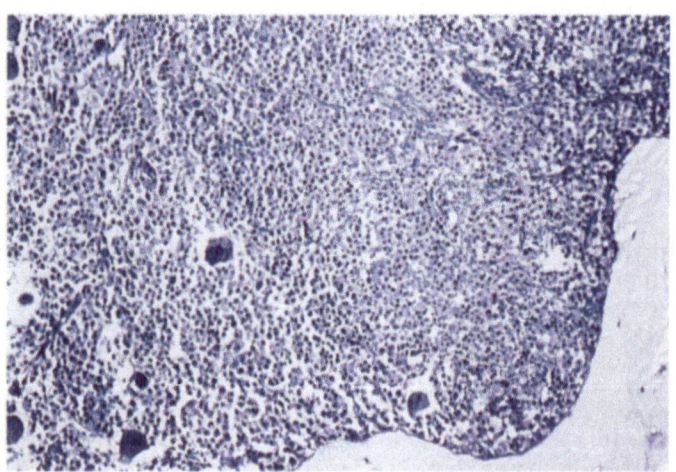

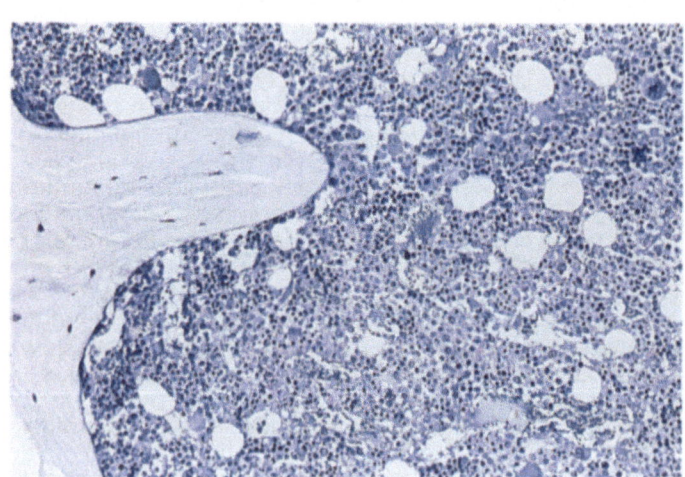

Fig. 7.4   The erythrocytic and granulocytic subtype

Fig. 7.5   The erythrocytic subtype

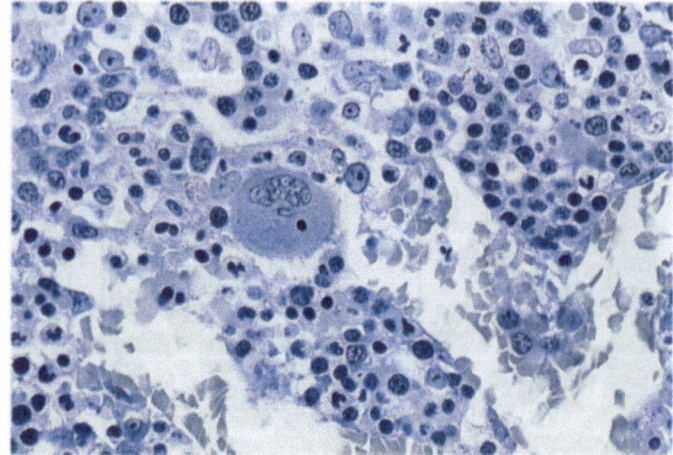

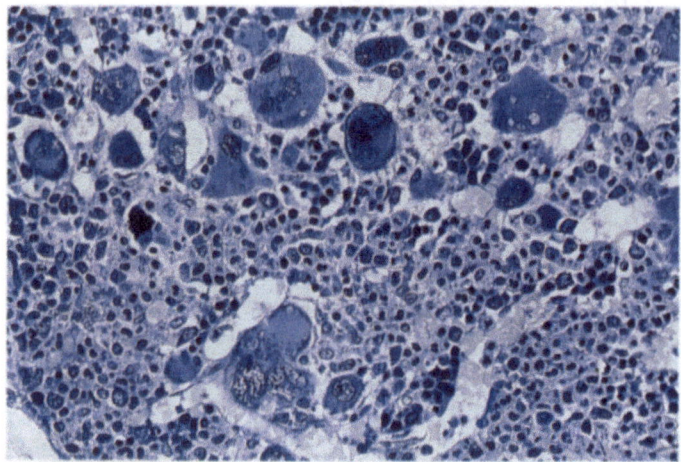

Fig. 7.6   Hyperplastic erythropoiesis, and megakaryocyte at engorged sinus, typical for PV

Figs 7.7–7.10   These figures illustrate some of the variation in size and nuclei of megakaryocytes that may be seen in PV. Note also engorged sinusoids

Fig. 7.7   Cluster of polymorphic megakaryocytes

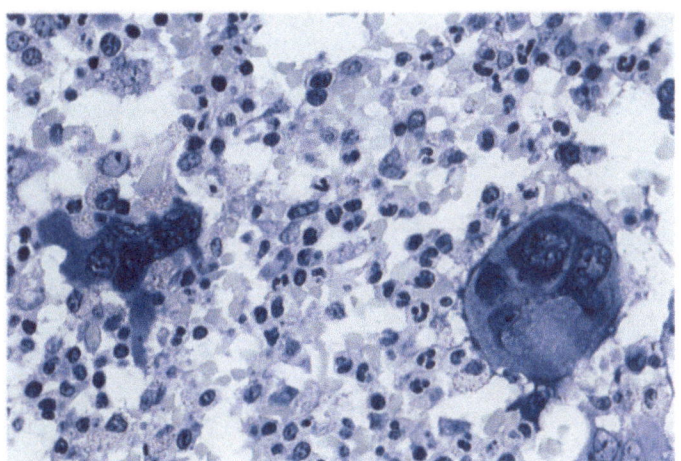

Fig. 7.8 Giant megakaryocyte in PV

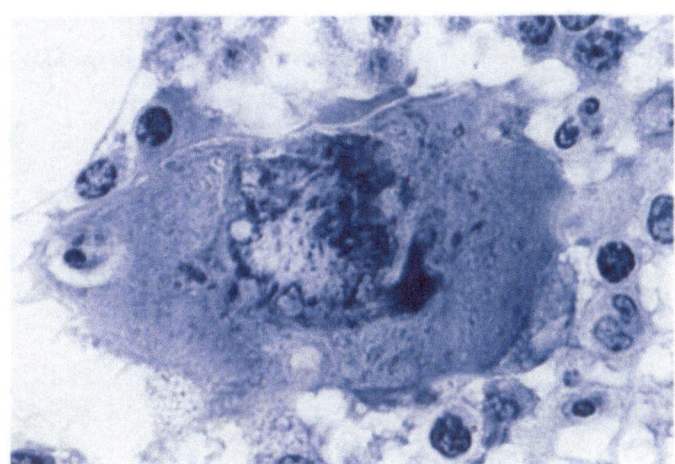

Fig. 7.9 Giant megakaryocyte with emperipolesis

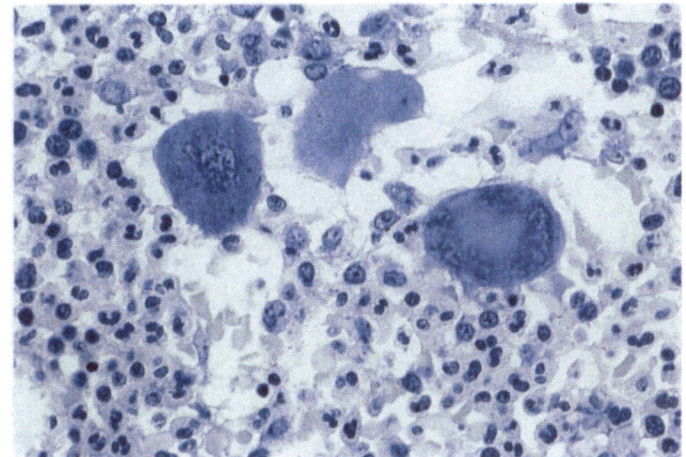

Fig. 7.10 Giant megakaryocytes. Note peripheral localization of nucleus in form of a ring in one megakaryocyte

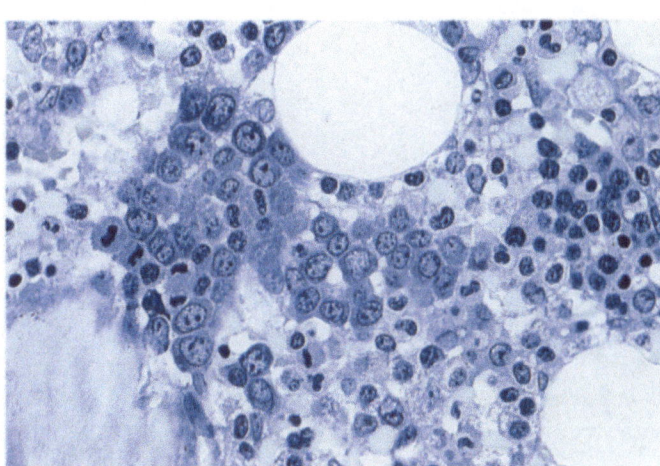

Fig. 7.11 Clusters of early erythroblasts at trabecular surface. Note mitotic figures

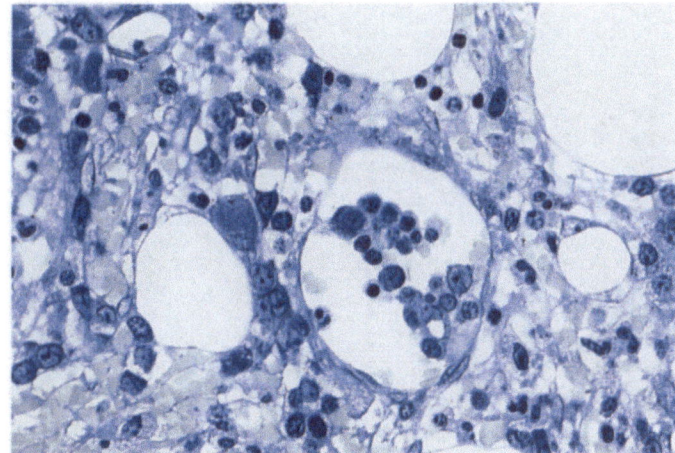

Figs 7.12 and 7.13 Bone biopsy sections showing intravascular haematopoietic precursors in PV

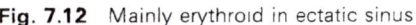

Fig. 7.12 Mainly erythroid in ectatic sinus

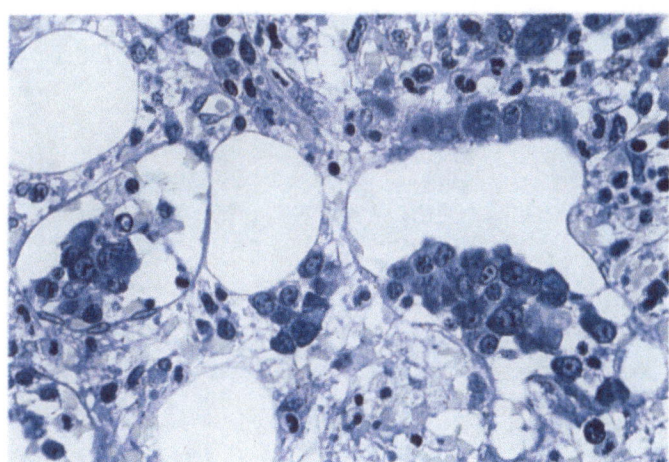

Fig. 7.13 Both erythroid and megakaryocytic precursors

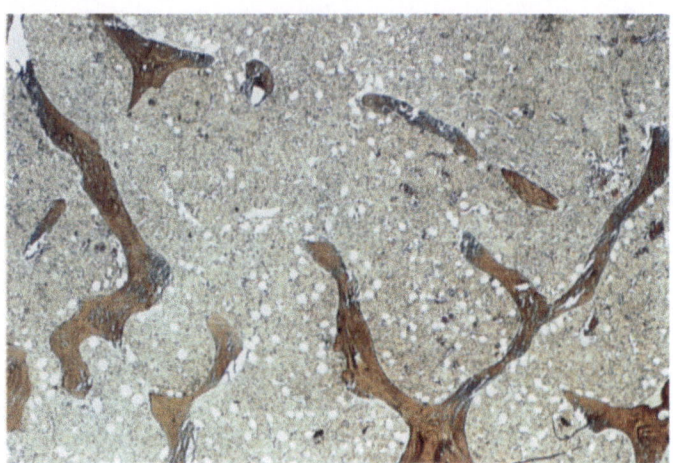

Fig. 7.14 Bone biopsy section of patient with PV showing trabecular osteopenia

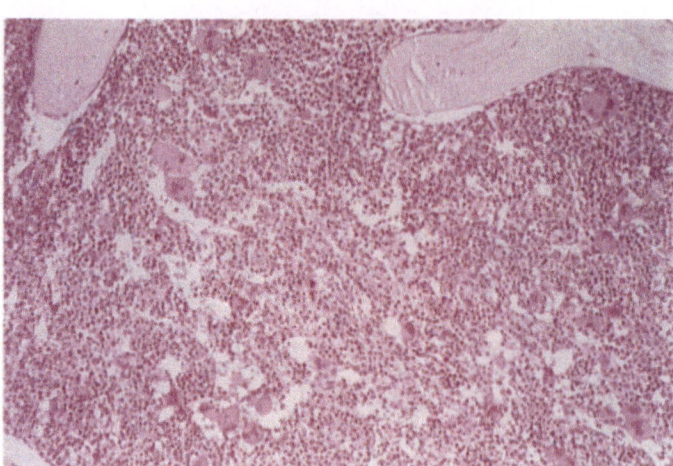

Fig. 7.15 Section of bone biopsy of patient with PV stained by Prussian blue; no demonstrable haemosiderin present

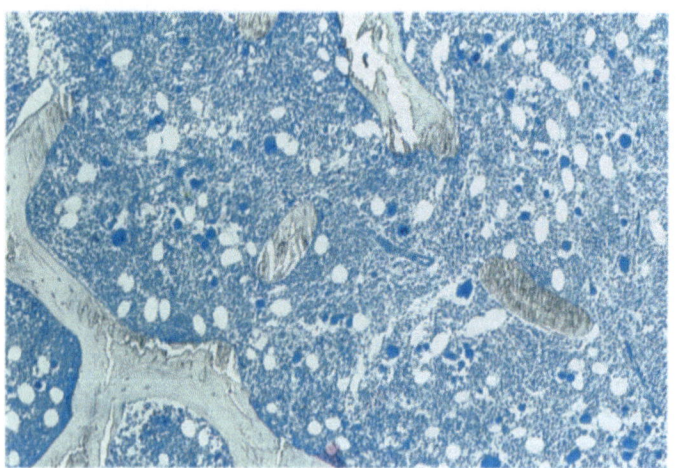

Fig. 7.16 Low-power view of section of bone biopsy of patient with thrombocytopenia who subsequently was shown to have PV (after splenectomy)

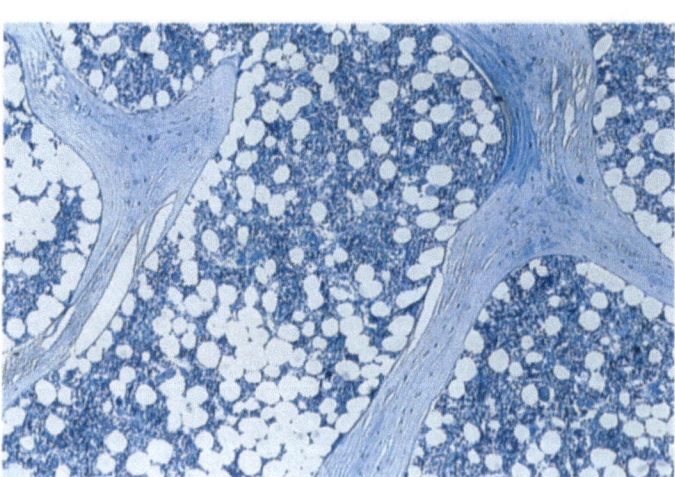

Fig. 7.17 Bone biopsy in case of PV without the typical histological picture

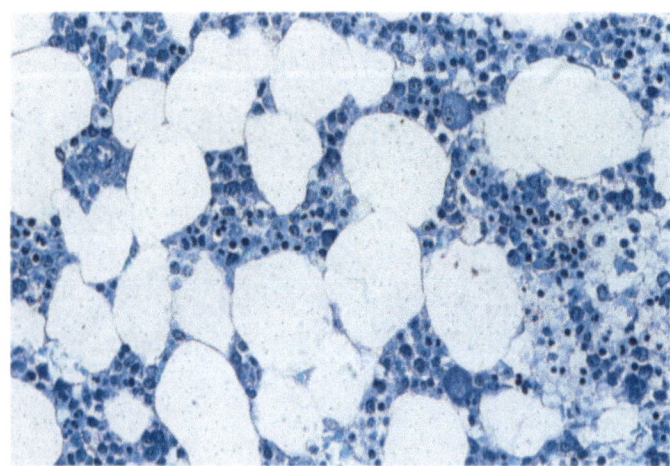

Fig. 7.18 Higher magnification of part of Fig. 7.17

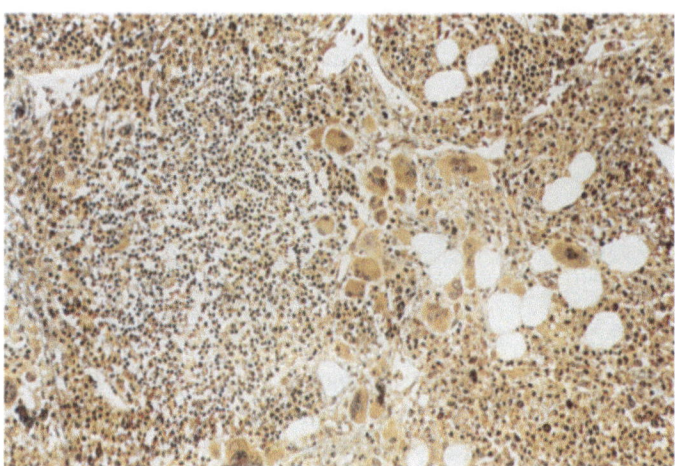

Fig. 7.19 Lymphoid cell aggregate in bone marrow in a case of PV. Note megakaryocytes at its periphery. Gomori

In the classic tri-linear PV there is an increase in overall cellularity with a corresponding decrease in fat cells; each of the hyperplastic cell lines is found in its normal location. Megakaryocytes range from giant to 'micro' forms, and show great variability in nuclear configuration; pyknotic nuclei, bare of cytoplasm, are also frequently present[10]. The megakaryocytes are dispersed singly and in clusters throughout the marrow. There is apparent hyperplasia and hyperaemia of sinusoids; iron stores are depleted, there is an increase in perivascular and paratrabecular reticulin fibres – and sometimes also in association with clusters of megakaryocytes. Lymphoid nodules (Fig. 7.19), plasmacytosis and trabecular osteopenia without evidence of increased osseous remodelling are also characteristic of PV. Development of myelofibrosis occurs mainly in cases with marked proliferation of megakaryocytes (types 1 and 2). In 'spent' or 'burned-out' PV the peripheral blood levels fall, and the bone marrow histology shows stromal changes, serous atrophy, fibrosis, increase in fat cells and reduced and dysplastic haematopoiesis. Further evolution to full-blown myelofibrosis/osteomyelosclerosis (Figs 7.20 and 7.21), to a blast crisis, or to another MPD, or even a malignant lymphoma (Fig. 7.22) have all been described[11,12].

Idiopathic thrombocythaemia (IT), also known as primary or essential thrombocythaemia, is a clonal disorder of a multi-potential stem cell. Analogous to PV there is independent colony growth *in vitro*[13]. Clinically, it is characterized by a sustained increase in the peripheral platelet count, often at levels of 1000×10^9/l or more. Though all cell lines are affected the disease is expressed primarily by hyperplasia of megakaryocytes resulting in the very high platelet counts[14-18]. However, the erythroid and granulocytic cell lines may at times show marked dysplastic features. The bone marrow may be hypo-, normo- or hypercellular (Figs 7.23–7.26) but hyperplastic and atypical megakaryocytes are always present, often forming clusters of pleomorphic cells showing considerable range in size and in nuclear configuration. The normal architectural pattern of the bone marrow is often preserved, with megakaryocytes lying adjacent to sinusoids or protruding into them (Figs 7.27–7.37). Since most are mature and functional megakaryocytes they shed their platelets directly into the blood stream (or portions of their cytoplasm or the whole megakaryocytes migrate into the sinusoids). Macrophages containing cellular debris or crystalline inclusions are also a feature of bone marrow histology in IT. Histological division into a diffuse and a clustered subtype has been made on the basis of megakaryocytic distribution – but the types may simply represent progressive megakaryocytic proliferation and accumulation. In some cases atypical megakaryocytes, especially small ones, may not be identified by histology, so that antibody reactions are required for their recognition[19,20].

It should be pointed out that the clinical syndrome of thrombocythaemia is found not only on the basis of a histological picture of IT in the bone marrow as described above[21]. A high platelet count, even to levels seen in IT (i.e. a million or over) may occur in PV, in the mixed form of CML and in MF/OMS (see below) and in promegakaryocytic myelosis[22] and in some cases of sideroblastic anaemia (Figs 7.38–7.47)[7]. Though a slow and fairly static course is typical for IT, the megakaryocytic hyperplasia may induce fibroblastic proliferation, and fibrillogenesis with resultant myelofibrosis at any time. Cases of megakaryocytic myelosis with both osteomyelosclerosis and osteolytic lesions have also been reported. Transition to an immature form may also occur, though less frequently[23,24]. This is usually signalled by a fall in the platelet count. Revised criteria for the diagnosis of IT have recently been published by the PV Study Group[25].

These are: platelet counts above IM ($> 1000 \times 10^9$/l), megakaryocytic hyperplasia in the bone marrow, with or without hyperplasia of the erythroid and the myeloid cell lines, Ph chromosome negative (though not always), increased reticulin in the bone marrow but not prominent fibrosis, no myeloid metaplasia, no increase in red cell mass, no iron deficiency, no previous myelosuppressive therapy, splenomegaly and hepatomegaly may be present. These criteria clearly illustrate the point made earlier: namely that the boundaries between the clinical entities of the CMPD are not sharp, there is overlap between them, and transitional forms occur. A secondary increase in megakaryocytes may be found in many conditions (see Chapter 3) but the polymorphism and clustering typical for megakaryocytes in the CMPD are generally not seen in the reactive states.

Chronic Myeloid Leukaemia (CML)

The Ph chromosome has been demonstrated in erythroid, myeloid and granulocytic cell lines, as well as in lymphocytes, indicating clonal origin in an early multi-potential precursor. Studies of bone biopsies have shown that they may be divided into two broad groups: the granulocytic and the granulocytic–megakaryocytic (Figs 7.48–7.50), that is expression primarily in a uni-linear or a bi-linear hyperplasia (Figs 7.51–7.56)[26]. In the uni-linear granulocytic type there are endosteal seams and perivascular cuffs of immature myeloid precursors, with mature granulocytes in the central inter-trabecular regions. Megakaryocytes may be increased, but are morphologically within normal limits, or small. There is eosinophilia and basophils are also increased, as are macrophages, many with crystalloid inclusions – the 'pseudo-Gaucher' cells[27]. The marrow is usually densely packed with few remaining fat cells. Plasma, mast and lymphoid cells and ineffective erythropoiesis with disruption of the erythrons and maturation arrest are also constant features. Reticulin, mainly perivascular, is increased[28], but a variable interstitial increase may also occur which in turn influences cellular percentages in smears of aspirates. Stainable iron is generally decreased in CML[29]. The trabeculae also undergo typical changes – they remain stout in the subcortical regions and attenuated in the deeper parts of the biopsy. Rare cases of CML have been described with granulocytic hyperplasia only of the neutrophilic, or the eosinophilic, or the basiphilic cell lines. Examples of immunohistology in the granulocytic type of CML are given in Figs 7.57–7.68. Moreover, electron microscopic studies have shown that leucocytes in CML may also have mixed granules, i.e. of more than one type[30].

In the mixed, bi-cellular type, there is both granulocytic and megakaryocytic hyperplasia – and this may be mainly of highly polymorphic megakaryocytes dispersed singly as well as clustered, or of small and micromegakaryocytes (Figs 7.69–7.75). Examples of immunohistology in the mixed type of CML are shown in Figs 7.76–7.80. With progression of disease, sequential biopsies have demonstrated: (1) transitions between these two types; (2) transformation to myelofibrosis mainly in the mixed type[31]; and (3) metamorphosis to a blast crisis, mainly in the unilinear granulocytic type, heralded by progressively wider endosteal seams of immature precursors (Figs 7.81–7.86)[3,7,32]. Phenotypic analysis in blast crisis in CML has shown that any cell line, including lymphoblastic, may be involved (Figs 7.87 and 7.88). Mixed types have also been reported.

Some studies of bone biopsies have shown that certain histological parameters have prognostic significance[32-34], though this was not the case in others[35]. Following aggressive chemotherapy the bone marrow is hypoplastic or aplastic, with dysplastic residual haematopoiesis (Figs

(Continued on p. 110)

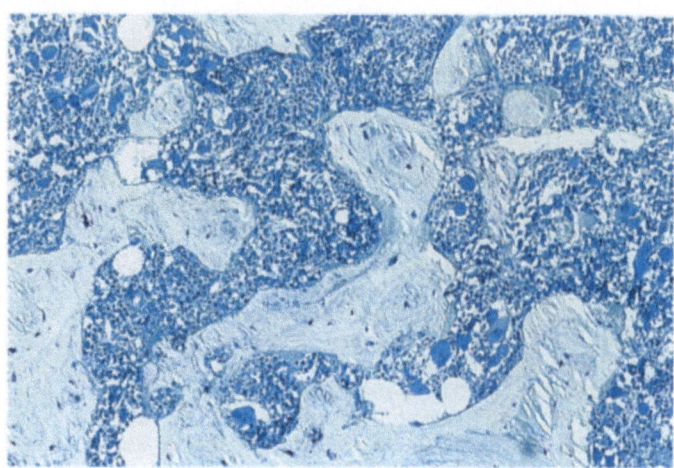

Fig. 7.20 Section of bone biopsy of patient with PV showing appositional new bone formation, indicating evolution to osteomyelosclerosis (OMS)

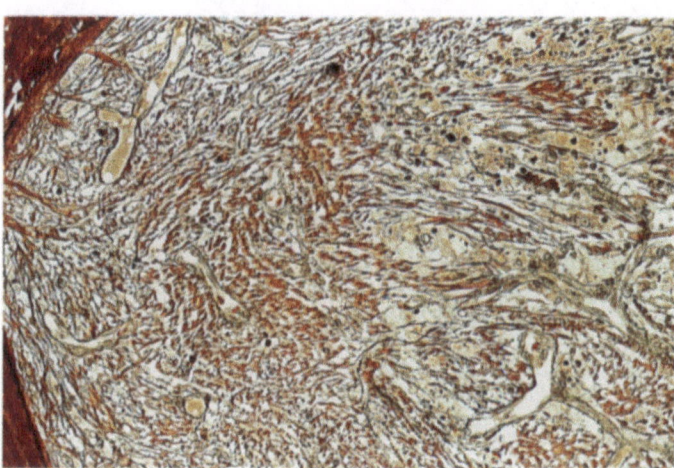

Fig. 7.21 Section of bone biopsy of patient with PV who developed MF. Note obliterative sclerosis of bone marrow

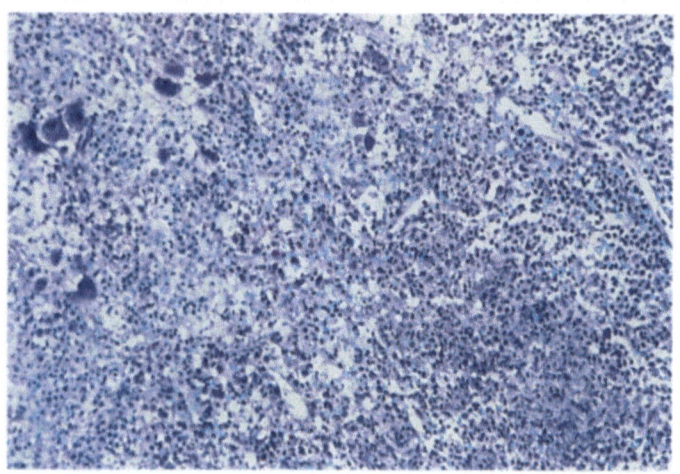

Fig. 7.22 Section of bone biopsy of patient with PV who developed a malignant lymphoma; note lymphoid cells right

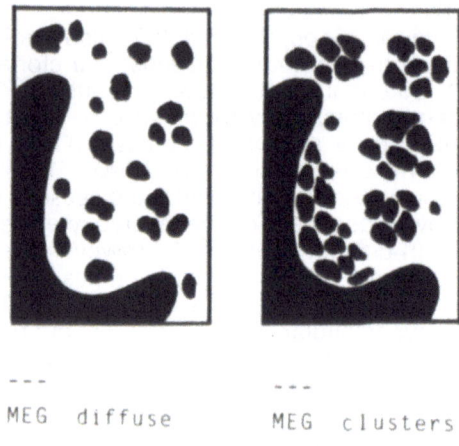

MEG diffuse   MEG clusters

Fig. 7.23 Sketch of bone biopsy in IT: dispersed and clustered pleomorphic megakaryocytes

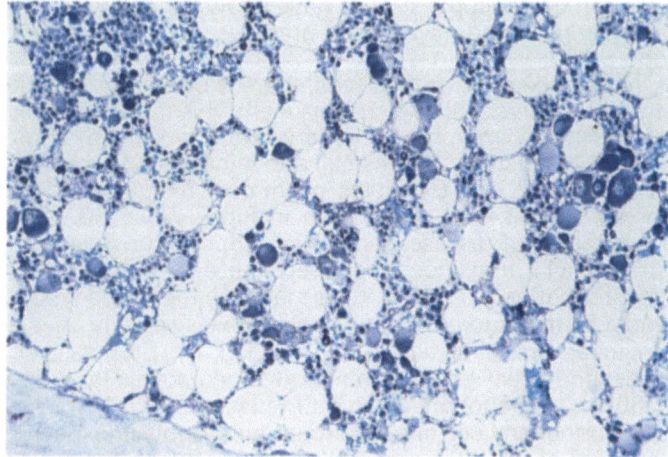

Figs 7.24–7.34 Sections of bone biopsies of patients with IT, demonstrating range in size, nuclear configuration, and topography of megakaryocytes

Fig. 7.24 Hypocellular bone marrow with megakaryocytic hyperplasia

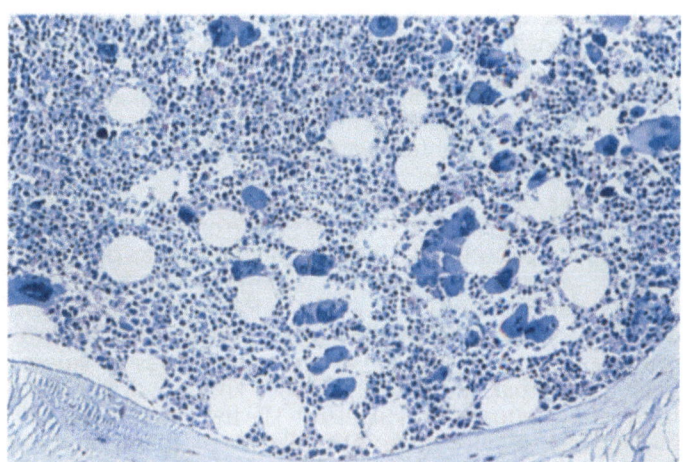

Fig. 7.25 Normocellular bone marrow with megakaryocytic hyperplasia

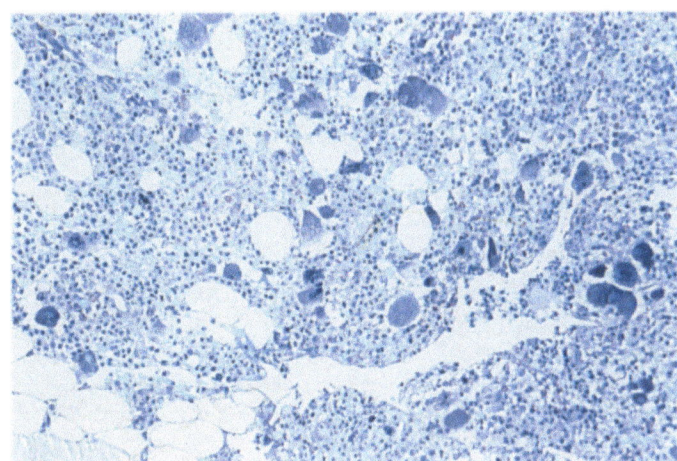

Fig. 7.26 Hypercellular bone marrow with megakaryocytic hyperplasia and clustering

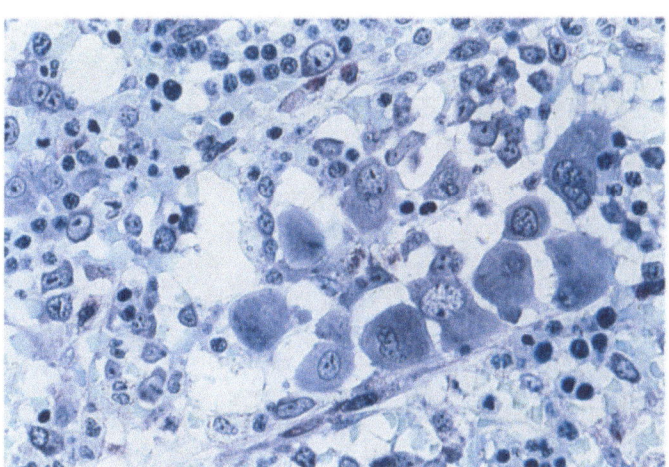

Fig. 7.27 Intravascular cluster of mainly immature megakaryocytes

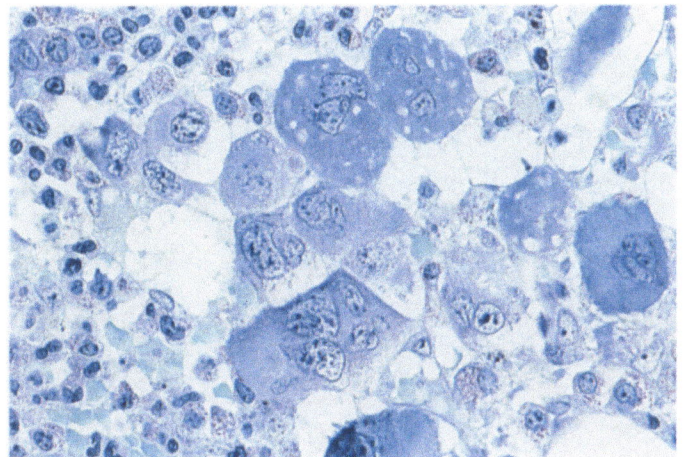

Fig. 7.28 Range in nuclear morphology of megakaryocytes in IT

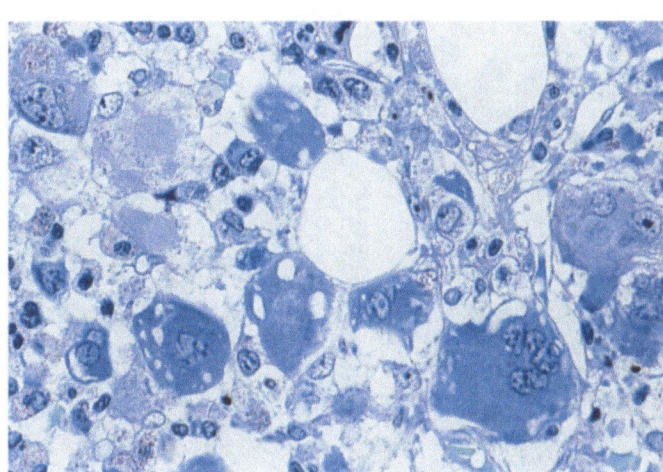

Fig. 7.29 Megakaryocytes with vacuolated cytoplasm

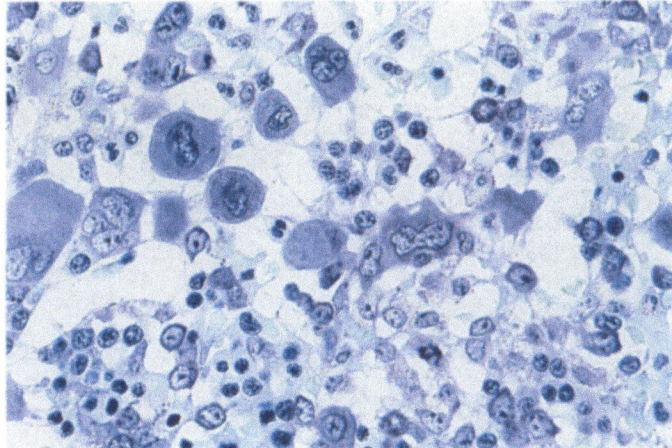

Fig. 7.30 Cluster of immature megakaryocytes in proximity to sinus

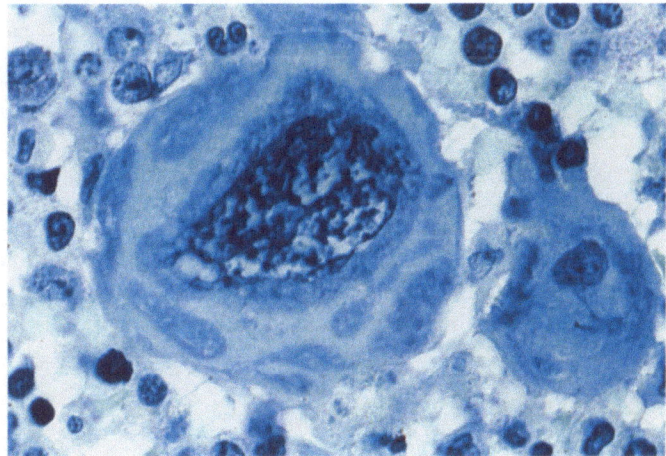

Fig. 7.31 The extreme hyperplasia of this megakaryocyte is highlighted by comparison with the cells around it

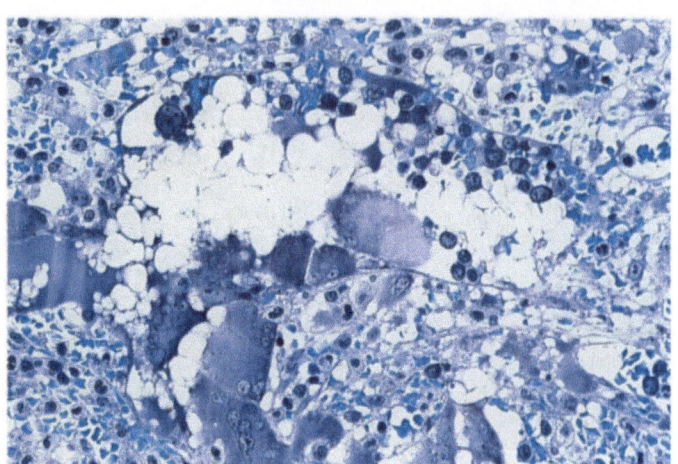

Fig. 7.32 Intra-luminal megakaryocytes lining the sinusoidal endothelium

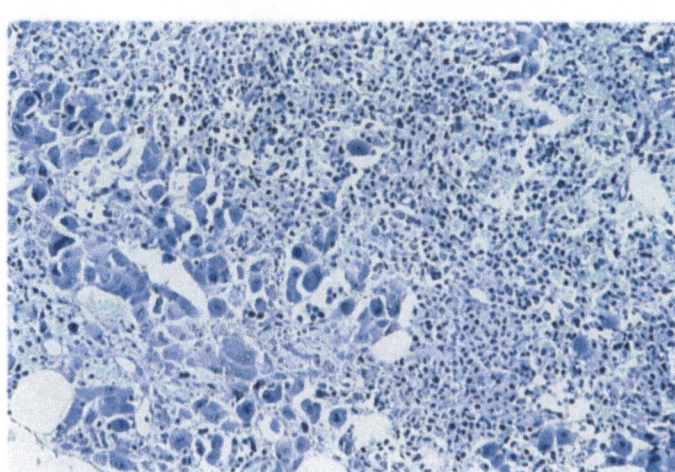

Fig. 7.33 'Compartmentalization' in the bone marrow in IT: megakaryocytes in one region, and other haematopoietic precursors in another

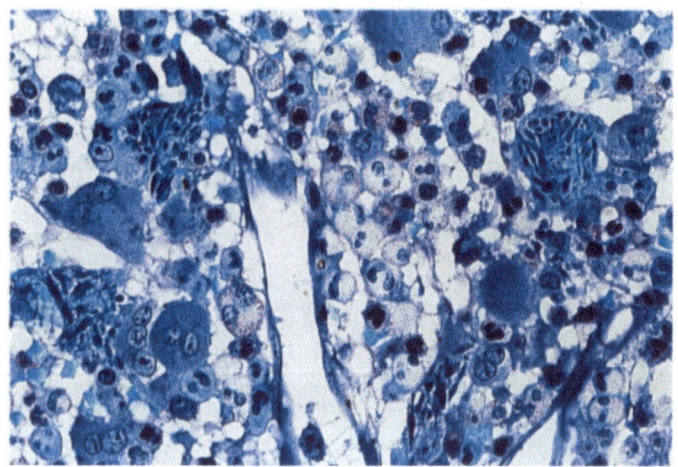

Fig. 7.34 Numerous crystal-containing macrophages in IT; these are found especially when there is also eosinophilic hyperplasia

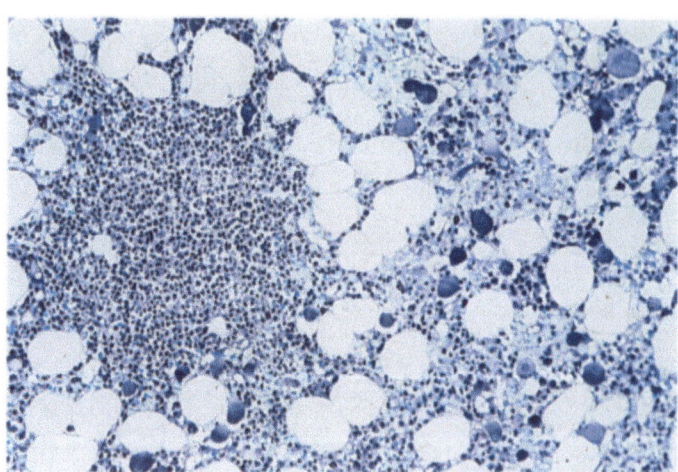

Fig. 7.35 Sections of bone biopsy of patient with IT; normocellular bone marrow, megakaryocytic hyperplasia and a lymphoid cell aggregate

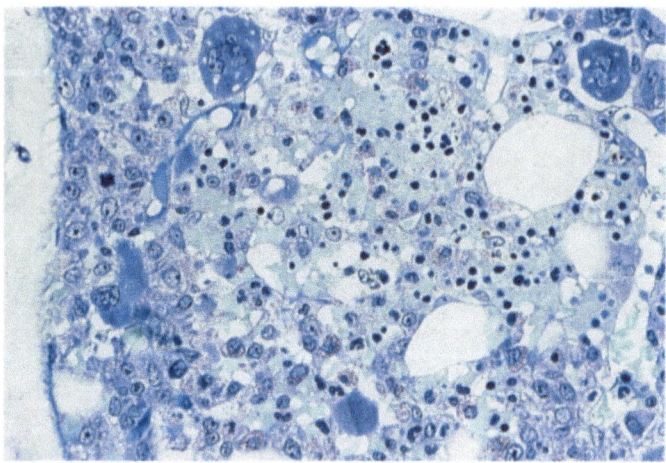

Fig. 7.36 Dyserythropoiesis in IT

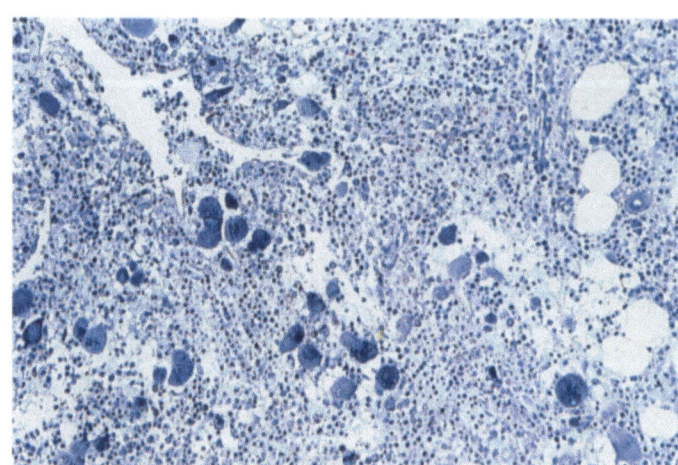

Figs 7.37–7.47 These illustrate the development of MF in IT
Fig. 7.37 Note incipient fibrosis in hypercellular bone marrow

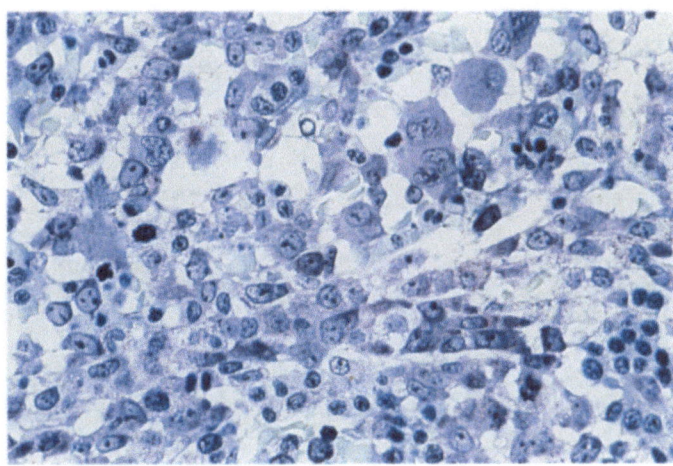

Fig. 7.38 Higher magnification of area from Fig. 7.37 showing incipient 'linear' effect, with developing fibrosis

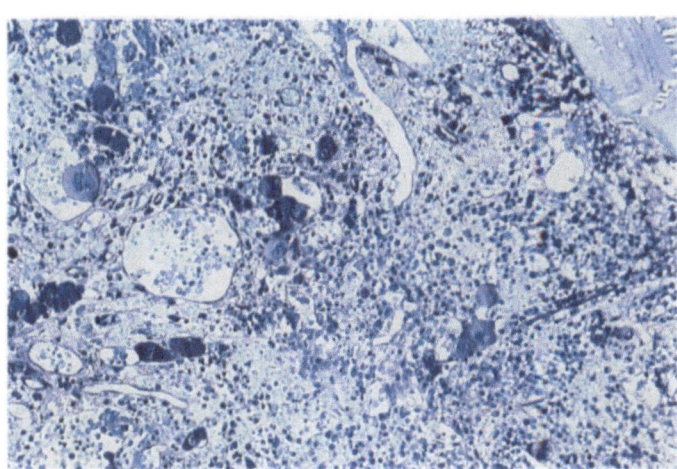

Fig. 7.39 Cellular bone marrow, but less dense as fibrosis develops

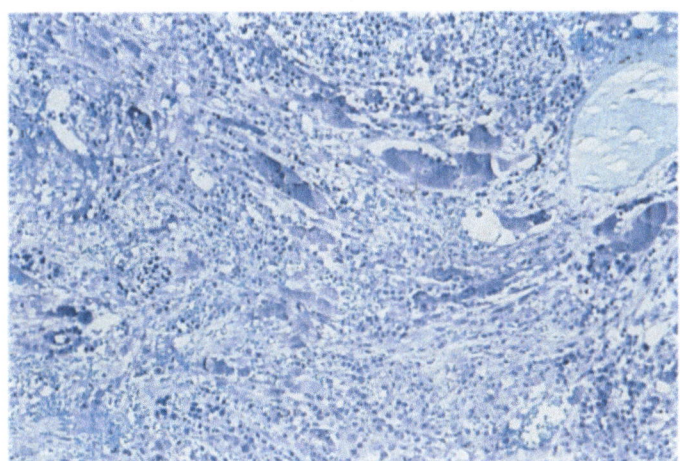

Fig. 7.40 Developing fibrosis in association with trabecular bone

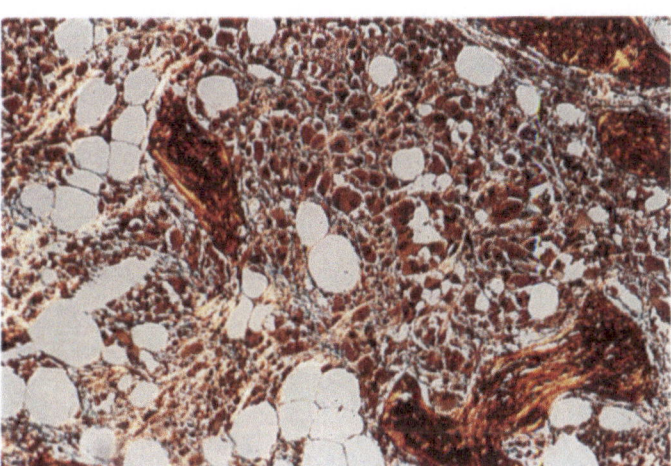

Fig. 7.41 Gomori's stain, viewed in polarized light, showing increase of fibres in the bone marrow

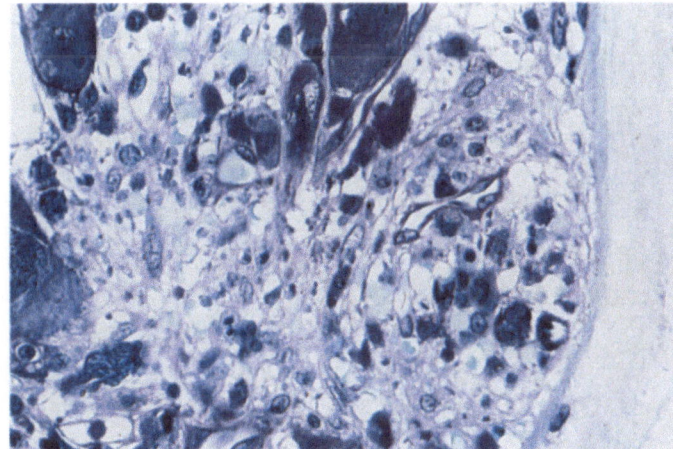

Fig. 7.42 Section of bone biopsy of patient with IT and decreasing platelet count. Note megakaryocytes within the marrow not in proximity to sinusoids, and platelets in the interstitium

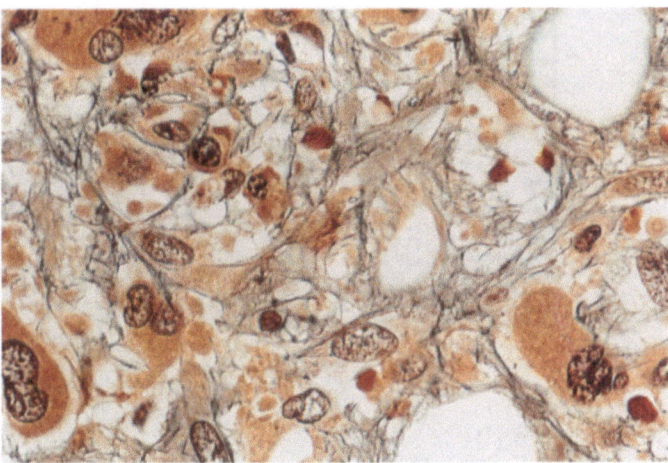

Fig. 7.43 Fine fibre network in association with megakaryocytes

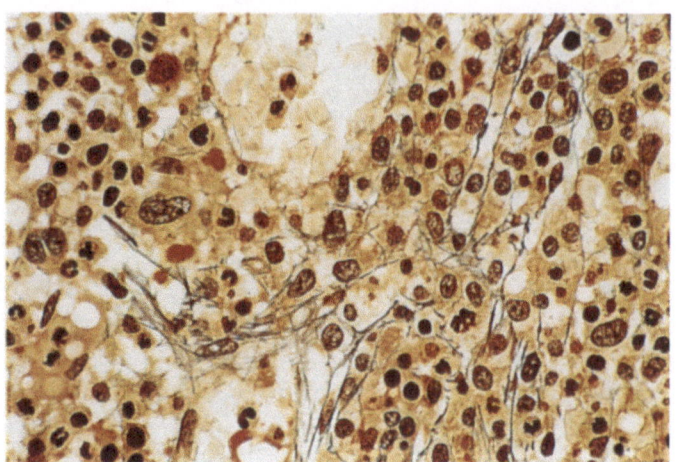

Fig. 7.44   Fibres between other haematopoietic elements

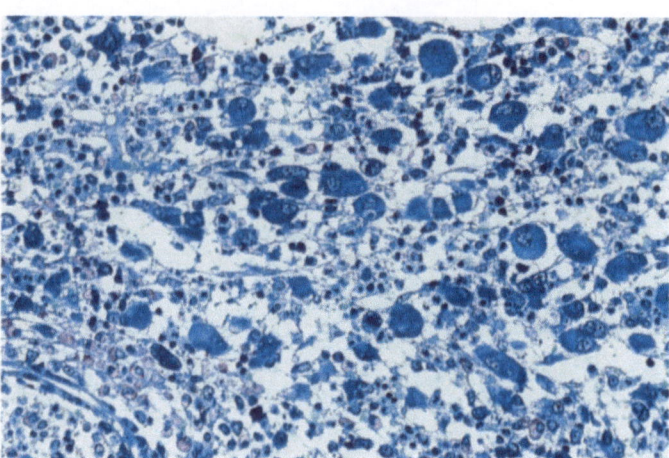

Figs 7.45 and 7.46   Transition to an immature form in IT with fall in peripheral platelet count; note few mature megakaryocytes

Fig. 7.45   Overview of hyperplastic megakaryocytes

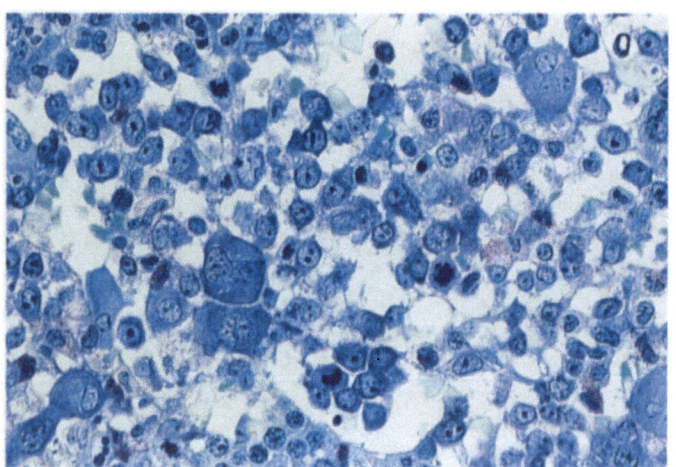

Fig. 7.46   Higher magnification illustrating mainly small, immature megakaryocytes

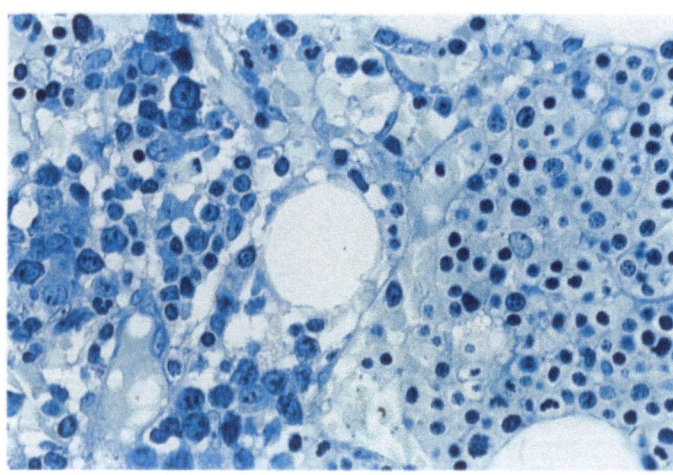

Fig. 7.47   Disorganization of erythropoiesis in IT with development of MF. Large erythroid islands with erythroblasts at similar stages of development

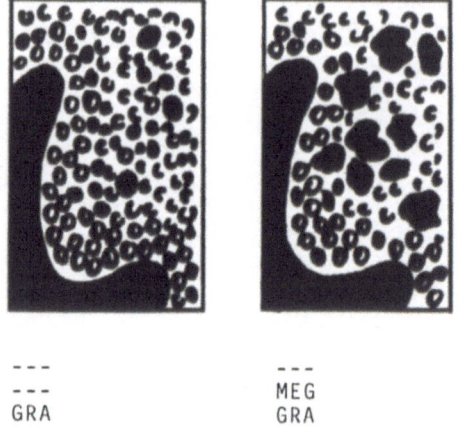

Fig. 7.48   Sketch of the granulocytic and mixed granulocytic-megakaryocytic types of CML

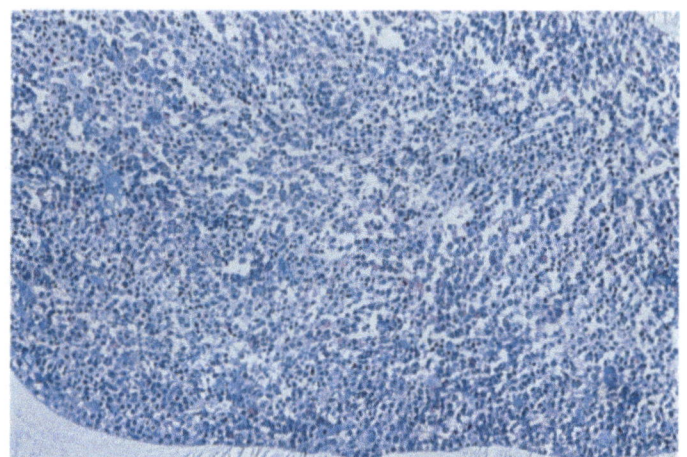

Fig. 7.49   Section of bone biopsy of patient with CML; bone marrow consisting mainly of hyperplastic granulopoiesis

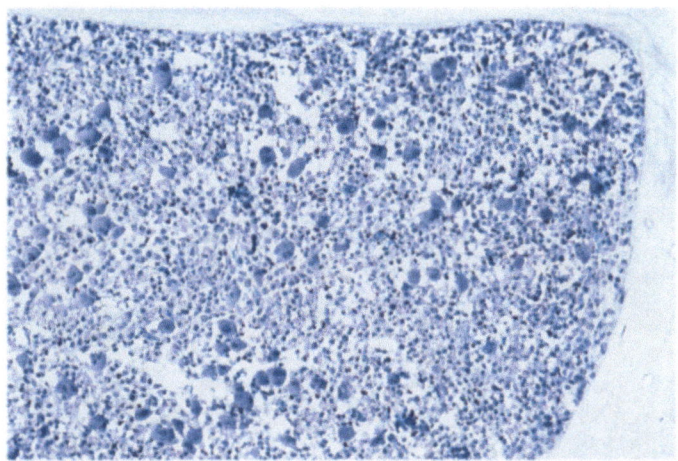

Fig. 7.50 Bone marrow showing the mixed granulo- and megakaryo-cytic hyperplasia, most of the megakaryocytes are small

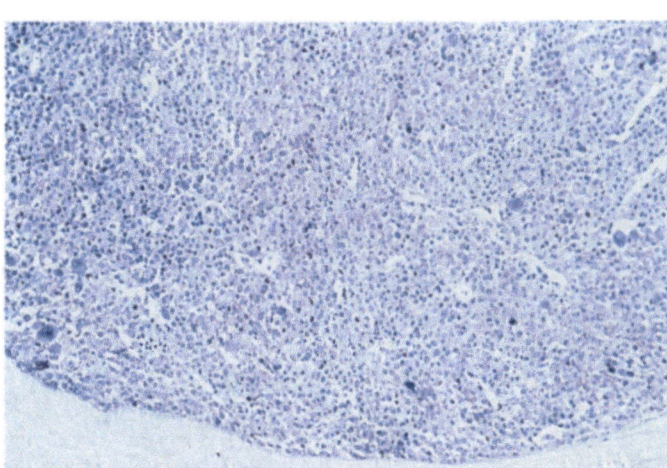

Figs 7.51 and 7.54 Densely packed marrow in mainly neutrophilic CML

Fig. 7.51 Low-power view

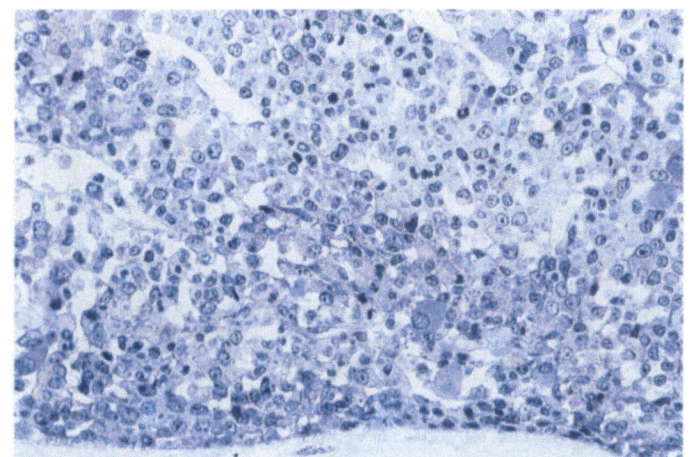

Fig. 7.52 High-power view showing immature cells at osseous surface

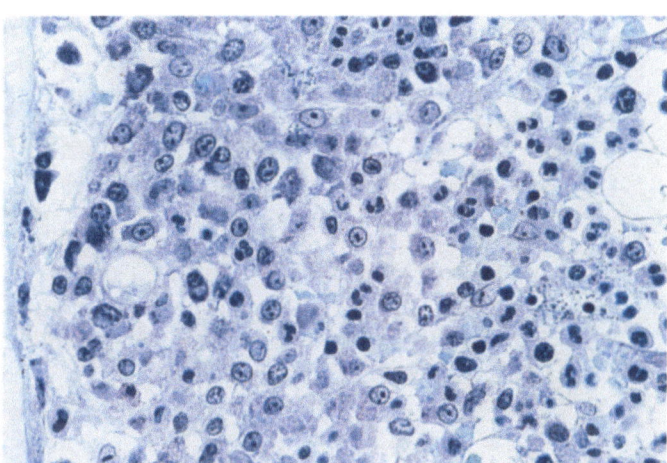

Fig. 7.53 Maturing granulocytes nearer the central marrow area

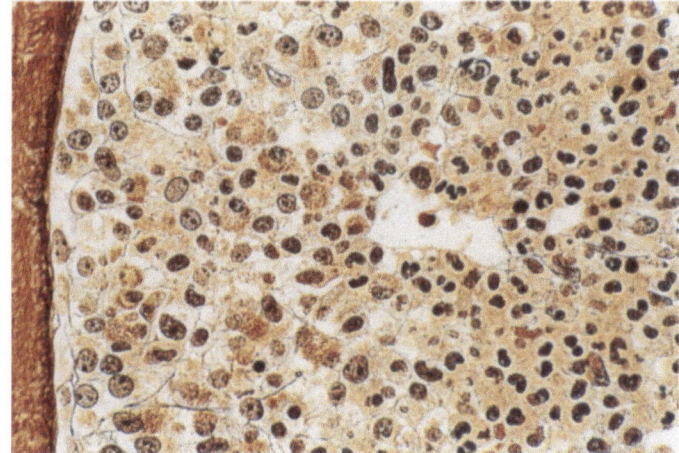

Fig. 7.54 Section stained with Gomori's stain – only a few fine reticular fibres are seen

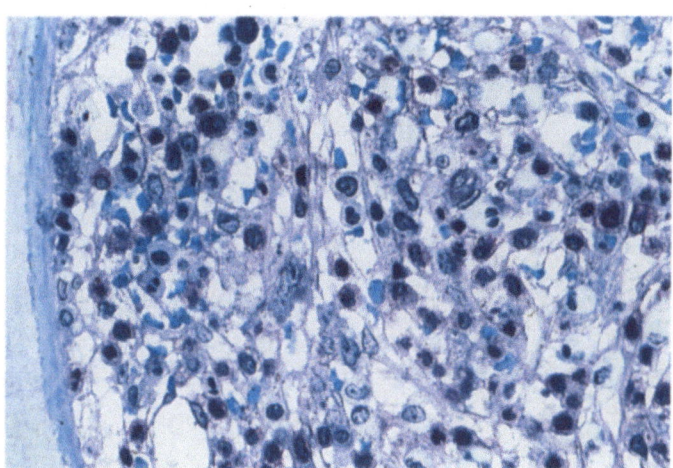

Fig. 7.55 Paratrabecular granulopoiesis – neutro-, eosino- and baso-philic precursors present

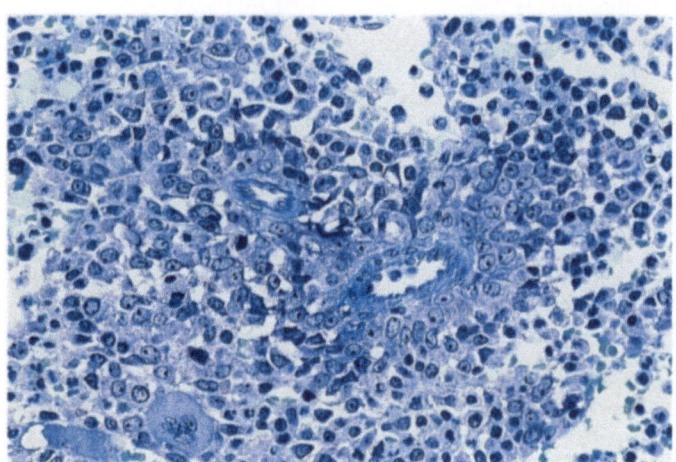

Fig. 7.56   Perivascular granulopoiesis in CML

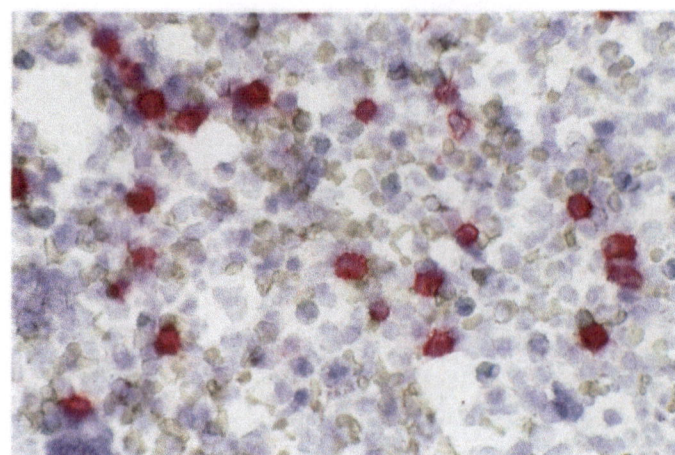

Figs 7.57–7.68   Immunohistochemistry in a case of CML; cryostat sections

Fig. 7.57   B lymphocytes identified by their reaction with CD22

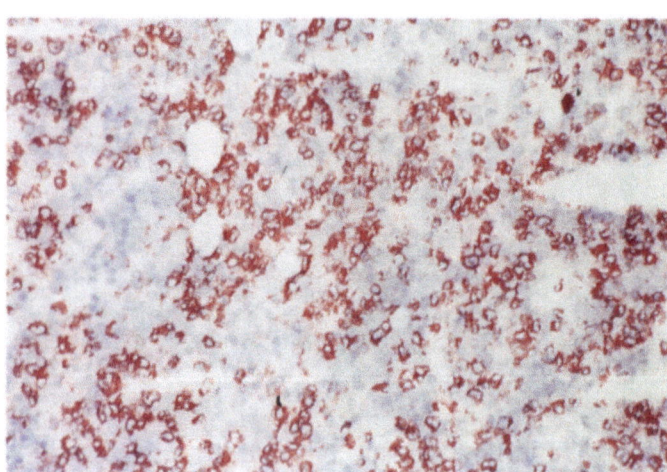

Fig. 7.58   Demonstration of reaction with VIM2 which reacts with myeloid and monocytic cells

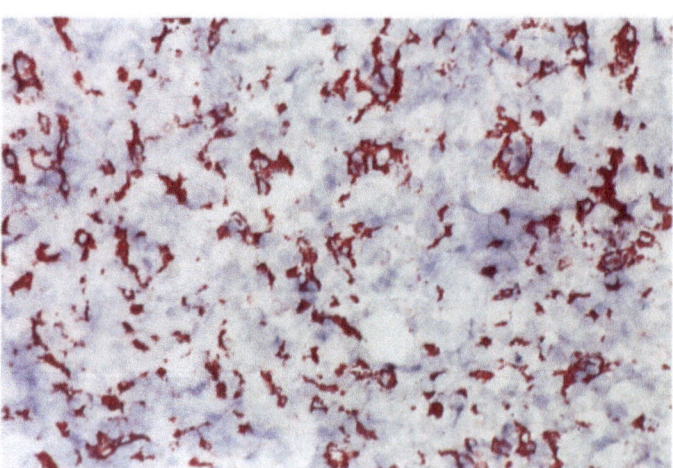

Fig. 7.59   Demonstration of monocytes and macrophages by the antibody KIM8

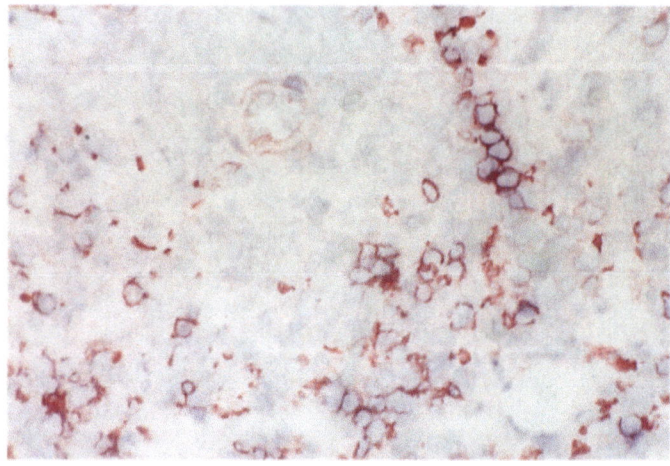

Fig. 7.60   Erythropoiesis demonstrated by the reaction to VIEG4

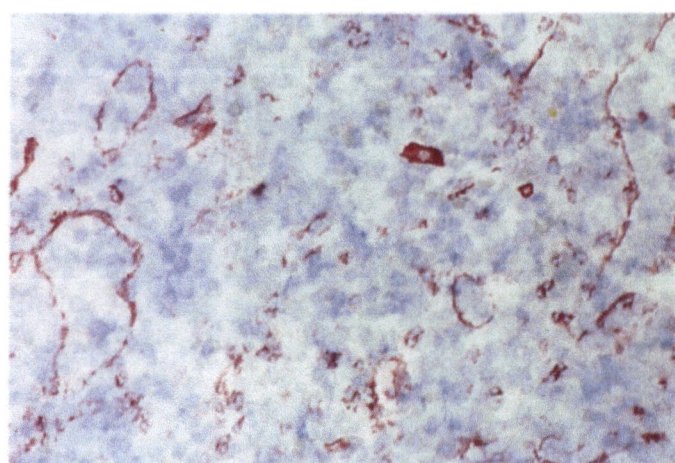

Fig. 7.61   Monocytes and endothelial cells recognised by the antibody VIMD2

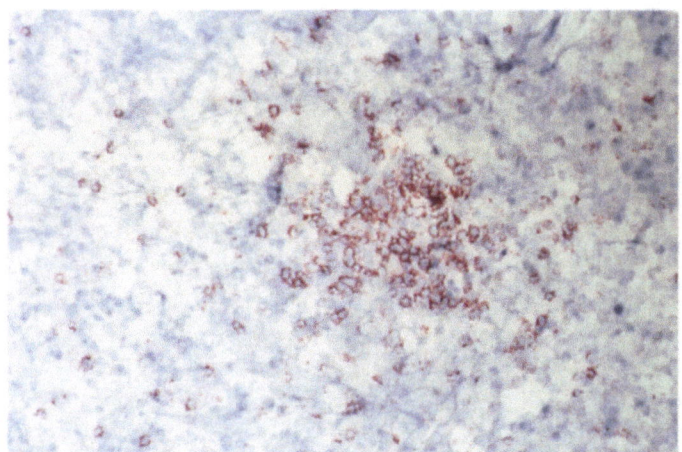

Fig. 7.62 Aggregate of T lymphocytes, positive with CD2

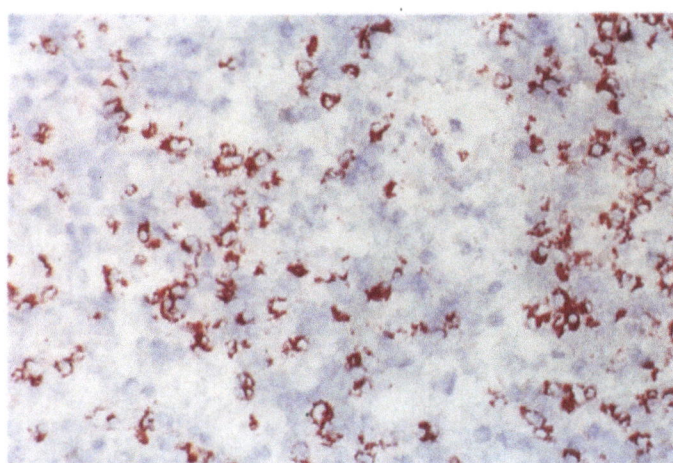

Figs 7.63–7.65 Same case as above, 2 months after bone marrow transplantation; bone biopsy taken during remission

Fig. 7.63 Demonstration of granulocytes of their reaction with VIM8

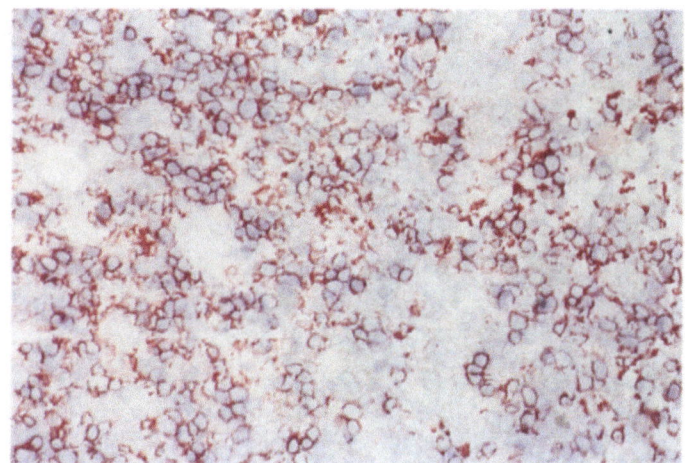

Fig. 7.64 Restitution of erythropoiesis demonstrated by reactivity with the antigen VIEG4

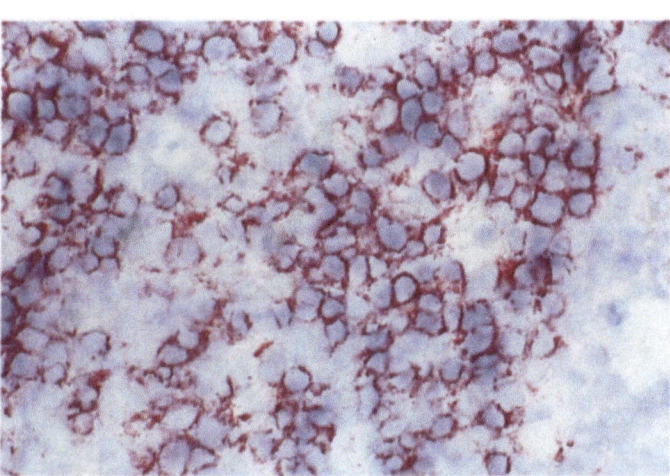

Fig. 7.65 Numerous precursors are positive with the antibody to transferrin receptor

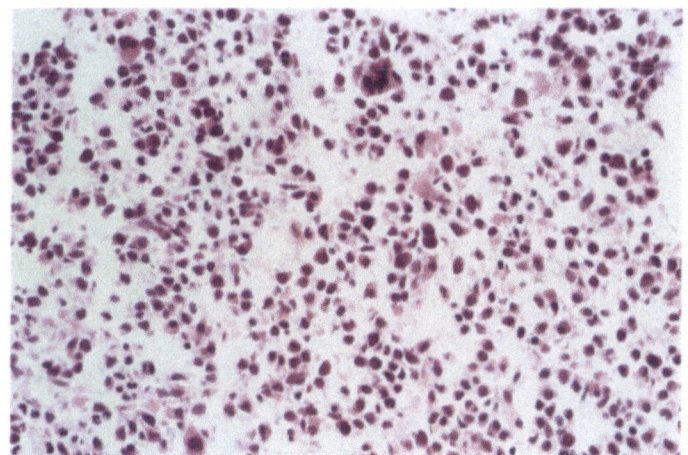

Fig. 7.66 Relapse 6 months after bone marrow transplantation. H&E

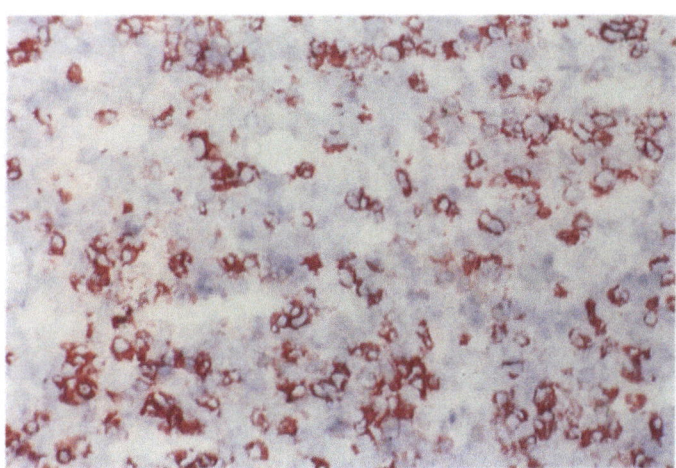

Fig. 7.67 Same as Fig. 7.66. Myelomonocytes stained by the antibody VIM2

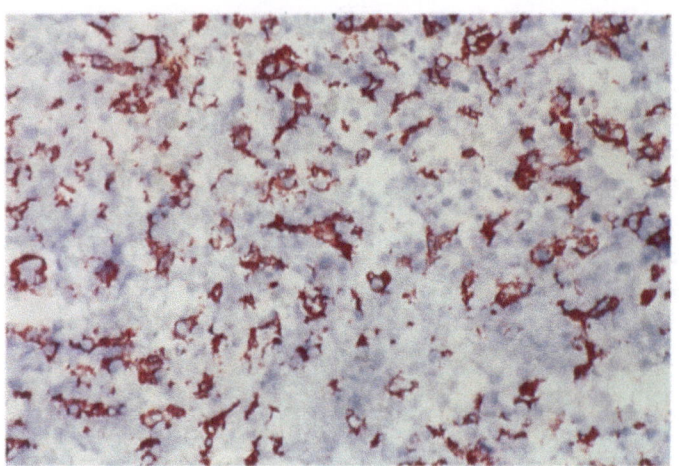

Fig. 7.68 Same as Fig. 7.66. Numerous monocytes and macrophages stained by the antibody KIM8, more than could be identified in the H&E-stained section (Fig. 7.66)

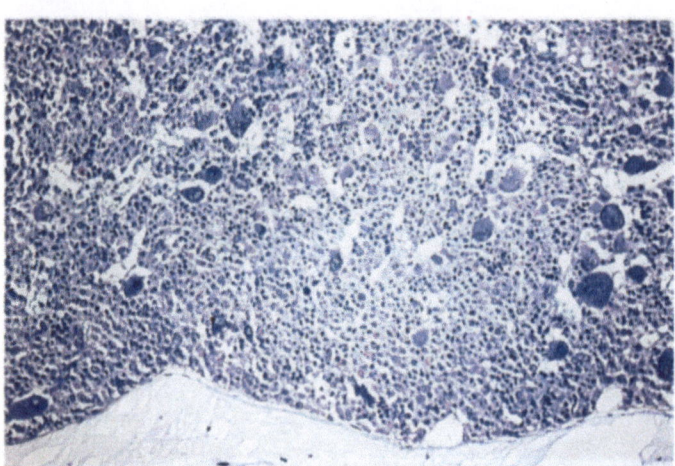

Figs 7.69–7.75 Bone marrow histology in the mixed granulocytic–megakaryocytic type of CML

Fig. 7.69 Note range in megakaryocyte size

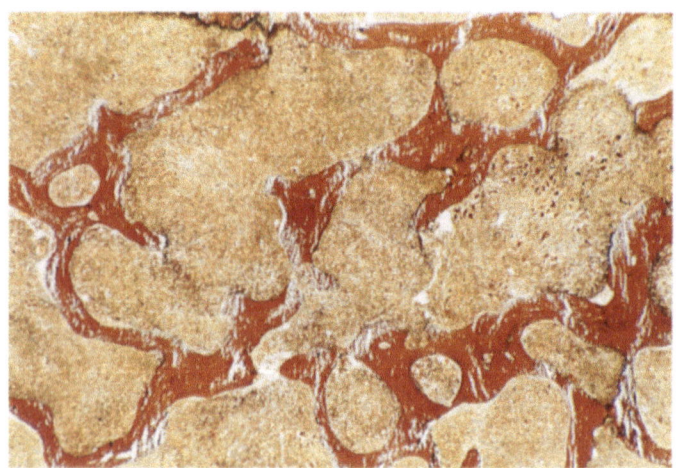

Fig. 7.70 Low-power view of section of patient with the mixed type of CML, showing uneven distribution of megakaryocytes. Gomori.

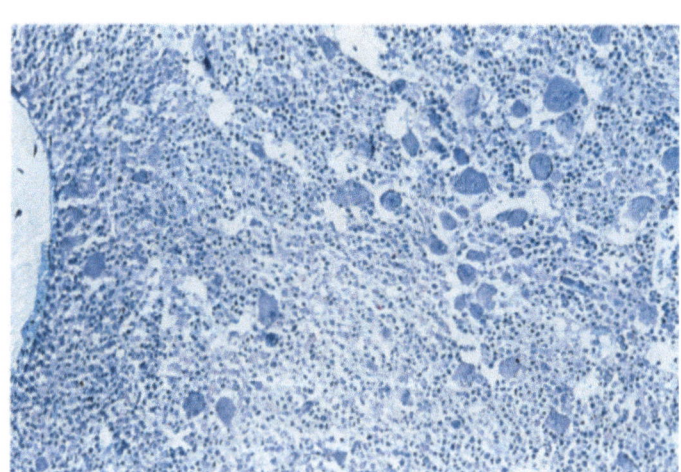

Fig. 7.71 Higher magnification of clusters of megakaryocytes

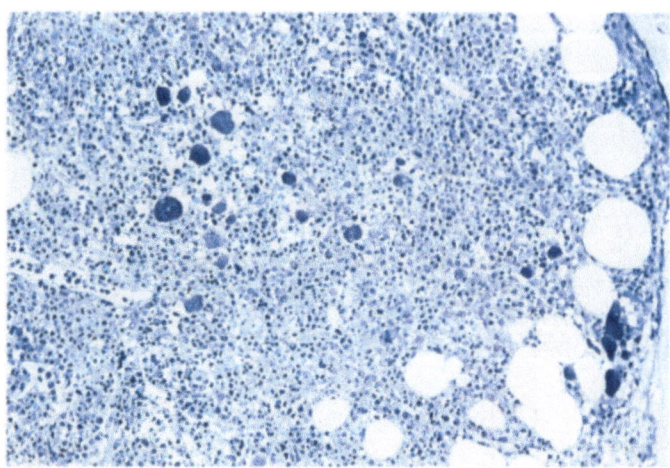

Fig. 7.72 Residual fat cells, and megakaryocytes at trabecular surface in CML

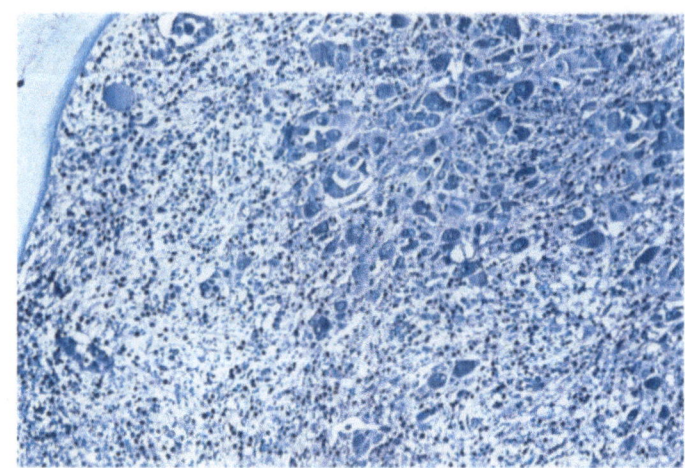

Figs 7.73 and 7.74 Transition to a more immature type in CML

Fig. 7.73 Granulopoiesis at trabecular surface

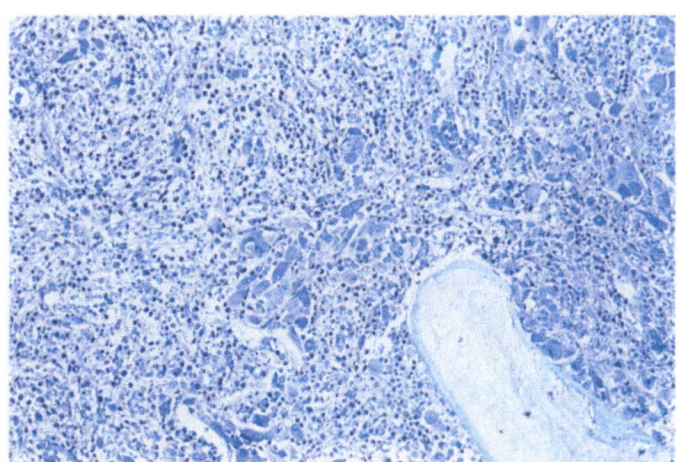

Fig. 7.74 Hyperplastic and immature megakaryocytes surrounding an ossicle

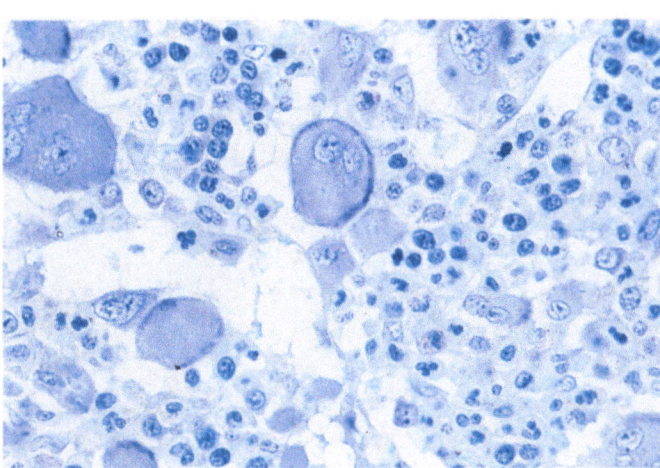

Fig. 7.75 Range in size of megakaryocytes. Note areas of variably stained cytoplasma

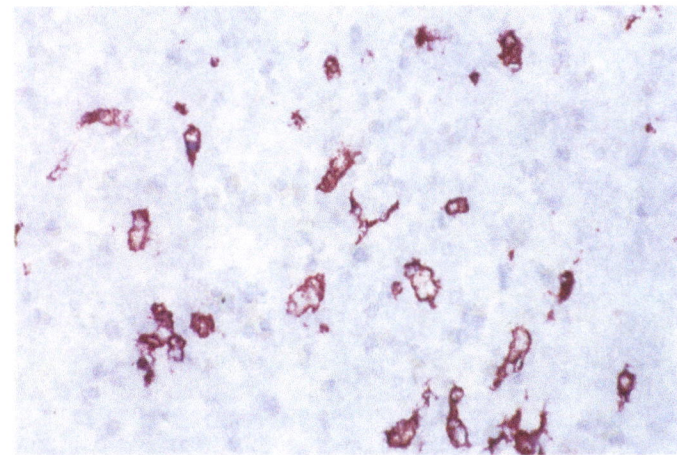

Figs 7.76–7.80 Immunohistochemistry in the mixed type of CML

Fig. 7.76 Demonstration of monocytes and macrophages by their reaction with KIM8

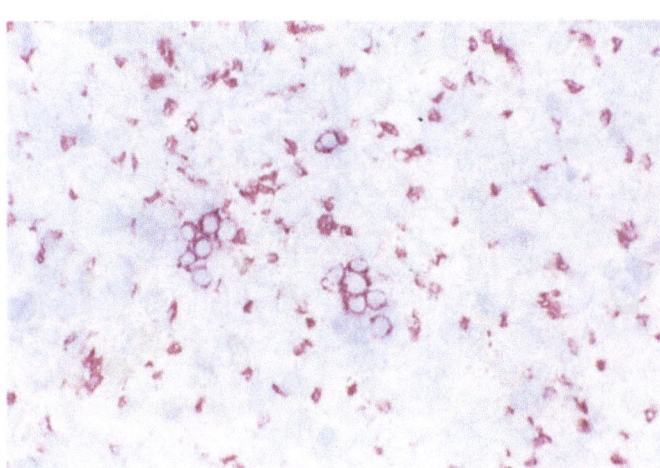

Fig. 7.77 Demonstration of residual erythropoiesis by staining with the antibody VIEG4

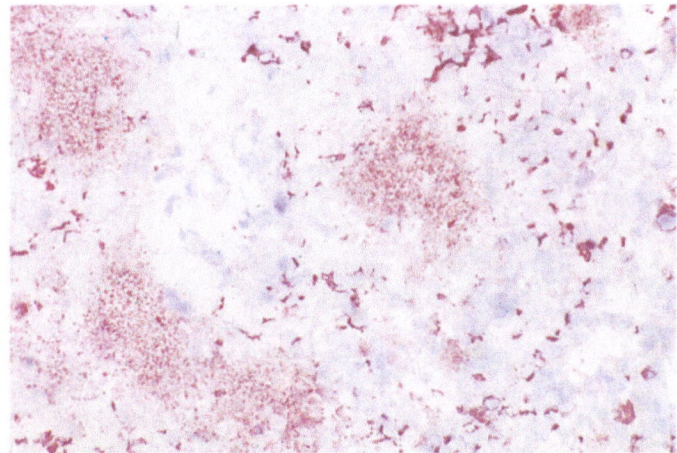

Fig. 7.78 Erythroid precursors stained by the antibody VIEG4. Note aggregates of erythrocytes in sinusoids

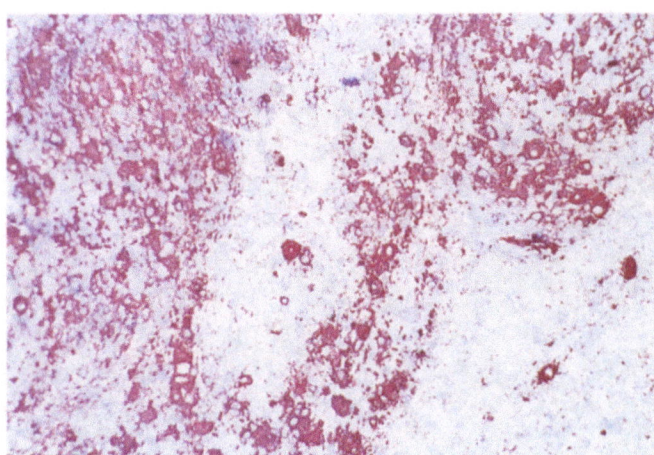

Fig. 7.79 Clusters of megakaryocytes demonstrated by reaction with the antibody VIPL1

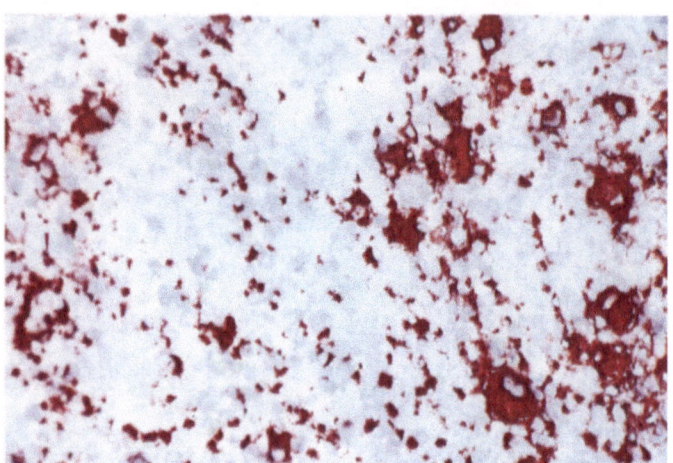

Fig. 7.80 Megakaryocytes and interstitial platelets demonstrated by the antibody VIPL1

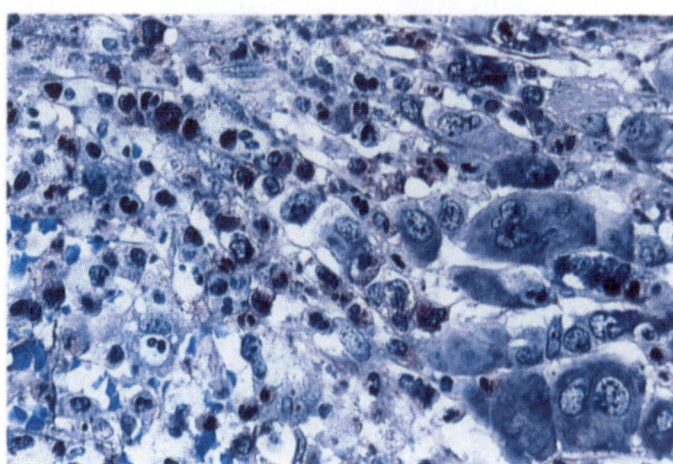

Figs 7.81–7.94 Evolution of CML
Fig. 7.81 Increasing hyperplasia of megakaryocytes

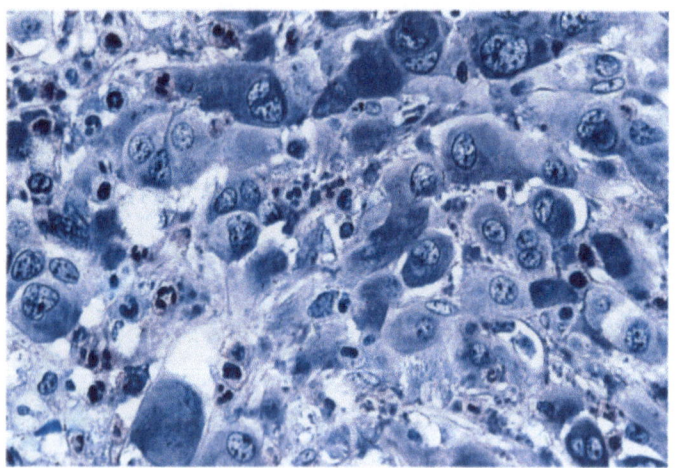

Fig. 7.82 Same case as in Fig. 7.81; the hyperplastic megakaryocytes include many mononuclear and immature forms

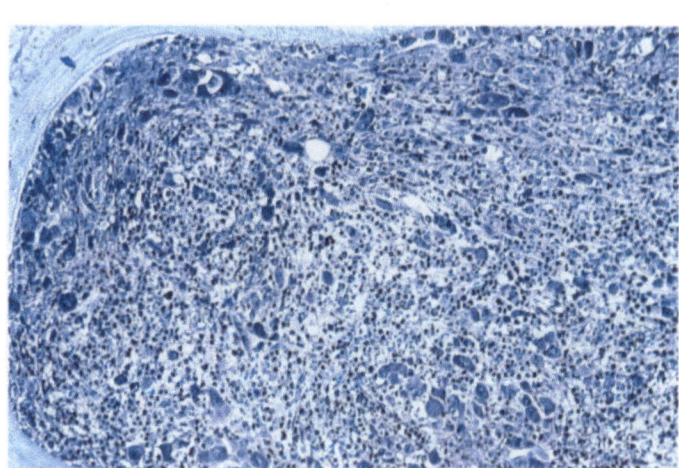

Fig. 7.83 Development of MF in mixed type of CML

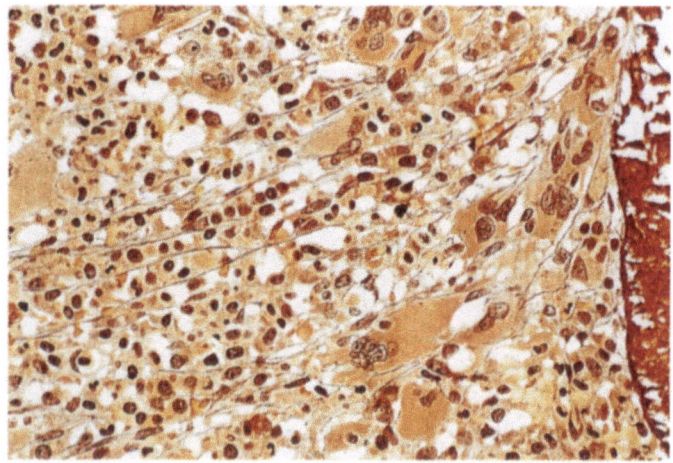

Fig. 7.84 Same case as in Fig. 7.83; higher magnification to show reticulin fibres

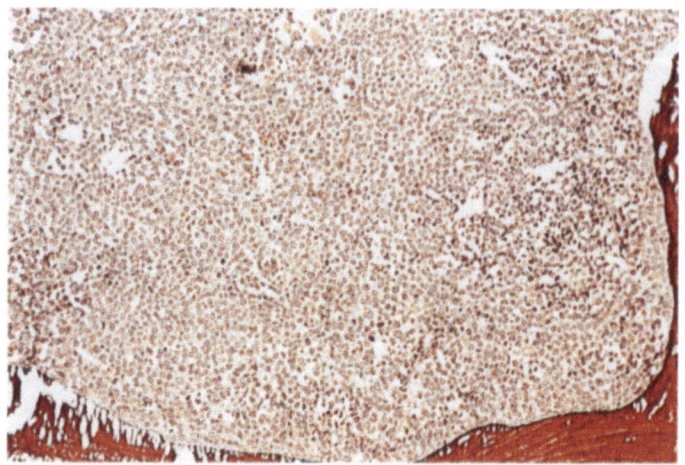

Fig. 7.85 Blast crisis in CML; the blasts extend from the trabecular surface to the central region of the marrow space

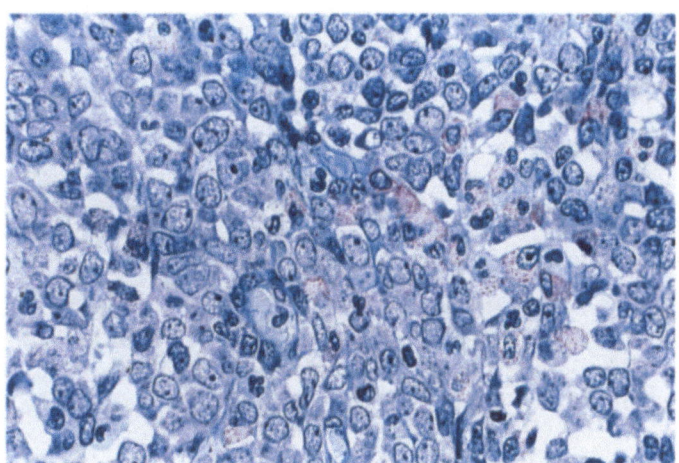

Fig. 7.86 Perivascular blasts in blast crisis

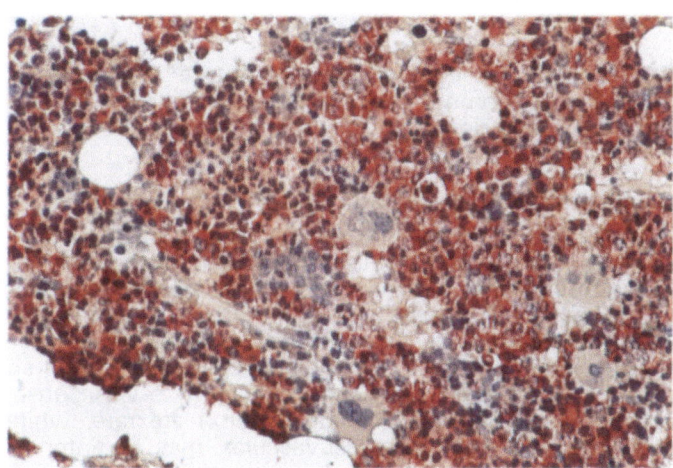

Fig. 7.87 Section of paraffin-embedded bone biopsy, Leder's stain demonstrating granulopoiesis in CML

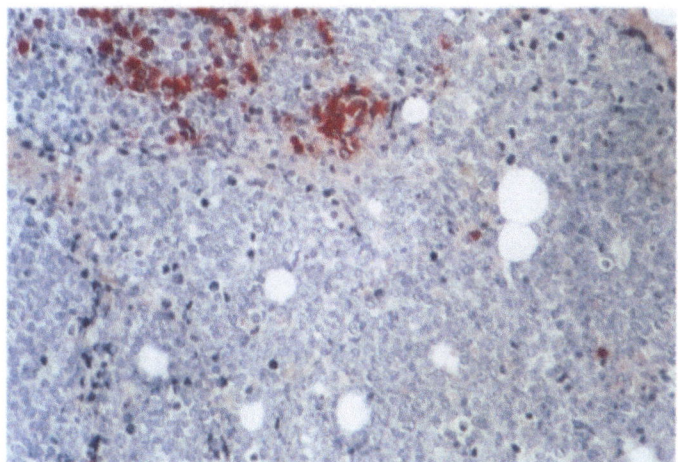

Fig. 7.88 Same case as Fig. 7.87; biopsy taken during blast crisis, lymphoid phenotype, section stained by Leder's stain. Few positive (myeloid) cells remain

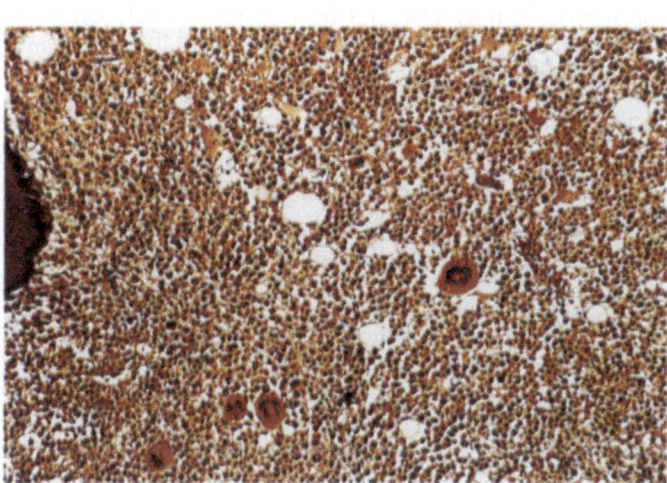

Fig. 7.89 Section of bone biopsy of patient with CML at presentation, stained by Gomori. There are few megakaryocytes, and reticular fibres are virtually absent

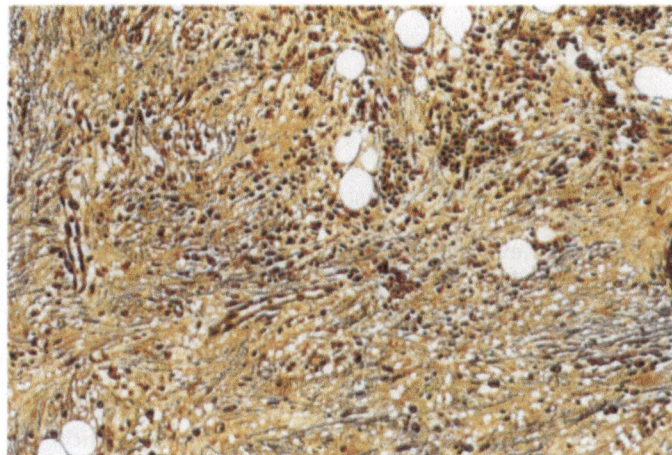

Fig. 7.90 Section of bone biopsy of same patient as Fig. 7.89 after chemotherapy, showing myelodysplasia with fibrosis

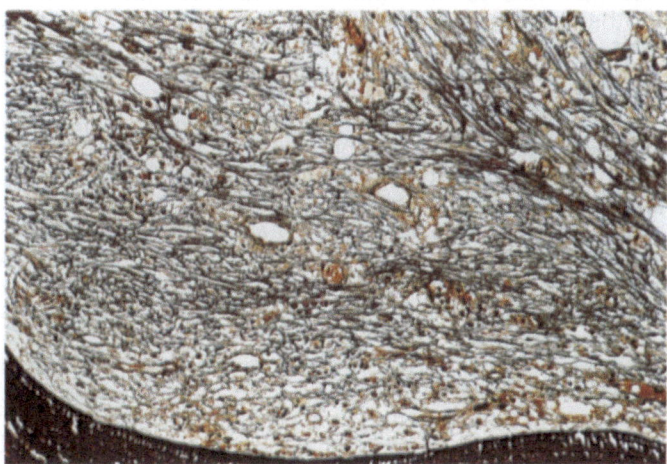

Fig. 7.91 Same patient as above, several months later, bone biopsy section showing obliterative myelofibrosis

7.89–7.93). Subsequent development of myelofibrosis may occur in some cases. Lymphoproliferative disorders have also been documented in patients with CML[36].

Differential Diagnosis of Bone Biopsies in CML

When only bone marrow histology is assessed, diagnostic difficulties may arise: the histological distinction between neutrophilic CML and a leukaemoid reaction, or between eosinophilic CML, the hyper-eosinophilic syndrome and reactive eosinophilia, may not be possible (Figs 7.94–7.96). However, in the reactive states fat cells are not so drastically reduced, the overall cellularity is less dense, macrophages with crystalloid inclusion are rare, while plasmacytosis, especially perivascular, may be intense. There is no basophilia, megakaryocytes are only moderately increased, without the morphological anomalies and clustering that may be seen in CML. Except in elderly patients with osteoporosis the trabecular bone structure is within normal limits. The abrupt transition from paratrabecular myeloblast seams to mature granulocytes occasionally seen in CML is not a feature of the reactive conditions. It may also not be possible, purely on bone marrow histology, to distinguish CML from the hyperplastic phase of MF. However, among other indications, the latter has a high leucocyte alkaline phosphatase (LAP) and few basophils in the peripheral blood.

Myelofibrosis/Osteomyelosclerosis (MF/OMS)

Myelofibrosis or myelosclerosis is taken to mean an increase in reticulin and collagenous fibres in the bone marrow (Fig. 7.97)[37]. The term osteomyelosclerosis is used when increased new bone formation – appositional, woven, or both – is also present in the histological sections of the bone marrow biopsy. Fibrosis in the bone marrow may be divided into five major groups, according to the aetiology or the stimulating agents[38]: as a consequence of (1) neoplastic myeloproliferative diseases, (2) neoplastic lymphoproliferative disorders, (3) extramedullary neoplasias growing in the bone marrow, (4) osseous disorders with augmented remodelling such as hyperparathyroidism and Paget's disease of bone, and (5) inflammatory reactions due to toxins, drugs, immune complexes and other unidentified aetiological agents. As indicated in the previous section, any of the myeloproliferative disorders – acute, subacute and chronic and the myelodysplasias – may give rise to myelofibrosis. Moreover, transition to another myeloproliferative disorder – for example a blast crisis, that is acute leukaemia – can also develop in established myelofibrosis/osteomyelosclerosis[39] (see also Figs 7.115–7.117 and 7.140–7.145).

In addition, those cases in the MPD with proliferation of megakaryocytes have a particular tendency to develop myelofibrosis/osteomyelosclerosis (Fig. 7.98). Generally, the development of fibrosis in the bone marrow runs a slowly progressive course over years. However, a rapidly progressive bone marrow fibrosis, often fatal, may also supervene in the course of other haematological malignancies, whether or not some degree of fibrosis was already present.

Fibrosis in the bone marrow may be roughly divided into three grades (Figs 7.99–7.115) depending on the degree of fibrosis present, and the same may be done for the increase in bone in osteomyelosclerosis. The increased bone present may be due to appositional osteoblastic new bone formation or to the formation of primitive woven bone within the marrow spaces, or by a combination of these processes. The mineralization of this new bone is variable – so that there may be a low or high proportion of osteoid present. Eventually, the normal trabecular structure may be completely replaced by a network of

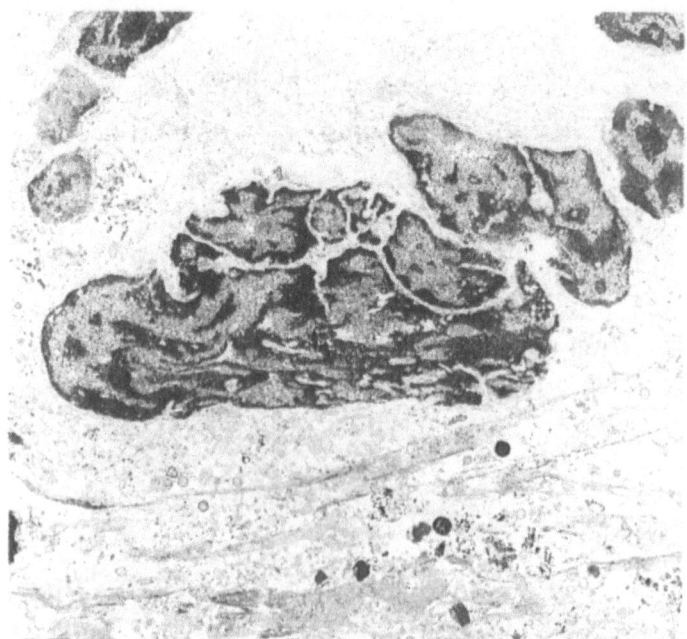

Fig. 7.105 Almost bare megakaryocyte nucleus. × 15 000

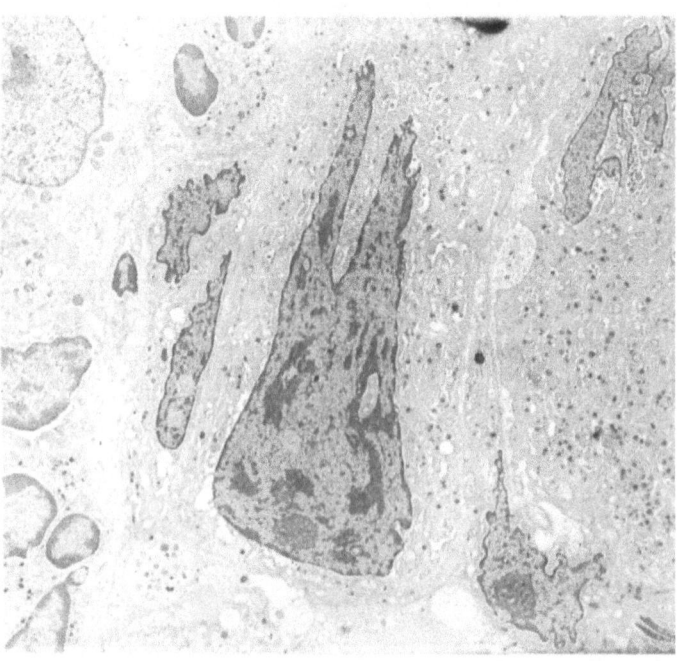

Fig. 7.106 Distortion of shape of megakaryocyte lying in fibrotic area. × 15 000

new bone. Osteolytic lesions may also occur[40] (Figs 7.118–7.133).

Fibrosis inevitably results in the disruption and eventual effacement of the normal architecture of the bone marrow. Initially areas of haematopoietic precursors are segregated into separate compartments by bands of connective tissue in the form of a diffuse network of coarse fibres (collagen Type III) and blood vessels. In addition to the hyperplasia and pleomorphism of megakaryocytes, the erythroid and myeloid precursors may show maturation inhibition, left shift and dysplastic features. Preservation of fat cells, in spite of a reduction in the amount of haematopoiesis, occurs especially in OMS, and there are differences in its distribution – paratrabecular in some cases and central intertrabecular in others. In MF the trabecular bone shows rarefaction without increased osteoclastic remodelling.

To some extent, bone marrow histology may reflect the

(Continued on p. 115)

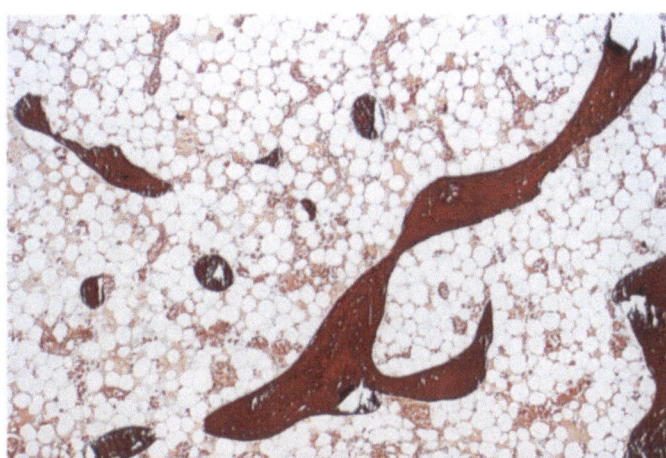

Fig. 7.92 Section of bone biopsy of patient with CML treated with chemotherapy showing aplastic bone marrow, stained with Gomori's stain, overview

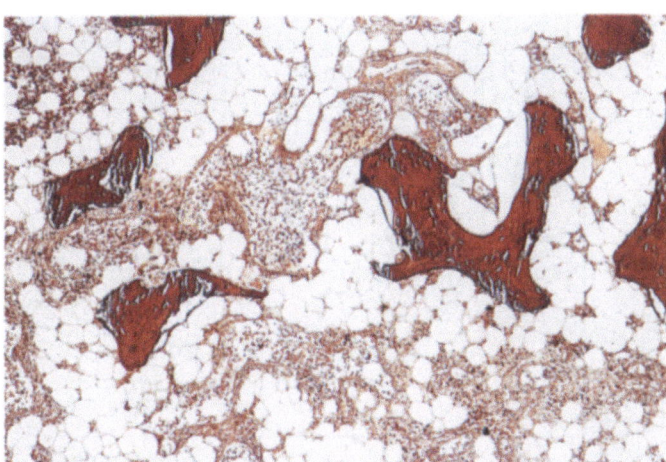

Fig. 7.93 Section of bone biopsy showing disorganization of marrow and ectatic sinusoids after therapy for CML, same case as in Fig. 7.92, higher magnification

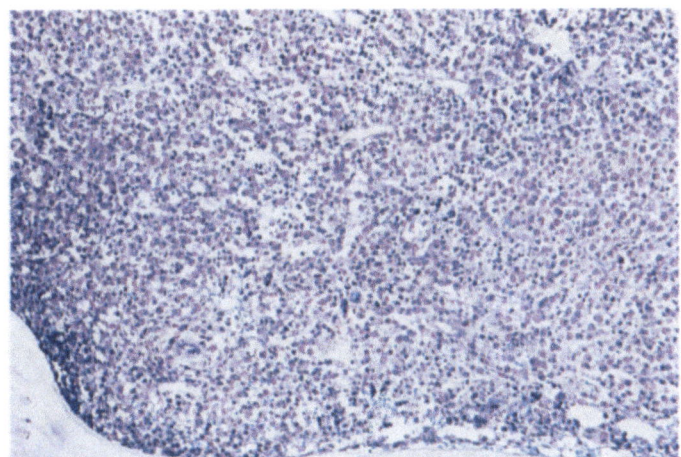

Fig. 7.94 CML with hyperplasia of the eosinophilic cell line

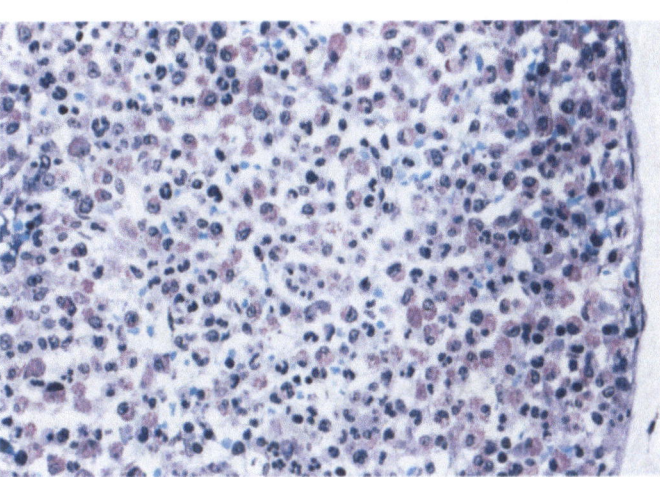

Fig. 7.95 Same as Fig. 7.94, showing immature eosinophilic precursors at the trabecular surface

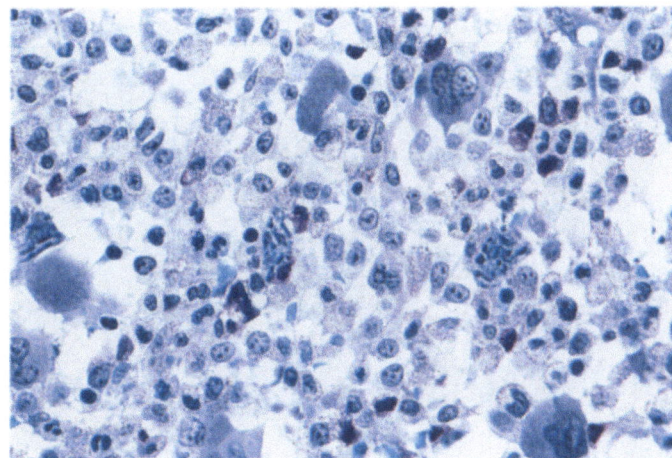

Fig. 7.96 Crystal-containing macrophages in CML

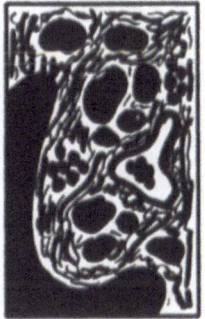

MFS   OMS

Fig. 7.97 Sketch of bone biopsy sections in full-blown MF and OMS. In MF there is myelofibrosis, while in OMS the marrow cavities are also decreased by the additional bone. There are polymorphous megakaryocytes, ectatic sinusoids and intravascular haematopoietic precursors in both MF and OMS

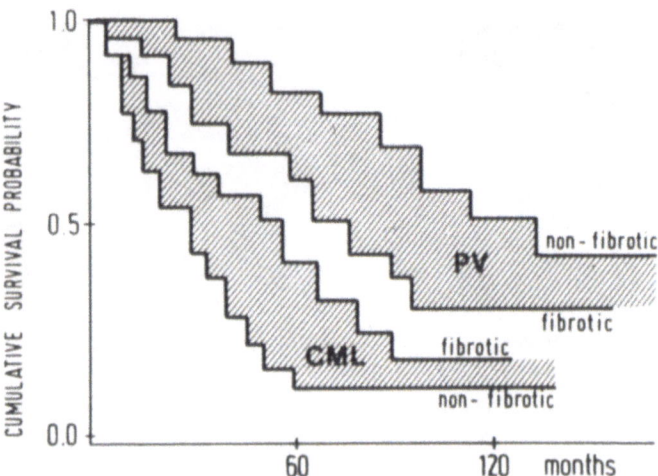

Fig. 7.98 Curves showing cumulative survivals of patients with PV and CML, based on the presence or absence of fibrosis in the initial bone biopsy

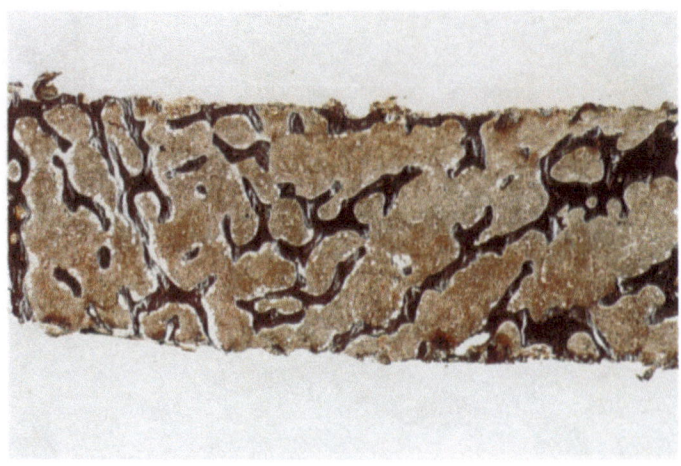

Figs 7.99–7.117 Sections of bone biopsies of patients with myelofibrosis

Fig. 7.99 Low power to show relatively normal trabecular bone structure, marrow with no residual fat cells, sections stained by Gomori's stain.

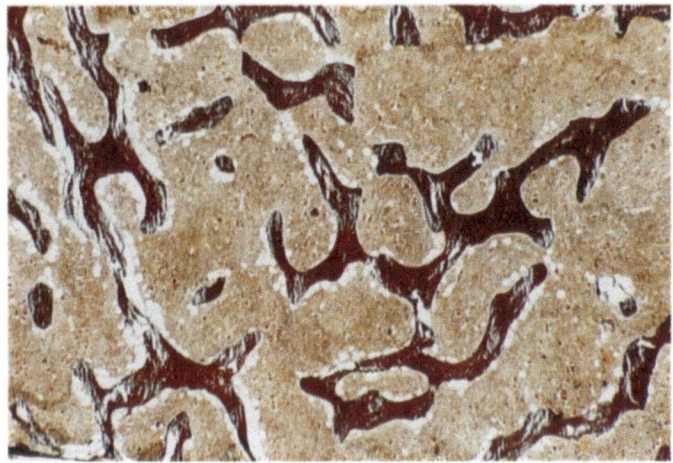

Fig. 7.100 Higher magnification of part of Fig. 7.99. Residual haematopoiesis and megakaryocytes dispersed in the bone marrow

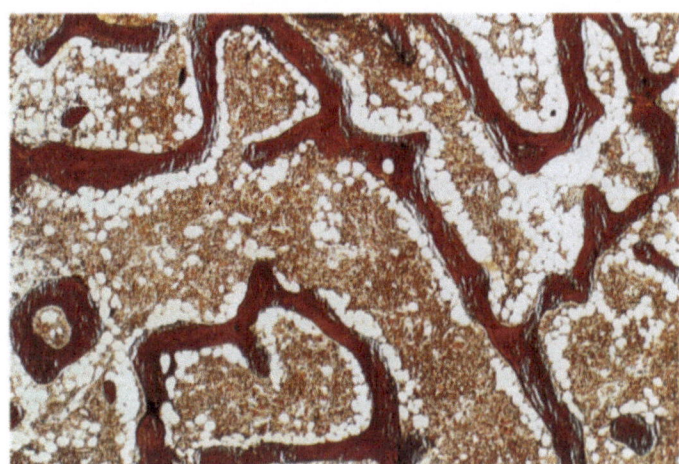

Fig. 7.101 Case of MF showing trabeculae surrounded by a layer of fat cells

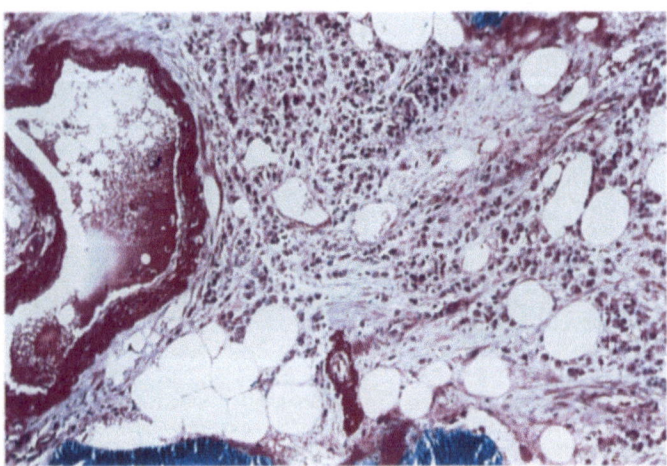

Fig. 7.102 Fibrotic marrow, with patchy residual haematopoiesis and sclerotic blood vessel. Ladewig

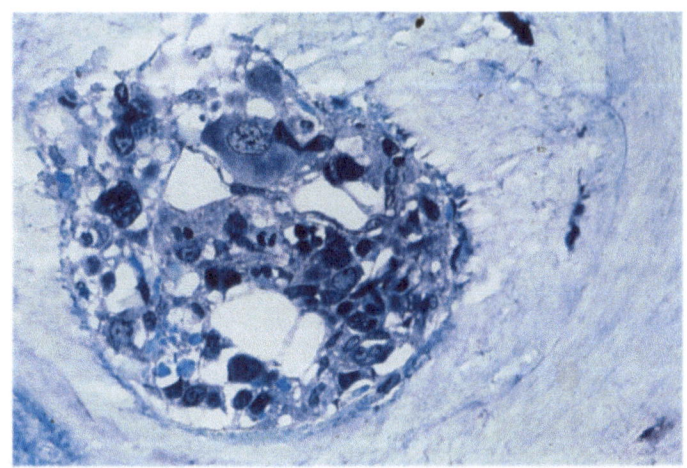

Fig. 7.103 Dysplastic haematopoiesis in Haversian canal in bone

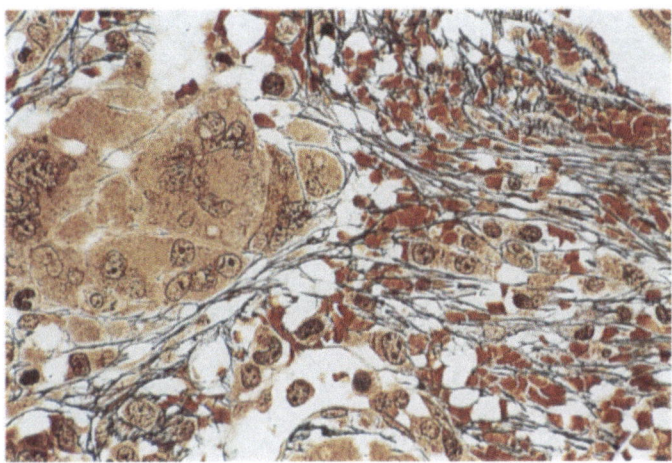

Fig. 7.104 Fibrotic and cellular areas in myelofibrosis; sections stained by Gomori's stain, note cluster of megakaryocytes, these could be mistaken for metastases

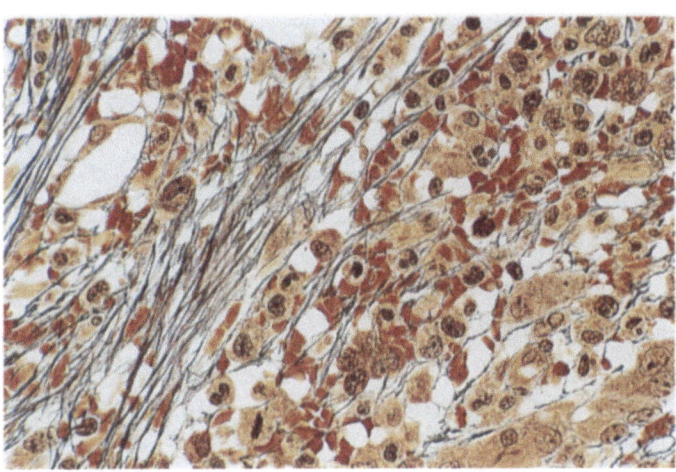

Fig. 7.107 Haematopoietic precursors located between bundles of fibres. Gomori

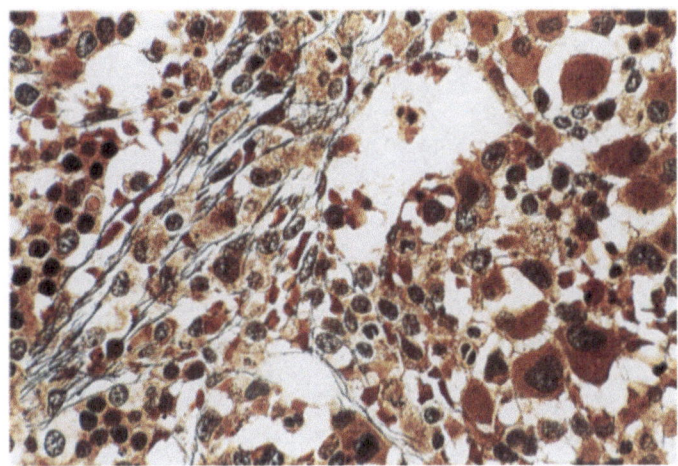

Fig. 7.108 Association of fibres with walls of sinusoids

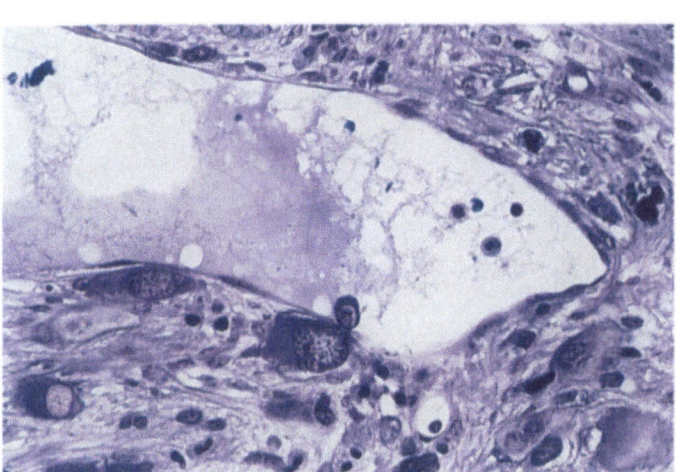

Fig. 7.109 Fibrotic bone marrow, some haematopoietic precursors among the fibres. Note part of megakaryocyte cytoplasm and nucleus migrating through sinus wall, section stained by toluidine blue

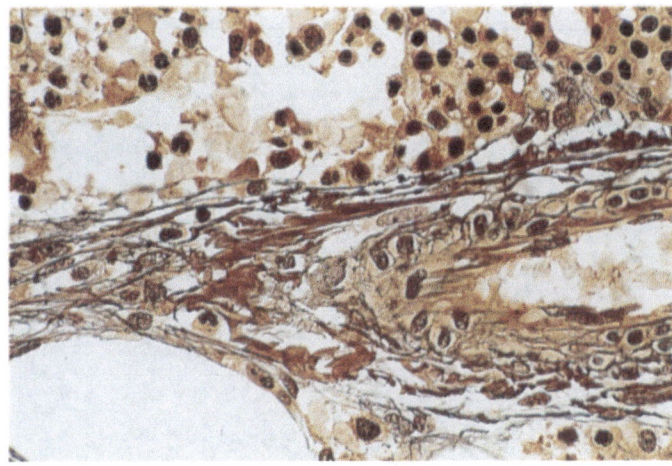

Figs 7.110 and 7.111 Fibrosis and sclerosis of blood vessels in MF
Fig. 7.110 Tangential cut through the blood vessel. Gomori

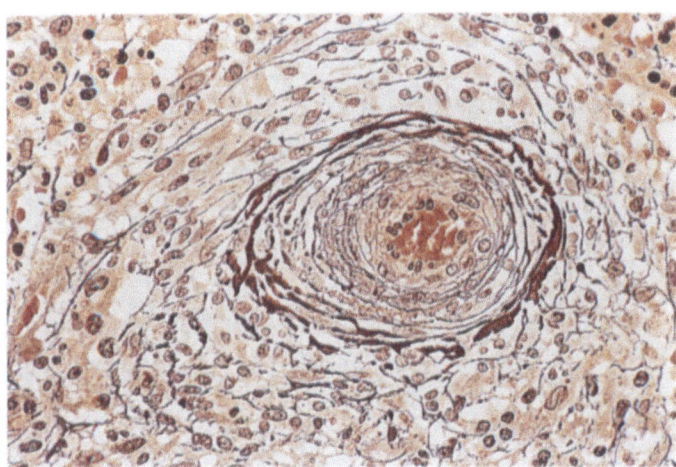

Fig. 7.111 Sclerosis of wall of small artery shown in cross-section

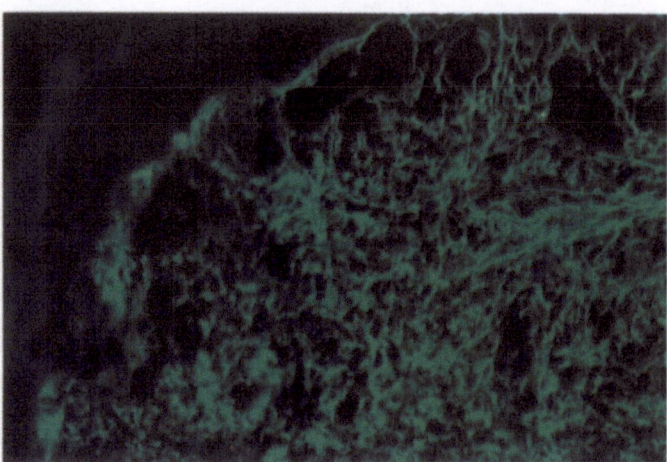

Fig. 7.112 Cryostat section of bone biopsy from patient with MF. FITC-labelled antibody to collagen Type III, collagen shows green fluorescence, some residual paratrabecular fat cells

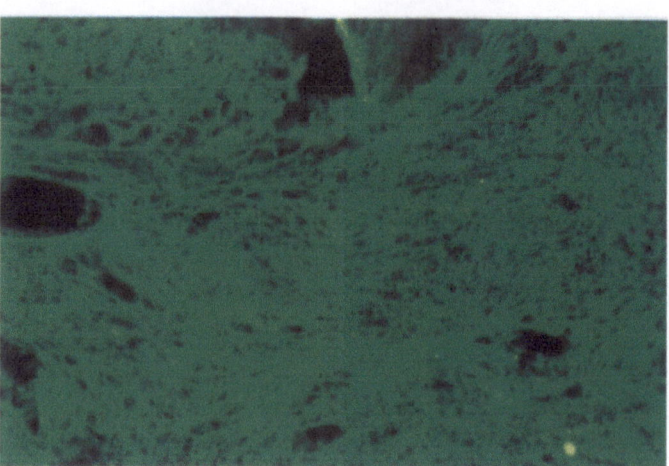

Fig. 7.113 Same as Fig. 7.112, illustrating bundles of collagenous fibres accompanying marrow cavities in MF

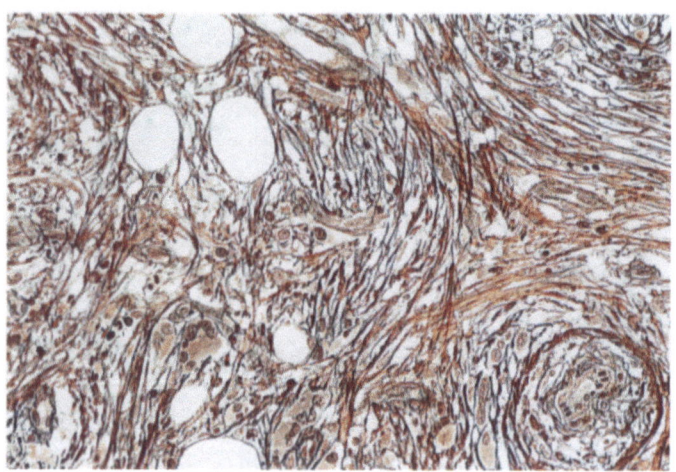

Fig. 7.114 Section of bone biopsy in MF illustrating replacement of most of haematopoietic and fat cells by fibrotic tissue. Gomori

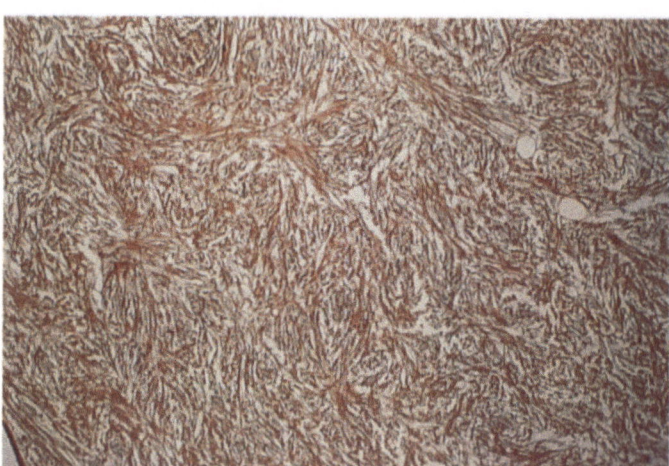

Fig. 7.115 Section of bone biopsy of 46 year old patient with pancytopenia and moderate splenomegaly: the whole biopsy showed obliterative fibrosis. Gomori

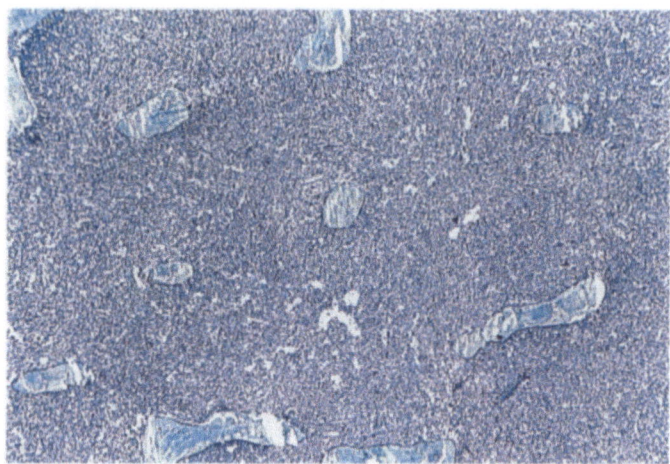

Fig. 7.116 Section of bone biopsy of same patient as above, taken 6 months later; cellular bone marrow consisting of sheets of blasts. Example of blast crisis in MF, overview

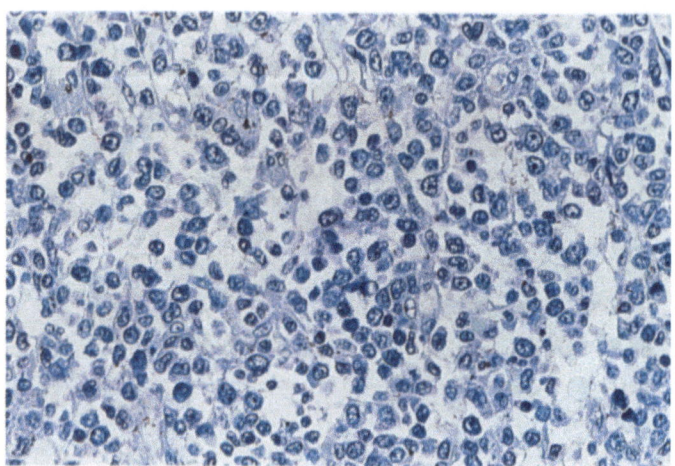

Fig. 7.117 Higher magnification showing the sheets of immature cells

stage of disease[41] and three histological stages have been described: (1) the hypercellular phase, (2) the patchy phase and (3) a phase of obliterative sclerosis. These correspond clinically: (1) to high peripheral blood values, (2) to progressive decrease in Hb, WBC and platelets, and finally (3) to pancytopenia with increasing transfusion requirements[42-45]. However, the histological stages are not sharply separated and may be found at the same time in different parts of the same BMB. Hence, it should be noted that marked differences in fibrosis and in haematopoiesis may be observed in the different marrow cavities.

Myelofibrosis is due to stimulation of fibroblasts and fibrillogenesis, and this is accompanied by additional stromal reactions. These include increased vascularization and blood flow. Ectatic sinusoids are nearly always present, containing haematopoietic precursors. There is infiltration with lymphocytes, plasma and mast cells, as well as macrophages with haemosiderin and crystalloid inclusions. Single or multiple lymphoid cell aggregates may be found. There may be areas of oedema and gelatinous degeneration. Some clusters of polymorphic megakaryocytes may still be found in the obliterative phase, even when the other cell lines may no longer be recognized.

It is now clear that fibrosis in the bone marrow is a secondary reactive phenomenon[46,47]. Among the contributing factors are release into the bone marrow stroma of megakaryocytic and platelet-derived growth factor (PDGF) and platelet Factor 4 – an inhibitor of collagenase[48-50]. In normal thrombogenesis, whole megakaryocytes, portions of their cytoplasm or platelets are shed directly into the blood stream. But when megakaryocytic hyperplasia involves their disintegration within the bone marrow, as well as deposition of platelets within the interstitium, these growth factors are released into the stroma and thus stimulate fibroblasts and fibrillogenesis[50]. The second postulated pathogenic mechanism is a chronic inflammatory reaction, possibly mediated by circulating immune complexes in some cases, and evidenced by the presence in the bone marrow of plasma, mast and lymphoid cells and nodules – all capable of producing growth factors[51,52]. A role for Vitamin D has also been postulated in idiopathic myelofibrosis[53]. Finally, it should be stressed that there is a close association between haematopoiesis, fibrosis and bone – and the exact mechanisms involved remain to be elucidated[54].

In some cases two concurrent conditions such as MF/OMS plus a lymphoproliferative disorder may be present in the bone biopsy[55].

Multi-parameter studies in two cases of OMS are illustrated in Figs 7.134–7.145.

Systemic Mastocytosis (Malignant Mastocytosis)

Mastocytosis is considered here as the mast cell is presumed to derive from the same precursor as the basophil, and therefore belongs to the myeloid series[56]. Two main types of systemic mastocytosis are distinguished: with and without involvement of the skin. Both are characterized by systemic mast cell proliferation[57-59]. The cutaneous variety has urticaria-pigmentosa-like lesions, and the diagnosis is made on biopsy of the skin. However, cutaneous manifestations may also appear years after the onset of systemic mastocytosis; or the latter may become manifest years after the onset of the skin lesions[60]. Involvement of the bone marrow occurs in over 70% of cases in both types, and may be accompanied by osteoporosis, osteolytic foci or osteosclerosis[60-66]. Mast cells, singly or in groups, may be present on the endosteal surface. The lesions are typical: mast cell granulomas with round or whorl-like configurations; located near bone and around blood vessels (Figs 7.146–7.160). They consist of mast cells,

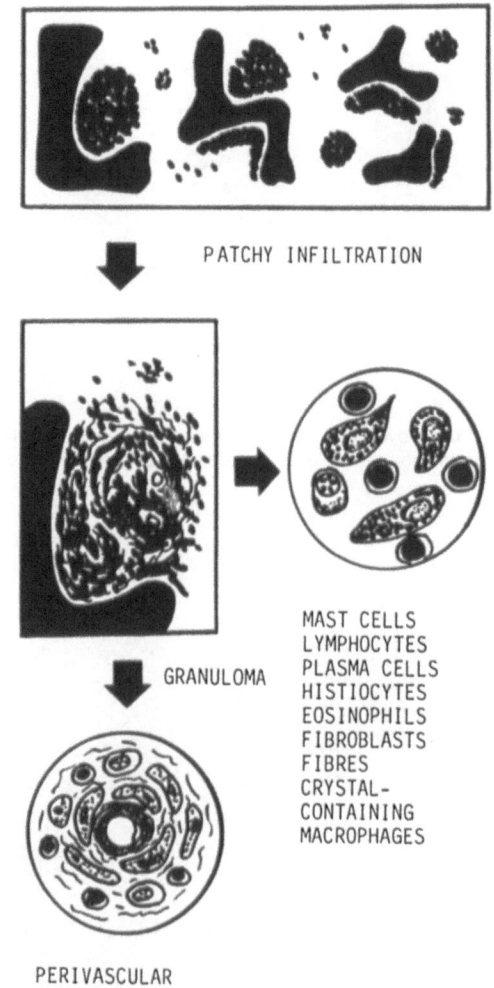

PATCHY INFILTRATION

GRANULOMA

MAST CELLS
LYMPHOCYTES
PLASMA CELLS
HISTIOCYTES
EOSINOPHILS
FIBROBLASTS
FIBRES
CRYSTAL-
CONTAINING
MACROPHAGES

PERIVASCULAR
INFILTRATION

Fig. 7.146 Sketch of systemic mastocytosis in the bone marrow. There is a patchy involvement: paratrabecular, intertrabecular and perivascular granulomas consisting of a heterogeneous cell population, though the majority are mast and lymphoid cells

lymphocytes, plasma cells, eosinophils and histiocytes and macrophages with crystalline inclusions – the Charcot–Leyden crystals, within a network of fibres and blood vessels[67,68]. The aggregates may be small or large and are usually multiple. The marrow between them consists of fat and haematopoietic tissue. In most cases, macrophages are increased, and phagocytosis may be quite prominent. Rarely, in early cases, the bone marrow may contain increased numbers of perivascular, paratrabecular and interstitial mast cells without the typical granulomas. Mastocytosis may also be diagnosed by increased levels of histamine metabolites in the urine[69,70]. Acute leukaemia may develop in the terminal phases. Mastocytosis may occur at any age, but is more common in adults, and is probably more frequently a cause of spinal osteoporosis than is suspected. Various myeloproliferative disorders may coexist with systemic mastocytosis, or develop subsequently in patients who already have SM[71-75].

It should be stressed that the manifestations of SM in the bone marrow biopsy are variable, with respect to the size, location and composition of the mast cell granulomas as well as the state of the trabeculae and of the residual haematopoiesis. There may be areas of oedema or of serous exudation as well as large areas of replacement by fat cells. In other regions there may be relative hyperplasia of blood cell precursors – for example a striking localized increase in megakaryocytes. When lymphoid nodules and lymphocytic infiltrations are extensive the picture may

(Continued on p. 123)

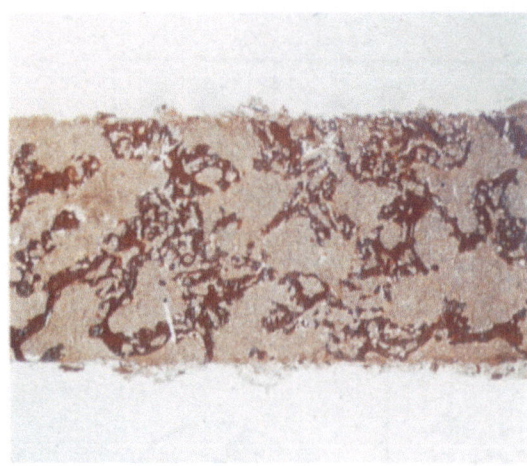

Fig. 7.118 Low-power overview of bone biopsy section in OMS. Note altered trabecular bone structure, and areas of sclerosis, Gomori

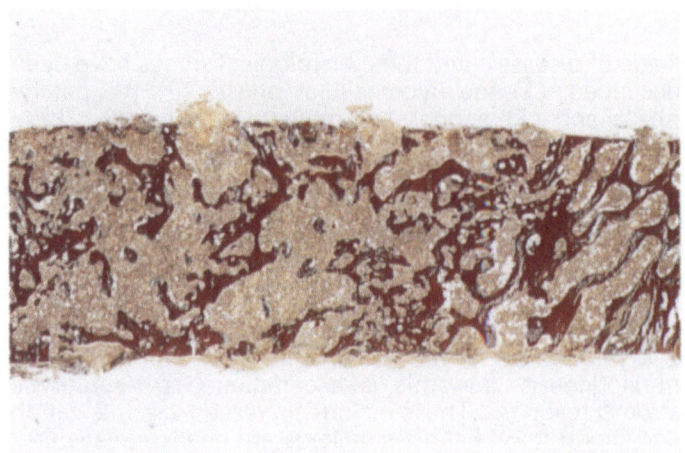

Fig. 7.119 Overview of bone biopsy section in OMS. There is greater variability in the pattern of the trabecular bone. Note preservation of the normal pattern in the subcortical region. Gomori

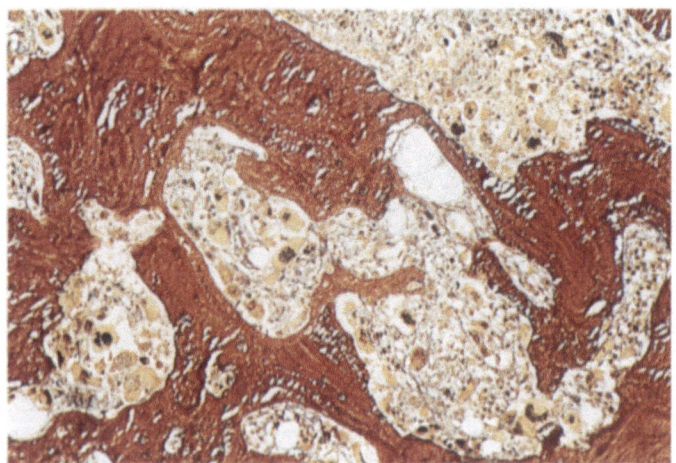

Fig. 7.120 Preservation of some haematopoiesis in the intertrabecular areas. Note hyperplasia of megakaryocytes

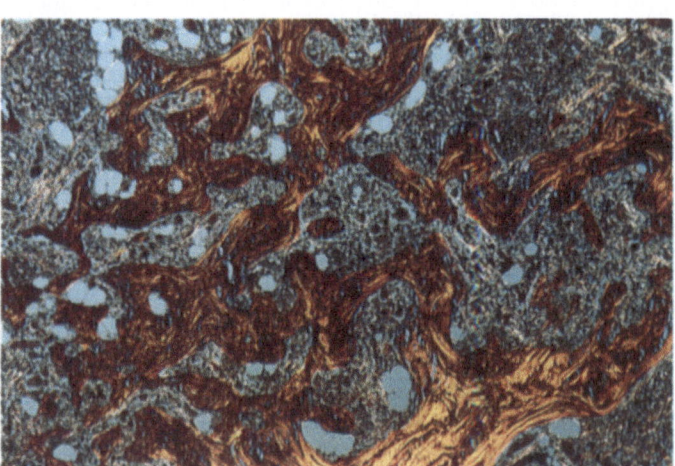

Fig. 7.121 Section of bone biopsy in OMS, Gomori's stain viewed in polarized light. There is relatively little fibrosis in the marrow

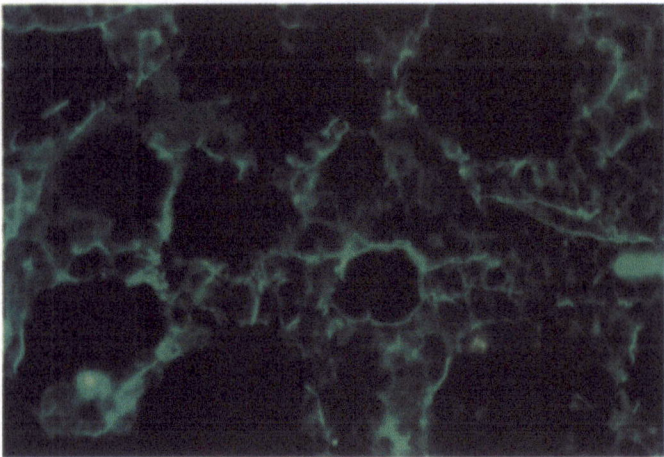

Fig. 7.122 Same case as Fig. 7.121. Cryostat section anti-collagen-type III antibody labelled with FITC – collagen fibres show green fluorescence; fibres between the marrow cells, rather than replacing them

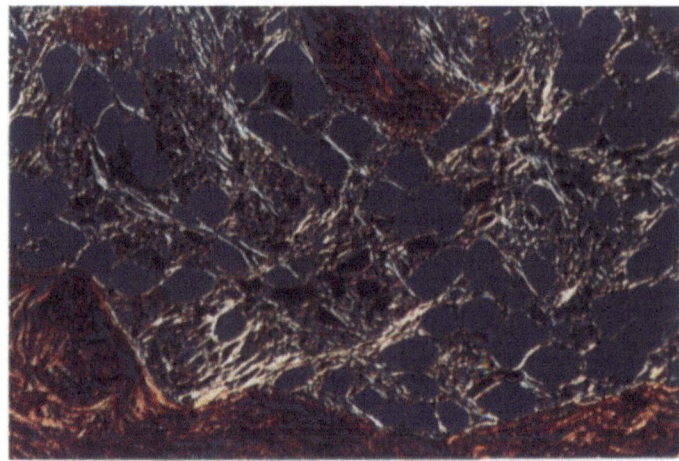

Fig. 7.123 Same cases as in Fig. 7.122, different area of same biopsy, from less sclerotic region, but showing more fibrosis. Gomori's stain, viewed in polarized light

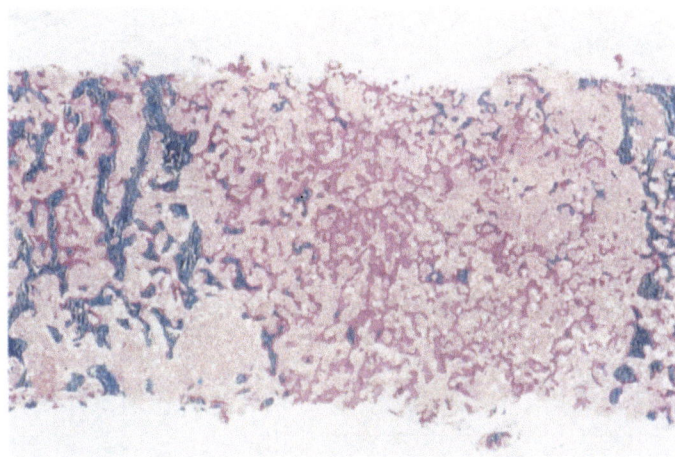

Fig. 7.124 Section of bone biopsy of patient with OMS, stained by Ladewig's stain. Calcified bone stains blue, osteoid red. Note large areas of osteoid, forming a network of bone, both in apposition to, and at a distance from, the calcified trabeculae

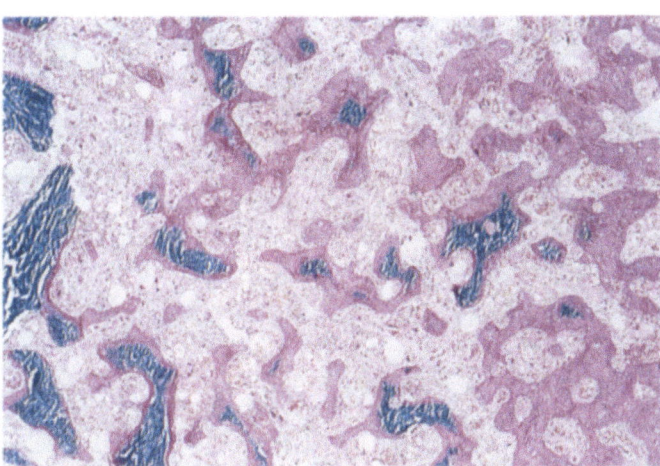

Fig. 7.125 Higher magnification of area from Fig. 7.124. Note megakaryocytic hyperplasia. Ladewig

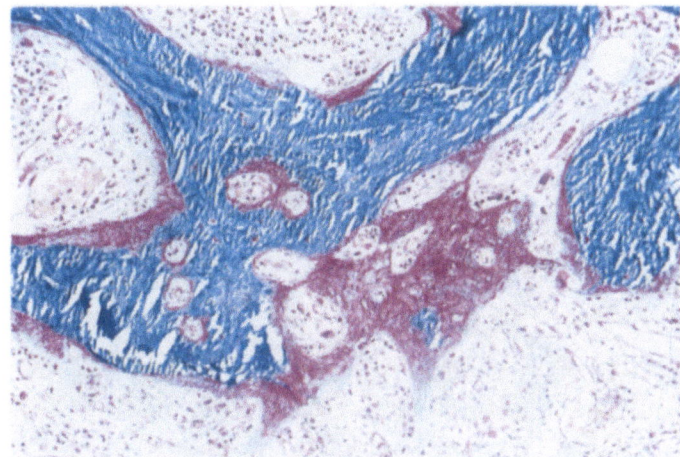

Fig. 7.126 Formations of primitive bone (red) enclosing marrow cells; Ladewig

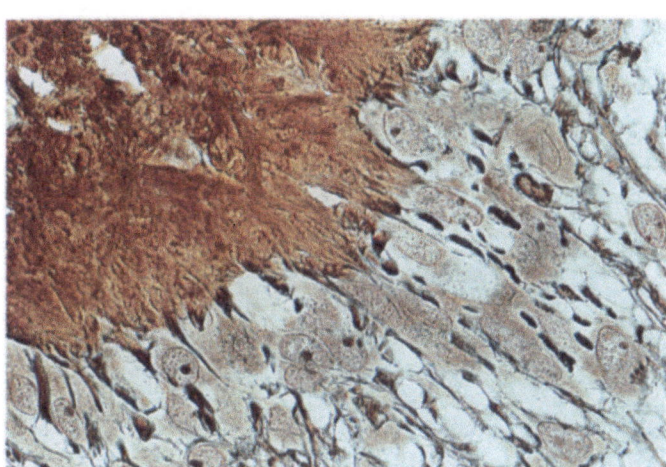

Fig. 7.127 Section of bone biopsy of patient with OMS showing osteoblasts at the trabecular surface and thick fibres radiating out from the bone. Gomori

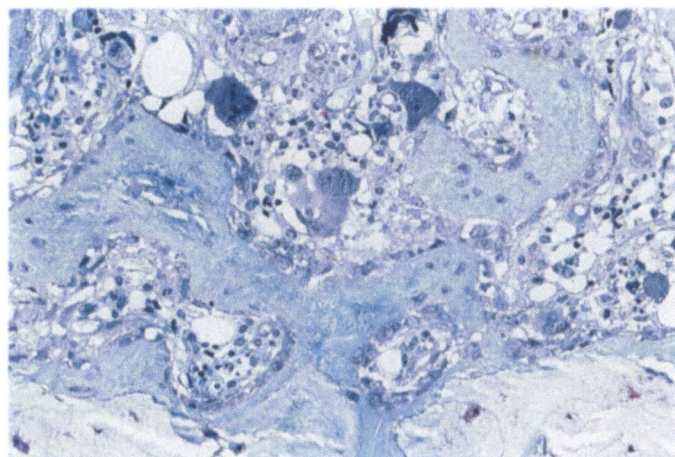

Fig. 7.128 Section showing sprouts of new bone covered by osteoblasts

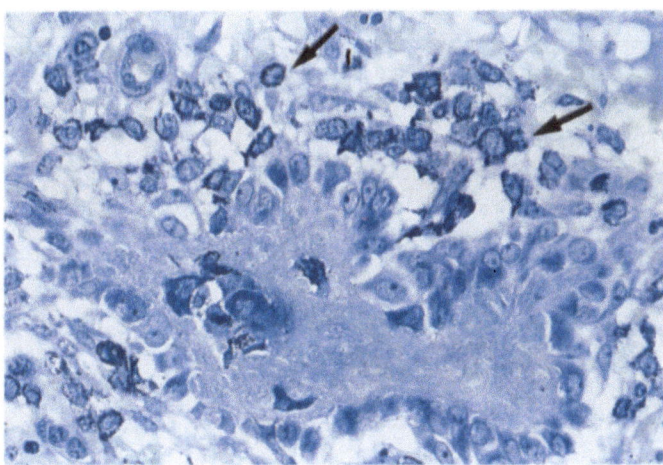

Fig. 7.129 High-power view of osteoblastic new bone formation. Note numerous mast cells associated with the osteoblasts

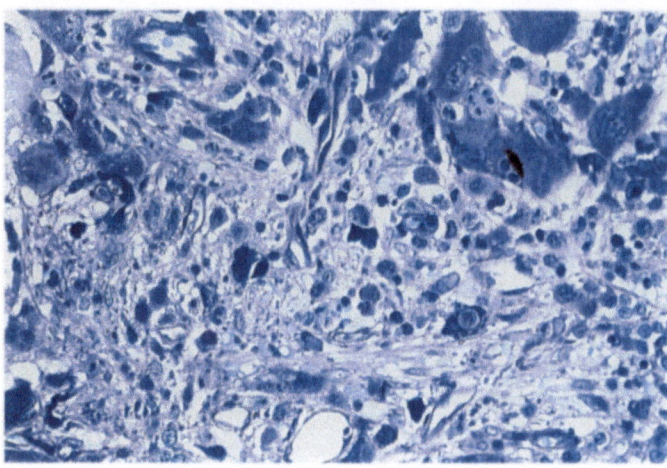

Fig. 7.130 Section showing megakaryocytes and fragments of mega-karyocyte cytoplasm in the interstitial connective tissue

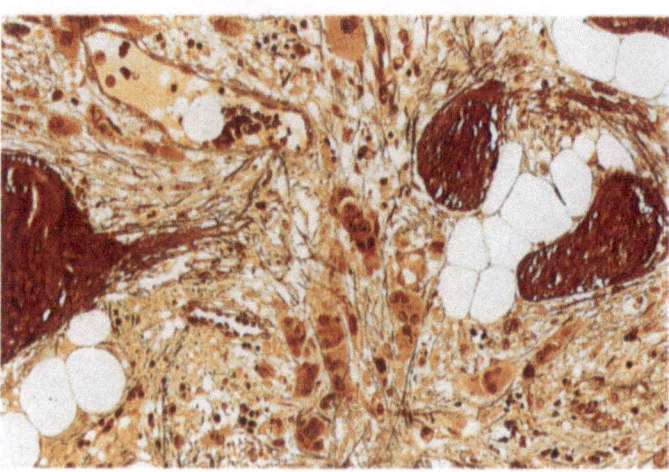

Fig. 7.131 Dysplastic megakaryocytes and paratrabecular fibrosis, also fibre bundles connecting ossicles

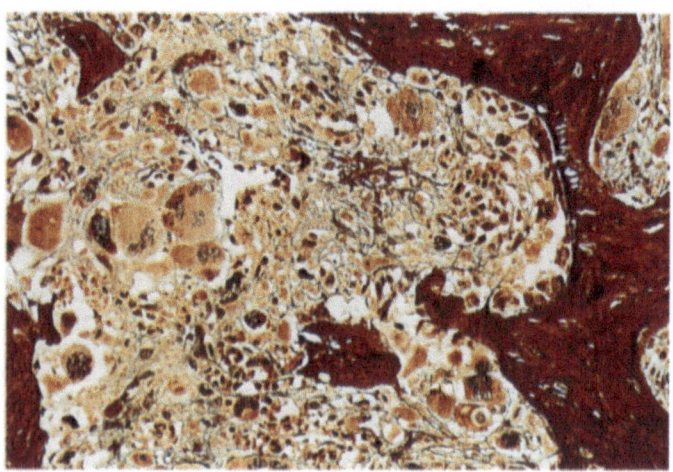

Fig. 7.132 Hyperplastic megakaryocytes and focal ossification in the marrow

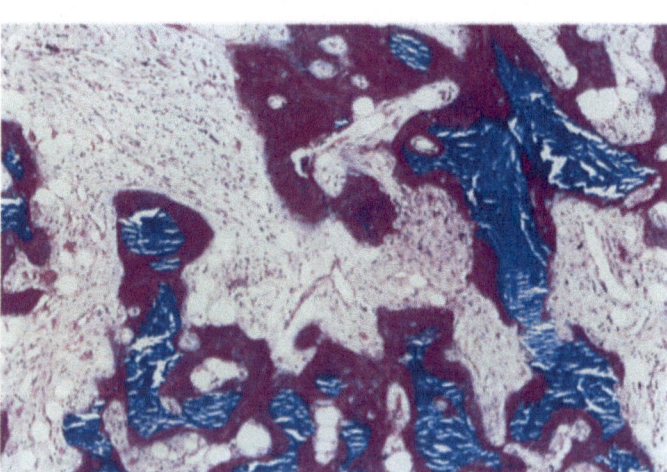

Fig. 7.133 Case of OMS, Ladewig's stain; marrow spaces contain loose connective tissue and blood vessels

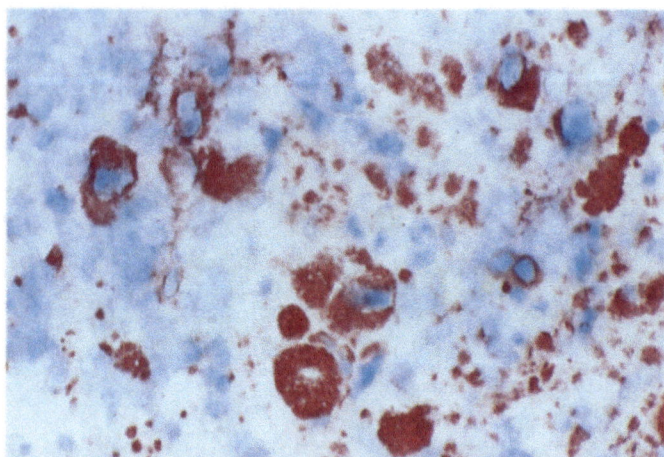

Figs 7.134–7.139 Immunohistochemistry on cryostat sections in OMS

Fig. 7.134 Demonstration of Factor VIII-related antigen (FVIII rag), megakaryocytes and platelets are stained, as well as endothelial cells

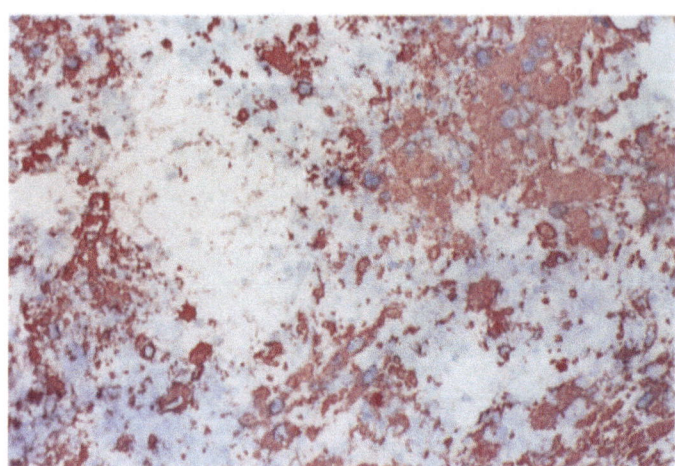

Fig. 7.135 Demonstration of megakaryocytic clusters and platelets by VIPL1

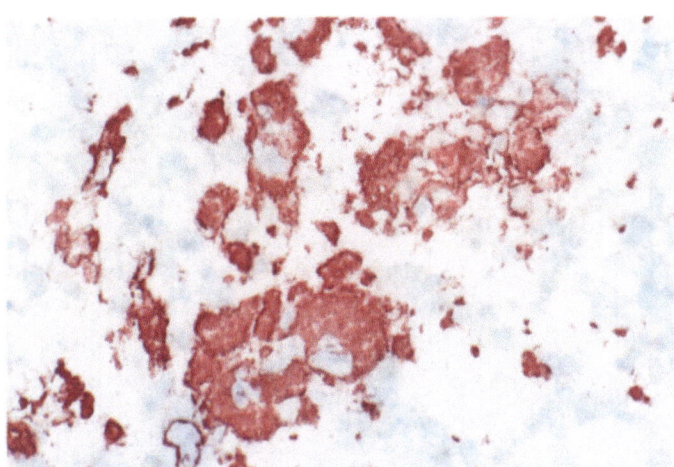

Fig. 7.136 Same as Fig. 7.135; higher magnification showing clusters of megakaryocytes, whose nuclei are not stained

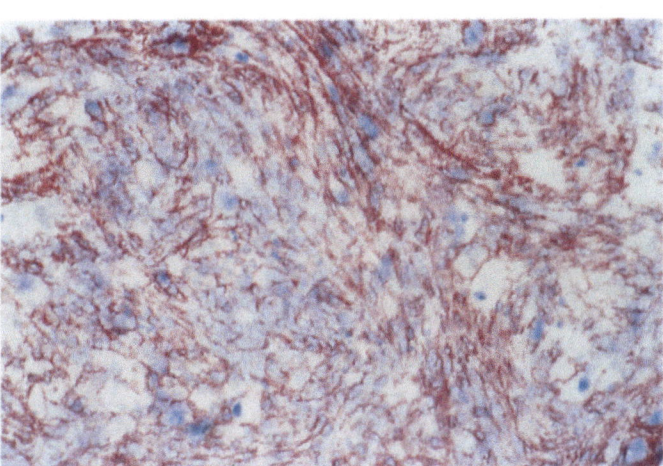

Fig. 7.137 Myelomonocytes, endothelial cells and fibroblasts are stained by the antibody My7

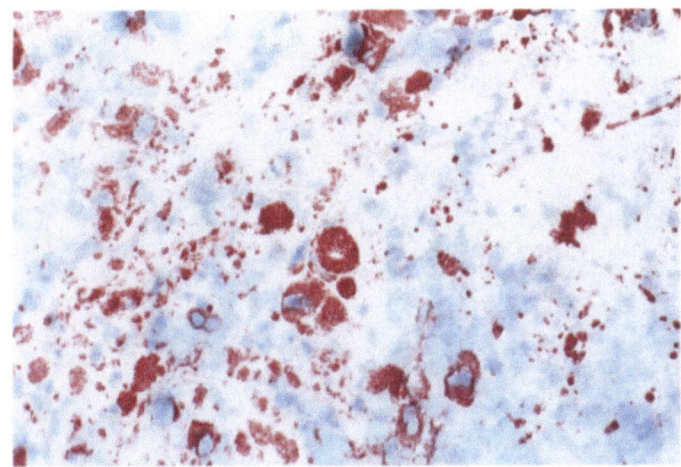

Fig. 7.138 Case of OMS, reaction with FVIII rag. Note very small positive cells; these would probably not have been identified as belonging to the megakaryocytic line in routine histology. Note positive sinusoidal endothelium

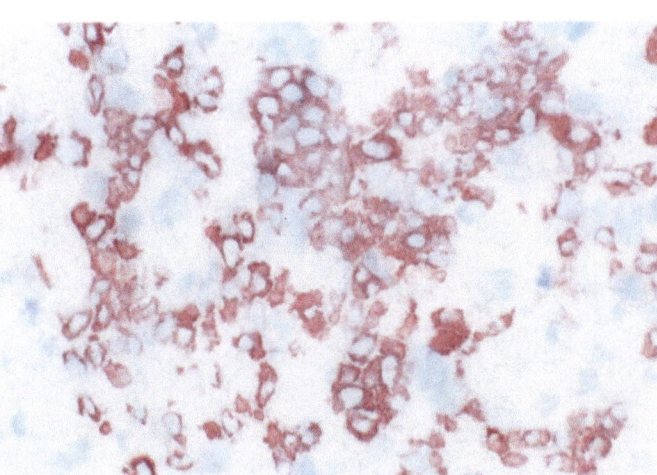

Fig. 7.139 Same case as in Fig. 7.138; non-fibrotic bone marrow area, myelomonocytes are stained by the antibody VIM2

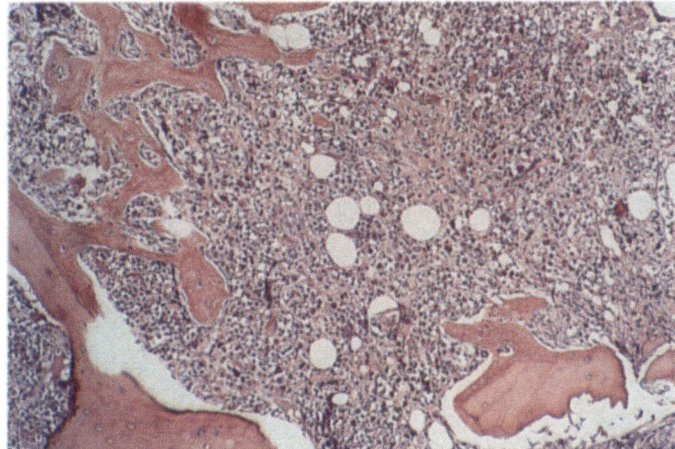

Figs 7.140–7.145 Sections of paraffin-embedded biopsies in OMS

Fig. 7.140 Cellular bone marrow, with patchy osteosclerosis

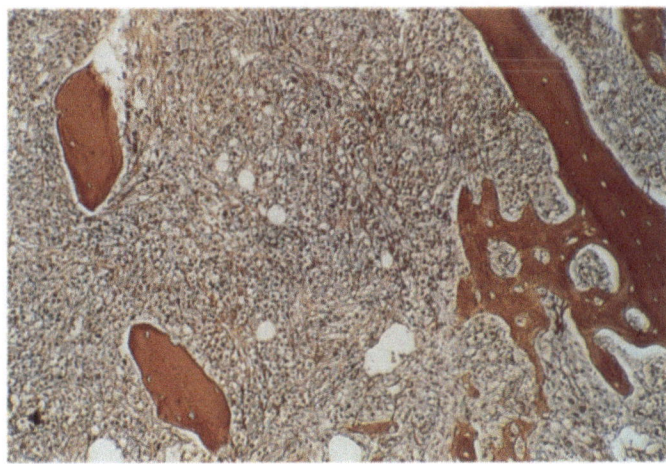

Fig. 7.141 Same case as above; stain for reticulin fibres, parallel section showing bone marrow fibrosis

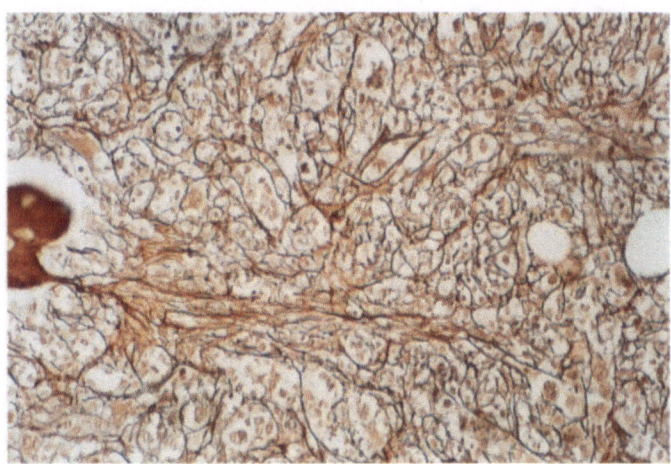

Fig. 7.142 Higher magnification showing attachment of fibre bundles to trabecular surface. Gomori

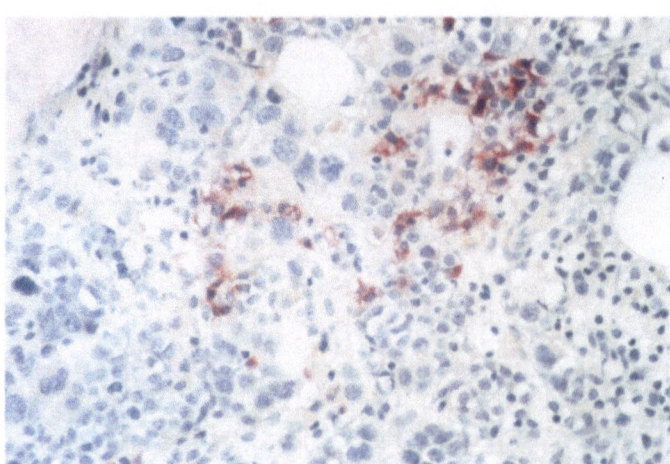

Fig. 7.143 Cellular, non-fibrotic area from same case as in Fig. 7.142, section stained by Leder's stain, there is mainly erythropoiesis; few positive myeloid cells present

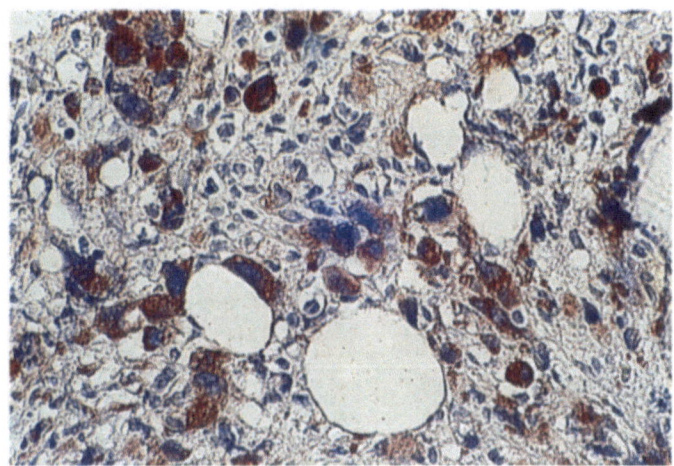

Fig. 7.144 Areas from same biopsy as Fig. 7.142; sections stained by antibody to FVIII rag. Note positively stained megakaryocytes and endothelial cells

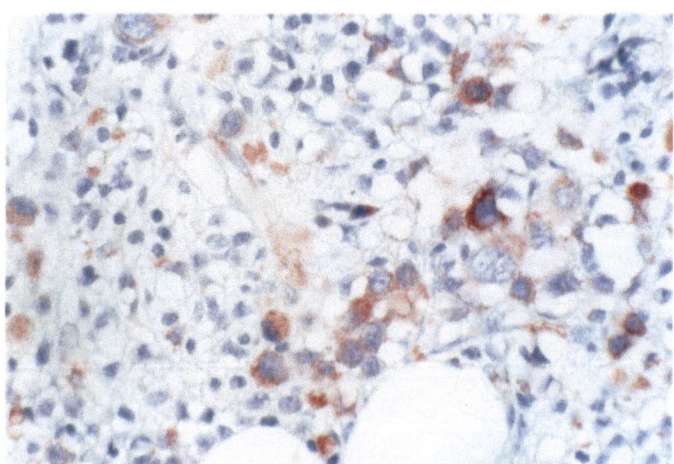

Fig. 7.145 As Fig. 7.144; many small cells are positively stained, indicating a greater hyperplasia of megakaryocytes than indicated in the corresponding H&E sections; development of mixed myeloid and megakaryoblastic acute leukaemia in OMS

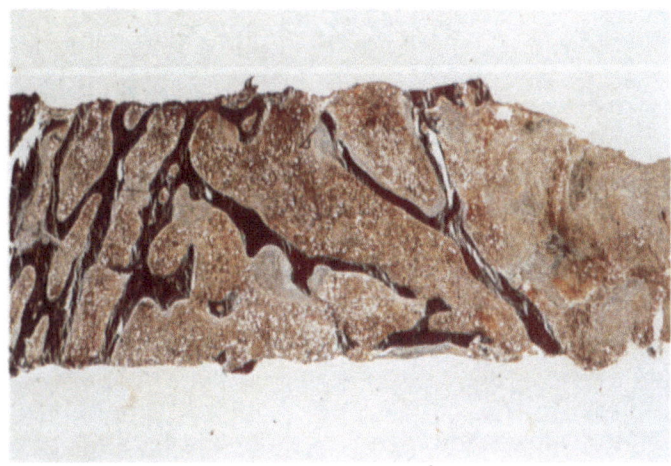

Figs 7.147–7.159 Sections of bone biopsies in systemic mastocytosis
Fig. 7.147 Stained by Gomori's stain. Note focal nature of the involvement

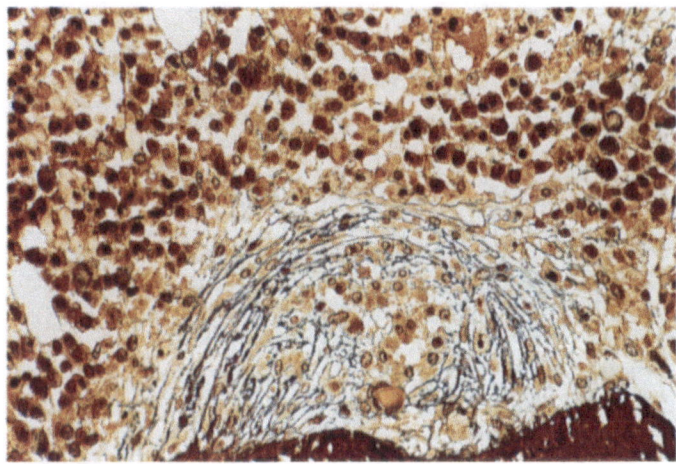

Fig. 7.148 Fibres of a mast cell granuloma attached to the bone. Gomori

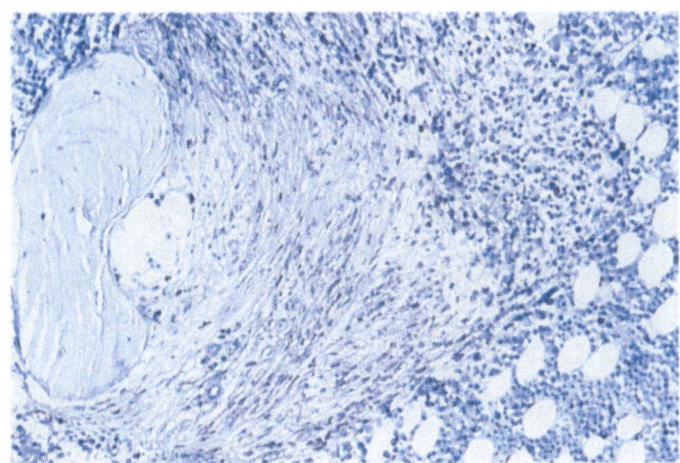

Fig. 7.149 Paratrabecular mast cell granuloma; fibrotic area near bone, cellular area at periphery

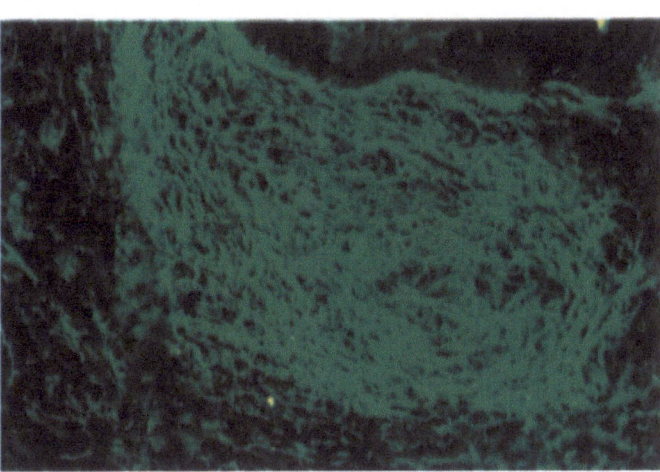

Fig. 7.150 Cryostat section; FITC-labelled antigen to collagen Type III; the mast cell granuloma shows green fluorescence

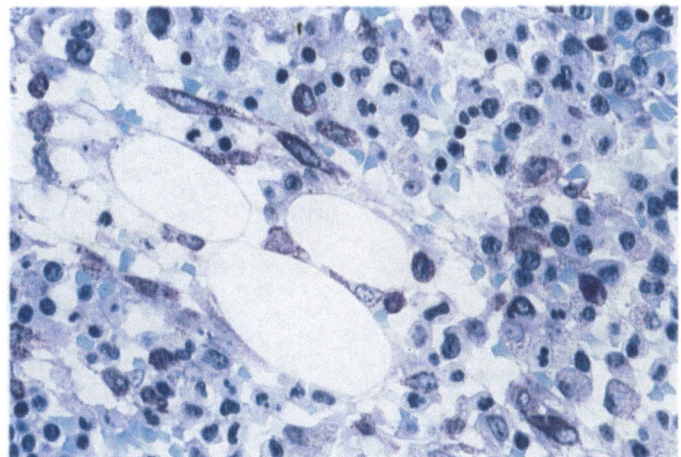

Fig. 7.151 Mast cells, both round and spindle-shaped, scattered among the marrow elements

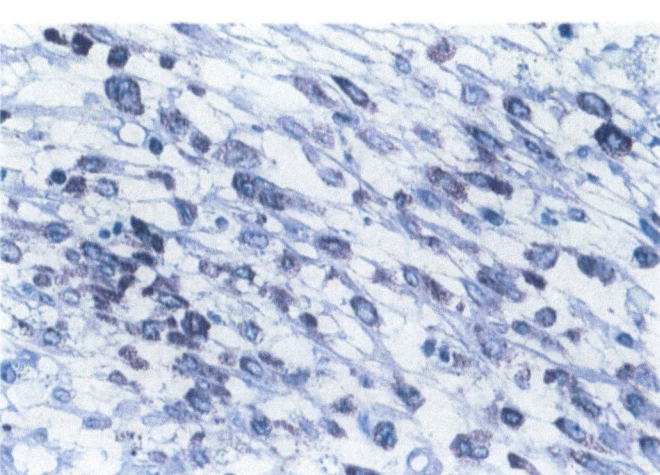

Fig. 7.152 Fibroblasts and mast cells from edge of a granuloma

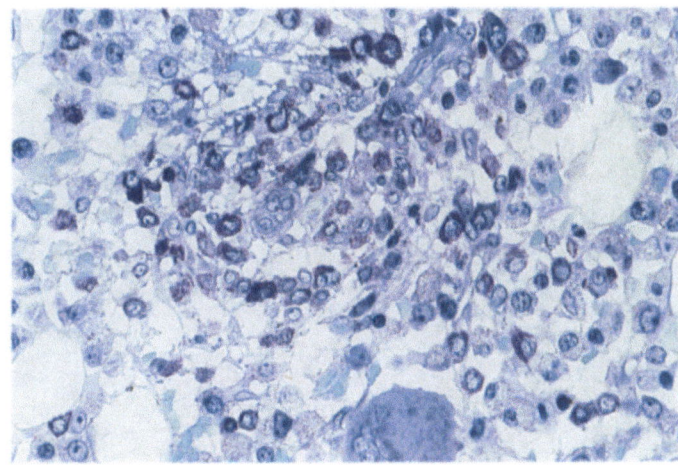

Fig. 7.153 Small mast cell granuloma around arteriole

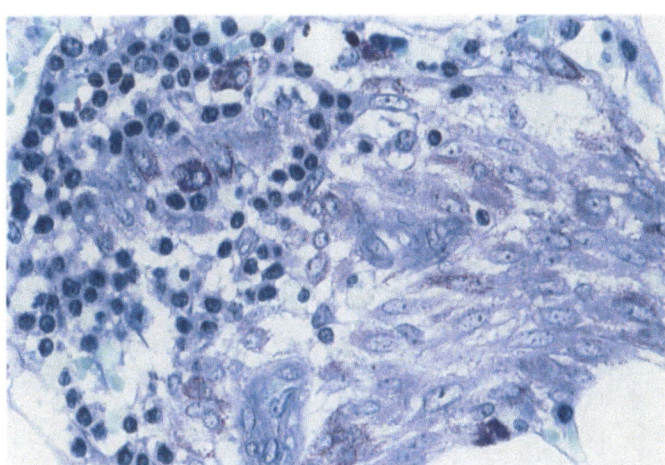

Fig. 7.154 Mast cells, fibroblasts and lymphoid cells. When few granules are present it may not be possible to distinguish between fibroblasts and mast cells

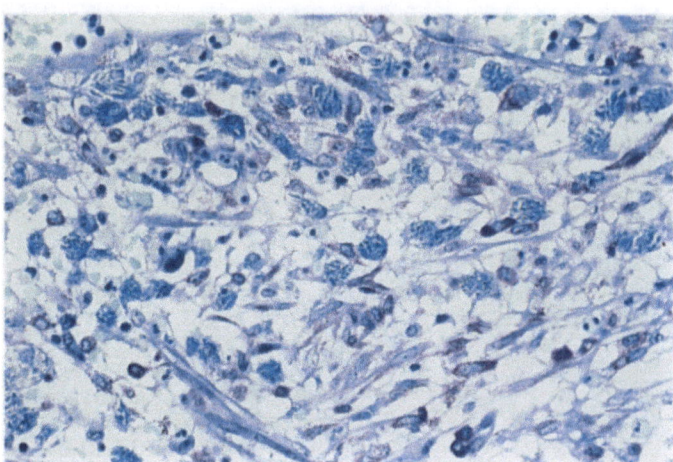

Fig. 7.155 Macrophages wih crystalloid inclusions and spindle-shaped mast cells

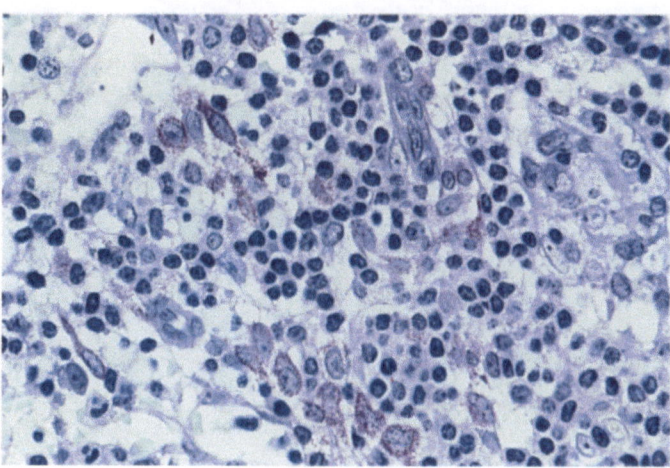

Fig. 7.156 Mast cell granuloma with high proportion of lymphocytes

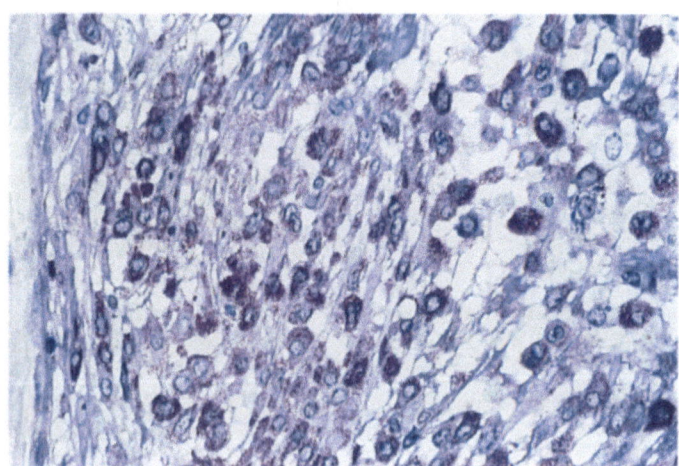

Fig. 7.157 Paratrabecular mast cell granuloma in patient with marked osteoporosis, and extensive bone marrow involvement

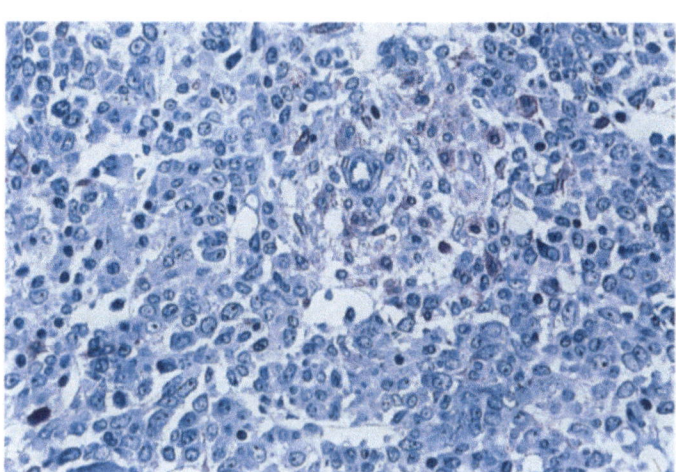

Fig. 7.158 Development of acute leukaemia in patient with systemic mastocytosis. Note perivascular granuloma surrounded by immature cells

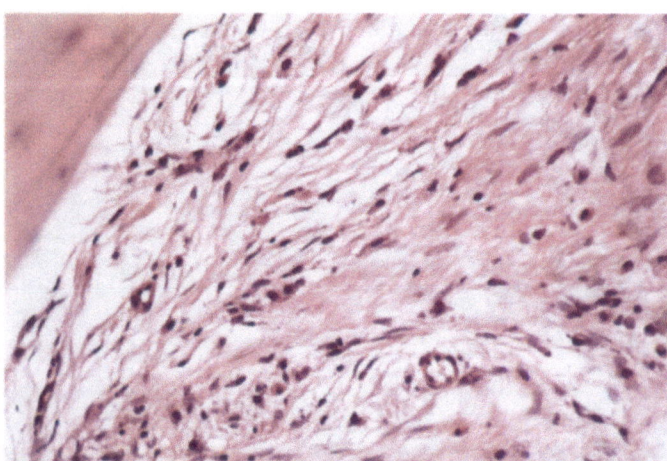

Fig. 7.159 Section of paraffin-embedded bone biopsy of patient with systemic mastocytosis, stained by H&E. Note fibrosis, but the mast cells could easily be missed

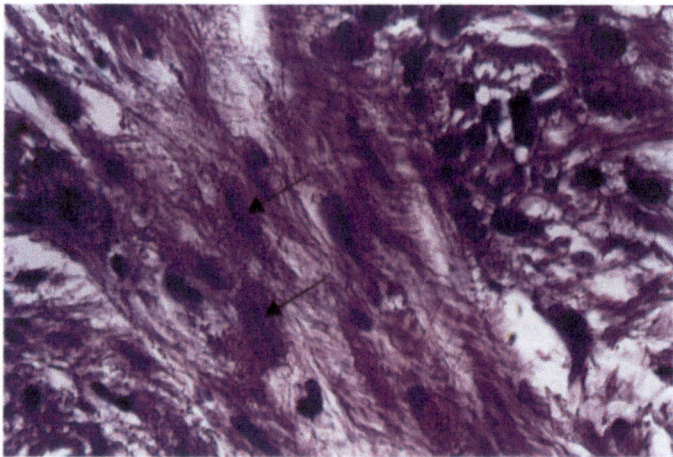

Fig. 7.160 Section parallel to that in Fig. 7.159 stained by toluidine blue, showing metachromatic staining of the mast cell granules

resemble that of marrow involvement by a lymphoma. The increased osseous remodelling, as evidenced by the changes in trabecular structure and the presence of osteoblasts and osteoclasts on the surface of the ossicles, may be accompanied by paratrabecular fibrosis, as in other conditions with activation of bone cells.

References

1. Frisch, B., Bartl, R., Burkhardt, R., Jäger, K. and Pappenberger, R. (1984). Bone marrow histology in the chronic myeloproliferative disorders: criteria for recognition, classification and prognostic evaluation. A study of 3500 biopsies. *Bibl. Haematol.*, **50**, 57

2. Georgii, A., Vykoupil, K. F. and Thiele, J. (1984). Classification of chronic myeloproliferative diseases by bone marrow biopsies. *Bibl. Haematol.*, **50**, 41

3. Frisch, B., Lewis, S. M., Burkhardt, R. and Bartl, R. (1985). *Biopsy Pathology of Bone and Bone Marrow*. London: Chapman and Hall

4. Gerwtiz, A. M. (1986). Human megakaryocytopoiesis. *Sem. Haematol.*, **23**, 27

5. Burkhardt, R., Bartl, R., Jäger, K., Frisch, B., Kettner, G., Mahl, G. and Sund, M. (1986). Working classification of chronic myeloproliferative disorders based on histological, haematological, and clinical findings. *J. Clin. Pathol.*, **39**, 237

6. Wolf, B. C. and Neiman, R. S. (1988). The bone marrow in myeloproliferative and dysmyelopoietic syndromes. In Hyun, B. H. (ed.), *Haematology/Oncology Clinics of North America. Bone Marrow Examination*, Philadelphia: W. B. Saunders, vol. 2

7. Frisch, B., Bartl, R. and Jaeger, K. (1989). Histologic diagnosis of chronic myeloproliferative disorders (CMPD). An update. *Haematol. Rev.* (In press).

8. Girard, P., Leonard, C., Quillard, J., Eydoux, P., Danel, P., Dommergues, J. P. and Tchernia, G. (1985). Myelofibrosis, myeloproliferative syndrome and monosomy C in children. *Eur. Pediatr. Haematol. Oncol.*, **2**, 13

9. Reid, C. D., Fidler, J. and Kirk, A. (1988). Endogenous erythroid cones (EEC) in polycythaemia and their relationship to diagnosis and the response to treatment. *Br. J. Haematol.*, **68**, 395

10. Kimura, H., Ohkoshi, T., Matsuda, S., Uchida, T. and Kariyone, S. (1988). Megakaryocytopoiesis in polycythemia vera: characterization by megakaryocytic progenitors (CFU-Meg) in vitro and quantitation of marrow megakaryocytes. *Acta Haematol. (Basel)*, **79**, 1

11. Najean, Y., Deschamps, A., Dresch, C., Daniel, M. T., Rain, J. D. and Arrago, J. P. (1988). Acute leukaemia and myelodysplasia in polycythemia vera. A clinical study with long-term follow-up. *Cancer*, **61**, 89

12. Ellis, J. T., Peterson, P., Geller, S. A. and Rappaport, H. (1986). Studies of bone marrow in polycythemia vera and the evolution of myelofibrosis and the second hematologic malignancies. *Sem. Haematol.*, **23**, 144

13. Juvonen, E., Partanen, S. and Ruutu, T. (1987). Colony formation by megakaryocytic progenitors in essential thrombocythaemia. *Br. J. Haematol.*, **66**, 161

14. Laszlo, J., Iland, H., Murphy, S., Peterson, P., Briere, J. and Rosenthal, D. (1983). Essential thrombocythaemia: Clinical and laboratory characteristics at presentation. *Clin. Res.*, **31**, 535A

15. Lahuerta-Palacios, J. J., Bornstein, R., Fernandez-Debora, F. J., Gutierrez-Rivas, E., Ortiz, M. C., Larregla, S., Calandre, L. and Montero-Castillo, J. (1988). Controlled and uncontrolled thrombocytosis. Its clinical role in essential thrombocythaemia. *Cancer*, **61**, 1207

16. Giles, F. J., Gray, A. G., Brozovic, M., Grant, I. R., Machin, S. J., Richards, J. D. M., Venutas, S., Singer, C. R. J., Yong, K. L., Davies, S. C., Hoffbrand, A. V., Mehta, A. B., Thomas, M. J. G. and Golstone, A. H. (1988). Alpha-interferon therapy for essential thrombocythaemia. *Lancet*, **2**, 70

17. Jand, J. H. and Demirjian, Z. H. (1988). A 44 year old woman with prominent thrombocytosis. *N. Engl. J. Med.*, **318**, 691

18. Thiele, J., Schneider, G., Hoeppner, B., Wienhold, S., Zankovich, R. and Fischer, R. (1988). Histomorphometry of bone marrow biopsies in chronic myeloproliferative disorders with associated thrombocytosis – features of significance for the diagnosis of primary (essential) thrombocythaemia. *Virchows Arch.*, **413**, 407

19. Thiele, J., Krech, R., Weinhold, St, Simon, K. G., Zankovich, R. and Fischer, R. (1987). The use of the anti-factor VIII method on trephine biopsies of the bone marrow for the identification of immature and atypical megakaryocytes in myeloproliferative diseases and allied disorders. A morphometric study. *Virchows Arch.*, **B54**, 89

20. Suda, J., Eguchi, M., Ozawa, T., Furukawa, T., Hayashi, Y., Kojima, S., Maeda, H., Tadokoro, K., Sato, Y., Miura, Y., Ohara, A. and Suda, T. (1988). Platelet peroxidase-positive blast cells in transient myeloproliferative disorder with Down's syndrome. *Br. J. Haematol.*, **68**, 181

21. Ludwig, H., Linkesch, W., Gisslinger, H., Fritz, E., Sinzinger, H., Radaszkiewicz, T., Chott, A., Flener, R. and Michsche, M. (1987). Interferon-alfa corrects thrombocytosis in patients with myeloproliferative disorders. *Cancer. Immunol. Immunother.*, **25**, 266

22. Burkhardt, R. (1988). Bone marrow in megakaryocytic disorders. In Hyun, B. H. (ed.), *Haematology/Oncology Clinics of North America. Bone Marrow Examination*. Philadelphia: W. B. Saunders, vol. 2

23. Verhest, A. and Monsiery, R. (1983). Philadelphia chromosome-positive thrombocythemia with leukemic transformation. *N. Engl. J. Med.*, **308**, 1603

24. Sedlacek, S. M., Curtis, J. L., Weintraub, J. and Levin, J. (1986). Essential thrombocythemia and leukaemic transformation. *Medecine*, **65**, 353

25. Murphy, S., Iland, H., Rosenthal, D. and Laszlo, J. (1986). Essential thrombocythemia: an interim report from the polycythemia vera study group. *Sem. Haematol.*, **23**, 177

26. Lorand-Metze, I., Vassallo, J. and Souz, C. A. (1987). Histological and cytological heterogeneity of bone marrow in Philadelphia-positive chronic myelogenous leukaemia at diagnosis. *Br. J. Haematol.*, **67**, 45

27. Kelsey, P. R. and Geary, C. G. (1988). Sea-blue histiocytes and Gaucher cells in bone marrow of patients with chronic myeloid leukaemia. *J. Clin. Pathol.*, **41**, 960

28. Lazzarino, M., Morra, E., Castello, A. *et al.* (1986). Myelofibrosis in chronic granulocytic leukaemia: clinico-pathologic correlations and prognostic significance. *Br. J. Haematol.*, **64**, 227

29. Sokal, J. I. and Sheerin, K. A. (1986). Decreased stainable marrow iron in chronic granulocytic leukemia. *Am. J. Med.*, **81**, 395

30. Schmidt, U., Mlynek, M. I. and Leder, L. D. (1988). Electron-micropscopic characterization of mixed granulated (hybridoid) leucocytes of chronic myeloid leukaemia. *Br. J. Haematol.*, **68**, 175

31. Thiele, J., Simon, K. G., Fischer, R. and Zankovich, R. (1988). Follow-up studies with sequential bone marrow biopsies in chronic myeloid leukaemia and so-called primary (idiopathic) osteomyelofibrosis. Evolution of histopathological lesions and clinical course in 40 patients. *Pathol. Res. Pract.*, **183**, 434

32. Islam, A. (1987). Prediction of impending blast cell transformation in chronic granulocytic leukaemia. *Histopathology*, **12**, 633

33. Lambertenghi-Deliliers, G., Pozzoli, E., Benazzi, E., Maiolo, A. T., Foa, P. and Polli, E. (1986). Bone marrow biopsy in chronic myeloid leukaemia: significance of some histological parameters. *Haematologica-(Pavia)*, **71**, 113

34. Dekmezian, R., Kantarjian, H. M., Keating, M. J., Talpaz, M., McCredie, K. B. and Freireich, E. J. (1987). The relevance of reticulin stain-measured fibrosis at diagnosis in chronic myelogenous leukaemia. *Cancer*, **59**, 1739

35. Rozman, C., Cervantes, F. and Feliu, E. (1989). Is the histological classification of chronic granulocytic leukaemia justified from the clinical point of view? *Eur. J. Haematol.*, **42**, 150

36. Zoumbos, N. C., Chrysanthopoulos, C., Starakis, J. and Kapatais-Zoumbos, K. (1987). K light chain myeloma developing in a patient with chronic neutrophilic leukaemia. *Br. J. Haematol.*, **65**, 504

37. Burkhardt, R., Bartl, R., Beil, E. *et al.* (1975). Myelofibrosis-osteomyelosclerosis syndrome. Review of literature and histomorphology. In *Advances in the Biosciences.* Oxford: Pergamon Press, vol. 16

38. Frisch, B. and Bartl, R. (1985). Histology of myelofibrosis and osteomyelosclerosis. In Lewis, S. M. (ed.), *Myelofibrosis. Pathophysiology and Clinical Management.* New York: Dekker

39. Pamphilon, D. H., Creamer, P., Keeling, D. H. and Prentice, A. G. (1987). Restoration of active haemopoiesis in a patient with myelofibrosis and subsequent termination in acute myeloblastic leukaemia: case report and review of the literature. *Eur. J. Haematol.*, **38**, 279

40. Herrera, A., Urbanitz, D., Rossner, A., Lingg, G. and Grundmann, E. (1986). Case report 402: Megakaryocytic myelosis with disseminated osteolysis and osteomyelosclerosis. *Skeletal Radiol.*, **15**, 672

41. Zankovich, R., Thiele, J., Modder, B., Steinberg, T., Simon, K. G., Fischer, R. and Diehl, V. (1988). So-called primary (idiopathic) osteomyelofibrosis/-sclerosis (OMF) within the scope of chronic myeloproliferative diseases. I. Initial clinical and histologic findings in 102 patients with special reference to early hyperplastic and advanced fibrosclerotic stages. *Med. Klin.*, **83**, 617

42. Gustavsson, P., Holm, J., Wahlin, A. and Norberg, B. (1985). Staging of idiopathic myelofibrosis. Significance of haemoglobin

value and reticulocyte count. *Acta Med. Scand.*, **218**, 487

43. Barosi, G., Berzuini, C., Liberato, L. N., Costa, A., Polino, G. and Ascari, E. A. (1988). A prognostic classification of myelofibrosis with myeloid metaplasia. *Br. J. Haematol.*, **70**, 397

44. Wolf, B. C. and Neiman, R. S. (1985). Myelofibrosis with myeloid metaplasia: pathophysiologic implications of the correlation between bone marrow changes and progression of splenomegaly. *Blood,* **65**, 803

45. Smith, R. E., Chelmowski, M. K. and Szabo, E. J. (1988). Myelofibrosis: A concise review of clinical and pathologic features and treatment. *Am. J. Hematol.*, **29**, 174

46. Moore, M. A. S. (1982). Pathogenesis of MF. In Hoffbrand, A. V. (ed.), *Recent Advances in Haematology.* Edinburgh: Churchill Livingstone

47. Castro-Malaspina, H. and Moore, M. A. S. (1982). Pathophysiological mechanisms operating in the development of myelofibrosis: role of megakaryocytes. *Nouv. Rev. Franc. Haematol.*, **24**, 221

48. McCarthy, D. M. (1985). Fibrosis of the bone marrow: content and causes (Annotation). *Br. J. Haematol.*, **59**, 1

49. Seyer, J. M. (1985). Mediators of increased collagen synthesis in fribrosing organs. *Fund. Appl. Toxicol.*, **5**, 228

50. Caen, J. P., Deschamps, J. F., Bodevin, E., Bryckaert, M. C., Dupuy, E. and Wasteson, A. (1987). Megakaryocytes and myelofibrosis in gray platelet syndrome. *Nouv. Rev. Fr. Haematol.*, **29**, 109

51. Chauvet, M., Hollard, D., Cousin, F. and Leger, J. (1987). Myelofibrosis. Pathology of the microenvironment. *Nouv. Rev. Fr. Haematol.*, **29**, 119

52. Hasselbalch, H., Nielsen, H., Berild, D. and Kappelgaard, E. (1985). Circulating immune complexes in myelofibrosis. *Scand. J. Haematol.*, **34**, 177

53. Eugster, C., Brun Del Re, G. P. and Bucher, U. (1987). The role of 1, 25-dihydroxy-vitamin D_3 ($1,25\,(OH)_2D_3$) in the treatment of idiopathic myelofibrosis. *Br. J. Haematol.*, **65**, 381

54. MacDougall, L. G., Pectifor, J. M. and Patel, J. M. (1987). Bone growth and haemopoiesis: steroid reversible anaemia, myelofibrosis and increased bone formation in a child. *Br. J. Haematol.*, **66**, 5–10

55. Subramanian, V. P., Gomez, G. A., Tin Han., Kim, U., Minowada, J. and Sandberg, A. (1985). Coexistence of myeloid metaplasia with myelofibrosis and hairy-cell leukaemia. *Arch. Intern. Med.*, **145**, 164

56. Schmidt, U., Mlynek, M. L. and Leder, L. (1988). Electron-microscopic characterization of mixed granulated (hybridoid) leucocytes of chronic myeloid leukaemia. *Br. J. Haematol.*, **68**, 175

57. Webb, Th. A., Chin-Yang Li and Yam, L. T. (1982). Systemic mast cell disease: A clinical and hematopathologic study of 26 cases. *Cancer,* **49**, 927

58. Korenblat, P. E., Wedner, H. J., Whyte, M. P. and Frankel, S. (1984). Systemic mastocytosis. *Arch. Intern Med.*, **144**, 2249

59. Rosenbaum, R. C., Frieri, M. and Metcalfe, D. D. (1984). Patterns of skeletal scintigraphy and their relationship to plasma and urinary histamine levels in systemic mastocytosis. *J. Nucl. Med.*, **25**, 859

60. Tharp, M. D. (1985). The spectrum of mastocytosis. *Am. J. Med. Sci.*, **289**, 119

61. Parwaresh, M. R., Horny, H. P. and Lennert, K. (1985). Tissue mast cells in health and disease. *Path. Res. Pract.*, **179**, 439

62. Stein, D. H. (1986). Mastocytosis: a review. *Pediatr. Dermatol.*, **3**. 365

63. Fallon, M. D., Whyte, M. P. and Teitelbaum, S. L. (1981). Systemic mastocytosis associated with generalized osteopenia. Histopathological characterization of the skeletal lesion using undecalcified bone from two patients. *Hum. Pathol.*, **12**, 813

64. Colver, G. B., Dawber, R. P. R., Smith, R., Ryan, T. J. and Wojnarowska, F. (1985). Osteoporosis and mastocytosis with late appearance of urticaria pigmentosa. *J. Roy. Soc. Med.*, **78**, 866

65. McKenna, M. J. and Frame, B. (1985). The mast cell and bone. *Clin. Orthop.*, **200**, 226

66. Case records of the Massachusetts General Hospital. Weekly clinicopathological exercises (1986). Case 38-1986. A 73-year-old man with diffuse osteoclerotic lesions. *N. Engl. J. Med.*, **315**, 816

67. Horny, H. P. and Kaiserling, E. (1988). Lymphoid cells and tissue mast cells of bone marrow lesions in systemic mastocytosis: a histological and immunohistological study. *Br. J. Haematol.*, **69**, 449

68. Travis, W. D., Li, C. Y., Bergstralh, E. J., Yam, L. T. and Swee, R. G. (1988). Systemic mast cell disease. Analysis of 58 cases and literature review. *Medicine,* **67**, 345

69. Olafsson, J. H. (1985). Cutaneous and systemic mastocytosis in adults. A clinical, histopathological and immunological evaluation in relation to histamine metabolism. *Acta Dermatol. Venereol.* (Suppl.), **115**, 1

70. Ridell, B., Olafsson, J. H., Roupe, G., Swolin, B., Granerus, G., Rodjer, S. and Enerback, L. (1986). The bone marrow in urticaria pigmentosa and systemic mastocytosis. Cell composition and mast cell density in relation to urinary excretion of tele-methylimidazole-acetic acid. *Arch. Dermatol.*, **122**, 422

71. Businco, L., Cantani, A., Businco, E. and Pepys, J. (1984). Systemic mastocytosis in a 5-year-old child: successful treatment with disodium cromoglycate. *Clin. Allergy*, **14**, 147

72. Kasimov, N. (1986). Mastocytosis in children. *Med. Sestra*, **45**, 41

73. Horny, H. P., Parwaresch, M.R. and Lennert, K. (1983). Basophilic leukaemia and generalized mastocytosis. *Verh. Dtsch. Ges. Pathol.*, **67**, 192

74. Vilter, R. W. and Wiltse, D. (1985). Preleukemia and urticaria pigmentosa followed by acute myelomonoblastic leukemia. *Arch. Intern. Med.*, **145**, 349

75. Travis, W. D., Chin-Yang Li., Yam, L. T., Bergstral, E. J. and Swee, R. G. (1988). Significance of systemic mast cell disease with associated hematologic disorders. *Cancer,* **62**, 965

Lymphoproliferations in the Bone Marrow

The bone marrow is an organ of lymphopoiesis, of passage in the migration of lymphoid cells, and in the maturation of plasma cells. With the increasing investigation of bone biopsies in recent years it has become evident that lymphoid cells, nodules, and follicles may frequently be encountered in bone marrow biopsies in a wide variety of reactive conditions as well as when involvement by malignant lymphomas is present. When dealing with possible bone marrow involvement by malignant processes of the lymphoid system, there are three main areas in which early or minimal involvement may be difficult to distinguish from reactive proliferations. These are reactive lymphocytosis, plasmacytosis and granulomas. Their differential diagnosis is briefly considered below. In addition, it should be stressed that knowledge of the clinical setting is essential for the correct interpretation of the biopsy findings (Figs 8.1–8.8).

Benign Lymphoproliferations in the Bone Marrow

Even under normal circumstances, lymphoid cells may constitute up to 20% of the population of nucleated cells in the bone marrow. However, there may be an absolute or a relative increase, the latter due to a reduction in haematopoietic tissue, as in some skeletal areas in advancing age, or in hypoplastic conditions.

Both B and T cells are found in the normal bone marrow[1], T cells 20–30%, B cells 70–80% of the lymphoid cells present, and there is a functional interaction between them, and in the regulation of haematopoiesis. Lymphoid cells are found in any of three forms in the bone marrow: (1) dispersed among the haematopoietic and fat cells; (2) in aggregates or nodules which may be intertrabecular or parasinusoidal (rarely paratrabecular), small or large, single or multiple; (3) nodules with germinal centres – lymphoid follicles, but these are the least frequent[2-4]. Nodules range in size from 0.1 to 2 mm, average 0.4 mm. They consist of small round lymphocytes with typical condensed chromatin and a narrow cytoplasmic rim, situated within a fine network of reticulin fibres, and

accompanied by some capillaries, histiocytes, plasma and mast cells and occasionally eosinophils. They may be surrounded by a layer of fat cells. Though lymphoid nodules may be found in any marrow, they are more often encountered in the older age groups, and more in females. Their occurrences in haematological and other conditions are dealt with in the appropriate sections. It should be remembered that the incidence of both malignant lymphomas and benign lymphoid nodules in the bone marrow is higher in the older age groups, and it may be difficult to distinguish early involvement by malignant lymphoma from such nodules. This applies particularly to bone marrow lymphocytosis[5] and early lymphocytic lymphomas with interstitial spread, and to multiple benign nodules and a nodular lymphocytic lymphoma. Demonstration of monoclonality may be required – but even that does not necessarily prove malignancy[6]; as a clonal but non-neoplastic expansion to an antigenic stimulus may also occur. Multiclonal lymphomas have also been described – for example in immunosuppressed patients. Moreover, evolution from polyclonal proliferation to a malignant has also been documented[7,8].

Increased bone marrow lymphocytes and lymphoid nodules are found in rheumatoid and autoimmune disorders, in viral infections (e.g. infectious mononucleosis and cytomegalovirus; and mumps, measles, chicken pox); protozoan infections – such as toxoplasmosis; and in other conditions. Consequently, the clinical setting must always be considered in the evaluation and interpretation of such biopsies. This is of particular importance with respect to patients with disorders of the immune system, in view of their association with lymphoproliferative disorders[9]. Lymphohistiocytic proliferations or aggregates have been found in the bone marrow of patients with various infections, as well as in patients with rheumatic and autoimmune diseases and immune deficiency syndromes; or as a reaction to drugs.

Reactive Bone Marrow Plasmacytosis and Multiple Myeloma

It may not be possible to make a histological distinction between (1) the plasmacytosis of chronic inflammatory or other diseases, (2) that of benign monoclonal gammopathy and (3) that of early or smouldering multiple myeloma. However, a monoclonal population may be

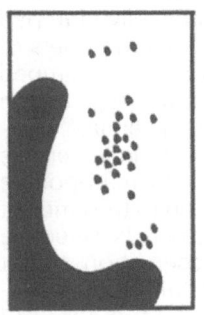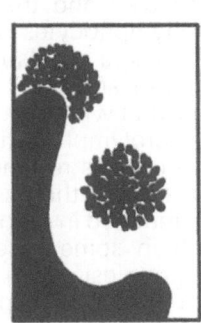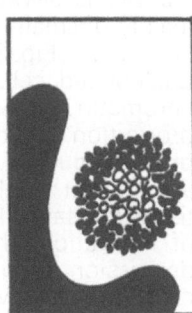

DIFFUSE
LYMPHOCYTES

LYMPHOID
NODULES

GERMINAL
CENTRES

Fig. 8.1 Lymphocytes in normal bone marrow: these may be found dispersed among the haematopoietic and fat cells, in aggregates, in nodules, and in follicles with germinal centres

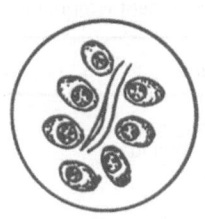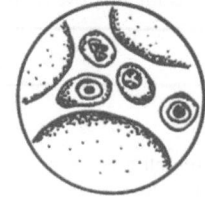

REACTIVE

NEOPLASTIC

Fig. 8.4 Perivascular reactive plasmacytosis and interstitial neoplastic plasmacytosis. Note nucleolated and somewhat pleomorphic plasma cells

identified by immunological investigation on imprints, cryostat or paraffin sections[10,11]. Though no single morphological feature of plasma cells is characteristic of a neoplastic clone, a high incidence of any of the following features within a population suggests malignancy: large nuclei, prominent nucleoli, cellular and nuclear pleomorphism, multinuclearity, crystalline or other inclusions and nucleocytoplasmic asynchronism.

The bone marrow histology is similar in the three conditions listed above. Small groups of plasma cells are found near blood vessels and among the haematopoietic and fat cells. In early MM there are also small paratrabecular and periarterial clusters of plasma cells.

Differential Diagnosis of Bone Marrow Involvement in Hodgkin's Disease and other Granulomatous Bone Marrow Infiltrates

Granulomatous infiltrates – small or large, single or multiple – may be found in rheumatic and autoimmune conditions, infections, allergies and immune deficiency states including acquired immune deficiency syndromes (AIDS); in angioimmunoblastic lymphadenopathy (AILD), in malignant histiocytosis (MH), and in systemic mastocytosis (SM). Lymphomatoid granulomatosis-like lesions have been described in 15% of 85 cases with malignant lymphomas[12].

The granulomas in some of these conditions may exhibit certain characteristic histological features: multinucleated giant cells in reactive or infectious bone marrow infiltrates, Reed–Sternberg and/or mononuclear Hodgkin cells in HD; arborization and whorl-like vascular patterns in AILD, together with deposition of PAS + interstitial material; concentric layers of mast cells, fibroblasts and lymphocytes in SM, and clusters and diffuse spread of histiocytes in malignant histiocytosis (MH). Should the biopsies be small, or the infiltrates single and small, or the characteristic features be absent, then purely histological distinction between these various entities is not possible.

Histology of Bone Marrow Involvement in the Malignant Lymphomas

Bone marrow biopsy has now been firmly established as an integral part of the investigation of patients with known or suspected malignant lymphomas. They are routinely taken to estimate stage of disease at initial diagnosis. Moreover, a bone marrow biopsy may be diagnostic in patients without peripheral lymphadenopathy[13,14], it may aid classification when inconclusive or divergent histologies are found at other sites. Recently magnetic resonance has been used to detect and estimate the extent of bone marrow involvement[15], and thus to complement bone marrow biopsy findings. The main histological parameters and their clinical correlations are given in Table 8.1.

Table 8.1 Bone marrow biopsies in malignant lymphomas

Parameter	Correlation
Involvement	Initial diagnosis
	Clinical staging
Predominant cell type	Classification
Proliferation pattern	Sub-grouping
Quantity	Histological staging
Haematopoiesis	Peripheral blood values
Bone structure	Hypercalcaemia, alkaline phosphatase levels
Cytological transformation	Accelerated clinical course
Sequential BMB	Effects of therapy, concurrent diseases

Classification of the Malignant Lymphomas

Morphological and immunological criteria, as well as enzymic reactions, have been utilized to classify the malignant lymphomas. In recent years these have been supplemented by increasingly refined immunological markers, cytogenetics, serological studies and the newer techniques of molecular biology[16–23]. However, as pointed out in the introduction to the updated Kiel classification[24], morphology remains the basis for lymphoma classification, at least in the foreseeable future. This refers mainly to lymph node histology, but applies equally well to the bone marrow, especially in view of the fact that there is a good correspondence between the two. In a study of the comparative histology of malignant lymphomas in lymph node and bone marrow[25] of 120 patients with classifiable infiltrations in both organs, congruence was found in 91/120 (76%) of the patients.

In most cases, malignant lymphomas involving the bone marrow are classifiable by histology[1,26]. In many patients the original diagnosis has already been established by lymph node biopsy, and the question is one of involvement for staging, or investigation of the other parameters listed in Table 8.1. In other cases a lymphoma is suspected on the basis of peripheral blood findings or results of imaging techniques. When the first histological diagnosis is by BMB, then immunological studies are usually also made on an aspirate taken with the biopsy, on biopsy imprints or on cryostat sections of part of the bone biopsy; or on sections of paraffin-embedded biopsies.

Bone marrow involvement in the malignant lymphomas, mainly of B-cell origin, showed six major types of spread, called growth patterns, which all merged into one pattern – the 'packed marrow' type with progession of disease and complete replacement of the marrow (Figs 8.9–8.20). The relatively infrequent T-cell lymphomas in the bone marrow show a diffuse, perivascular and/or intravascular spread[1,23]. Nodular involvement is rare.

The manifestations of the malignant lymphomas in the bone marrow will be briefly described; the order followed here is that of the updated Kiel classification. The phenotypic identification as B or T cell-derived is made on the basis of marker studies[20,27]. An example of bone marrow involvement in a patient with lymph node established T-zone lymphoma is illustrated in Figs 8.21–8.25.

Chronic Lymphocytic Leukaemia (CLL)

Lymphocytic = B-cell chronic leukaemia (CLL) and prolymphocytic (P-CLL)

CLL is the commonest leukaemia and malignant lymphoma; it involves the pathologic systemic accumulation of long-lived lymphocytes (Figs 8.26–8.32). The bone marrow is always involved and the infiltration consists mainly of small round lymphocytes with heavily clumped chromatin (Fig. 8.31). There are also variable numbers of nucleolated cells – these are larger, have less clumped chromatin and a somewhat wider rim of cytoplasm: a high proportion indicates prolymphocytic leukaemia. Lymphoid nodules with structures resembling follicle centres are present in about 25% of the cases. Haematopoietic tissue and fat cells are reduced in proportion to the amount of infiltration; though in some cases there is selective depression of haematopoiesis with preservation of fat cells; or selective inhibition of a particular cell line – e.g. erythroid or megakaryocytic (Figs 8.33–8.35). But erythroid hyperplasia is present when CLL is complicated by haemolysis. A network of reticulin fibres is present in the infiltrations (Fig. 8.36) and a few mast and plasma cells are also found. There is trabecular osteopenia without increased remodelling. Though rare cases of B-CLL with osteoblastic or osteolytic lesions have been reported

(Continued on p. 133)

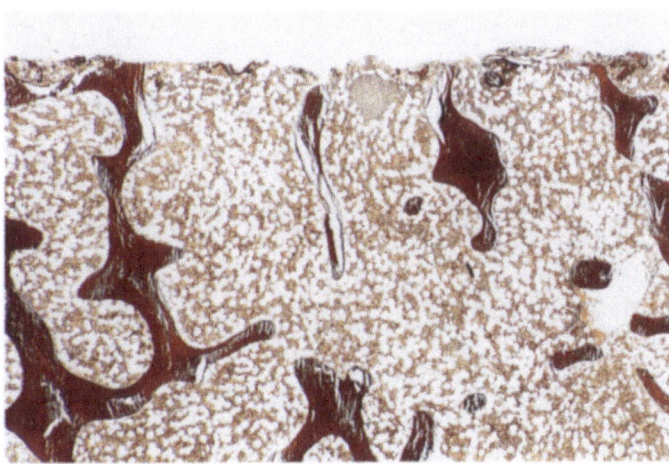

Fig. 8.2 Bone biopsy section showing single lymphoid nodule, top, right of centre. Gomori

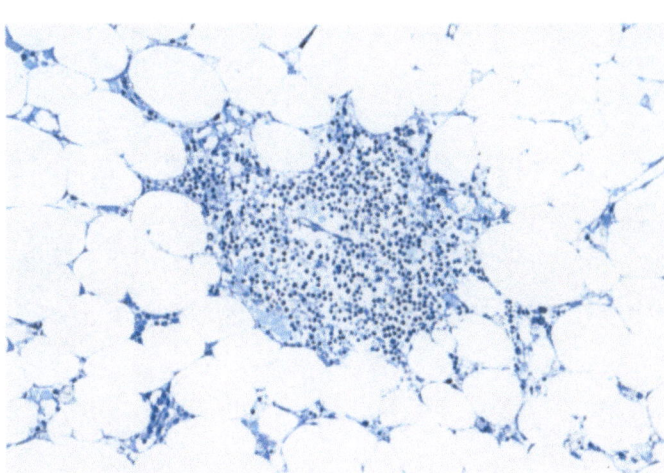

Fig. 8.3 Lymphoid nodule in hypocellular bone marrow

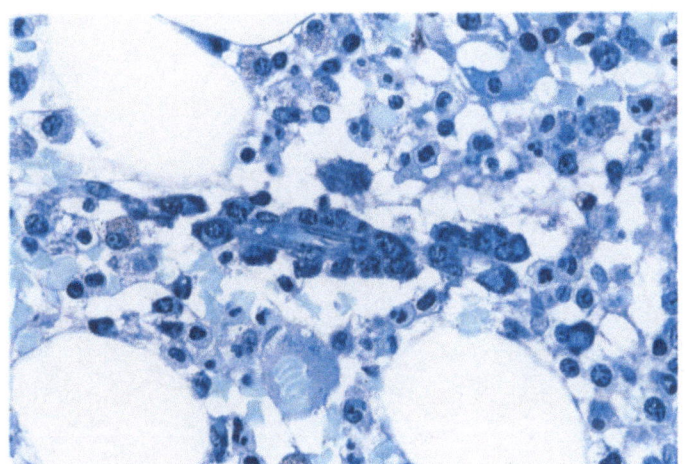

Fig. 8.5 Reactive perivascular plasma cytosis

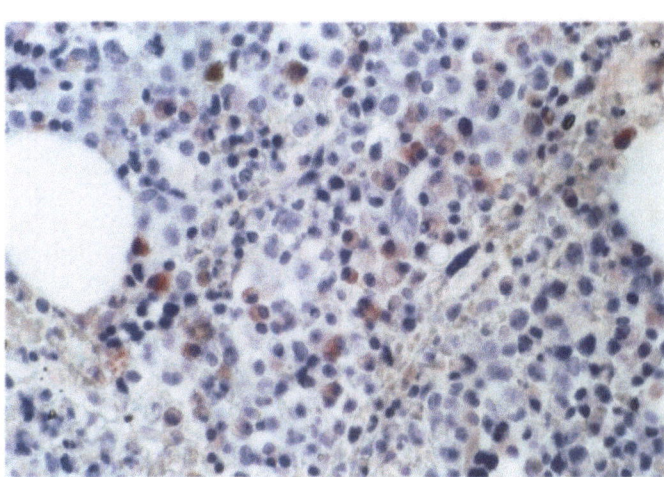

Fig. 8.6 Reactive interstitial plamacytosis in bone biopsy of patient with pyelonephritis. Plasma cells positive for kappa light chain, paraffin section

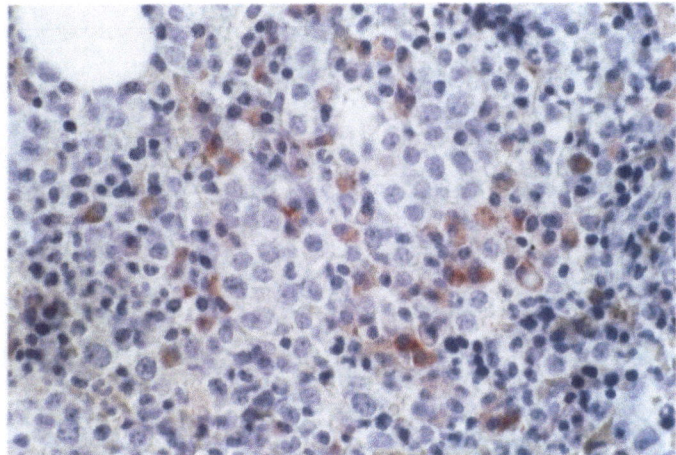

Fig. 8.7 Same patient as in Fig. 8.6. Plasma cells positive for lambda light chain

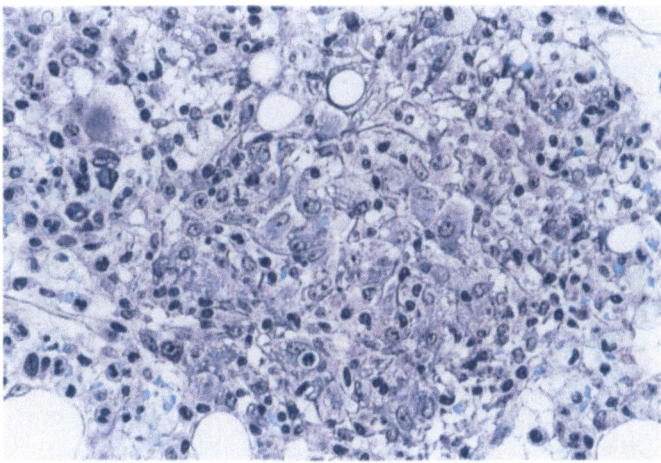

Fig. 8.8 Bone biopsy section of patient with AIDS showing an epithelioid cell granuloma

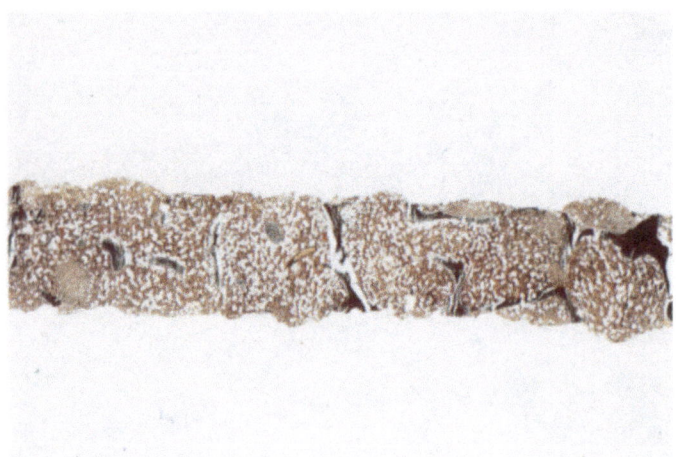

Figs 8.9–8.20 These illustrate the six types of spread or growth patterns of lymphoproliferations in the bone marrow, all low-power overviews, stained by Gomori's stain

Fig. 8.9 Minimal nodular infiltration

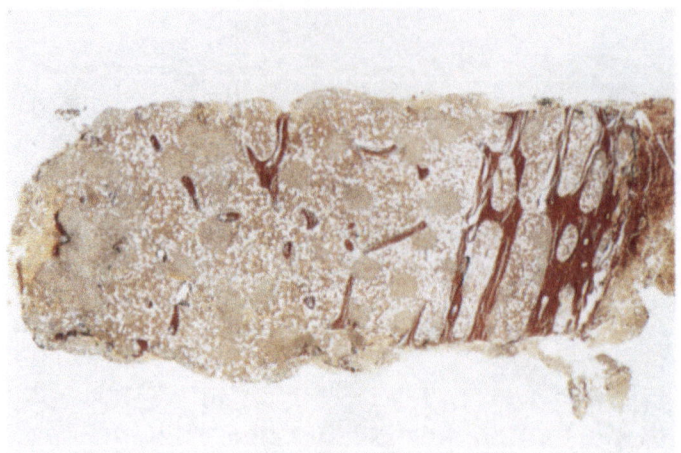

Fig. 8.10 Multiple small nodules. Note osteoporosis

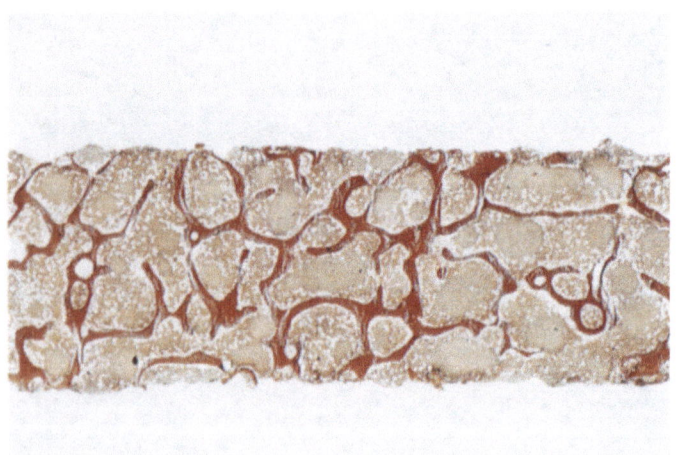

Fig. 8.11 Extensive infiltration by larger nodules, some confluent

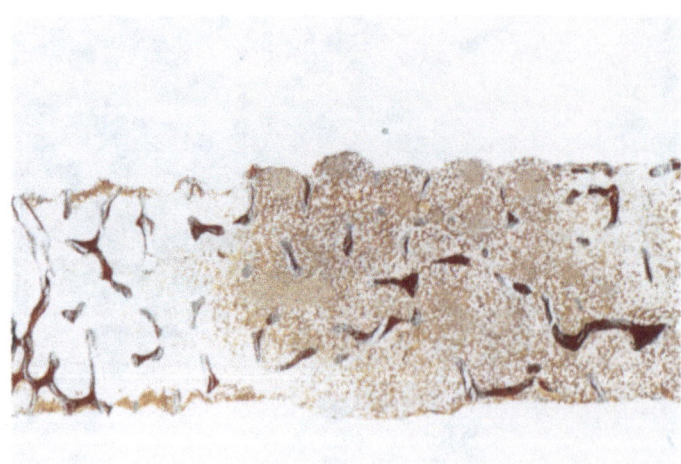

Fig. 8.12 Focal marrow involvement in hypocellular bone marrow

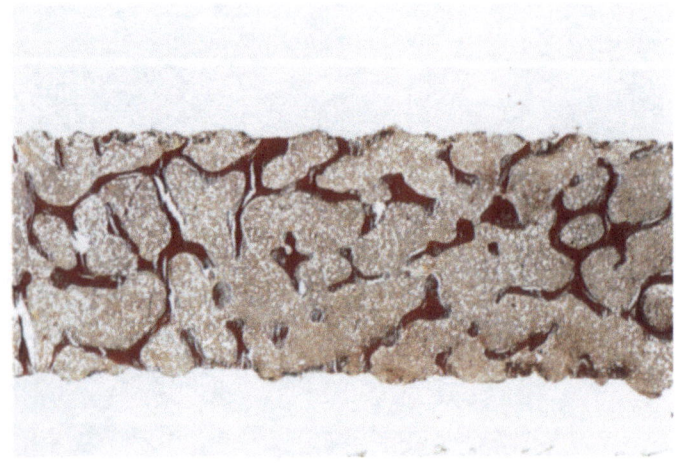

Fig. 8.13 Diffuse and nodular infiltration

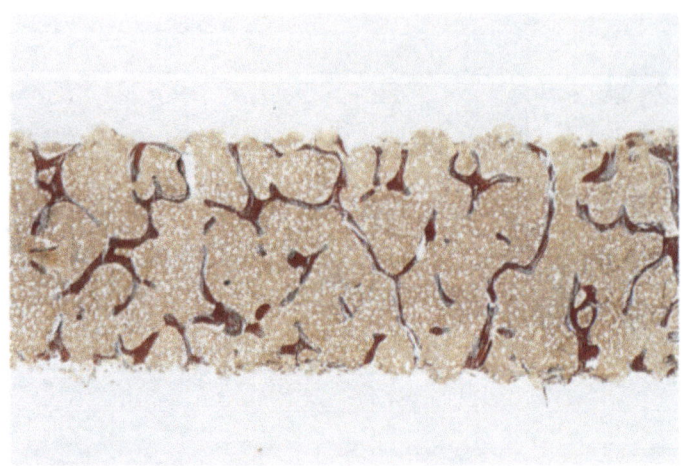

Fig. 8.14 Diffuse interstitial involvement without nodules

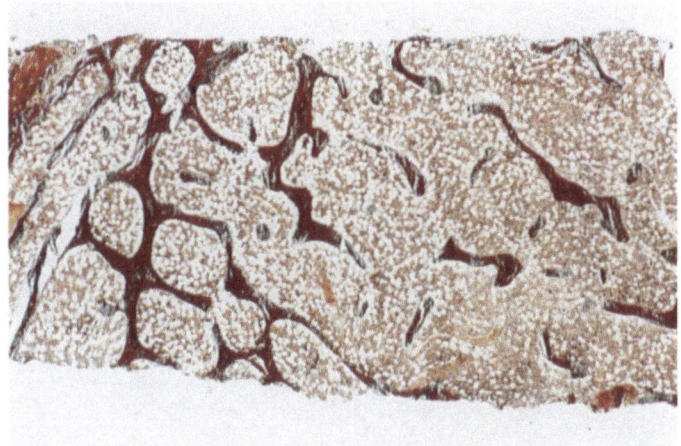

Fig. 8.15 Minimal interstitial infiltration in a normocellular bone marrow; cannot be identified at low magnification

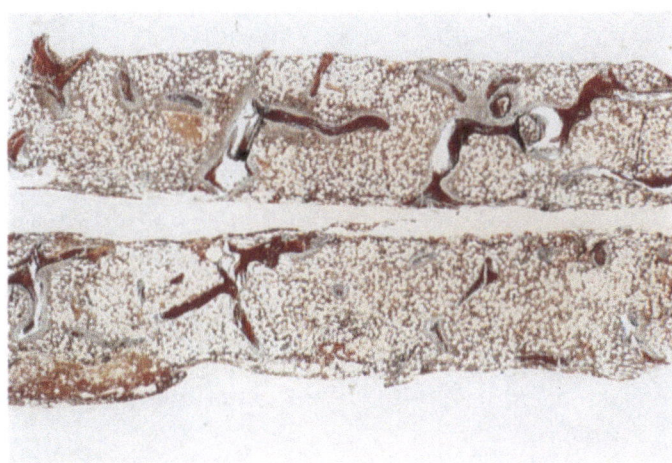

Fig. 8.16 Paratrabecular infiltration

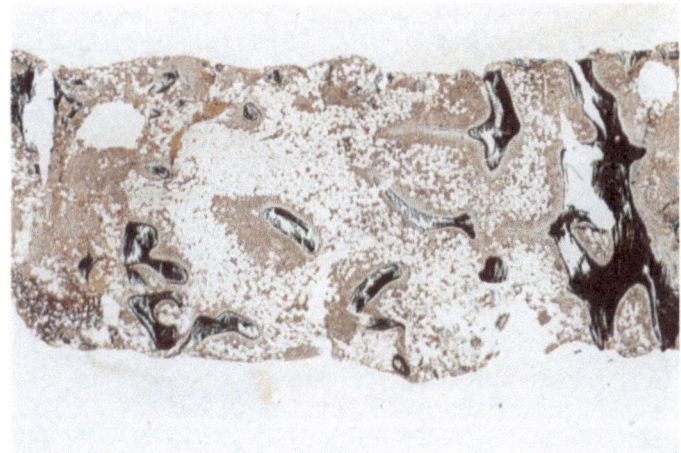

Fig. 8.17 More extensive paratrabecular infiltration with osteoporosis and hypocellular bone marrow

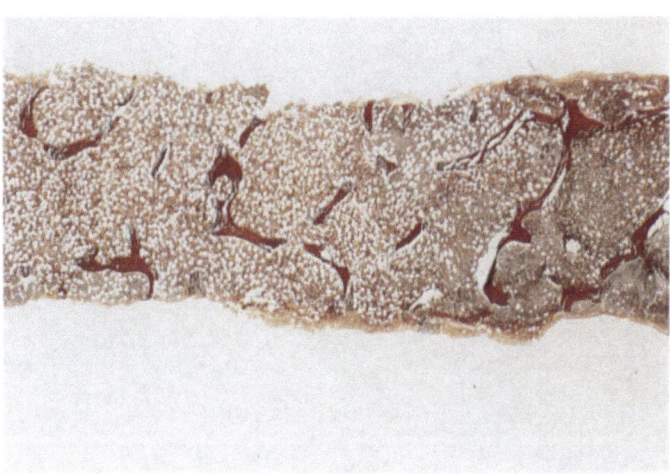

Fig. 8.18 Focal patchy involvement at one end of the biopsy (right)

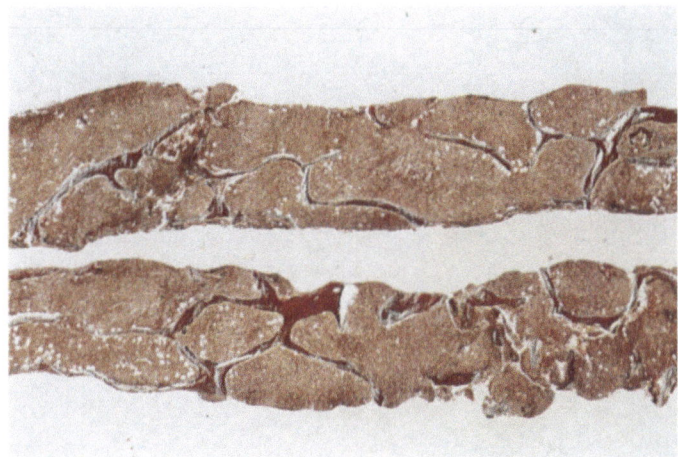

Fig. 8.19 Complete replacement of the bone marrow in lower section

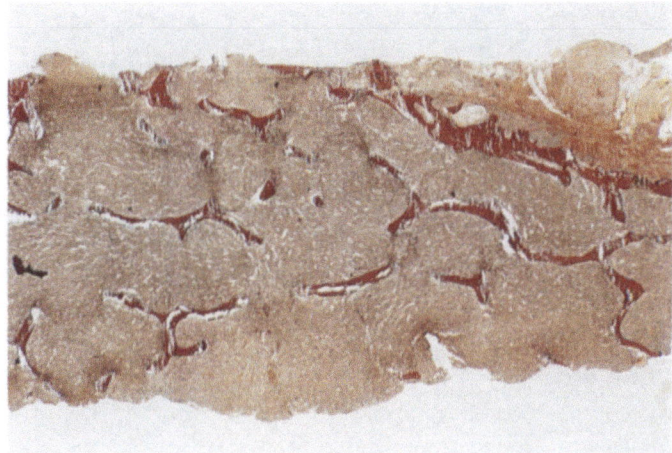

Fig. 8.20 Packed marrow pattern with attenuation of trabecular bone, cortex and periosteum, right side

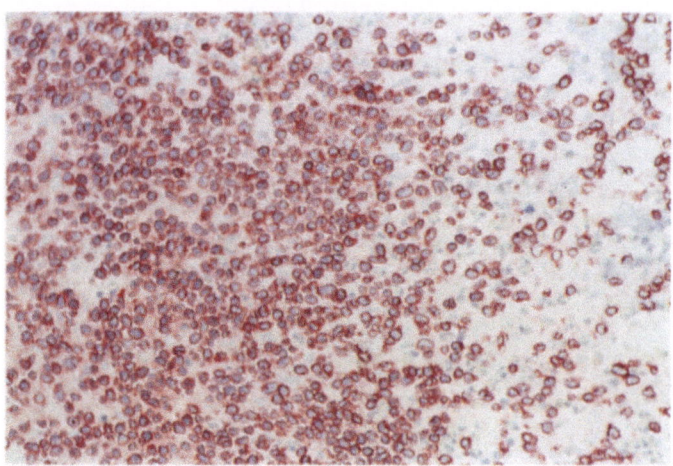

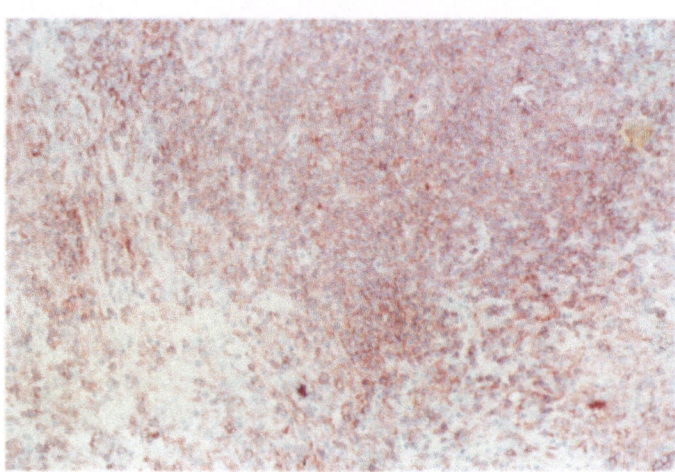

Figs 8.21–8.25 Cryostat sections of patient with T zone lymphoma, showing nodular infiltration in the bone marrow

Fig. 8.22 Reactivity of lymphocytes with Leu 3a (CD4)

Fig. 8.21 Neoplastic lymphoid cells stained by Leu 4 (CD 3)

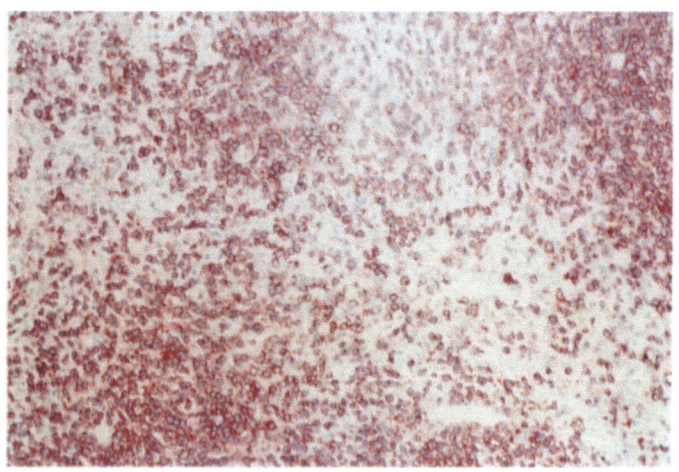

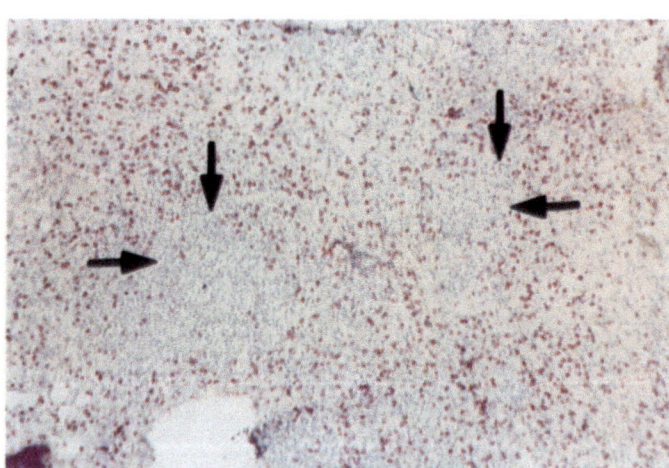

Fig. 8.23 Demonstration of neoplastic T lymphocytes by Leu 1 (CD5)

Fig. 8.24 No reactivity with Leu 2a (CD9) within the nodules. Leu 2a-positive cells around the neoplastic nodules

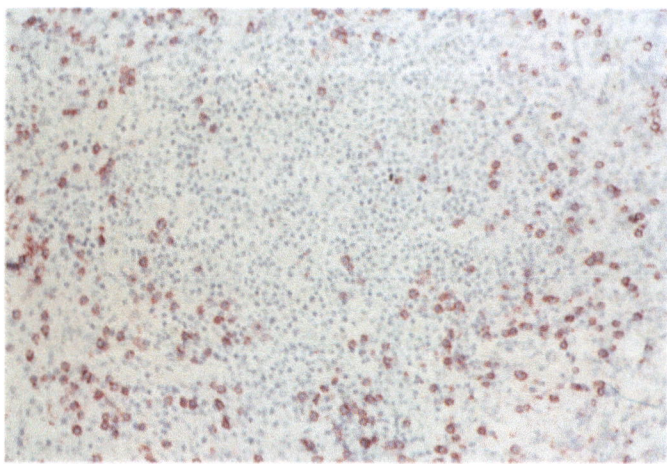

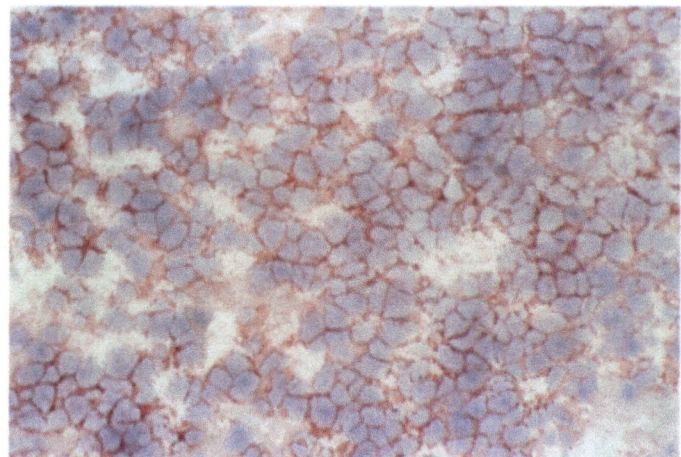

Fig. 8.25 Negative nodule surrounded by CD9-positive lymphocytes

Fig. 8.26 B-CLL with lymphocytes positive to HLA-DR-antigen. Cryostat section

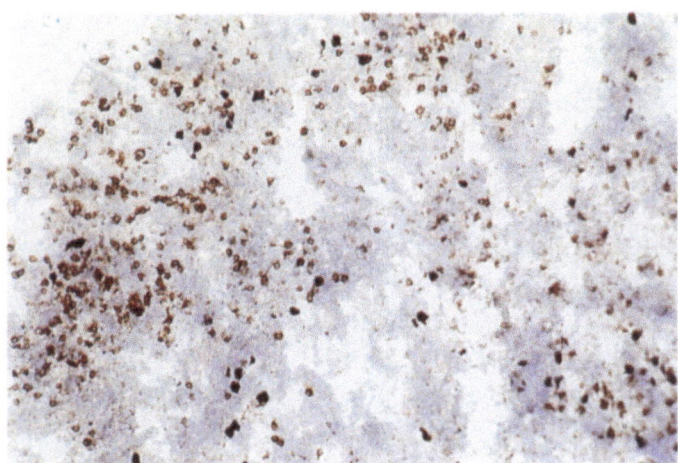

Fig. 8.27 T cells in B-CLL. Cryostat section

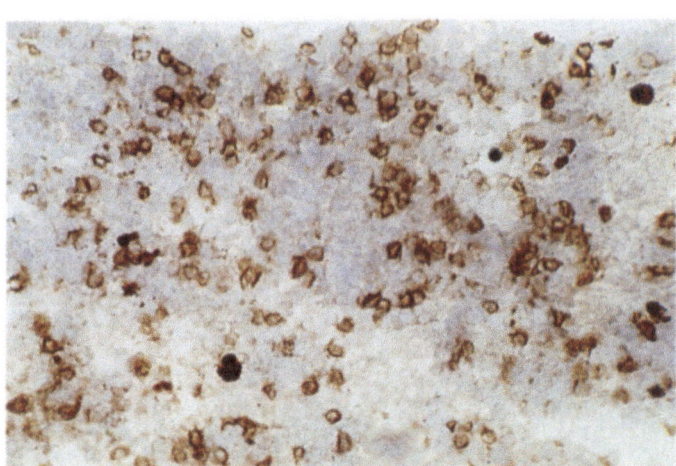

Fig. 8.28 High magnification of T cell aggregates in B-CLL. These cannot be identified in routine histology. Cryostat section.

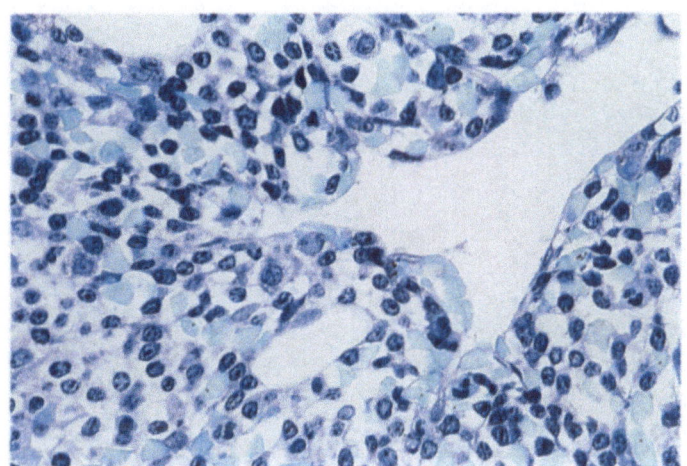

Fig. 8.29 Perisinusoidal spread of lymphocytes in T-CLL

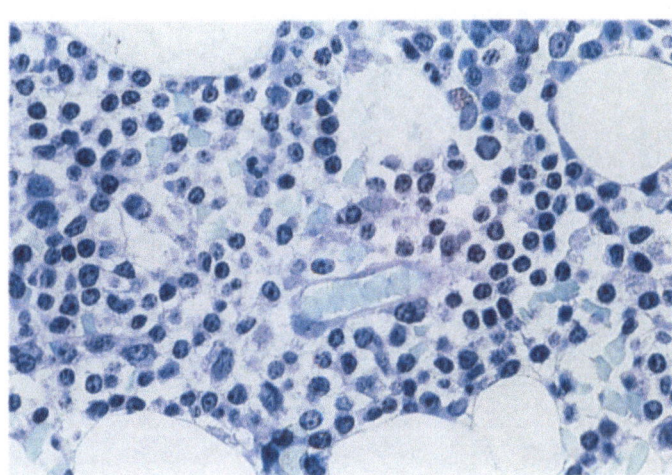

Fig. 8.30 Perivascular and interstitial spread of lymphocytes in T-CLL

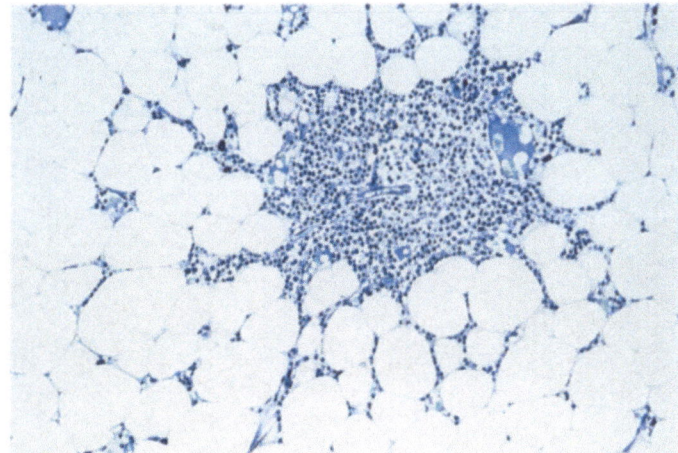

Fig. 8.31 CLL nodule with extensions between the fat cells – typical for lymphomatous nodule

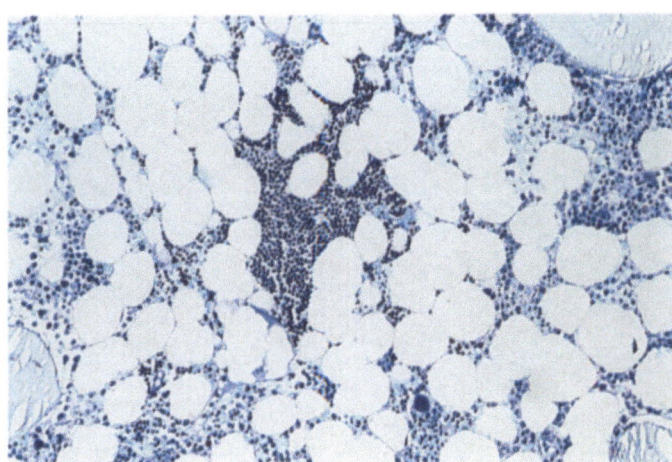

Fig. 8.32 Diffuse infiltration in hypocellular bone marrow in CLL

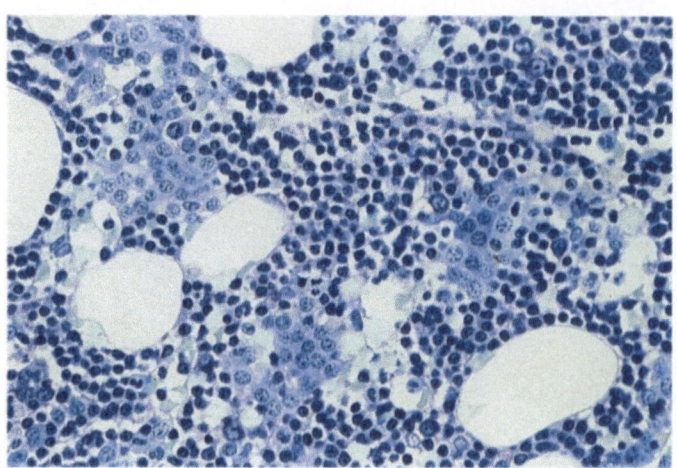

Fig. 8.33 CLL, diffuse type, with groups of erythroid precursors showing maturation arrest and megaloblastoid features

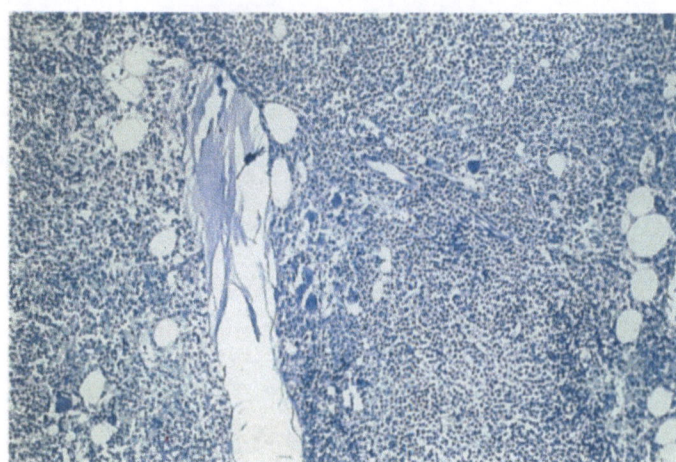

Fig. 8.34 Bone biopsy section of 68-year-old patient with CLL whose Hb decreased steadily. There is paratrabecular myelopoiesis and megakaryocytes but no erythroid precursors – CLL with pure red cell aplasia

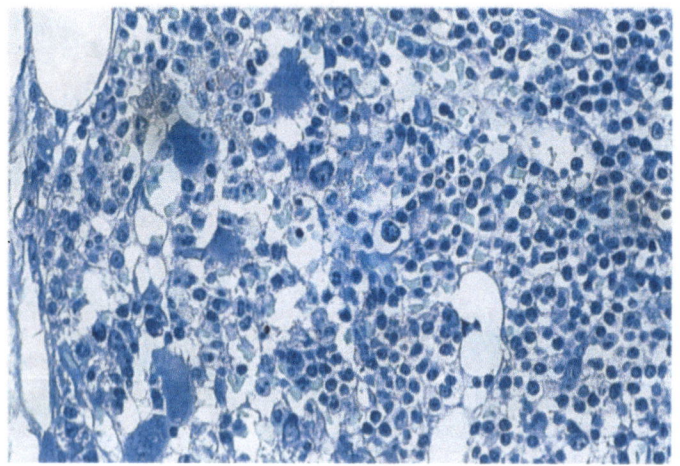

Fig. 8.35 High magnification to show myeloid cells and megakaryocytes

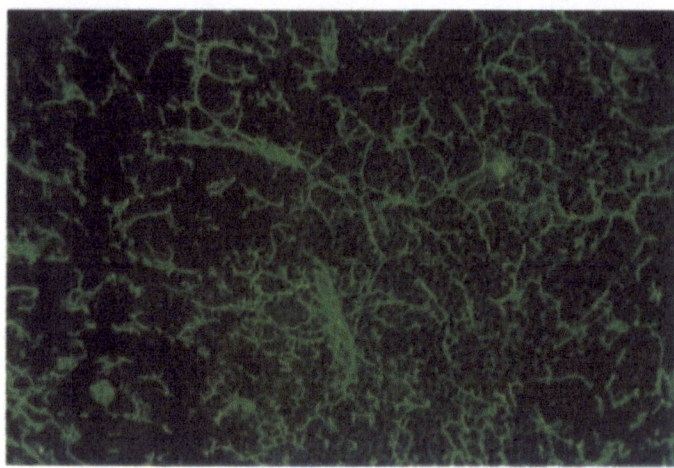

Fig. 8.36 Cryostat section reacted with antibody to collagen type III, diffuse fibrosis in case of CLL, packed marrow

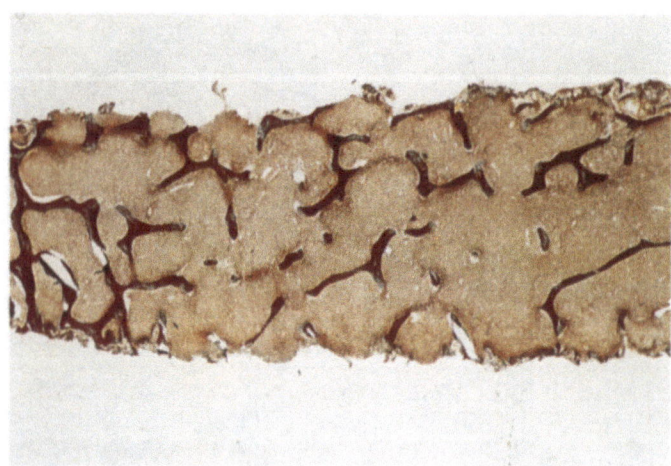

Fig. 8.37 Packed marrow pattern with mainly normal trabeculae. Gomori

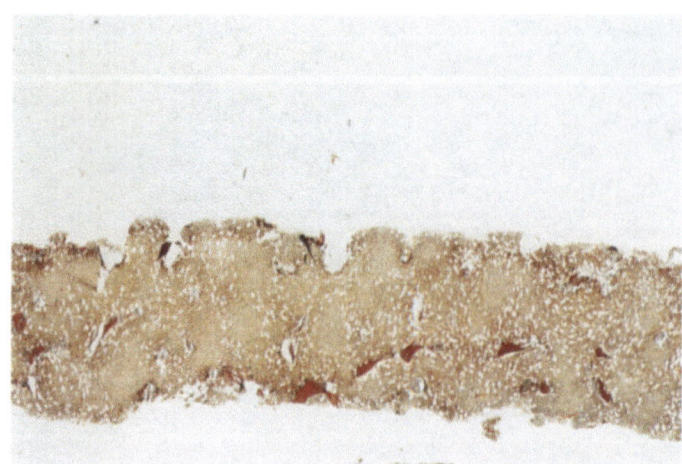

Fig. 8.38 CLL with marked osteopenia in the packed marrow. Gomori

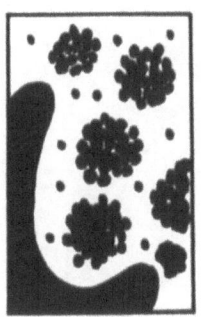 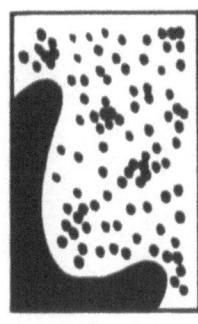 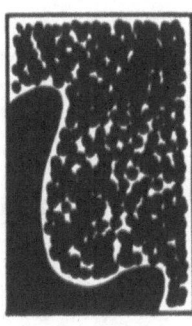

NODULAR INTERSTITIAL PACKED

Fig. 8.40 The three main proliferation patterns of CLL in the bone marrow

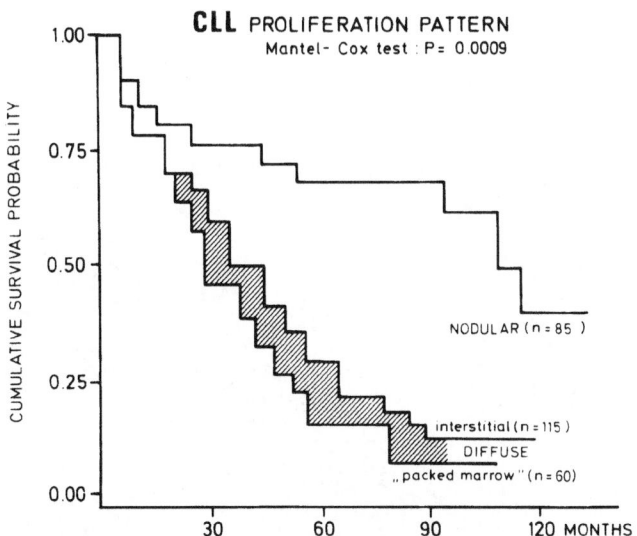

Fig. 8.49 Survival curves of patients with CLL on the basis of the initial proliferation patterns in the bone biopsy

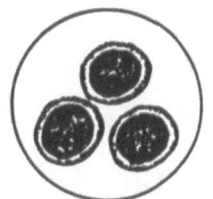 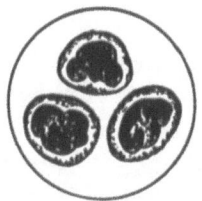 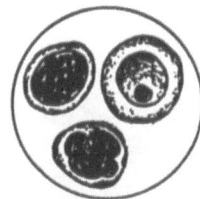

SMALL ROUND NOTCHED MIXED

Fig. 8.50 Main types of lymphocytes in CLL showing range in cell size and nuclear configuration

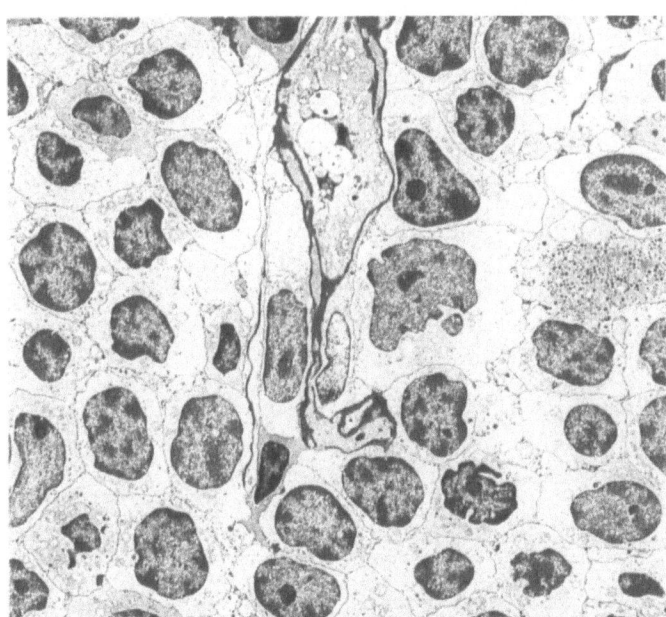

Fig. 8.54 Mainly small, round lymphocytes in CLL. EM × 10 000

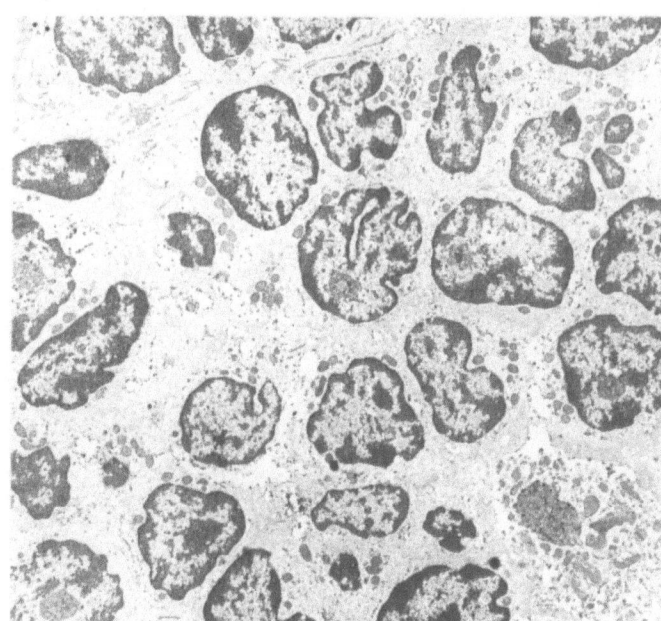

Fig. 8.55 Mainly notched lymophocytes in CLL. EM × 15 000

(Figs 8.37–8.39), marked osteoclastic activation is more characteristic of the T-cell lymphoproliferations. B-CLL is a clonal proliferation of lymphoid cells which appear mature morphologically, but are maturationally immature, and do not necessarily represent the neoplastic counterpart of the circulating peripheral blood B lymphocyte[28,29]. Occasionally, CLL B lymphoid cells may mature, leading to clinical multiple myeloma[30].

B-CLL demonstrates three main patterns of spread in the bone marrow: (1) nodular, (2) interstitial, and (3) packed marrow (Figs 8.40–8.48). These three bone marrow patterns have prognostic significance at all clinical stages (median survivals of 90, 46 and 28 months respectively) (Fig. 8.49). The favourable prognosis of an initial nodular growth pattern in the bone marrow has been confirmed in several reports[31–33], and recently reviewed by Frisch and Bartl[34]. Close study of the growth patterns in sequential biopsies, especially by means of the Gomori stain for reticulin fibres, showed that both nodular and interstitial patterns eventually progressed to the packed marrow type (Fig. 8.48). CLL could also be classified into three histological types on the basis of four cellular characteristics: small round nuclei, notched nuclei, large round nuclei and presence of nucleoli (Figs 8.50–8.55). These three types are small round, small notched and mixed with median survivals of 53, 26 and 28 months respectively. A long survival in B-CLL has also been correlated with a surface IgMk phenotype[35].

Estimation of the quantity of infiltration[34,36] in the biopsy could be used for histological staging and correlated with the clinical stages, according to the staging systems most widely used[34,37]. In most cases histological progression – i.e. increase in tumour cell burden – reflects the clinically advanced stages, especially when clinical stages 3 and 4 are combined to form the group of 'bone marrow failure'. This is also indicated by the correlation between tumour cell burden in the BMB, peripheral lymphocytosis and the platelet counts; i.e. increases in tumour cell burden are

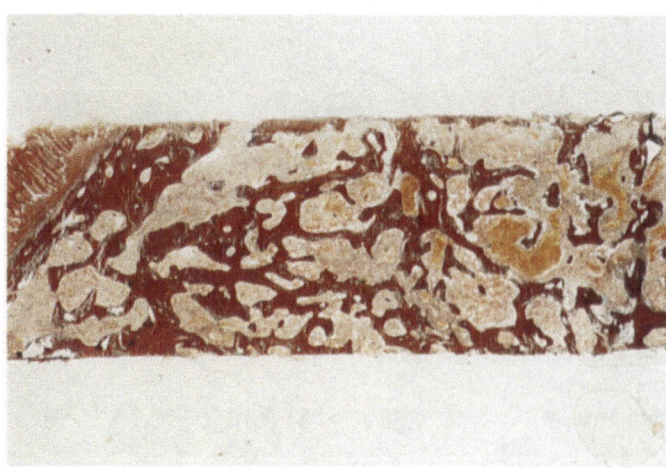

Fig. 8.39   CLL with osteosclerosis. Gomori

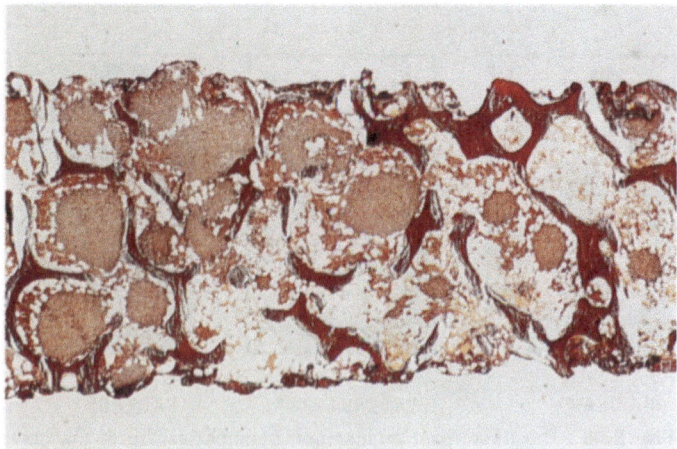

Fig. 8.41   Variably sized nodules in hypocellular bone marrow in CLL. Gomori

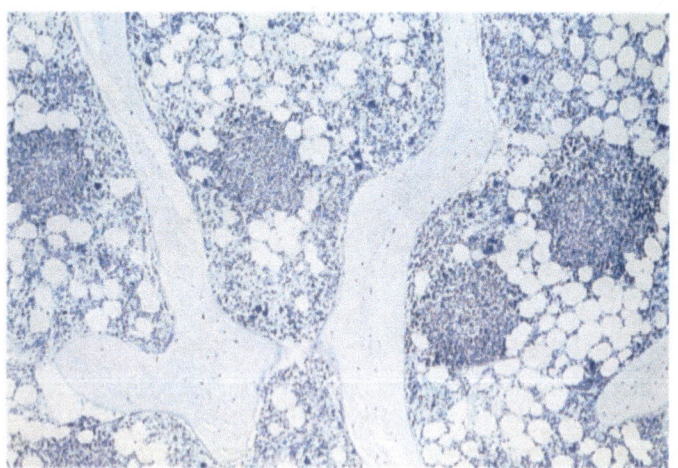

Fig. 8.42   Well-delineated nodules in hypo- to normocellular marrow with haematopoiesis in CLL

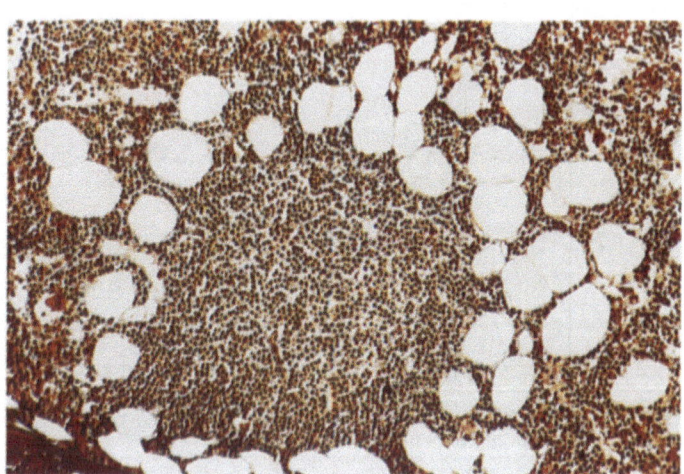

Fig. 8.43   Nodule surrounded by fat cells in CLL: Gomori

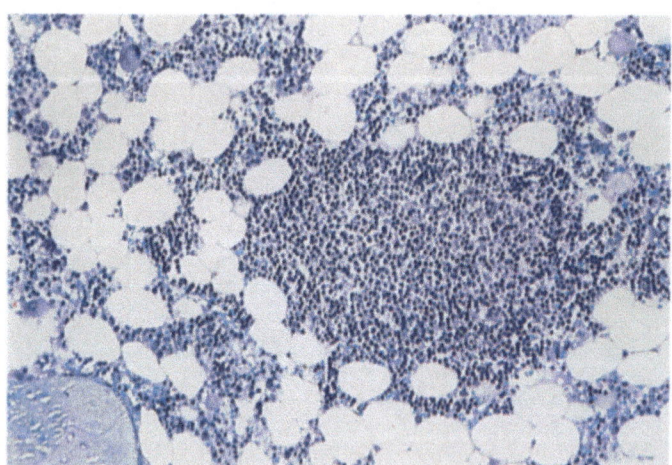

Fig. 8.44   Nodular and diffuse involvement in CLL

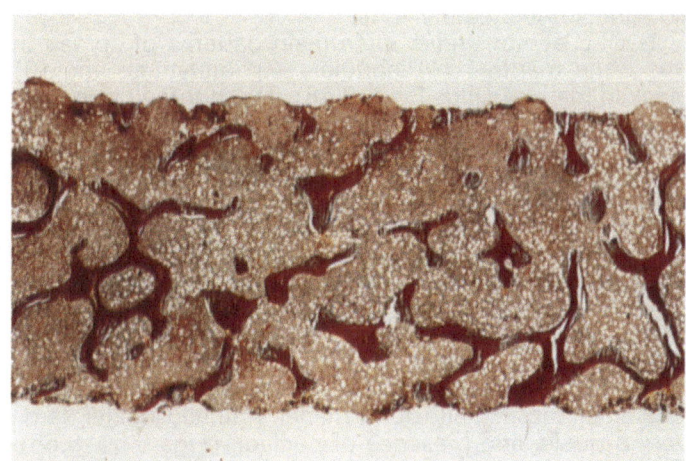

Fig. 8.45   Progressive accumulation of lymphocytes in the diffuse type. Gomori

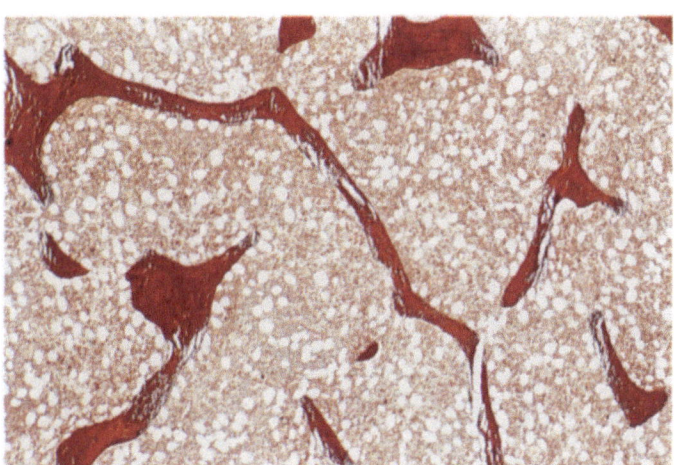

Fig. 8.46 Loose interstitial infiltration with preservation of fat cells. Gomori

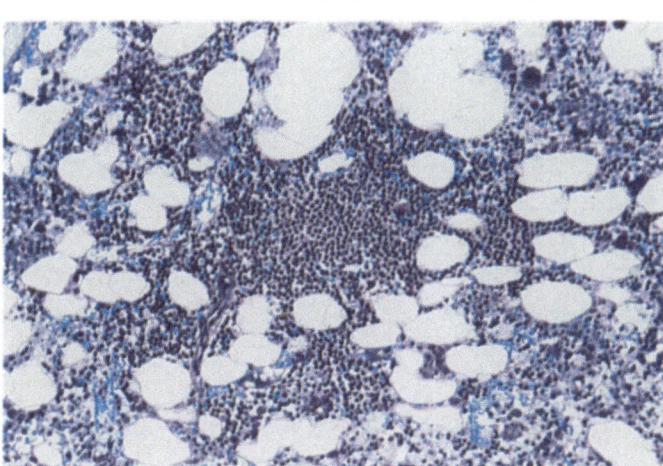

Fig. 8.47 Nodular and diffuse pattern showing lymphoid cells together with some haematopoietic elements among the fat cells surrounding the nodule

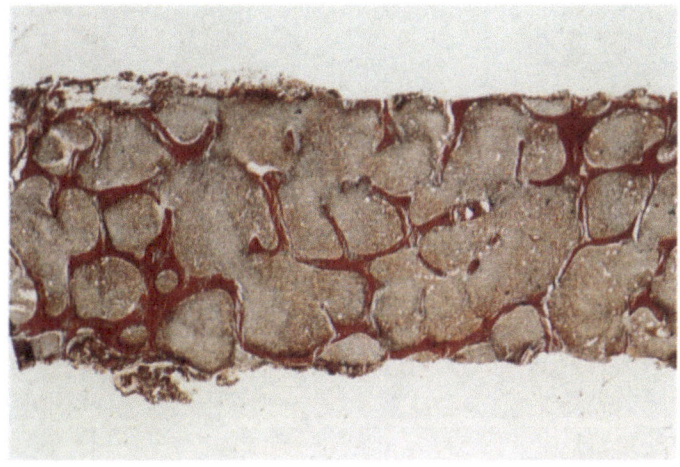

Fig. 8.48 Packed marrow with replacement of both haematopoietic and fatty tissue. Gomori

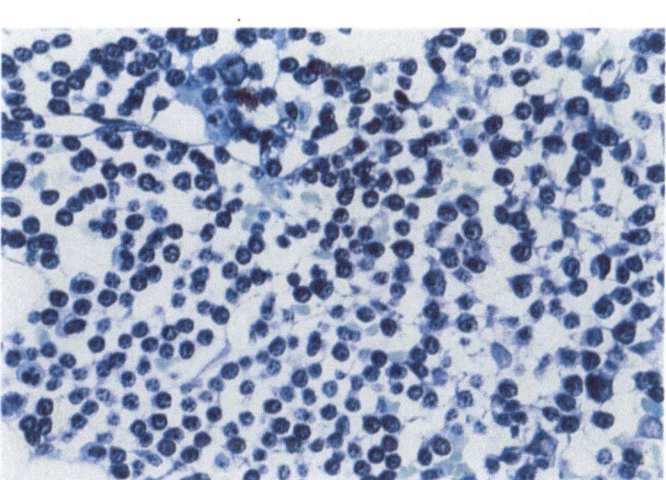

Fig. 8.51 CLL nodular, composed mainly of small round lymphocytes

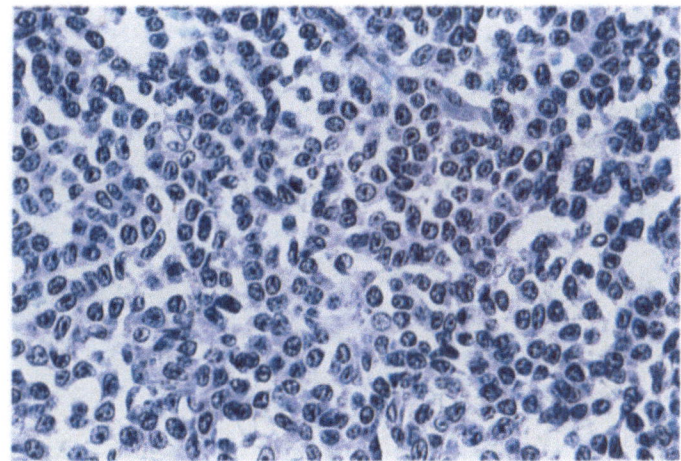

Fig. 8.52 CLL diffuse, notched lymphocytes

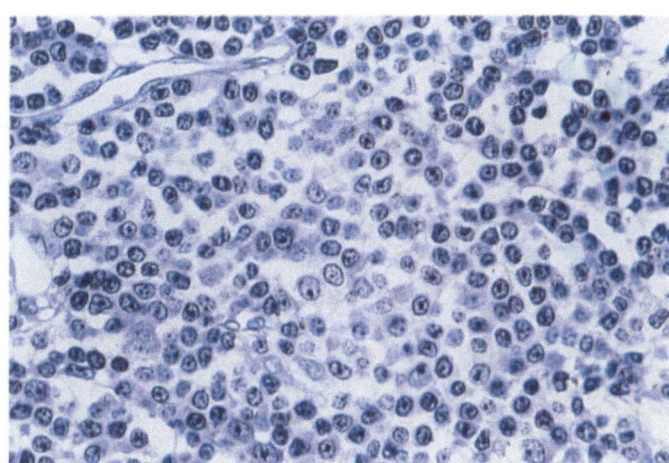

Fig. 8.53 CLL diffuse, mixed type consisting of small round, notched, and larger lymphocytes with nucleoli

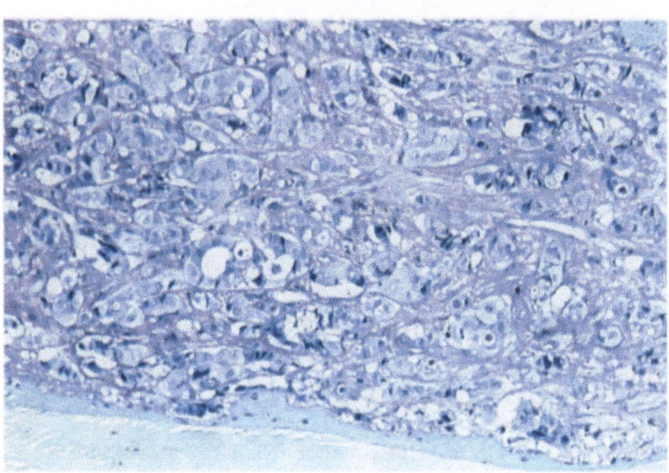

Fig. 8.56 Patient with CLL and prostatic cancer, no lymphocyte infiltration, only metastasis

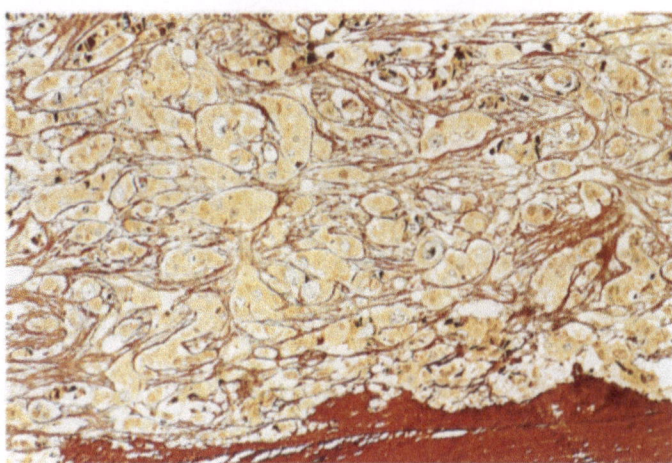

Fig. 8.57 Same biopsy as in Fig. 8.56. Extensive fibrosis. Gomori

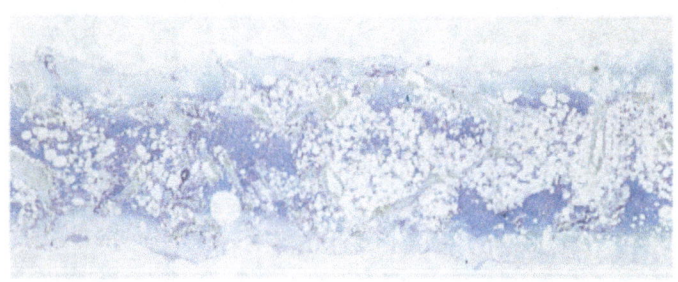

Figs 8.58–8.63 Post-chemotherapy bone marrows of patients with CLL

Fig. 8.58 Low-power view showing haemorrhagic empty bone marrow

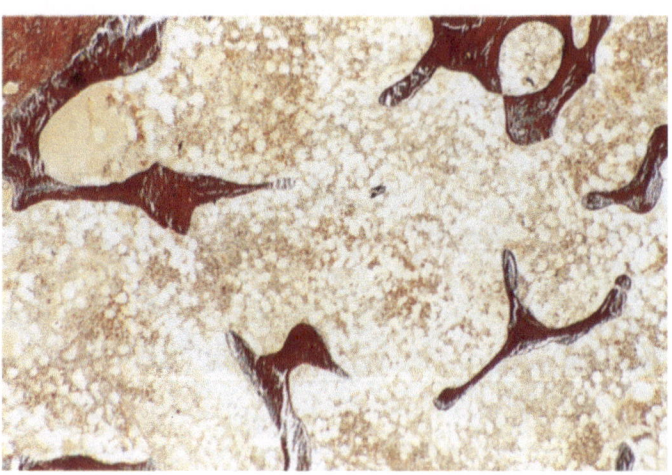

Fig. 8.59 Haemorrhage and degeneration and fatty bone marrow. Gomori

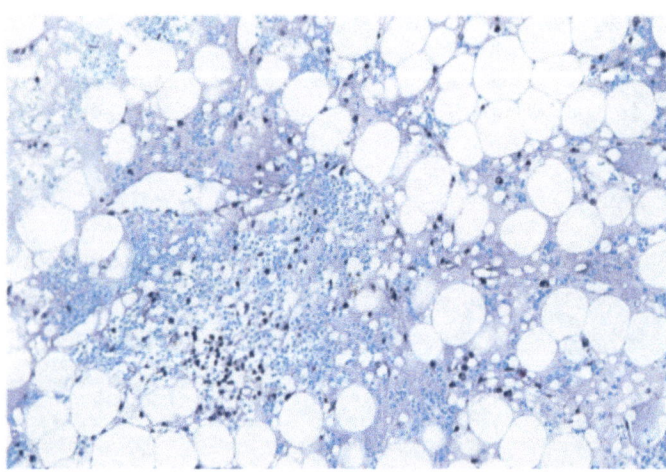

Fig. 8.60 Serous atrophy and fat cells. No haematopoietic tissue

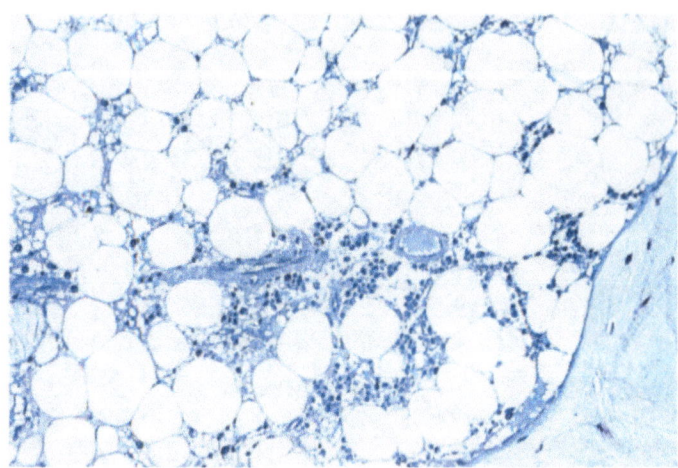

Fig. 8.61 Inflammatory cells in fatty bone marrow

accompanied by increases in the lymphocyte count and decreases in the platelet counts and haemoglobulin. Both growth patterns and the proliferative cell system reflect the aggressivity of the disease and have clinical and prognostic relevance[34,38,39]. Terminal transformations of CLL into acute forms (e.g. Richter's syndrome) were recognized in BMB in their initial stages. Moreover, the simultaneous presentation of CLL with multiple myeloma, polycythaemia vera, and myeloblastic leukaemia has been described. The association of CLL with erythraemic myelosis has also been reported[30,40,41]. Figures 8.56 and 8.57 demonstrate replacement of the bone marrow and the lymphoid infiltration in a case of CLL by metastatic carcinoma. Post-chemotherapy bone marrows in CLL are shown in Figs 8.58–8.63.

Prolymphocytic CLL

The lymphoid cells are small to medium with moderate amounts of cytoplasm and a high proportion of nucleolated cells; generally a packed marrow pattern is observed (Fig. 8.64). There is a positive acid phosphatase reaction in the lymphoid cells when the test is performed on smears, imprints and cryostat sections.

Early CLL, and smouldering CLL

Occasionally bone biopsies and peripheral blood counts are taken during the initial phases for other reasons, and the patients subsequently developed the full-blown clinical and histological pictures of CLL. In these retrospectively diagnosed early cases, which at the time did not fulfil the criteria for CLL, the lymphoid cells were dispersed between fat and haematopoietic elements and around the sinusoids in the interstitial pattern while a few aggregates were present in the nodular pattern (Fig. 8.65). The quantity in both cases was low. In 'smouldering CLL' the initial tumour cell burden was also minimal, usually of the nodular type, and remained so for long periods, without disease progression. A benign variant of CLL, called benign monoclonal B cell lymphocytosis corresponding to stage 0 CLL, which remained static for long periods, has been described[5].

It should be pointed out that the purely morphological distinction between benign lymphoid nodules and bone marrow lymphocytosis on the one hand, and early lymphomatous infiltrations on the other hand, may not be possible and immunohistology may be required.

T-cell CLL with a nodular growth pattern in the bone marrow has not been reported. The cases reported so far have shown interstitial, diffuse, perivascular and packed marrow types; a few lymphoid cell aggregates may also be present. The nuclei are often convoluted and the cytoplasm more abundant than that of B cell CLL. The T cell origin must be established by means of immunological studies on peripheral blood, smears of aspirates, imprints of the biopsies, cryostat sections, or on paraffin sections of decalcified bone biopsies.

Hairy Cell Leukaemia (HCL)

This is now classified as a malignant lymphoma of B-cell lineage, on the basis of immunologic, enzyme and electron microscopic studies (Figs 8.66–8.68)[42–45]. Nevertheless, recent studies have demonstrated reactivity of hairy cells with an antibody usually restricted to early thymocytes and Langerhans cells, thereby again introducing an element of ambiguity into the postulated derivation of hairy cells[43]. Both clinical course and therapeutic response are highly variable, which has led some observers to the conclusion that HCL represents a spectrum rather than a single disease entity[44,45]. Involvement of the bone marrow is nearly always present (Figs 8.69–8.71). Initially there is

a patchy infiltration, interstitial and perivascular, of small to large clusters or aggregates of hairy cells. Subsequently, large areas of the bone marrow may be completely replaced by hairy cells. There is variable preservation of fat cells, and of islands of haematopoietic tissue. These lymphoid cells have round to oval to indented or convoluted nuclei[45]; they usually have fairly abundant cytoplasm with lateral, long, interdigitating extensions – the processes which give them their name of 'hairy' cells (Fig. 8.72). There are rod-like cytoplasmic inclusions in about half of the cases – visible as bars or circles under oil in the light microscope. On electron microscopy the typical ribosome lamellar complexes may be seen (Figs 8.73–8.75). However, these are not specific, as they have been found in a wide variety of diseases; and in benign plasma cells[46].

The hairy cells are situated within a characteristic background, except in the early cases as described above. This microenvironment consists of a reticular fibre network which also encloses lymphocytes, plasma and mast cells, extravasated erythrocytes and precursors of red and white cells and megakaryocytes (Figs 8.76 and 8.77). Erythropoietic islands showing maturation arrest and megaloblastoid features are often present within a hairy cell infiltrate (Fig. 8.78). There are also numerous small blood vessels, histiocytes or reticular cells and fibroblasts.

The loose network of widely separated cells is typical of hairy cell infiltration in the bone marrow, in contrast to other lymphomatous infiltrations in which the cells are more densely packed together. In some cases, especially early ones with minimal infiltrations, the differential diagnosis includes other malignant lymphomas and monocytic infiltrates.

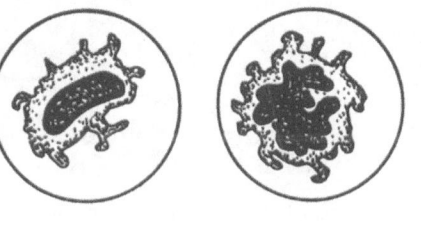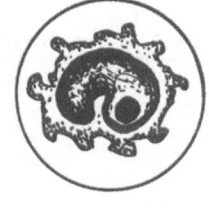

OVOID   CONVOLUTED   INDENTED

Fig. 8.79 Schematic representation of the three main configurations of hairy cell nuclei: ovoid, convoluted and indented

When examined under high magnification, hairy cell nuclei display a wide range of size and configuration with three main types: ovoid, convoluted and indented (Figs 8.79–8.82). Usually one type predominates in each individual case. The ovoid type has the best, and the indented type has the least, favourable prognosis. These three cell types are more easily distinguished in sections of plastic-embedded BMB than in haematoxylin and eosin-stained sections of decalcified and paraffin-embedded BMB. The reaction for tartrate-resistant acid phosphatase can be performed on peripheral blood smears (not indicated if the lymphocyte count is low), on smears of aspirates or on imprints of the biopsy, especially in cases of 'dry tap' on attempts at aspiration. Studies on the evolution of the disease have shown that the hairy cell burden in the bone marrow correlates with the clinical course, and a rapid increase of tumour mass indicated an unfavourable prognosis. Transformation of the mainly ovoid to the indented type also signalled a rapid progression. These findings have been supported by a recent report of a blastic variant of HCL[47]. HCL must be differentiated from B cell CLL, cleaved type (centrocytic) lymphomas, myelomonocytic and monocytic infiltrations, monocytoid B cell lymphomas and splenic B cell lymphomas with 'villous' lymphocytes in the peripheral blood[48,49]. Reduction in the amount of hairy cell mass, and repopulation by haematopoietic

(Continued on p. 142)

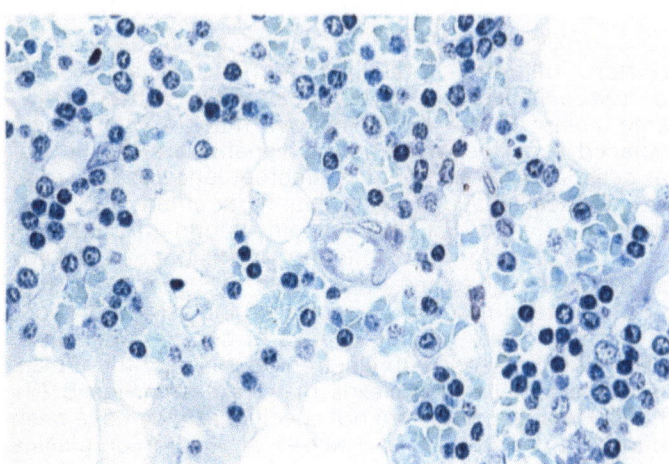

Fig. 8.62   Residual infiltration in the diffuse type of CLL

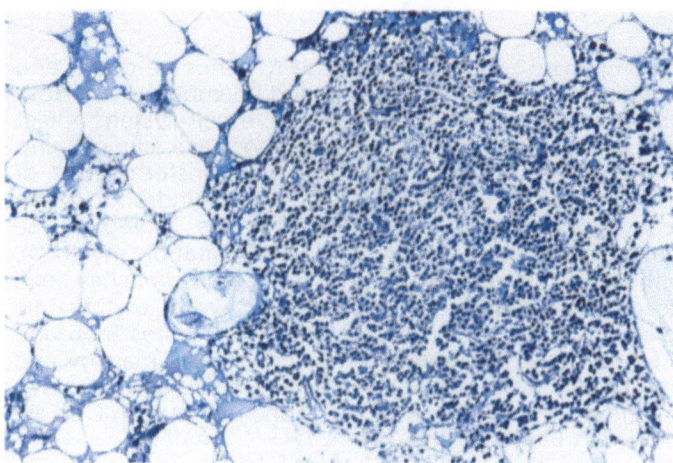

Fig. 8.63   Residual paratrabecular nodule in the nodular type of CLL

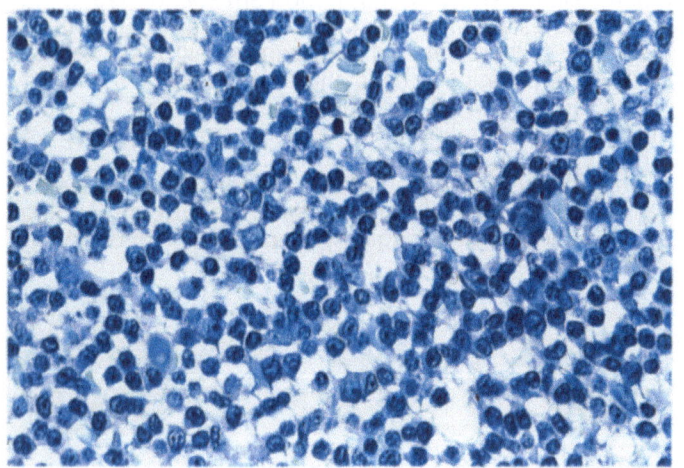

Fig. 8.64   Case of prolymphocytic CLL: packed marrow, many of the lymphocytes have nucleoli

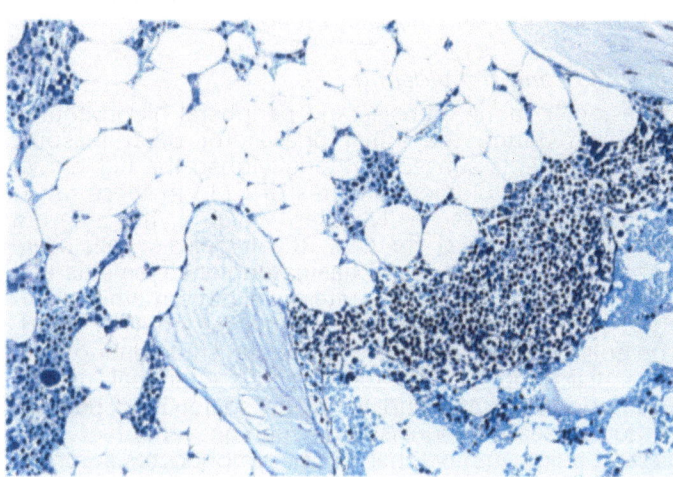

Fig. 8.65   Case of 'smouldering' CLL with lymphocyte aggregate in hypocellular bone marrow

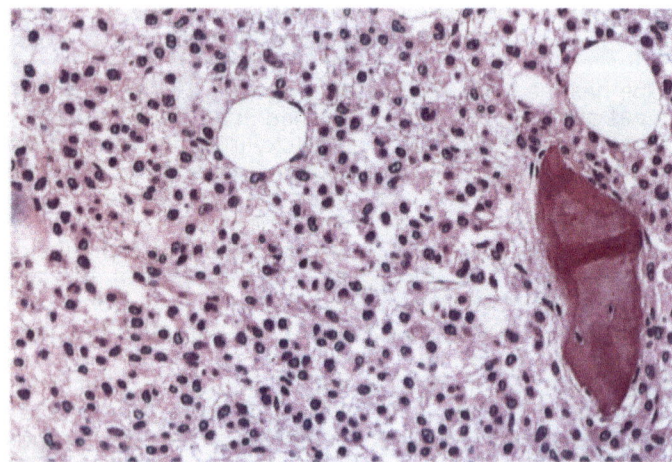

Fig. 8.66   Section of bone biopsy of patient with HCL. H&E

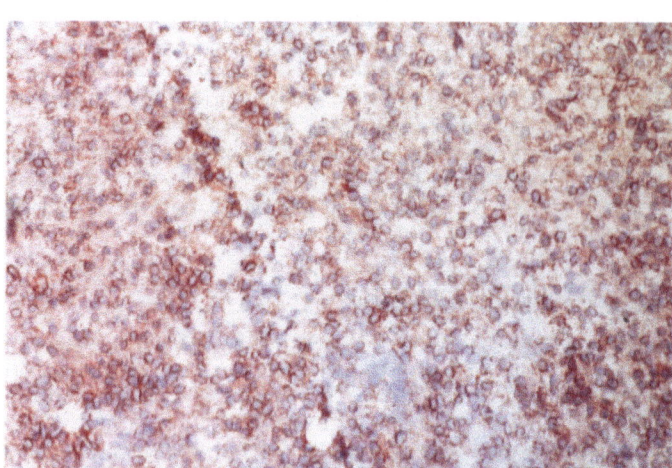

Fig. 8.67   Cryostat section of same patient as in Fig. 8.66. Hairy cells stained by CD2. Residual haematopoietic cells negative

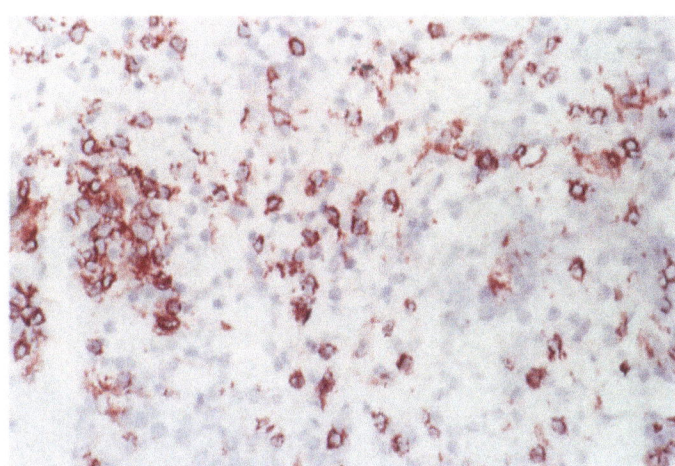

Fig. 8.68 Cryostat section of same patient as in Fig. 8.66. T-lymphocytes, monocytes and macrophages stained by LEU 3a

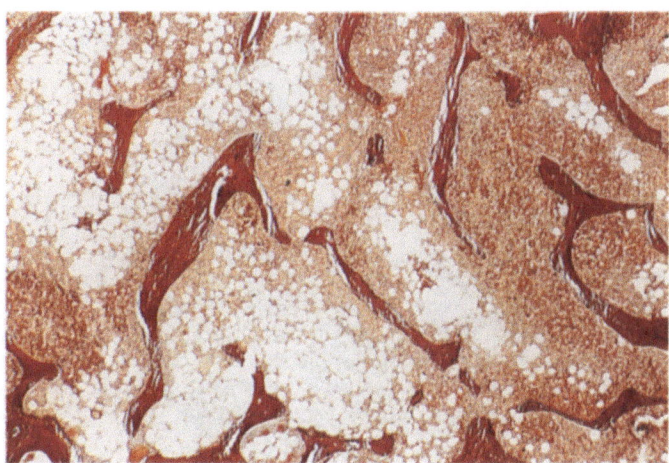

Fig. 8.69 Patchy growth pattern in a patient with HCL. Gomori

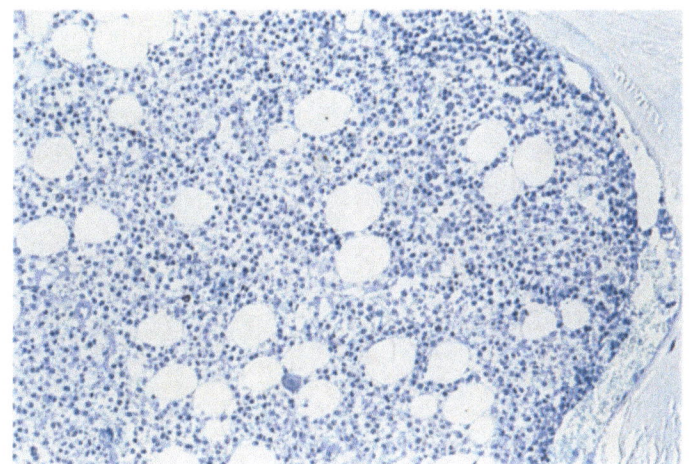

Fig. 8.70 Diffuse interstitial infiltration in HCL

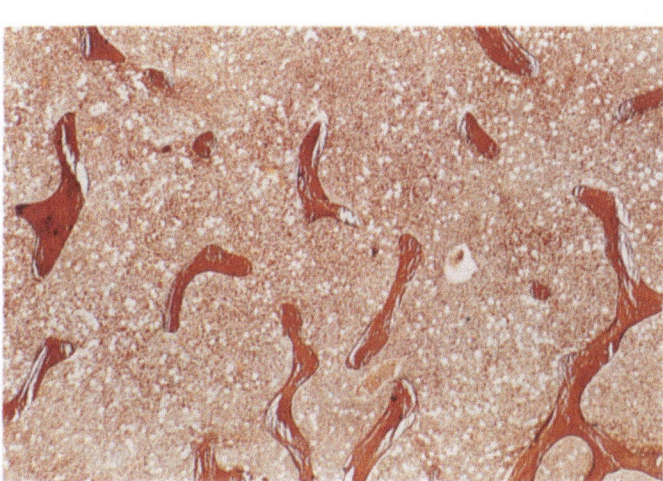

Fig. 8.71 Packed marrow type in HCL

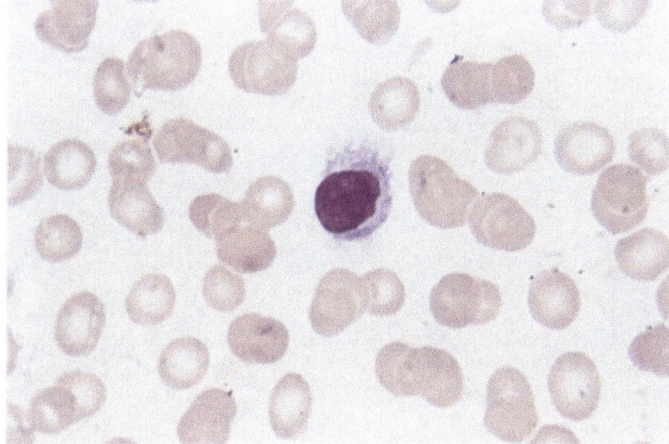

Fig. 8.72 Peripheral blood smear, showing a typical hairy cell

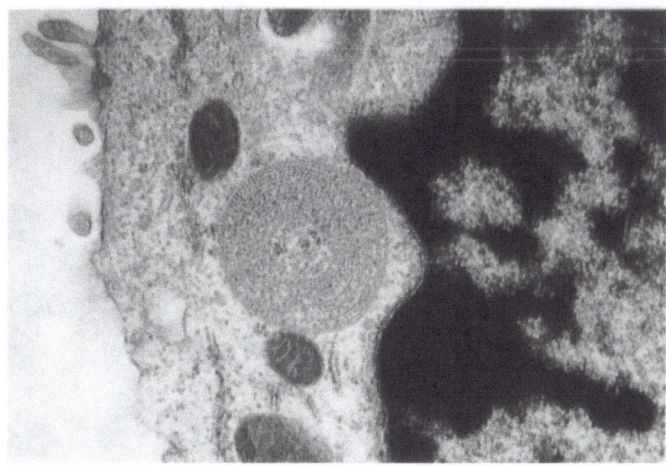

Fig. 8.73 Electron micrograph of hairy cell, demonstrating a characteristic circular ribosome lamellar complex. × 75 000

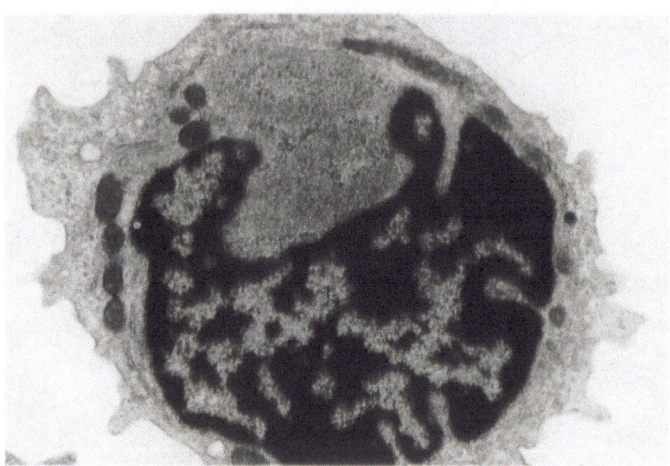

Fig. 8.74 Hairy cell with cytoplasmic villi and two ribosome lamellar complexes. EM × 20000

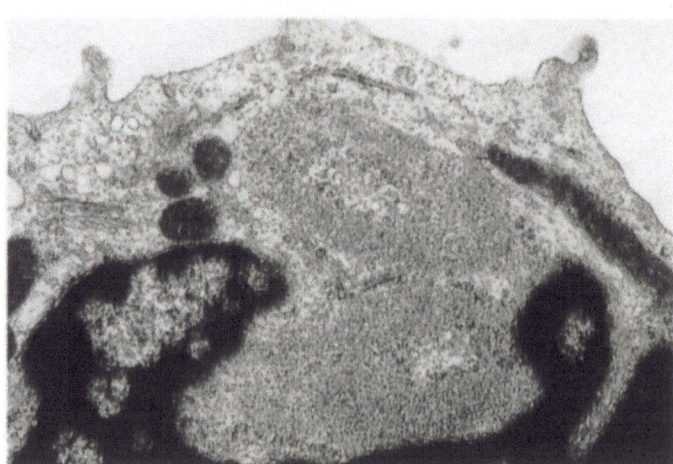

Fig. 8.75 Higher magnification of Fig. 8.74 showing structural details of the two ribosome lamellar complexes. EM × 75000

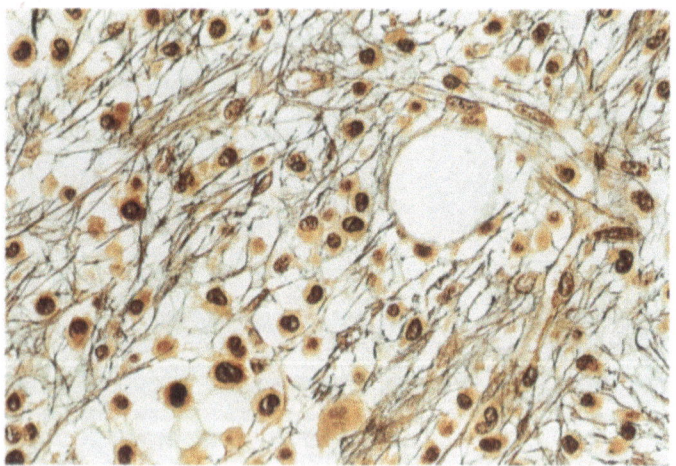

Fig. 8.76 Bone biopsy of patient with HCL, section stained by Gomori to show delicate reticular network and hairy cell infiltration

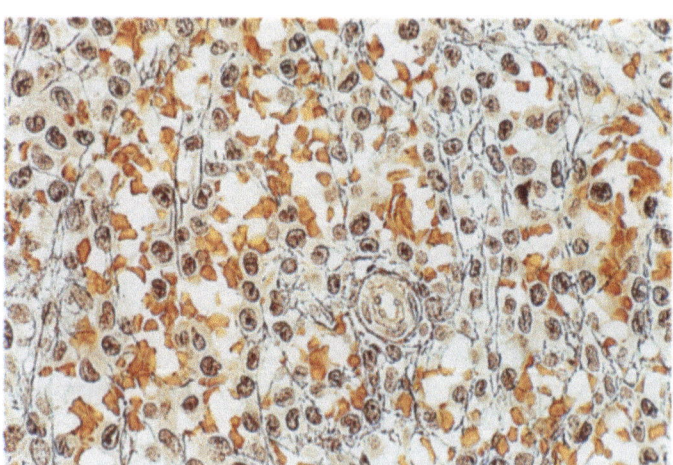

Fig. 8.77 Section of bone biopsy in case of HCL to illustrate the typical appearance of the infiltrated marrow: a loose infiltration of hairy cells within a fine reticular network and with numerous erythrocytes. Gomori

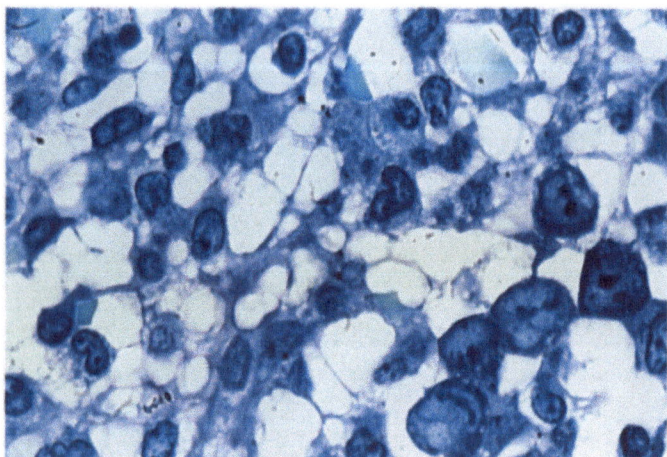

Fig. 8.78 Cluster of early erythroblasts within hairy cell infiltration

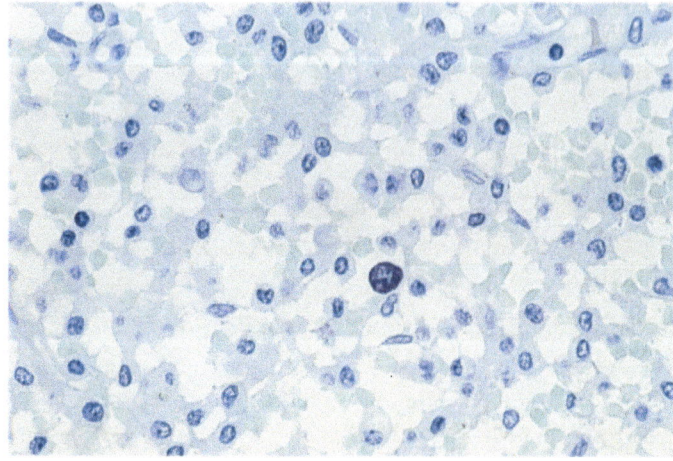

Figs 8.80–8.82 High magnifications to illustrate the three types of hairy cell nuclei: ovoid, convoluted and indented

Fig. 8.80 Ovoid cell type of HCL

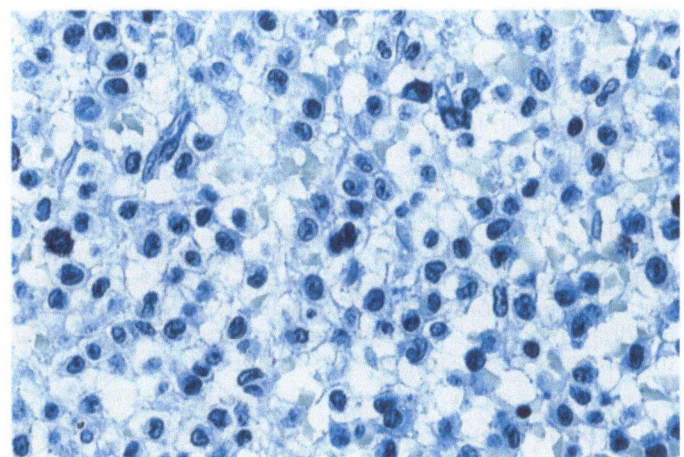

Fig. 8.81 Convoluted cell type of HCL

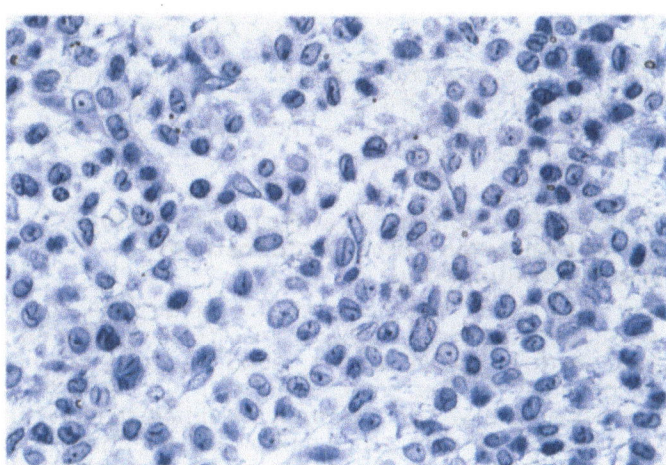

Fig. 8.82 Indented cell type of HCL

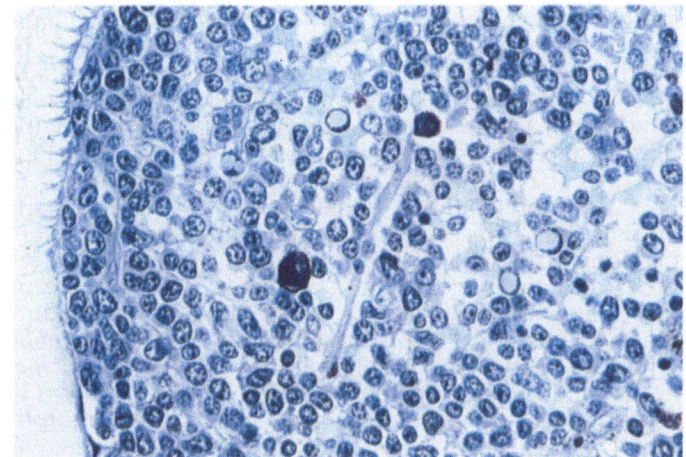

Fig. 8.83 Bone biopsy section of patient with WM, showing replacement of bone marrow by the infiltration including cells with intranuclear inclusions (Dutcher bodies)

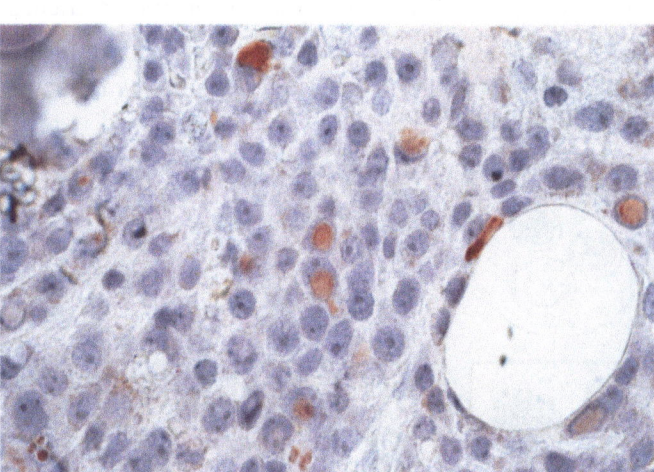

Fig. 8.84 Section of paraffin-embedded bone biopsy in WM showing cells with intranuclear secretion stained by antibody to IgM

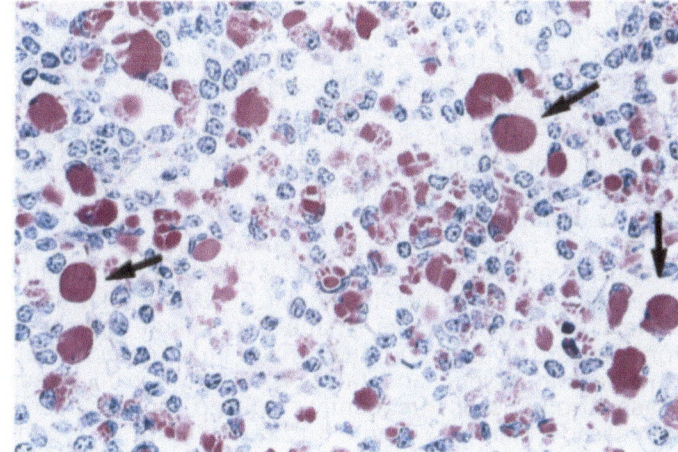

Fig. 8.85 Intranuclear PAS-positive material in WM; the cells resemble signet-ring cells (arrowed)

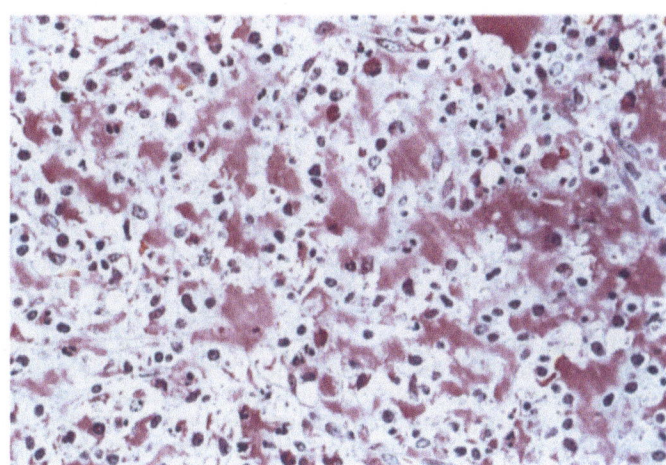

Fig. 8.86 Interstitial amorphous deposits in WM Ladewig

elements, has been demonstrated in some patients in response to therapy with interferon[50]. The occurrence of HCL with myeloid metaplasia and myelofibrosis has also been described[51].

Malignant Lymphoma Lymphoplasmacytic/cytoid (Immunocytoma, Waldenström's Macroglobulinaemia)

This is a B cell lymphoma of low-grade malignancy secreting monoclonal IgM, or IgG (Figs 8.83–8.86). Bone marrow involvement is found in about 80% of the patients[52,53]. The predominant cell type is a small lymphocyte with variable plasmacytoid differentiation, but there is a wide spectrum of lymphoid cells, ranging from small lymphocyte to plasma cell. In a typical case there are nuclear inclusions, consisting of immunoglobulins, the so-called Dutcher bodies (PAS+) in a variable number of the infiltrating cells. Three proliferation patterns are recognized: (1) nodular with multiple nodules adjacent to sinusoids and trabeculae; (2) interstitial/nodular in which there is a loose interstitial infiltration in addition to the nodules; and (3) packed marrow in which there is complete replacement of haematopoietic and fat cells (Figs 8.87–8.89). EM and immunohistology often reveal the plasmacytoid nature of cells identified as lymphocytes in the light microscope.

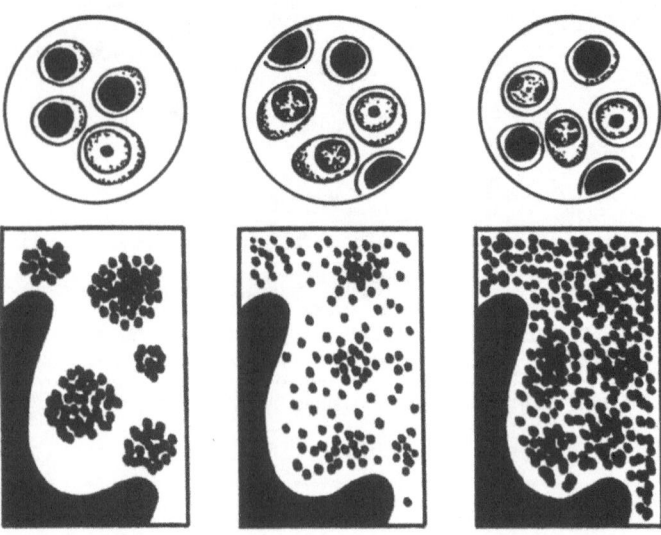

LYMPHO-   LYMPHO-   POLYMORPHOUS
PLASMACYTOID   PLASMACYTIC

Fig. 8.90 Bone marrow involvement in the three types of Waldenström's macroglobulinaemia

There are three histologic subdivisions (Fig. 8.90), comparable with the subtypes recognized in the lymph nodes: (1) lymphoplasmacytoid, (2) lymphoplasmacytic and (3) polymorphous (Figs 8.91–8.93). However, as in the lymph nodes, there is some overlap between them. The first generally has a nodular pattern, the second an interstitial/nodular pattern with numerous plasma and mast cells, and the third usually presents with a packed marrow pattern whose cell population consists of lymphocytes, plasma cells, centrocytes, centroblasts and immunoblasts. These types are characterized by differences in growth patterns, clinical features, anatomic extent and median survivals. Bone marrow mast cells are increased in all types. Haematopoietic precursors are located within the infiltrates as well as between them. Hyperplastic and ectatic sinusoids with sclerosis of the endothelium, and prominent histiocytes, are especially characteristic of the lymphoplasmacytic type. The blood vessels in any case of immunocytoma may be filled with a homogeneously stained PAS+ material (Fig. 8.94).

In the evolution of disease conversion of an immunocytoma to an immunoblastic lymphoma has also been described (Figs 8.95 and 8.96). Diagnostic difficulties may arise in the absence of PAS+ inclusions, and when the infiltration is minimal. The picture may resemble nodular lymphoid hyperplasia, or CLL. However, mast cells are more numerous in immunocytoma. Immunohistology is required in borderline cases. Post-therapy sections of bone biopsies of patients with WM showing residual interstitial, perivascular and paratrabecular infiltrations are shown in Fig. 8.97–8.99.

Malignant Lymphoma Plasmacytic, Multiple Myeloma (MM)

Most plasma cell neoplasias show systemic spread when first diagnosed (90% of the cases)[54–56]. A minority of patients have solitary, multifocal or sarcomatous-like plasmacytomas without involvement in the initial iliac crest biopsy; consequently a negative BMB does not exclude the possibility of multiple myeloma. When clinically indicated, sequential biopsies should be performed. The morphological diagnosis of MM is still based on percentages of plasma cells in an aspirated marrow sample[54–56], in spite of the fact that equal or even higher numbers of plasma cells may be present in other, non-neoplastic conditions. The monoclonal or polyclonal nature of the plasma cells may be determined by immunohistology (Figs 8.100–8.102). Moreover, a morphological classification of MM has not yet been widely adopted, though many authors have described plasmacytomas with different cytological features[57]. Myelomas may be divided into two broad groups: plasmacytic – primarily 'mature' plasma cells, and plasmablastic – predominantly 'immature' plasma cells[58,59]. Further subdivisions could be made when cellular size, cytoplasmic structure and nuclear configuration are considered (Figs 8.103–8.110): (1) Marschalko, (2) small cell, (3) cleaved, (4) polymorphous, (5) asynchronous, and (6) blastic. These types may be combined into three prognostic grades, comparable to the malignant lymphomas: low-grade types 1 and 2; intermediate-grade types 3, 4 and 5; high-grade malignancy, type 6[60]. Some nucleolated plasma cells are present even in minimal infiltrations, and their presence constitutes a diagnostic parameter for multiple myeloma[60]. Their presence is possibly also correlated with the plasma cell labelling index, which also constitutes a significant prognostic index[61]. Accumulations of secretions within the cytoplasm of the plasma cells may occur in all cases of MM. Mostly these appear as the characteristic Russell bodies, though they may also have a crystalline or needle-like shape (Figs 8.111–8.118).

Though most cases of MM are characterized by osteolytic lesions – which may present as foci or as generalized osteoporosis or both[62], cases of osteosclerotic MM have also been reported (see below) (Figs 8.119–8.120).

In early bone marrow involvement, plasma cells are dispersed among the other marrow elements in addition to small clusters in paratrabecular or perivascular areas. In later stages the clusters expand to form large aggregates or sheets (myelomas), and finally may replace both the haematopoietic and fat cells. Even in early cases, haematopoiesis is frequently reduced and fat cells increased (Figs 8.121 and 8.122). Erythropoiesis with maturation inhibition is a constant feature. A fine fibre network interweaves the infiltrated areas, but coarse fibrosis is rare (Figs 8.123 and 8.124). However, the presence of fibrosis may interfere with bone marrow aspiration and lead to inconclusive results[63]. Some lymphocytes are scattered among the plasma cells and lymphoid cell aggregates or nodules are found in about

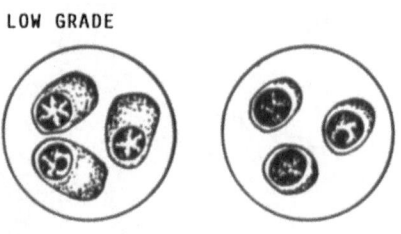

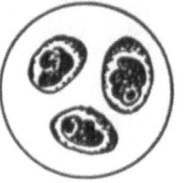 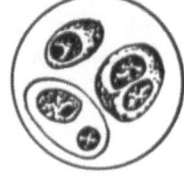 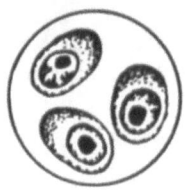

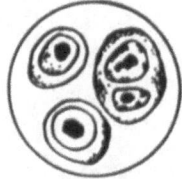

Fig. 8.103 Schematic representation of the types of plasma cells in the three histological grades of malignancy

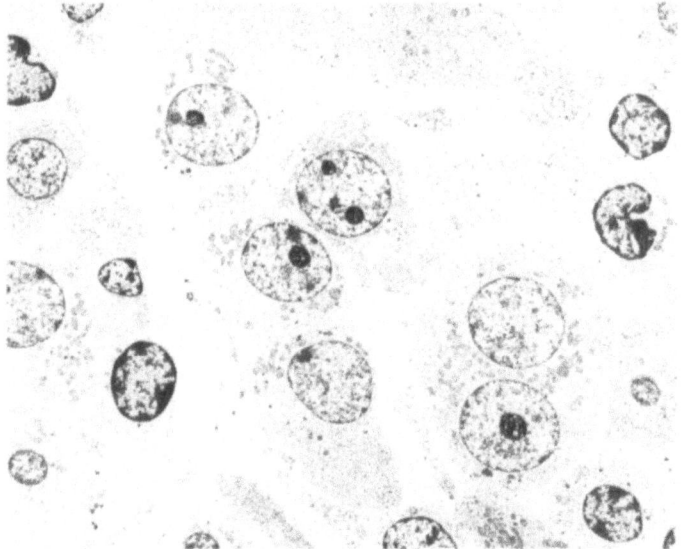

Fig. 8.111 Plasma cells at different maturation stages in MM. EM × 5000

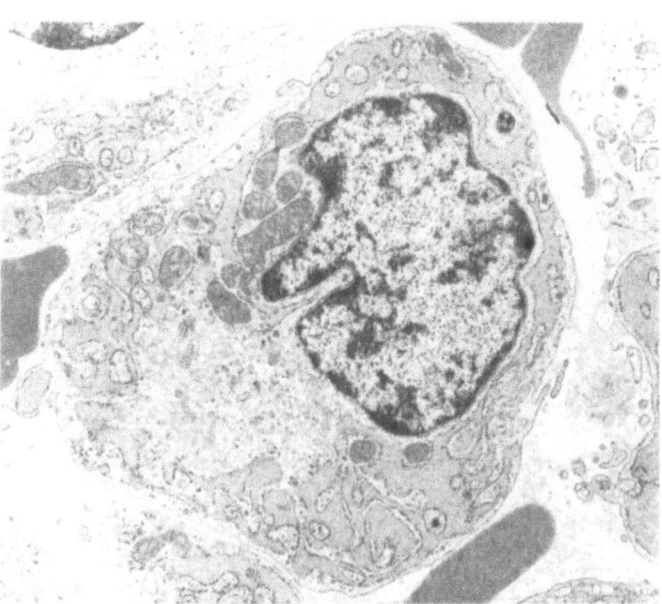

Fig. 8.112 Myeloma cell with cleaved nucleus and dilated endoplasmic reticulum. EM × 25 000

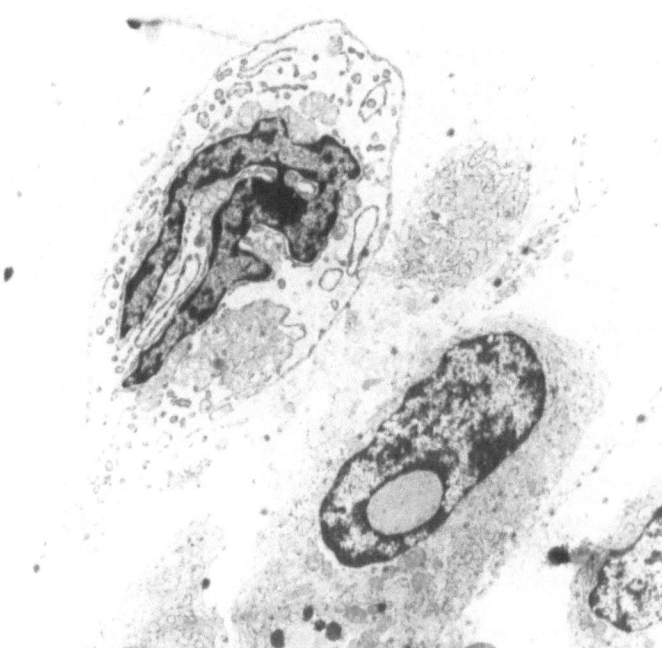

Fig. 8.113 Myeloma cells, one with Dutcher body, the other with invagination of cytoplasm and organelles into the nucleus. EM × 20 000

and nodular[64], or diffuse and nodular[65]. The quantity of the plasma cell burden may be used for histological staging of MM, to supplement any clinical staging system used.

The lytic bone lesions characteristic for multiple myeloma and the accompanying hypercalcaemia and hypercalciuria have now been successfully treated with diphosphonates[66]. These are inhibitors of osteoclasts, hence a bone biopsy may be required.

Non-secretory Multiple Myeloma

It has been estimated that in 1–5% of cases a paraprotein cannot be detected, and the diagnosis is based on multiple lytic bone lesions, osteoporosis and bone marrow plasmacytosis[67]. However in 8/9 cases tested, immunoperoxidase staining revealed the presence of a monoclonal immunoglobulin in the plasma cells. Similarly, bone marrow plasma cells of 4/5 patients with non-secretory MM

10% of the cases (Fig. 8.125). Osteoclastic and some osteoblastic remodelling are prominent adjacent to the infiltrated areas (Figs 8.126 and 8.127). Altogether six architecture patterns have been observed in BMB: (1) interstitial (the commonest), (2) interstitial/sheets, (3) interstitial/nodular, (4) nodular, (5) focal sarcomatous-like and (6) packed marrow (Figs 8.128 and 8.129). A nodular pattern is associated with coarse fibrosis. Other studies have described three patterns: diffuse, interstitial

(Continued on p. 150)

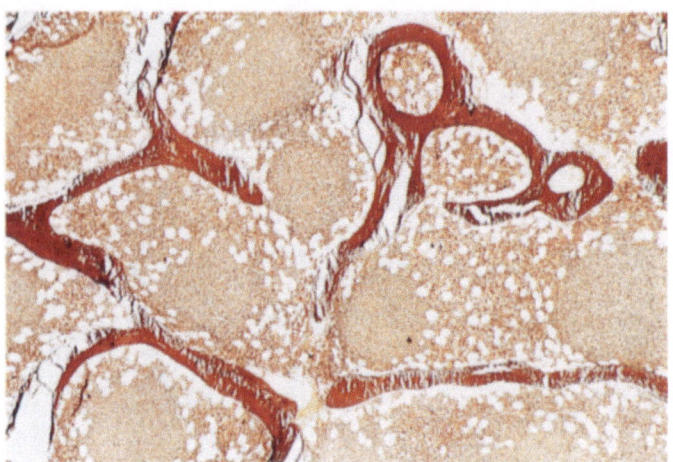

Fig. 8.87   Nodular proliferation pattern in WM. Gomori

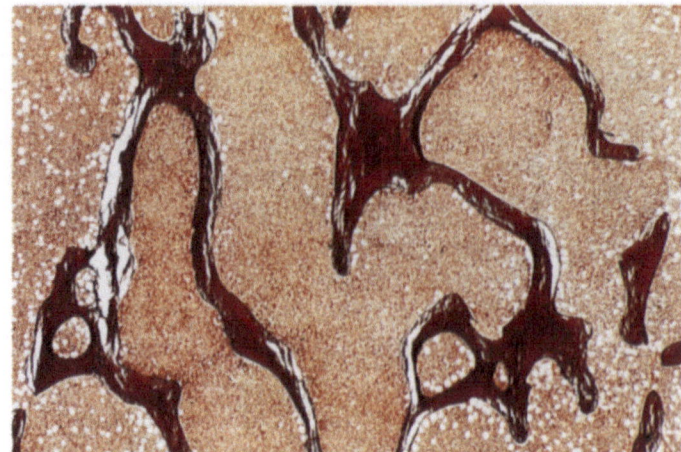

Fig. 8.88   Interstitial/nodular pattern in WM. Gomori

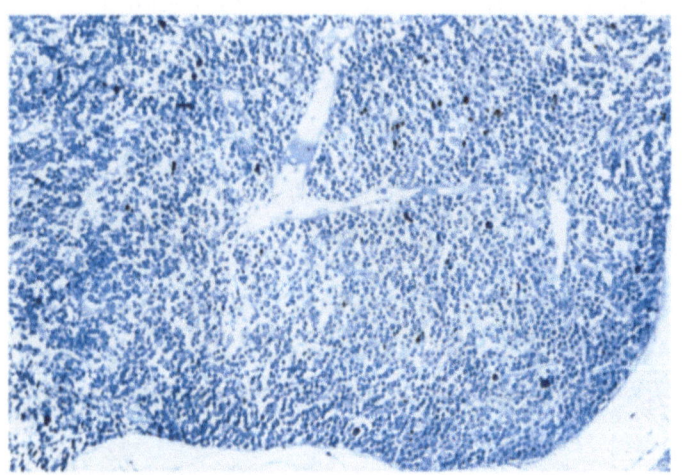

Fig. 8.89   'Packed marrow' in WM

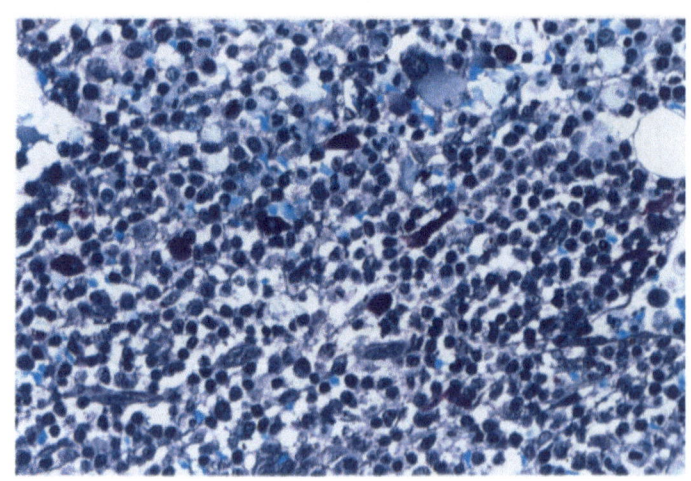

Fig. 8.91   Lymphoplasmacytoid type in WM

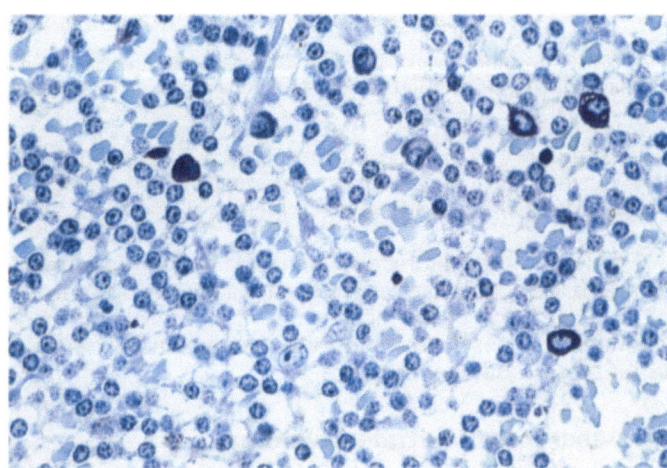

Fig. 8.92   Lymphoplasmacytic type of WM. Note mast cells

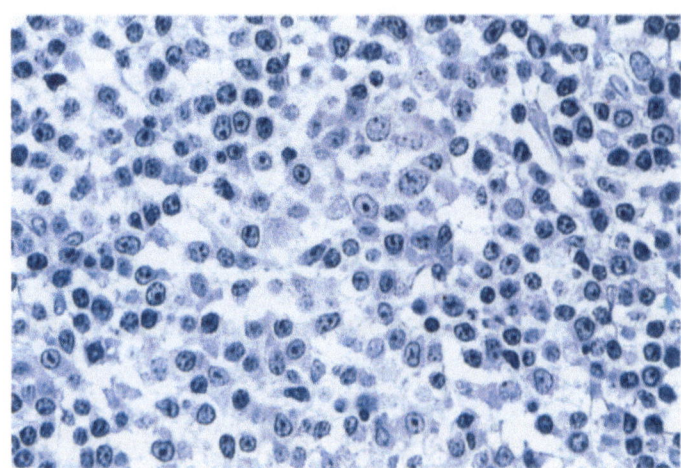

Fig. 8.93   Polymorphous type of WM

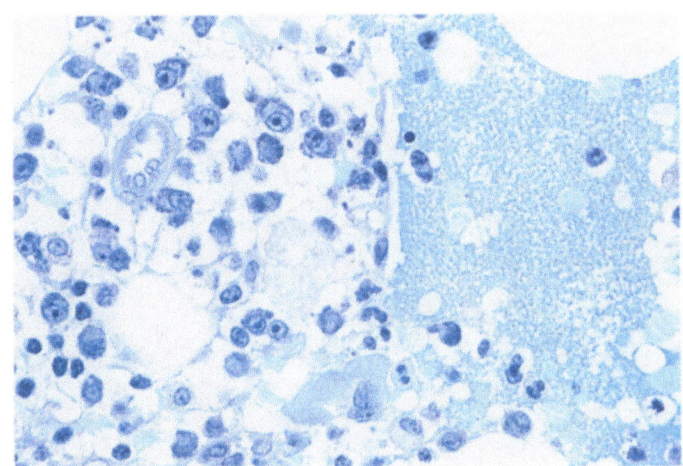

Fig. 8.94 Case of WM with cryoglobulinaemia. Note nucleolated plasma cells

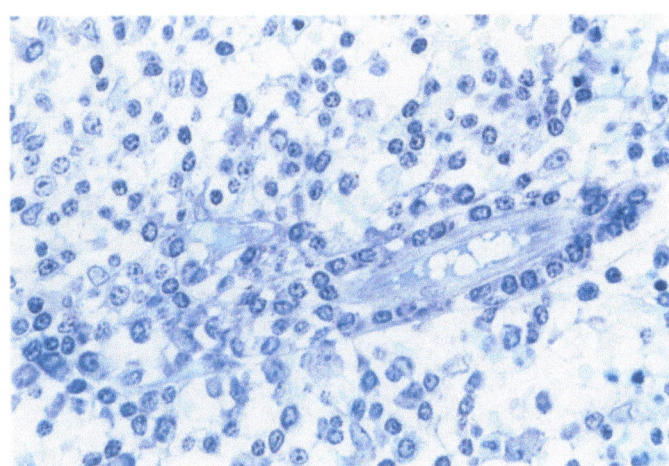

Fig. 8.95 Case of WM before transformation to multiple myeloma

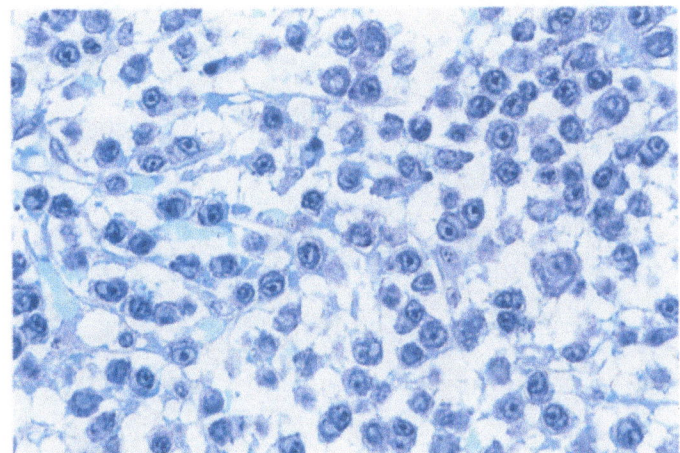

Fig. 8.96 Same case of WM as in Fig. 8.95, developing into multiple myeloma

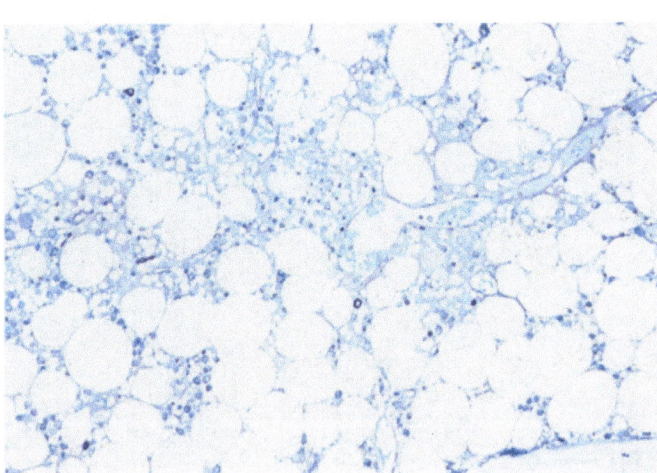

Fig. 8.97 Bone biopsy of patient with WM after therapy, showing atrophic marrow and minimal infiltration

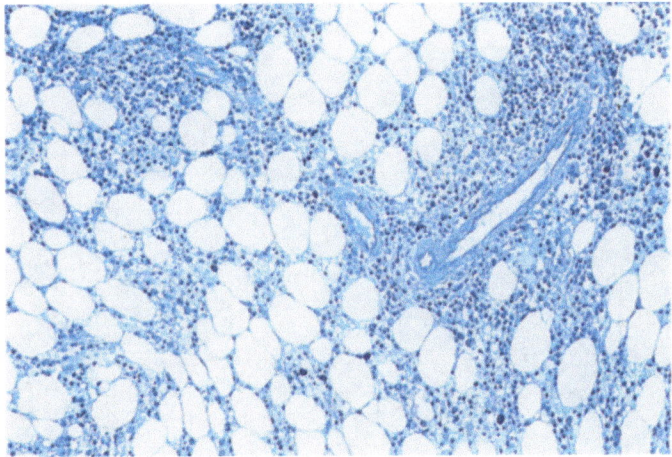

Fig. 8.98 Bone biopsy of patient with WM after therapy, showing perivascular infiltration

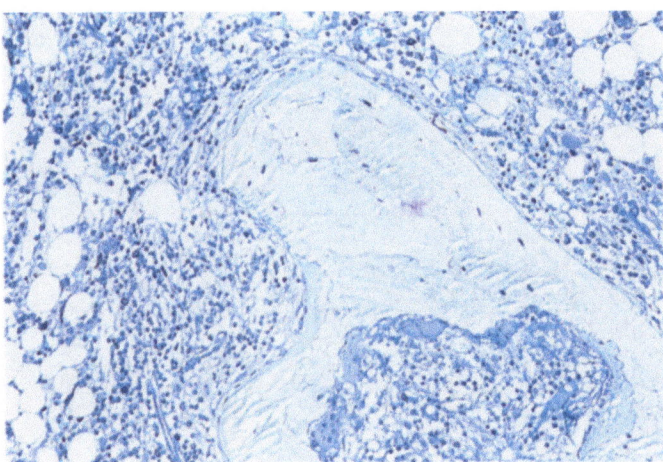

Fig. 8.99 Bone biopsy of patient with WM after therapy with residual lymphoid cells within paratrabecular network of fibres. Note osteoclasts

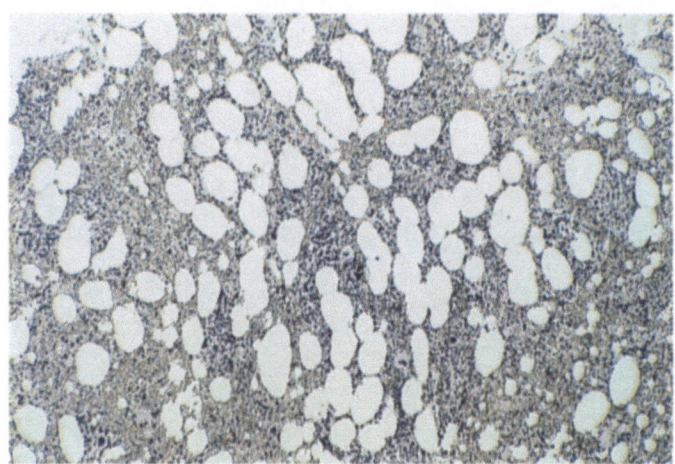

Fig. 8.100 Decalcified paraffin-embedded bone biopsy section of patient with MM showing no reaction with antibody to kappa light chain

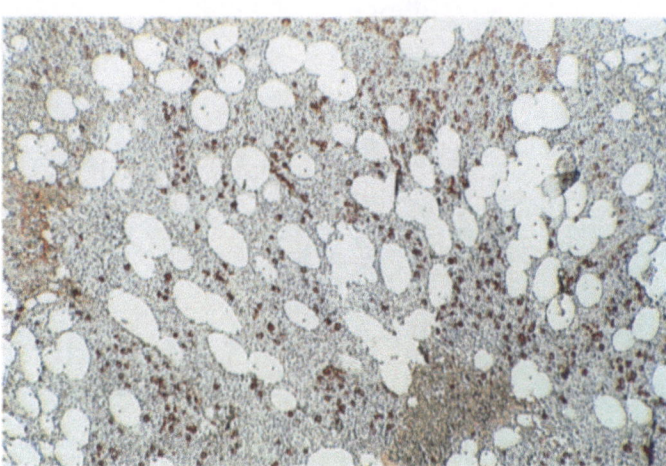

Fig. 8.101 The same biopsy as Fig. 8.100. Plasma cells stained by antibody to lambda light chain

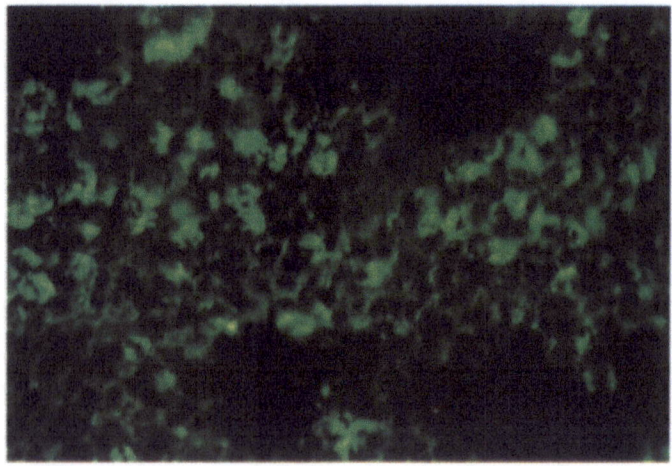

Fig. 8.102 Cryostat section: reaction with antibody to IgG labelled with FITC; plasma cells show green fluroescence, case of MM

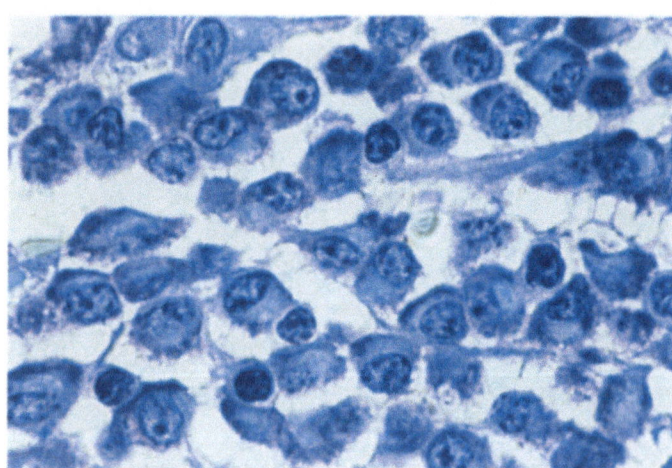

Fig. 8.104 Marschalko type plasma cell in MM. These resemble benign mature plasma cells

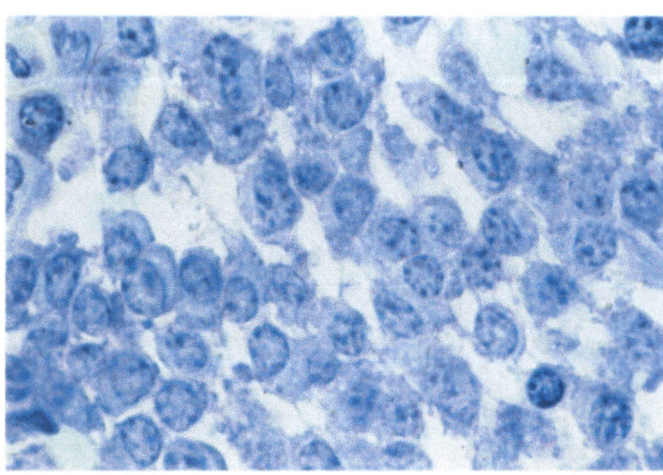

Fig. 8.105 Small cell type in MM

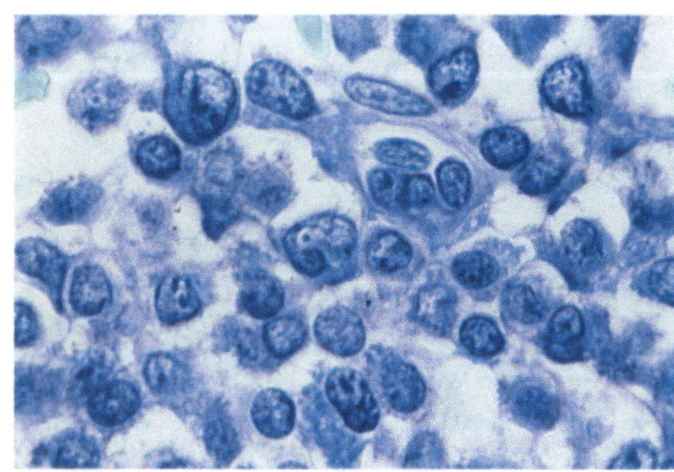

Fig. 8.106 Cleaved cell type in MM

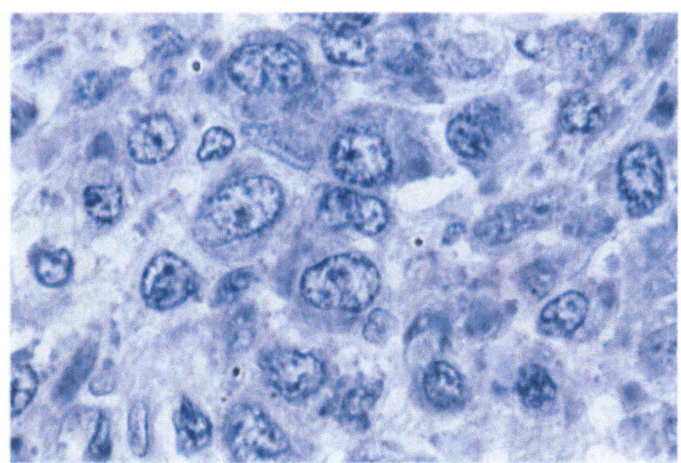

Fig. 8.107   Polymorphous cell type in MM

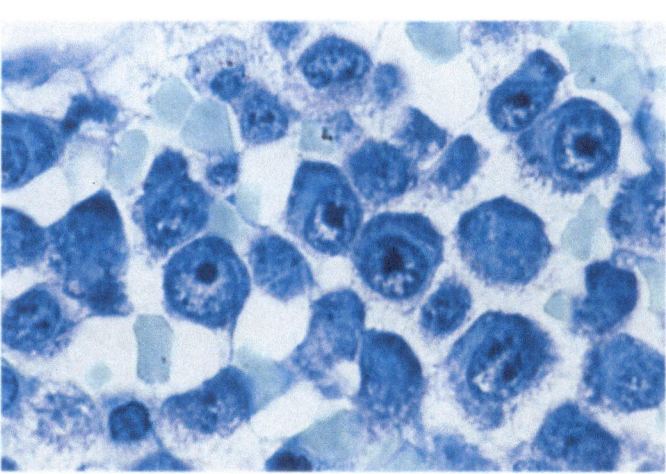

Fig. 8.108   Asynchronous cell type in MM

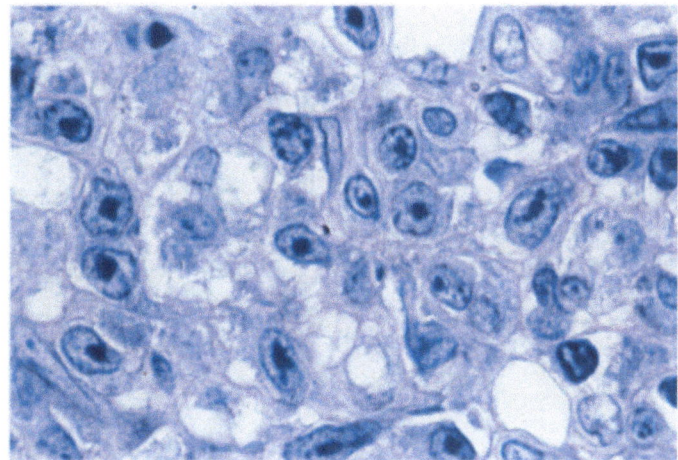

Fig. 8.109   Blastic cell type in MM

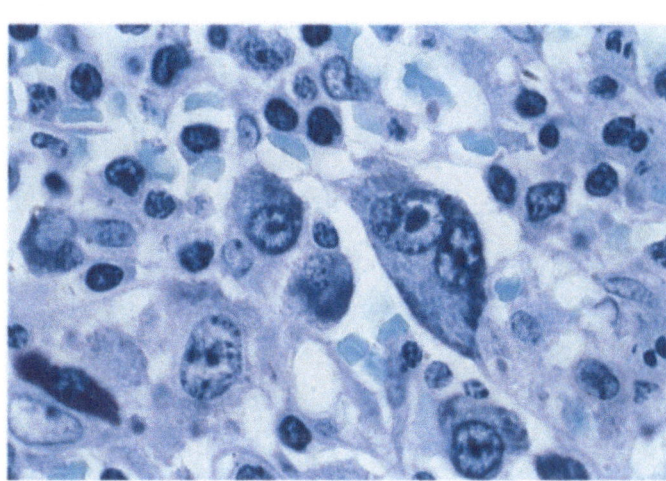

Fig. 8.110   Pleomorphic blastic cell type with giant binucleate plasma cell in MM

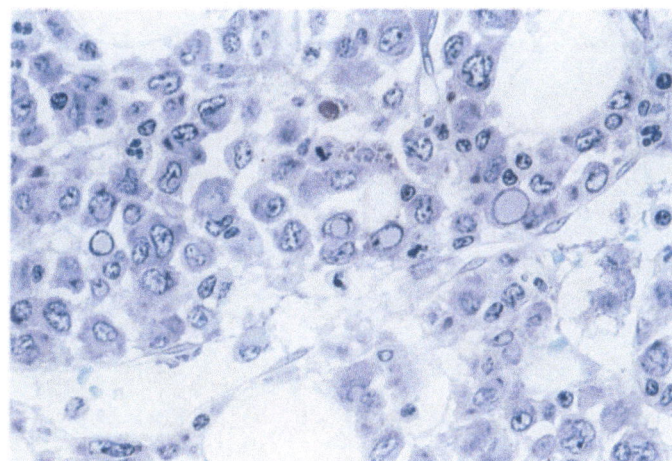

Fig. 8.114   Intra-nuclear inclusion in plasma cells in MM – Dutcher bodies

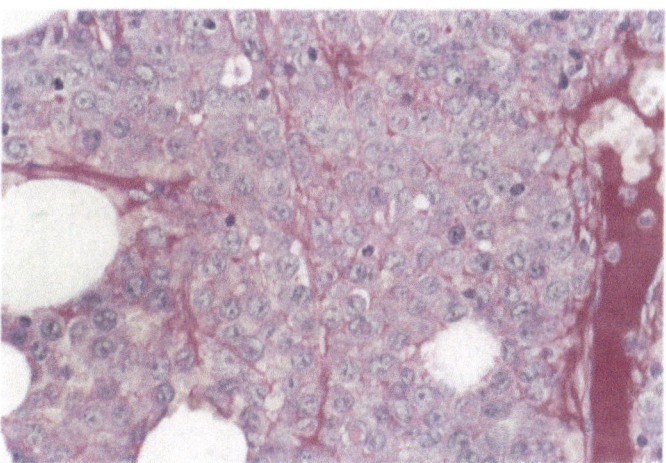

Fig. 8.115   Paraffin section in MM, intranuclear, interstitial and intra-vascular PAS-positive material. PAS

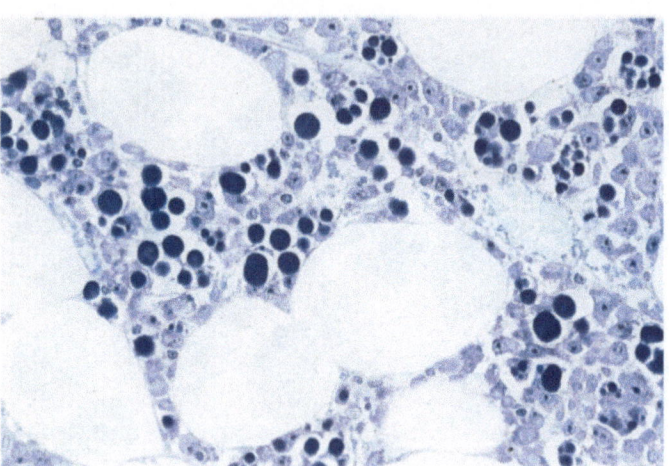

Fig. 8.116   Numerous plasma cells with Russell bodies

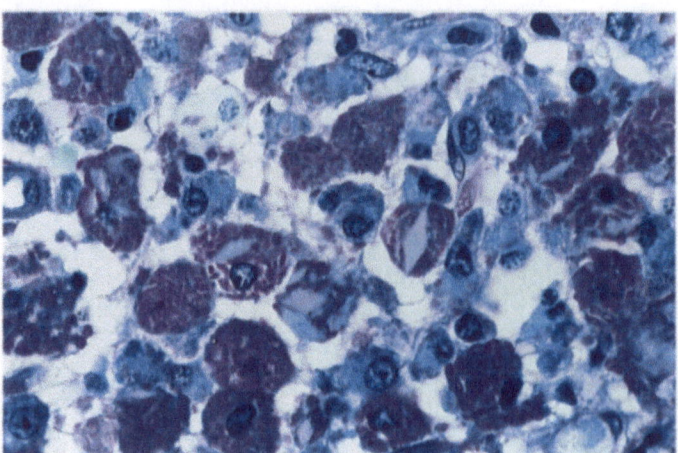

Fig. 8.117   Plasma cells with abundant cytoplasm and cytoplasmic crystals

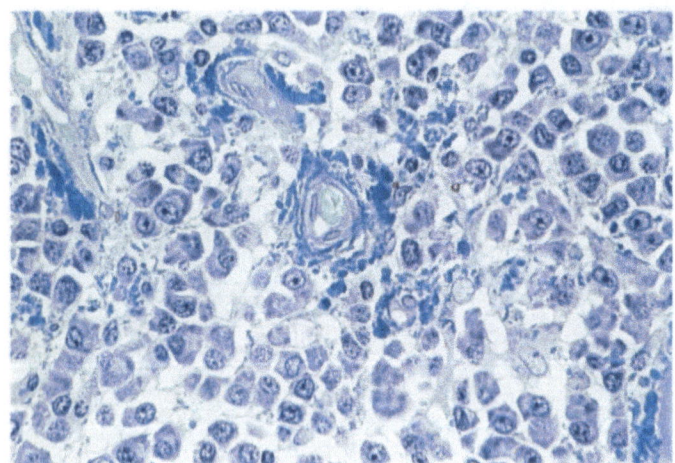

Fig. 8.118   Case of MM with perivascular and interstitial amyloidosis

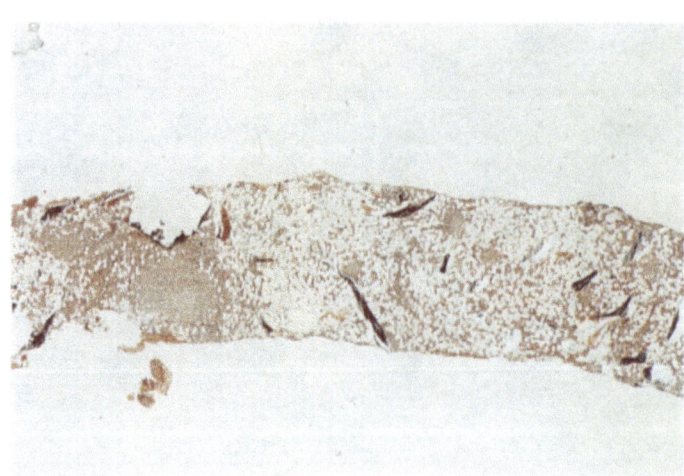

Fig. 8.119   Focal infiltration, fatty marrow and marked osteopenia in MM. Gomori

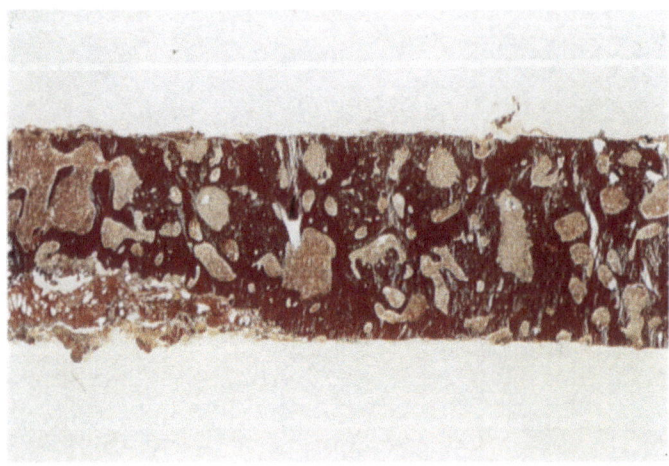

Fig. 8.120   Marked osteosclerosis in MM. Gomori

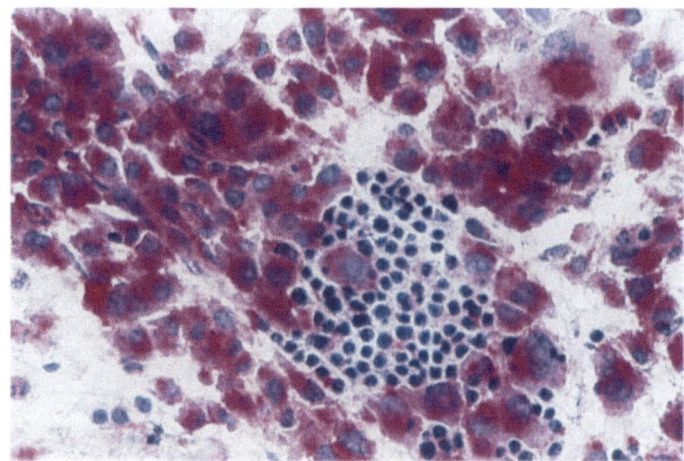

Fig. 8.121   Cryostat section incubated for demonstration of acid phosphatase activity (red). Note aggregate of lymphoid cells within sheet of plasma cells

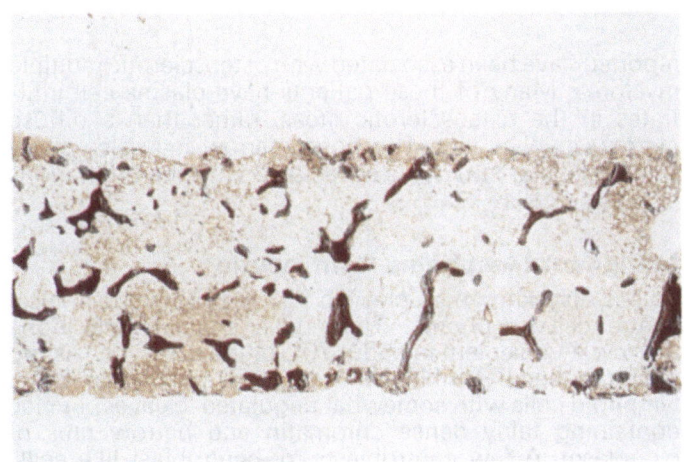

Fig. 8.122 MM with almost total atrophy in the bone marrow. Gomori

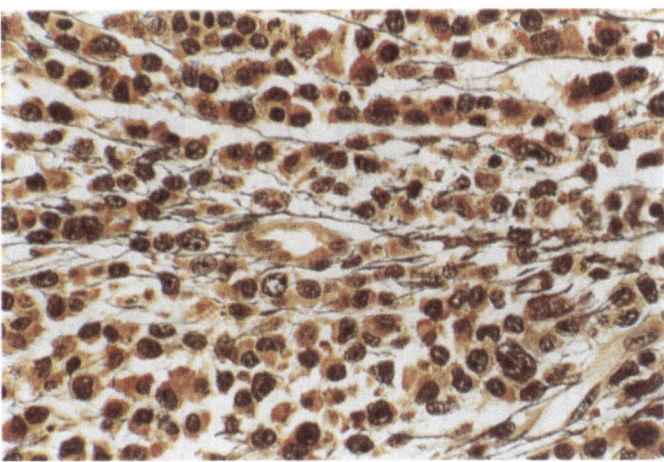

Fig. 8.123 Section of bone biopsy showing fibrosis in areas of myelomatous infiltrations, plasmacytic type. Gomori

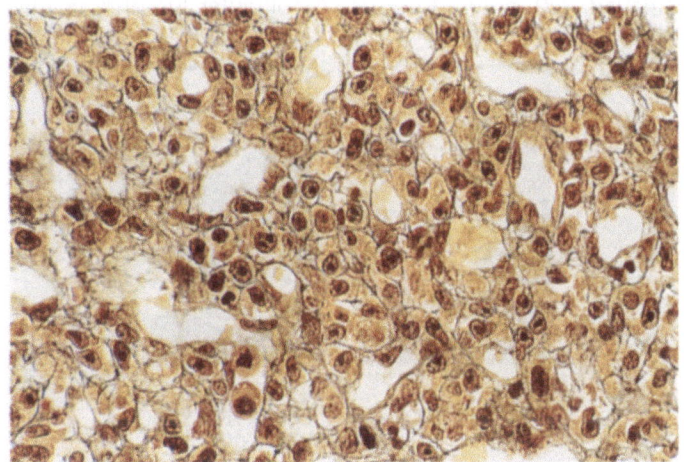

Fig. 8.124 Fine reticulin fibrosis in MM, blastic type. Gomori

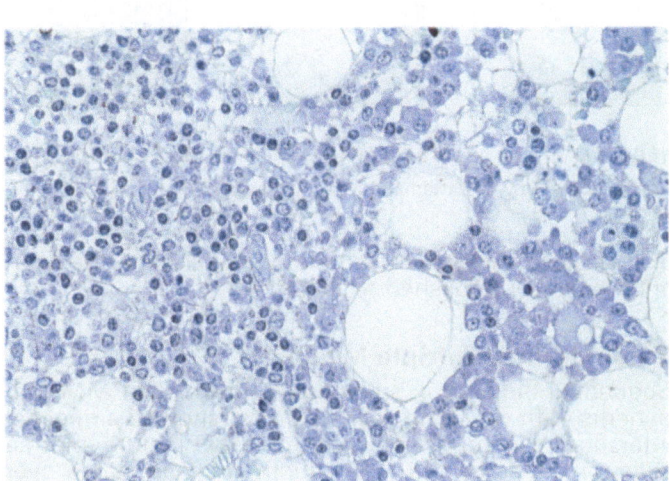

Fig. 8.125 Lymphoid cell nodule in multiple myeloma

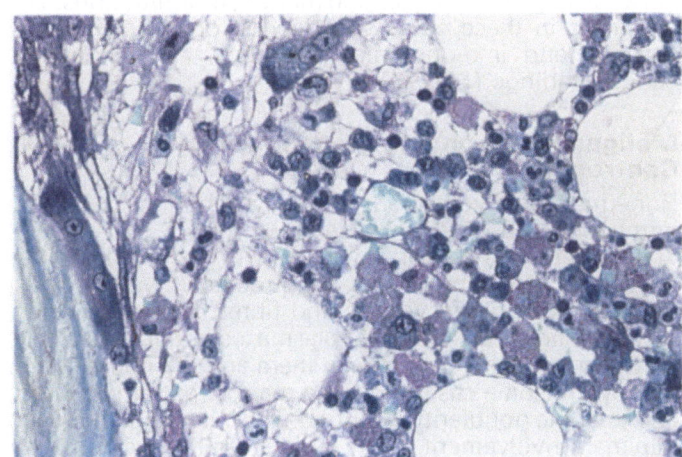

Fig. 8.126 Osteoclast on bone near myelomatous infiltration

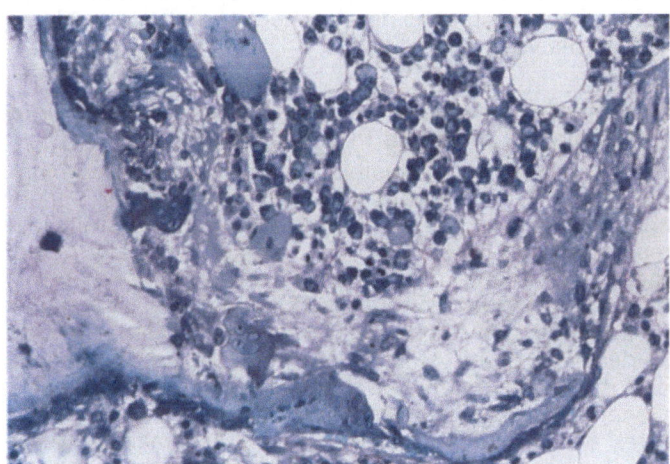

Fig. 8.127 Trabeculae with marked osseous remodelling

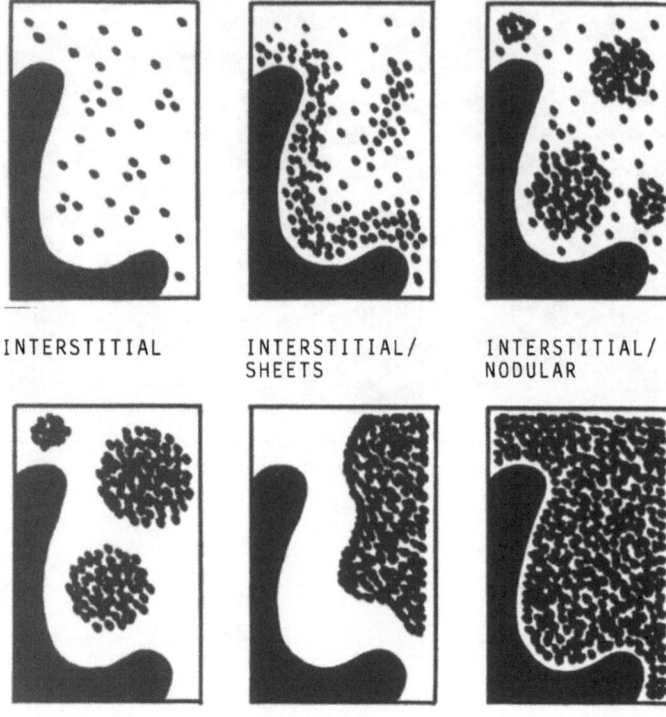

INTERSTITIAL   INTERSTITIAL/   INTERSTITIAL/
                      SHEETS   NODULAR

NODULAR   SARCOMATOUS   PACKED MARROW

Fig. 8.128 Growth patterns in MM

also showed the presence of monoclonal light chains in another series published recently[68].

Smouldering Multiple Myeloma

Sequential biopsies in smouldering or indolent MM (i.e. patients with very long survival times) showed a minimal interstitial infiltration of predominantly mature plasma cells, or the small cell type which remained stable over long periods (Figs 8.130–8.132).

Follow-up in Multiple Myeloma

Sequential biopsies (Figs 8.133–8.138) are also useful to monitor therapy, especially to document residual infiltration, marrow atrophy, fibrosis, development of myelodysplasia, acute leukaemia (Fig. 8.139) or another malignancy. For example the development of multiple myeloma in patients with sarcoidosis[69].

Castleman's Disease (Angio-follicular Lymphoid Hyperplasia), and the POEMS Syndrome

Based on lymph-node histology, two subtypes are recognised: the hyaline vascular type and the plasma-cell variant characterised by sheets of plasma cells in the interfollicular regions (Figs 8.140 and 8.141). It is still not clear whether these are variants of the same disease process or two distinct disorders[70]. There are both localized and multicentric forms of Castleman's disease; the latter shows evidence of multisystem involvement including anaemia and thrombocytopenia, and bone marrow involvement[71]. Generalized lymphadenopathy with morphological features of the multicentric variant of Castleman's disease has also been observed in AIDS[72]. Moreover, there appears to be a link between Castleman's disease and plasma cell dyscrasias, and several cases of the plasmacytic type of Castleman's disease have had the features of the POEMS syndrome (polyneuropathy, organomegaly, endocrinopathy, M-proteins and skin changes)[73]. However, it should be noted that most cases of the POEMS syndrome so far

reported have been associated with osteosclerotic multiple myeloma. Many of these patients have plasma cell infiltrates in the osteosclerotic areas, rather than a diffuse marrow involvement. The bone marrow may also show small follicular structures associated with the infiltrations of plasma cells[73].

Malignant Lymphoma Centrocytic

This is also known as cleaved cell lymphoma, or follicle centre cell lymphoma. There is a characteristic bone marrow involvement in about 70% of the cases, consisting of paratrabecular infiltrations of small to medium-sized lymphoid cells with somewhat angulated 'cleaved' nuclei, containing fairly dense chromatin and narrow rims of cytoplasm. A few centroblasts, or centroblast-like cells, are often present (Figs 8.142–8.148). These infiltrations are generally enmeshed within a fairly dense network of coarse fibres, radiating out from the trabeculae, and which stops at the boundary between the infiltration and the central, residual haematopoietic tissue. According to size and nuclear morphology, three subtypes are distinguished: (1) small centrocytic, cleaved; (2) large centrocytic, cleaved; (3) polymorphous. A follicular lymphoma may also undergo conversion to a blastic type[74,75].

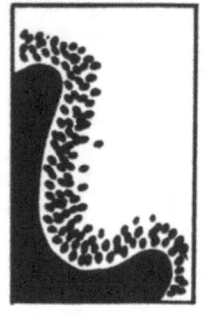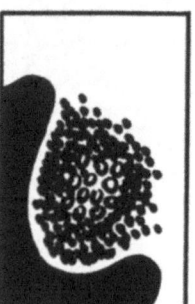

CENTROCYTIC   CENTROBLASTIC/
                     CENTROCYTIC

Fig. 8.142 Bone marrow involvement in centrocytic and centroblastic/centrocytic lymphomas, showing the characteristic paratrabecular and nodular patterns

In BMB with a packed marrow the morphological distinction between centrocytes and CLL of the B2 notched or the T CLL types, or immunocytoma, may not be possible. The same holds true for the distinction between large centrocytes and monocytic infiltrations. The diagnosis in these cases will depend on supplementary enzymic and immunological methods, as well as the clinical findings (Figs 8.149–8.151).

Malignant Lymphoma Centroblastic/ Centrocytic

Bone marrow involvement in this lymphoma is relatively infrequent – about 20% of the cases (Figs 8.152–8.160). The pattern is nodular: follicles with germinal centres consisting of centroblasts, centrocytes, lymphocytes, reticular cells, blood vessels and fibres. At the periphery of the follicles eosinophils, plasma cells and mast cells may form a transition between them and the normal bone marrow. In some cases a packed marrow pattern is found, and then the nodularity is blurred. The distinction between minimal involvement and nodular immunocytoma or benign lymphoid nodules or follicles is not possible on histology alone.

Malignant Lymphoma Centroblastic

Involvement is relatively rare (20%) and shows a packed marrow pattern (Fig. 8.161). The characteristic nuclear

(Continued on p. 156)

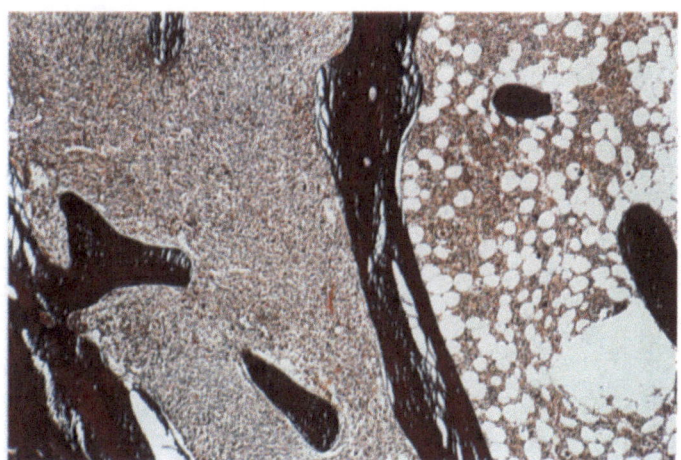

Fig. 8.129 Sarcomatous type in MM. Gomori

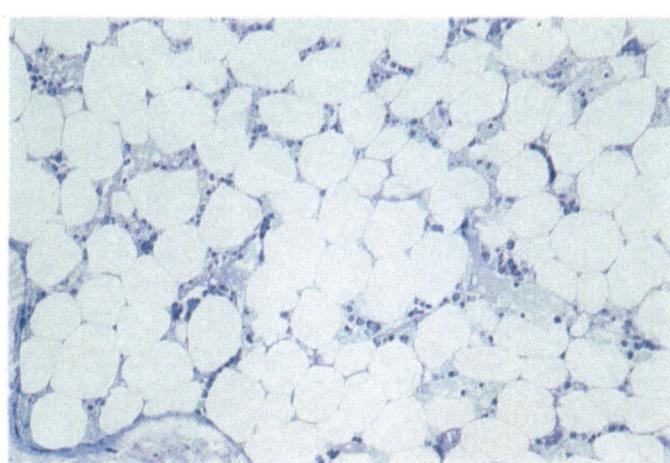

Fig. 8.130 Interstitial infiltraion beyween fat celis in hypocellular bor e marrow (smouldering variant of MM)

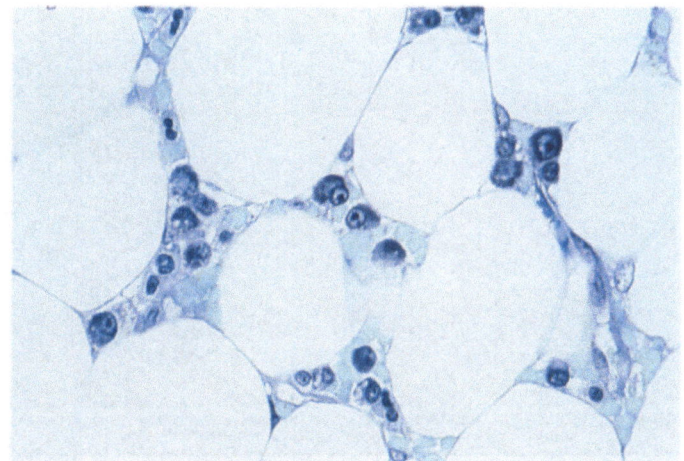

Fig. 8.131 Higher magnification of the biopsy in Fig. 8.130, showing a few nucleolated plasma cells between the fat cells

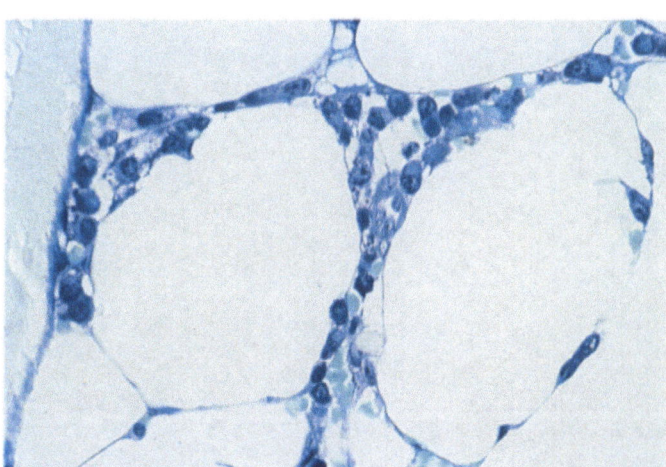

Fig. 8.132 Smouldering MM with minimal interstitial infiltration, small cell type

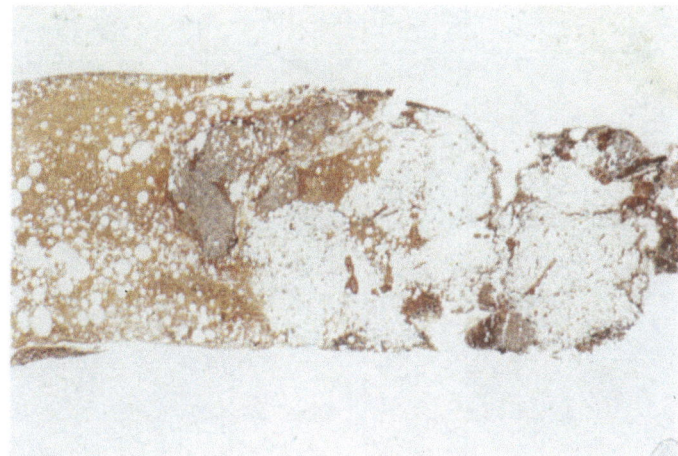

Fig. 8.133 Section of bone biopsy of patient with MM after chemotherapy; there are areas of haemorrhage, fat cells and residual infiltration in a previously packed bone marrow. Gomori

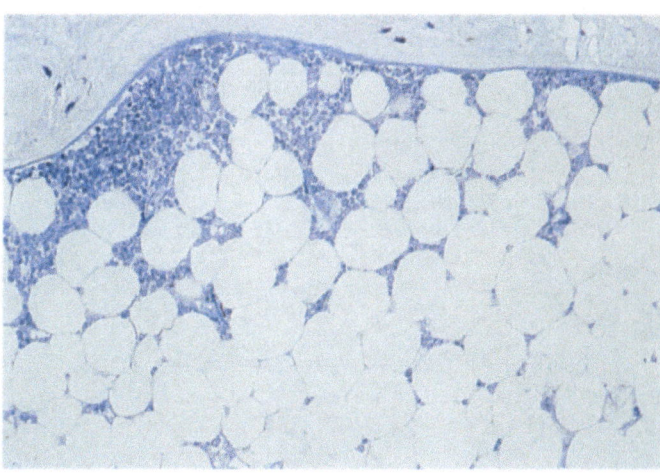

Fig. 8.134 Residual paratrabecular infiltration after chemotherapy

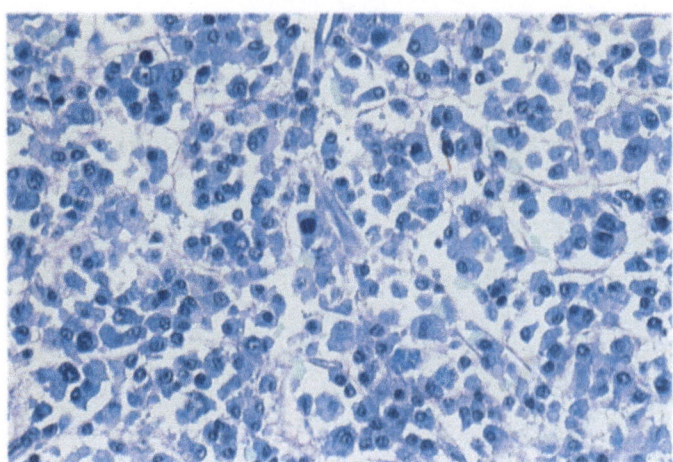

Fig. 8.135   Bone biopsy in MM, packed marrow type, pre-treatment

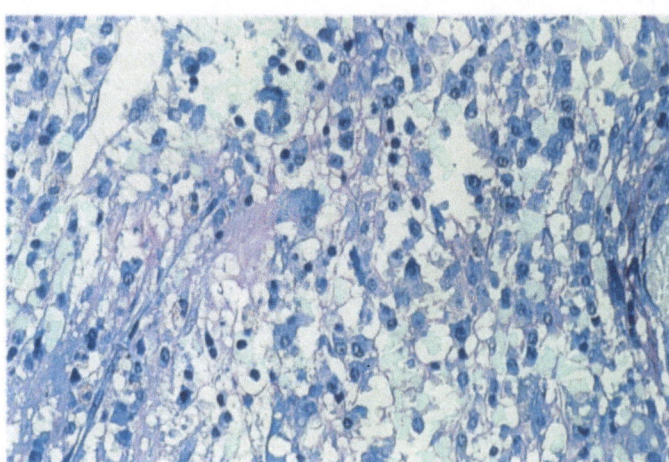

Fig. 8.136   Same patient as Fig. 8.135, after 6 weeks of therapy, with incipient fibrosis

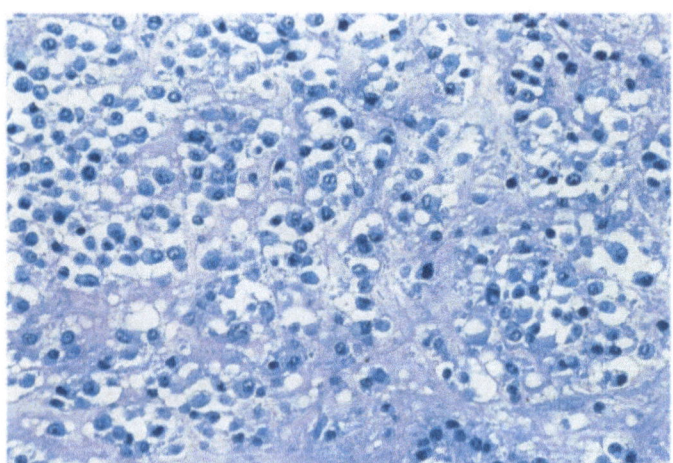

Fig. 8.137   Same patient as Fig. 8.135, after 3 months of therapy, with coarse fibrosis and residual infiltration

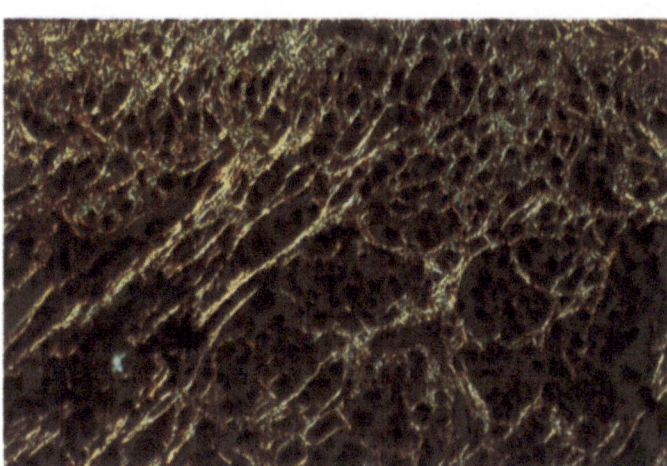

Fig. 8.138   Same biopsy as Fig. 8.136, with coarse fibrosis, in polarized light. Gomori

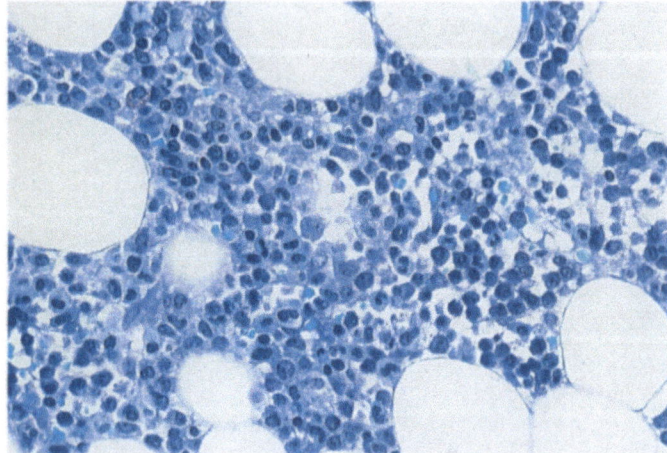

Fig. 8.139   Bone biopsy section of patient with MM who developed acute leukaemia. Note infiltrations of both plasma and immature myeloid cells

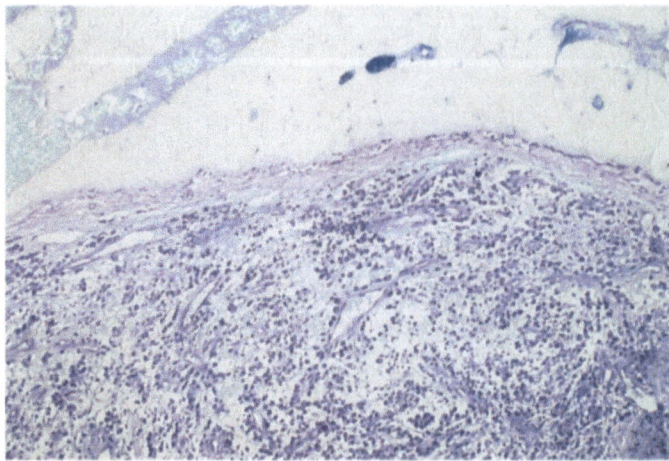

Fig. 8.140   Bone biopsy of patient with Castleman's disease and osteoblastic lesions on X-ray. Dense infiltration of bone marrow. Note osteoblasts on bone

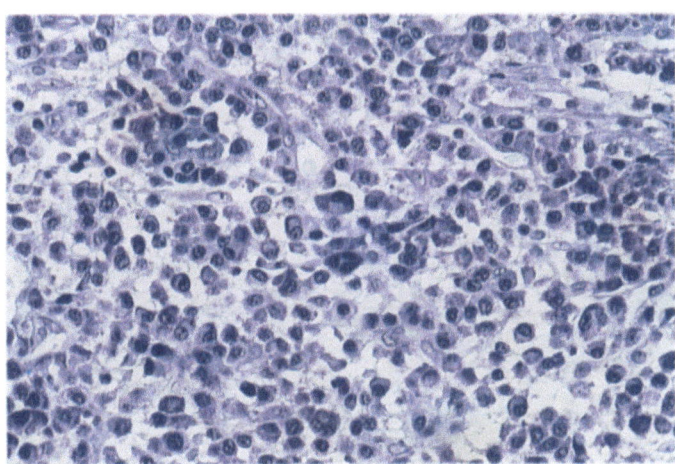

Fig. 8.141 Same biopsy as Fig. 8.140. Dense plasmacytic infiltration with no residual haematopoiesis

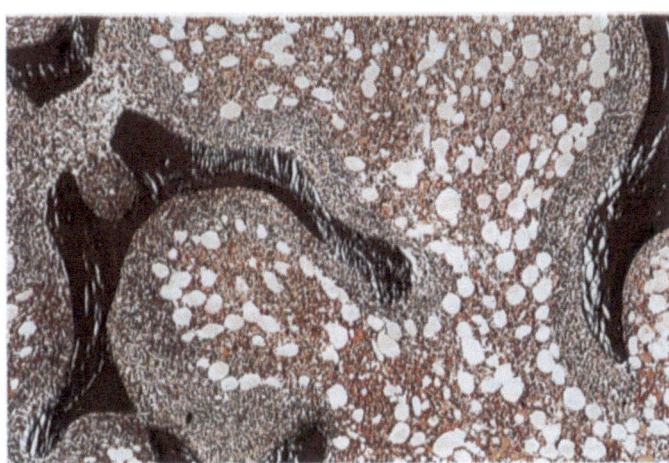

Fig. 8.143 Paratrabecular proliferation pattern in centrocytic lymphoma. Gomori

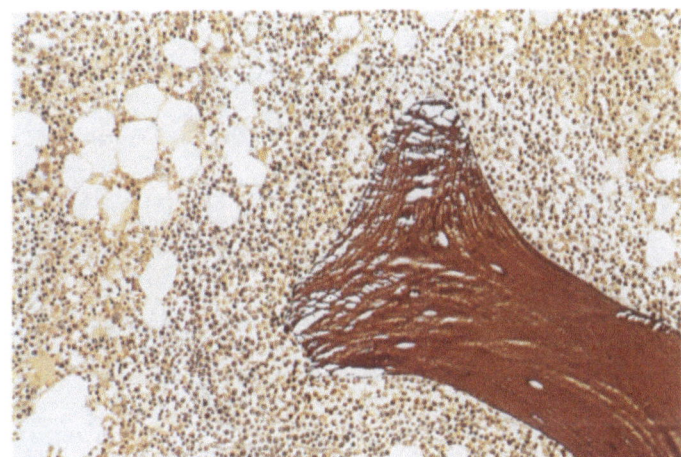

Fig. 8.144 Trabecula enveloped by centrocytic infiltration, extending between fat and marrow cells. Gomori

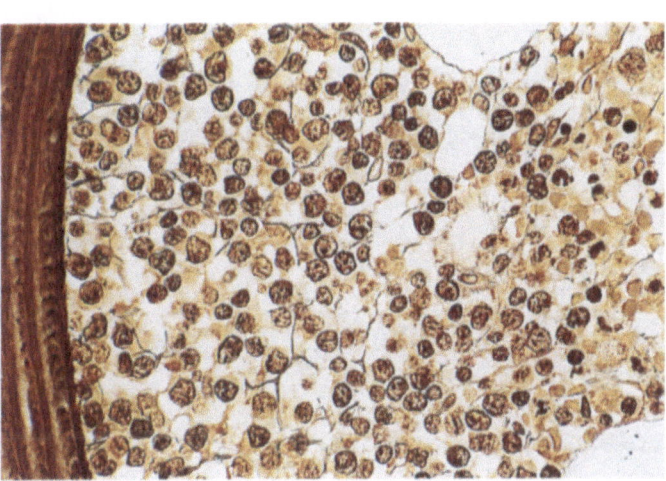

Fig. 8.145 High magnification of area in Fig. 8.144, illustrating delicate reticulin fibres between centrocytes. Note cleaved nuclei. Gomori

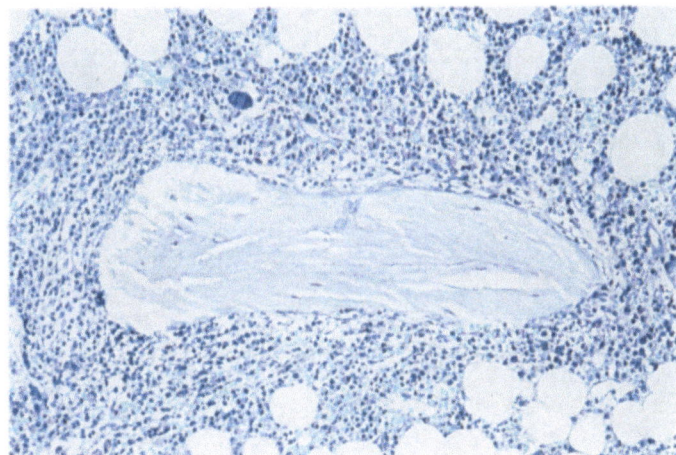

Fig. 8.146 Paratrabecular seam of centrocytes mixed with haemato-poietic cells

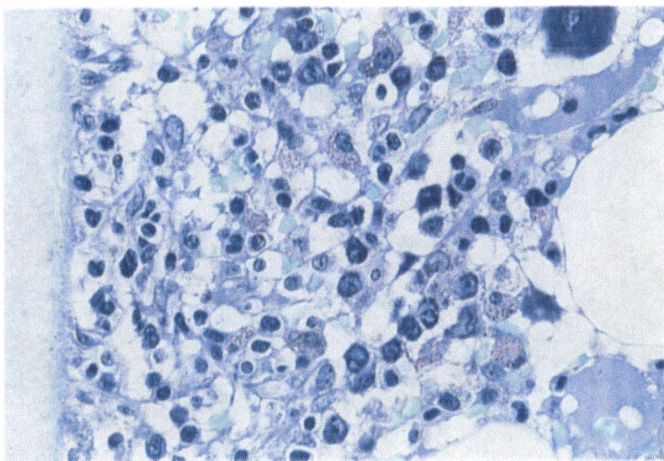

Fig. 8.147 High-power view of biopsy in Fig. 8.146, showing paratra-becular centrocytes, neutrophils, eosinophils and plasma cells

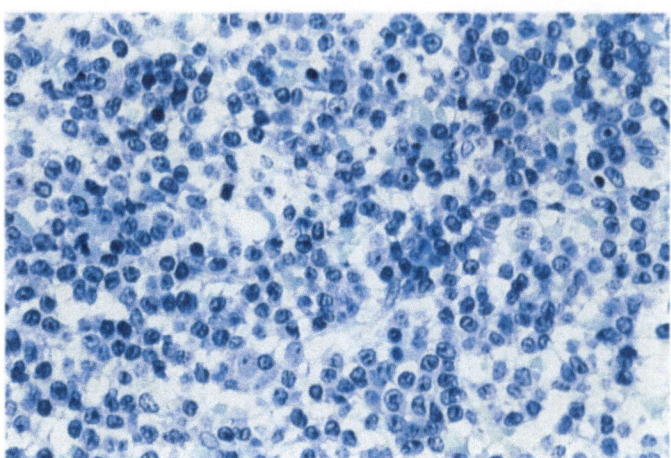

Fig. 8.148 Centrocytes in case of packed marrow

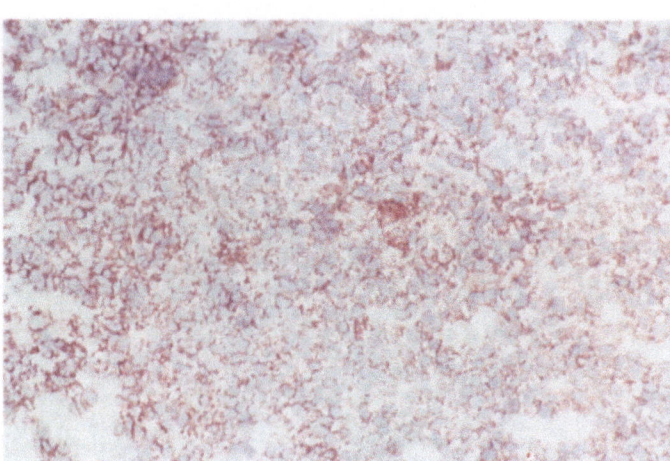

Fig. 8.149 Cryostat section of bone biopsy of patient with centrocytic lymphoma, packed marrow, showing reactivitiy with antibody to IgM

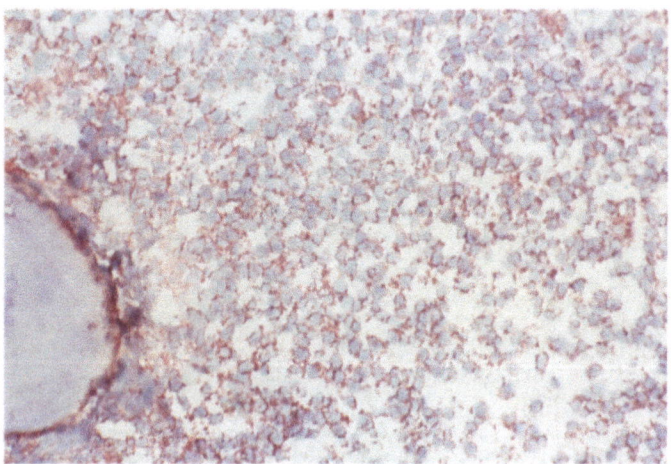

Fig. 8.150 Cryostat section of same biopsy as in Fig. 8.149, showing positive reaction with the antibody to lambda light chain

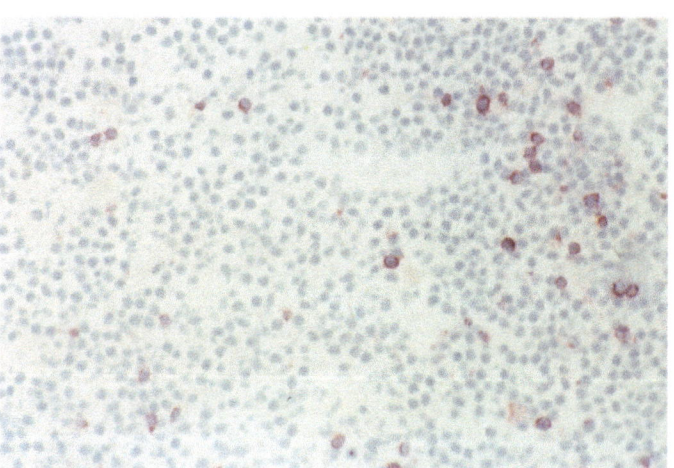

Fig. 8.151 Cryostat section of same biopsy as in Fig. 8.149, illustrating T cells as shown by their staining with Leu 4 (CD3)

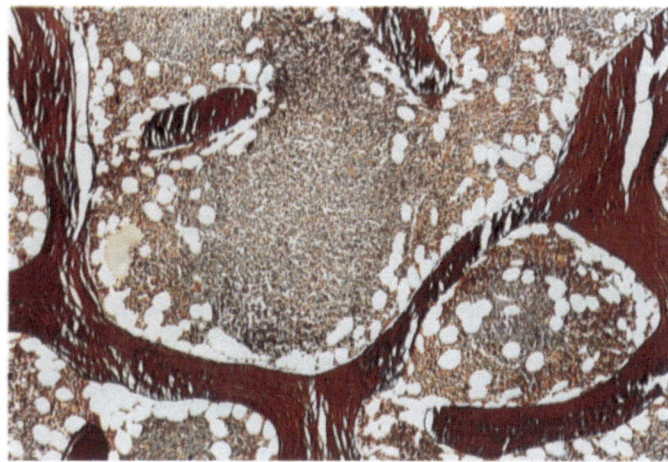

Fig. 8.152 Nodular infiltration in CB/CC lymphoma. Gomori

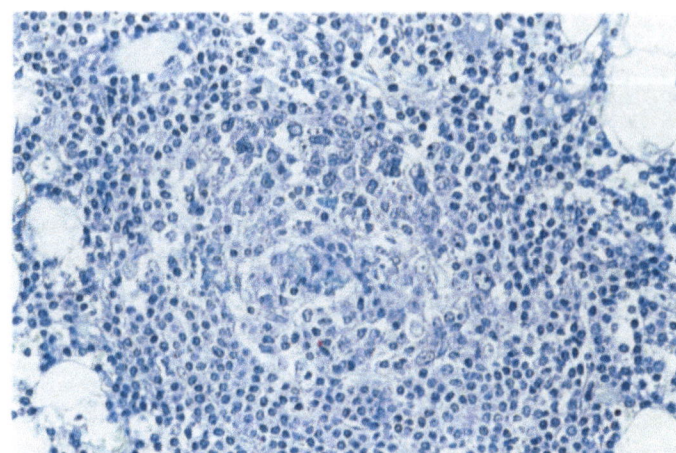

Fig. 8.153 Higher magnification in CB/CC, showing lymphoid follicle with germinal centre

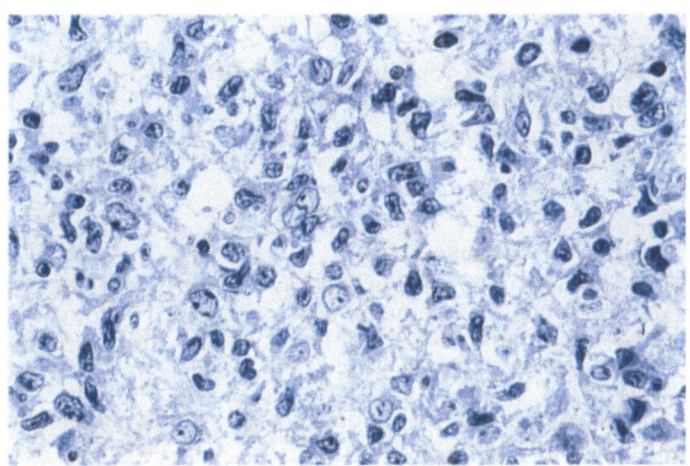

Fig. 8.154 Mixture of centroblasts and centrocytes in CB/CC

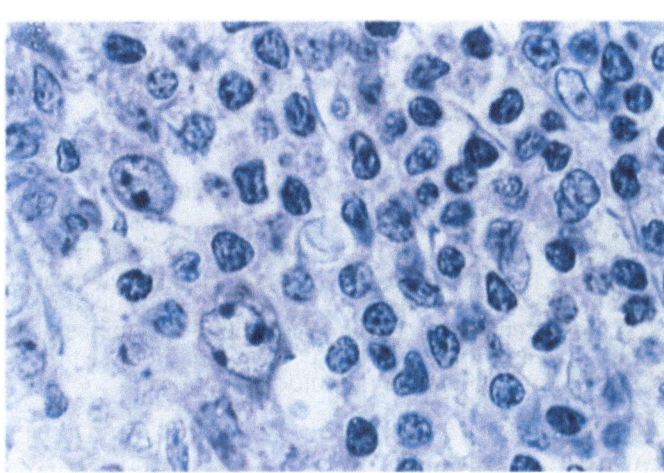

Fig. 8.155 High-power view to show the characteristic nuclei of the centroblasts with nucleoli at the nuclear membrane

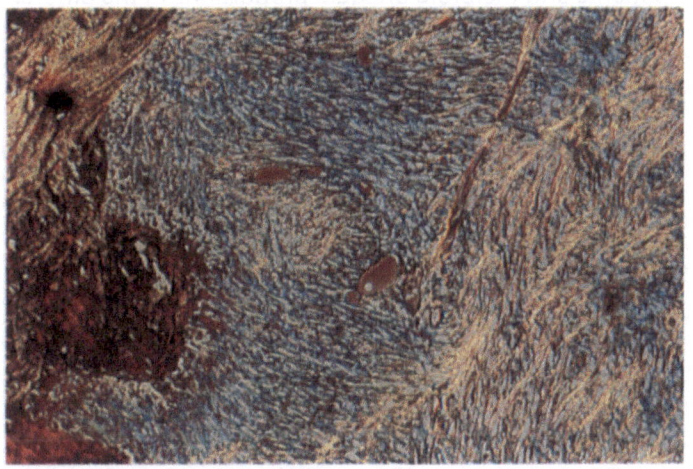

Fig. 8.156 Coarse fibrosis in bone biopsy of patient with CB/CC, packed marrow. Gomori, polarized light

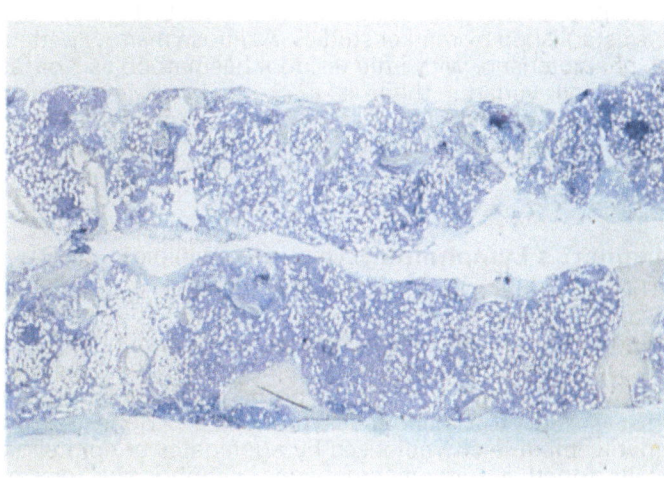

Fig. 8.157 Bone biopsy of patient with CB/CC after therapy, with residual nodules

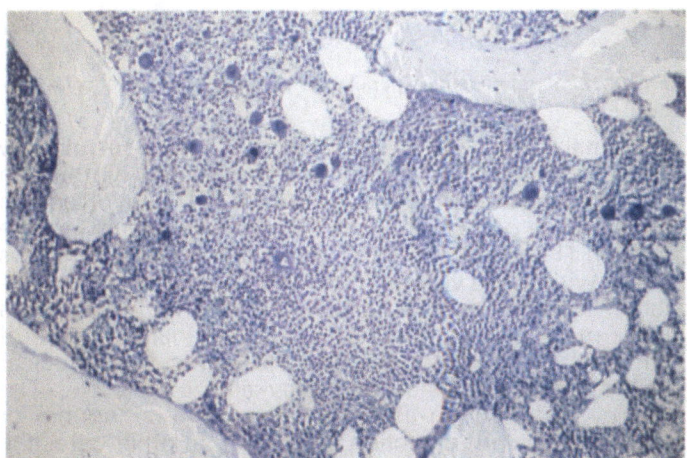

Fig. 8.158 Bone biopsy of patient with PV who developed a CB/CC lymphoma. Note residual lymphoid nodule and megakaryocytes

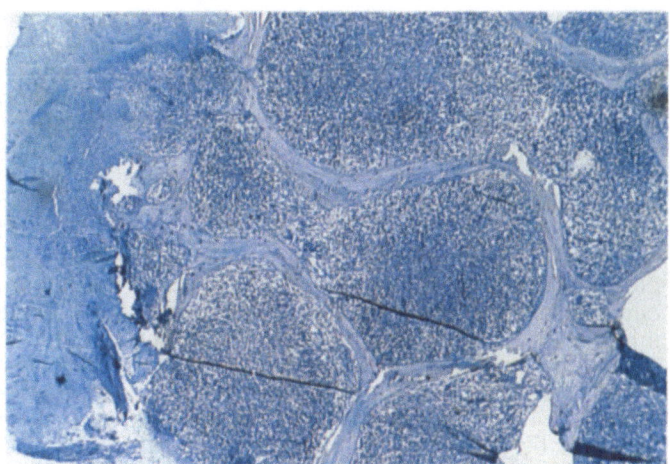

Fig. 8.159 Section of bone biopsy of patient with CB/CC lymphoma. Most of the intertrabecular tissue is necrotic, note the outlines of the follicles

structure and the nucleoli indicate the cell type so that little difficulty is encountered.

Malignant Lymphoma Immunoblastic

In this lymphoma also, the bone marrow is infrequently involved (Figs 8.162–8.164). When it occurs the marrow is usually packed, to the exclusion of haematopoietic and fat cells. B immunoblasts have round nuclei with prominent central nucleoli and basophilic cytoplasm. In contrast, T immunoblasts are polymorphic, but definitive identification requires immunological studies[14].

Burkitt Lymphoma

Marrow involvement is rare; it is a subtype of the small non-cleaved follicle centre cell lymphoma.

Malignant Lymphoma Lymphoblastic (adult patients) (see also section on acute leukaemia)

The phenotype (e.g. common ALL, B ALL, T ALL) must be established by marker studies. A diffuse marrow pattern is characteristic, with little residual haematopoiesis or fat. In T-cell variants there is a pronounced perivascular infiltration of lymphoid cells with oval, notched or convoluted nuclei, and variable amounts of cytoplasm (Figs 8.165–8.172).

Lennert's Lymphoma (Lympho-epithelioid)

This is classified with the T-cell lymphomas (Figs 8.173–8.175)[76]. Nevertheless, a few patients had a B-cell phenotype, though these lymphomas were morphologically indistinguishable from their T-cell counterparts. This lymphoma is thought to mark the border between Hodgkin's disease and the malignant lymphomas[77]. Bone marrow involvement is characterized by aggregates of epithelioid cells together with macrophages, lymphocytes, plasma cells, immunoblasts and sometimes eosinophils. Occasional Hodgkin's or Reed–Sternberg-like cells may be found.

Angioimmunoblastic Lymphadenopathy with Dysproteinaemia (AILD) (Lymphogranulomatosis X)

This is now also classified with the T-cell lymphomas (Figs 8.176–8.182). However, AILD is considered (by some investigators) to occupy a position, at least initially, somewhere between benign lymphoid proliferation and clonal lymphoid transformation[78]. Studies with monoclonal antibodies have shown a variable antigenic profile in frozen sections of lymph node biopsies in AILD; but expression of the proliferation-associated antigen recognized by the antibody Ki67 in more than 25% of lymphoid cells is thought to constitute an unfavourable prognostic marker in AILD. Bone marrow involvement occurs in about half of the cases. There are usually multiple infiltrates consisting of a heterogeneous cell population including immunoblasts, lymphocytes, centrocytes, plasma cells and eosinophils within a reticular framework[79–81]. Interstitial deposits of PAS+ material may or may not be pronounced. Marked vascular proliferation may result in arborizing capillaries, which form whorl-like arrangements together with reticulin fibres.

Other T-cell lymphomas such as mycosis fungoides and Sezary syndrome rarely spread to the bone marrow except in advanced stages of disease. Bone marrow manifestations in peripheral T-cell lymphomas have recently been described[23,82,83].

(Continued on p. 162)

Histologically Unclassifiable Malignant Lymphomas in the Bone Marrow

In a small percentage of cases the lymphoid infiltrations in the bone marrow cannot be classified without multiparameter enzyme and marker studies.

Hodgkin's Disease (HD)

The origin or derivation of the typical Hodgkin or Reed–Sternberg cells still remains controversial[84–86]; though in some cases immunological phenotyping of Hodgkin's cells revealed a B-cell origin[87,88]. Recent studies have shown that involvement of the bone marrow is low at initial presentation (6%) in patients with stage I and stage II disease and in nodular sclerosis (1%, 2% and 4% respectively). A higher incidence (22%) has been found in patients with the lymphocytic depletion type in the lymph node biopsy. However, since one of the criteria for systemic spread (stage IV) is involvement of the bone marrow, a bone marrow biopsy is an integral part of the initial investigation of patients with HD[2]. Various factors may influence the rate of detection: (1) selection of patients and therefore unequal proportions in the different lymph node histologies and clinical stages; (2) biopsy techniques, size and histological preparation; and (3) differences in the interpretation of the histological findings[1].

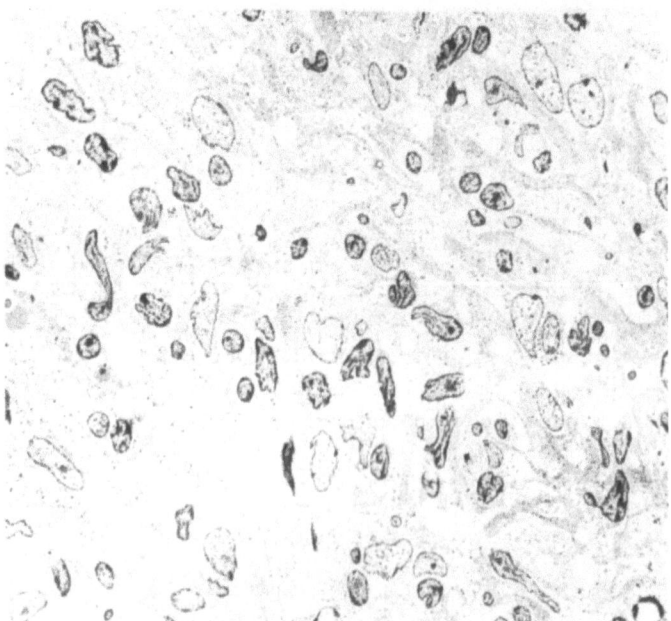

Fig. 8.185 Heterogenous population of lymphoid and reticular cells in HD. EM × 2000

To make the initial diagnosis of HD in the bone marrow (Figs 8.183–8.185), Reed–Sternberg cells within an appropriate stromal setting are required. The involved foci may replace part or all of the normal bone marrow in the section (Figs 8.186–8.190). Such foci consist of fibrous tissue with blood vessels (often with prominent endothelial cell nuclei) within which are eosinophils, plasma cells, macrophages, histiocytes and a variable degree of lymphocytic infiltration. Mononuclear HD cells, bi-nuclear HD cells, and lacunar cells may also be present. The marrow in the non-involved areas may be normal or hyperplastic with reduction in fat cells. In other cases the normal marrow between the foci may be replaced by a loose connective tissue stroma containing fibres, lymphoid plasma and mast cells, and some haematopoietic precursors. Small, epithelioid cell clusters may also be found. The lesions in involved biopsies range from small paratrabecular foci to large, patchy areas of lymphogranulomatous tissue.

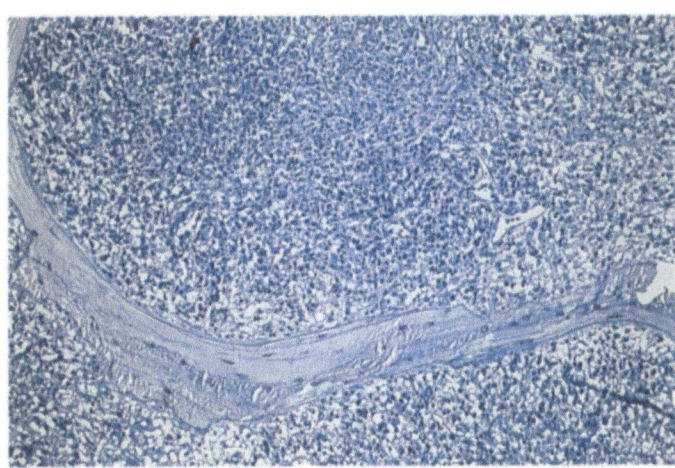

Fig. 8.160 Higher magnification of the same biopsy as in Fig. 8.159. Small area with viable cells

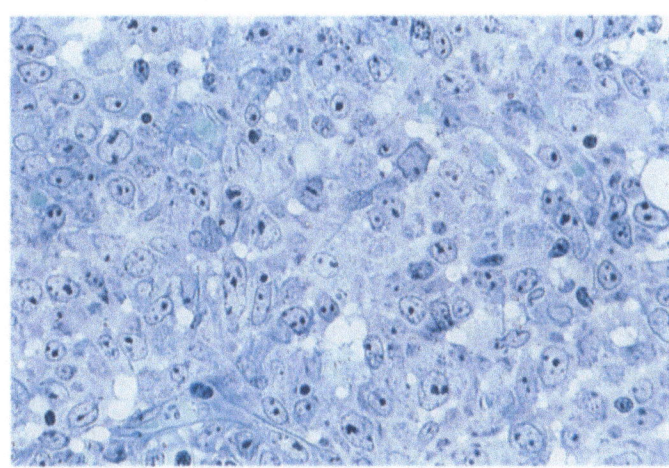

Fig. 8.161 Dense bone marrow infiltration in CB lymphoma, packed marrow type

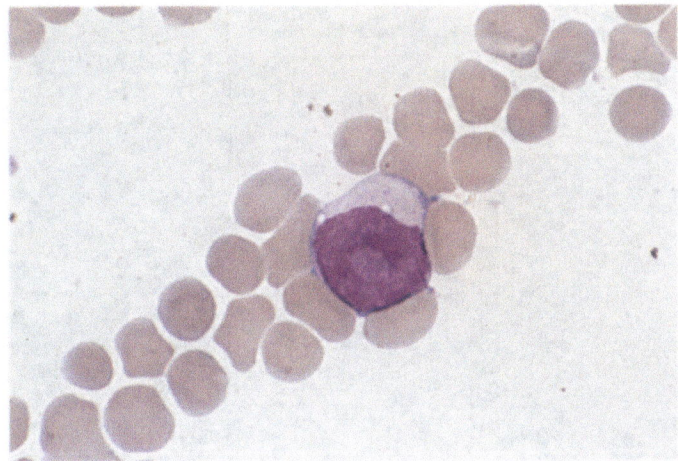

Fig. 8.162 Immunoblast with large central nucleolus in peripheral blood smear of patient with IB lymphoma

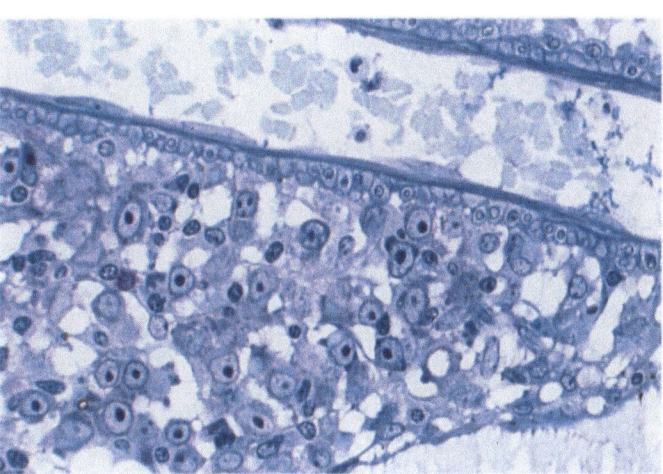

Fig. 8.163 Bone biopsy same patient as in Fig. 8.162, showing infiltration of monomorphic immunoblasts

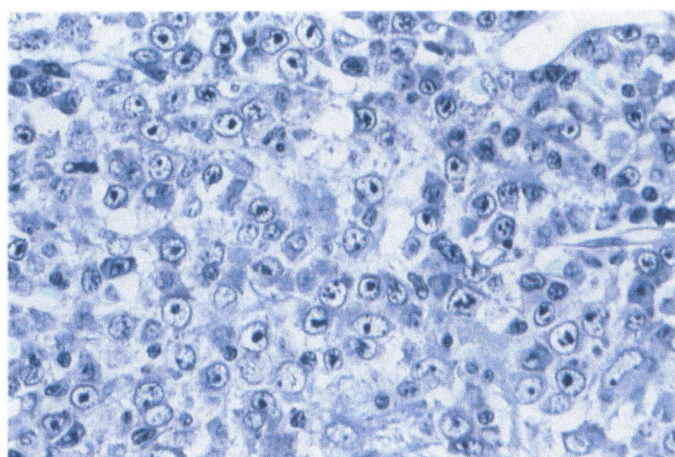

Fig. 8.164 Bone biopsy of patient with immunoblastoma, characterised by pleomorphic immunoblasts

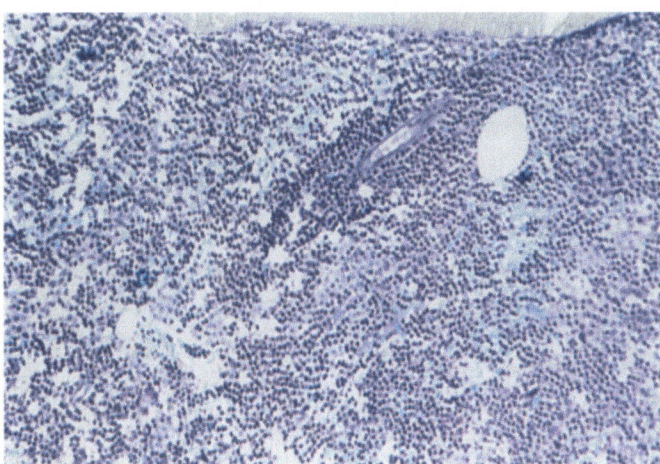

Fig. 8.165 Extensive bone marrow involvement in T-lymphoblastic lymphoma

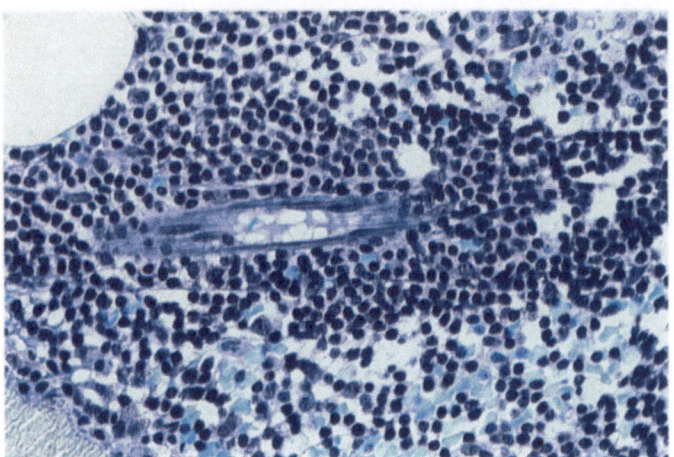

Fig. 8.166 High-power view from the section in Fig. 8.165, showing dense perivascular infiltration

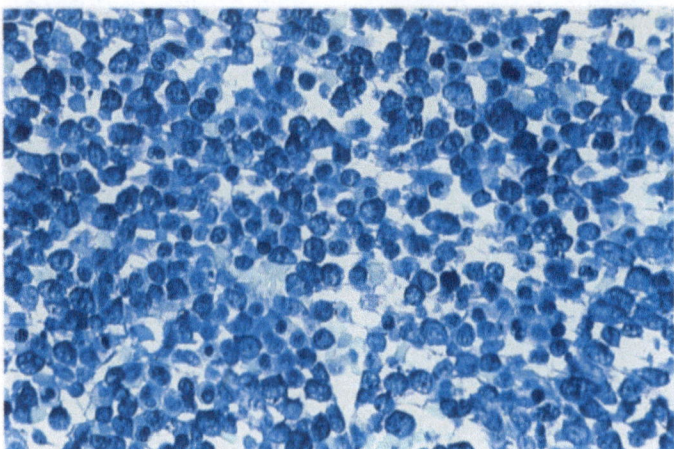

Fig. 8.167 Bone marrow involvement in patient with mediastinal T-cell lymphoma, packed marrow

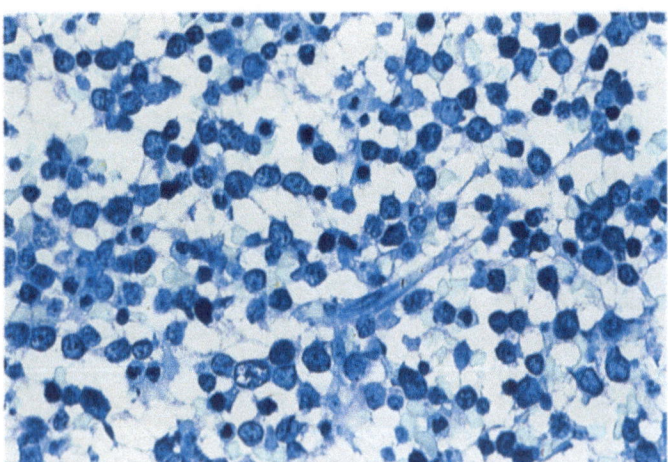

Fig. 8.168 The same patient as in Fig. 8.167, illustrating diffuse infiltration by small lymphoid cells with high nucleo-cytoplasmic ratio and round, oval or notched nuclei with one or two small nucleoli

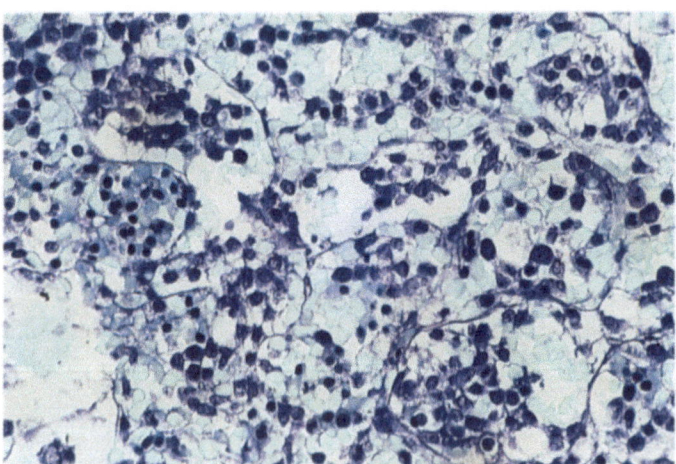

Fig. 8.169 Sections of bone biopsy of patient with T-cell lymphoma; initially mainly intravascular involvement in the bone marrow, which progressed to a packed marrow pattern within a few months' time. There is disruption of the sinusoidal walls, disorganization of the bone marrow architecture and marked vascular proliferation

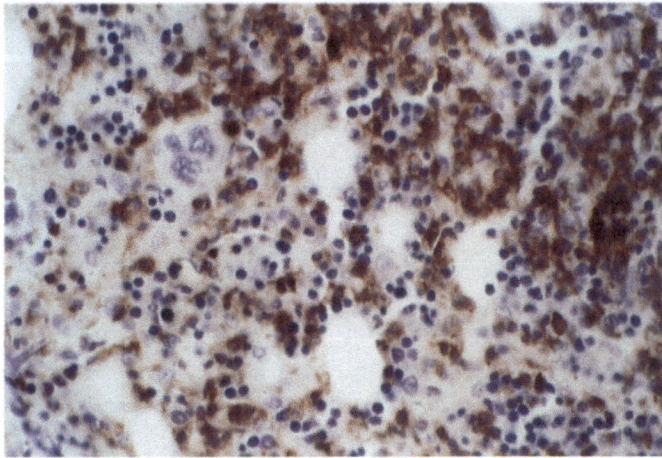

Fig. 8.170 The same case as in Fig. 8.169. Paraffin section stained by UCHLI (a pan T cell marker)

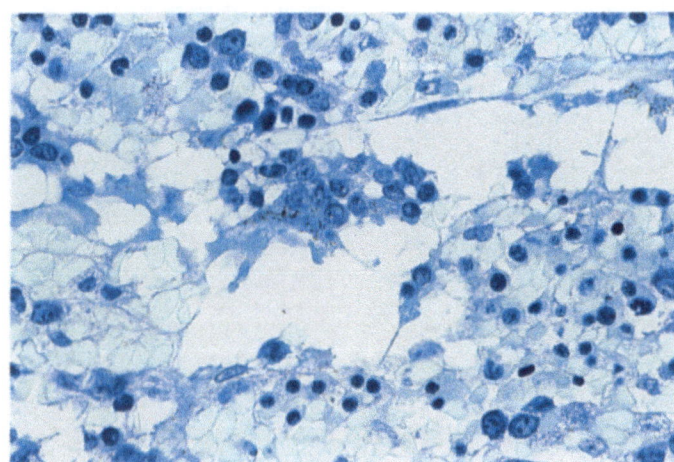

Fig. 8.171 The same case as in Fig. 8.169. Intravascular cluster of T cells, with residual haematopoiesis

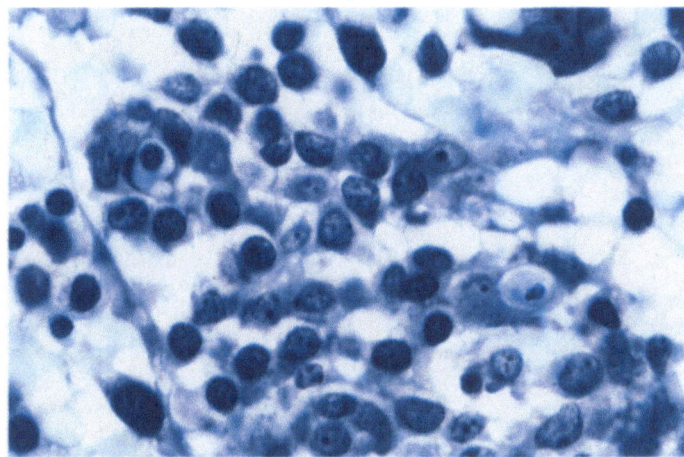

Fig. 8.172 The same case as in Fig. 8.169. Higher magnification to show details of nuclei

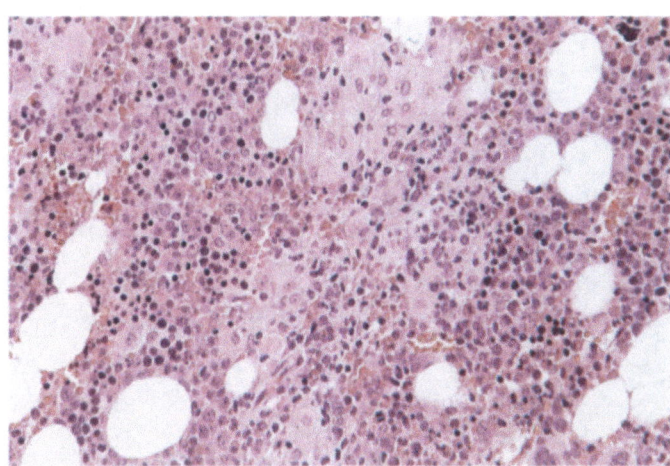

Fig. 8.173 Paraffin section showing epithelioid cell granuloma in patient with Lennert's lymphoma. H&E

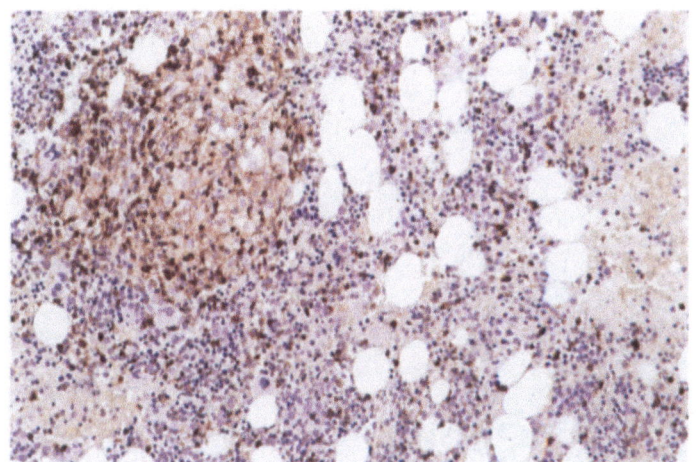

Fig. 8.174 The same case as in Fig. 8.173. Section showing UCHL I positive T cells within and around a granuloma

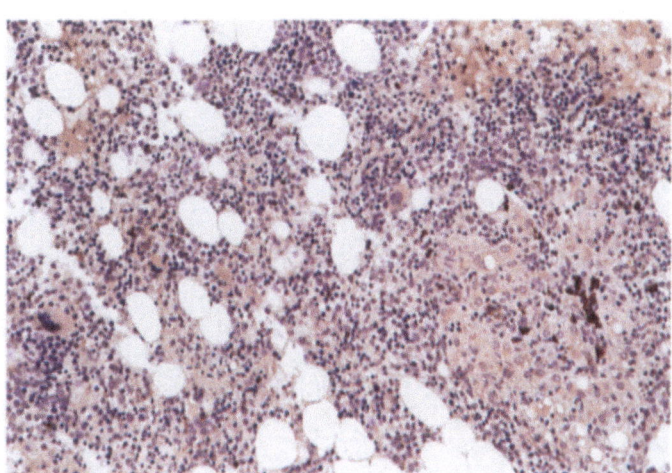

Fig. 8.175 The same case as in Fig. 8.173. Very few B cells, as shown by staining with the antibody MB2

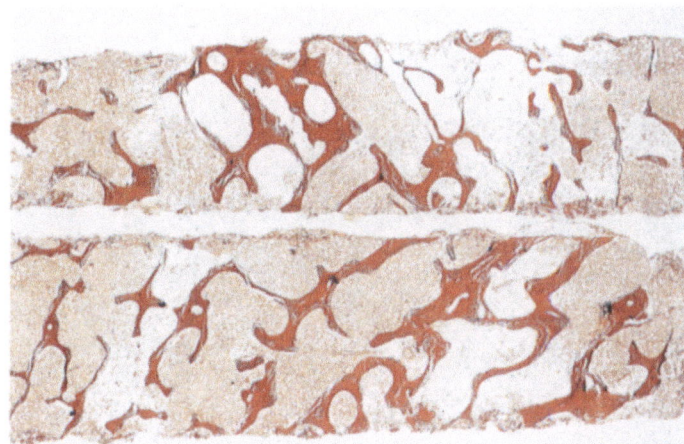

Fig. 8.176 Patchy bone marrow involvement in AILD. Gomori

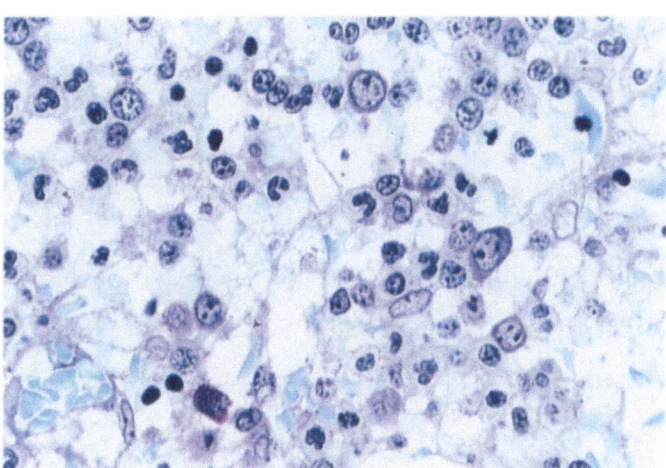

Fig. 8.177 Heterogeneous cell population in an involved area in AILD

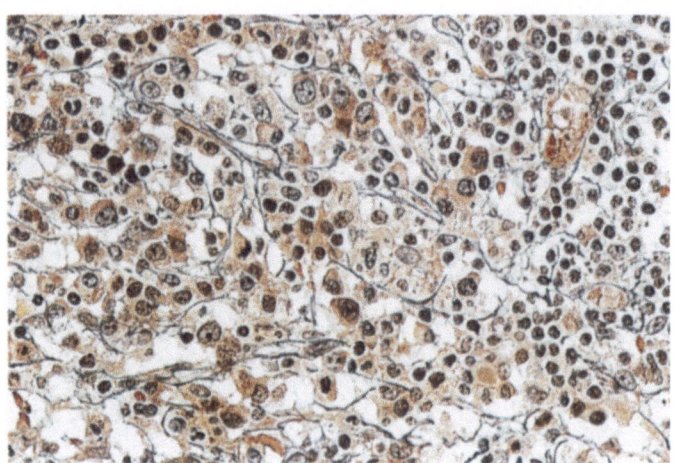

Fig. 8.178 Reticular fibre network in AILD. Gomori

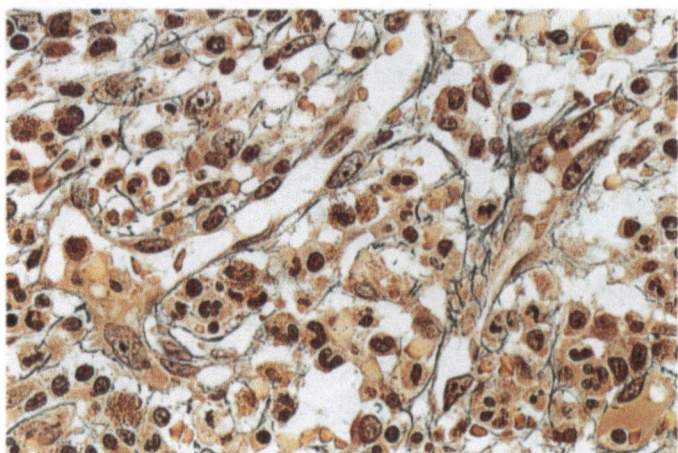

Fig. 8.179 Prominent vascular proliferation in AILD. Gomori

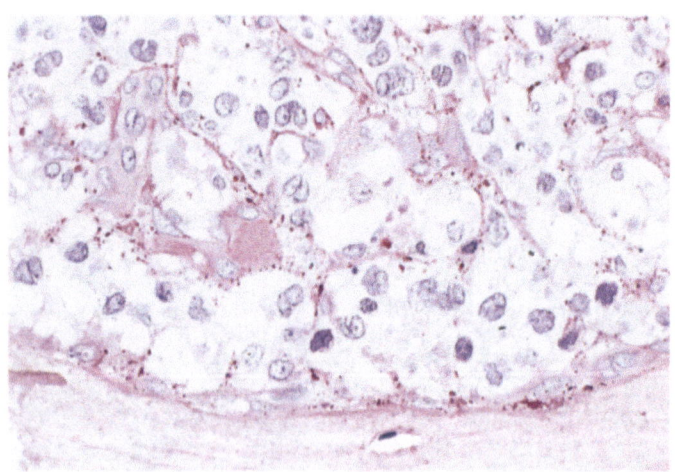

Fig. 8.180 Interstitial deposits of PA5-positive material in AILD. PAS

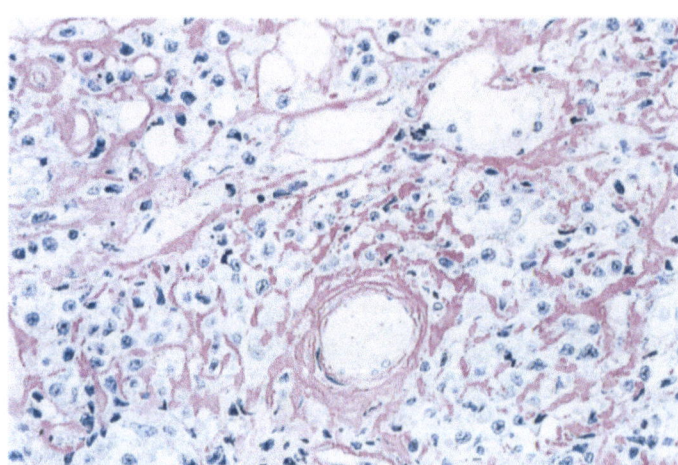

Fig. 8.181 Perivascular and marked intercellular deposits of PAS-postive material. PAS

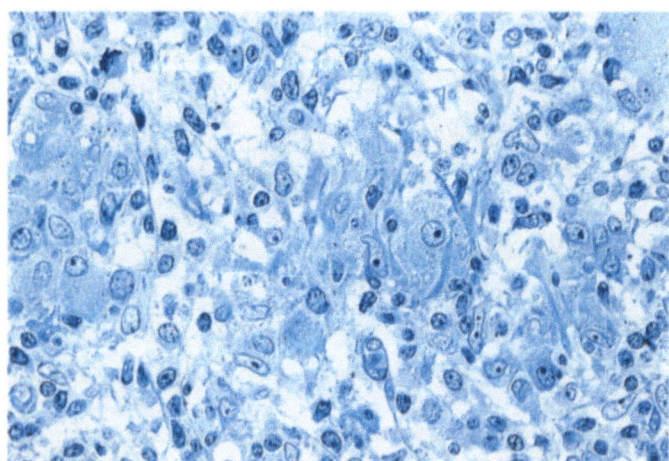

Fig. 8.182 Numerous epithelioid cells in bone marrow of patient with lymphogranulomatous X

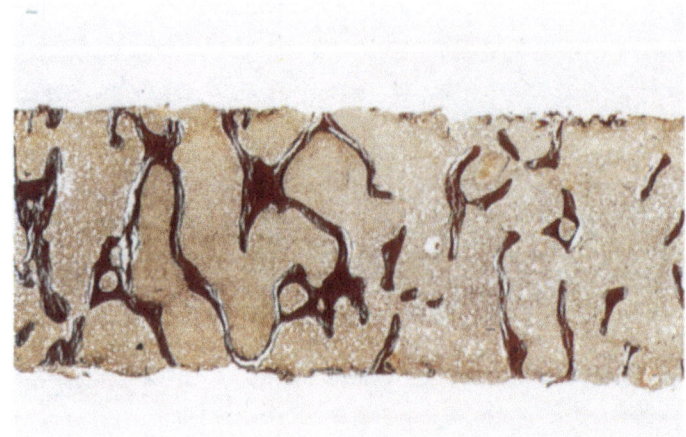

Fig. 8.183 Focal involvement of bone marrow in HD. Gomori

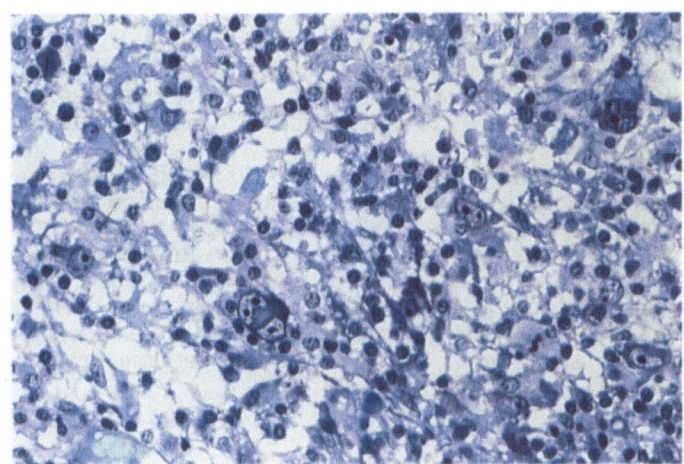

Fig. 8.184 Case of primary involvement of the bone marrow in HD. Note mononuclear Hodgkin's and Reed–Sternberg cells

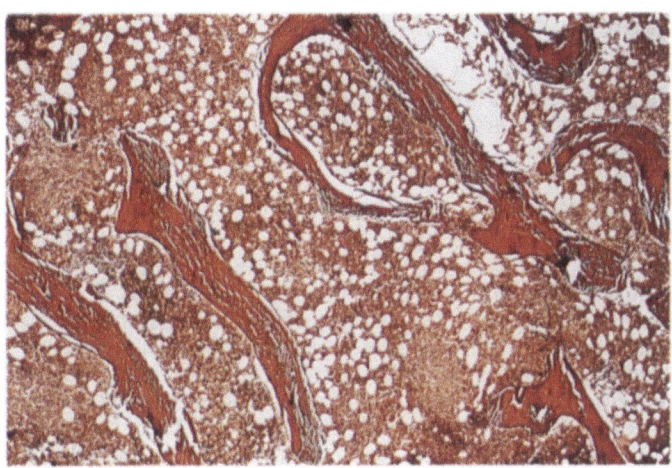

Fig. 8.186 Minimal nodular infiltration of the bone marrow in HD. Gomori

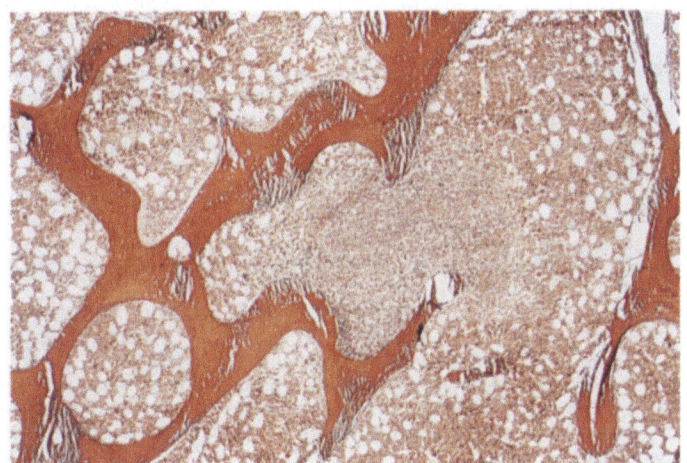

Fig. 8.187 Single paratrabecular infiltration in HD. Gomori

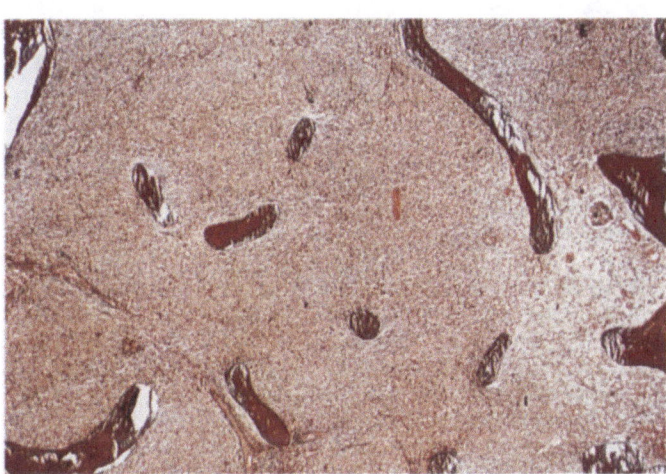

Fig. 8.188 Packed marrow in HD with marked osteopenia. Gomori

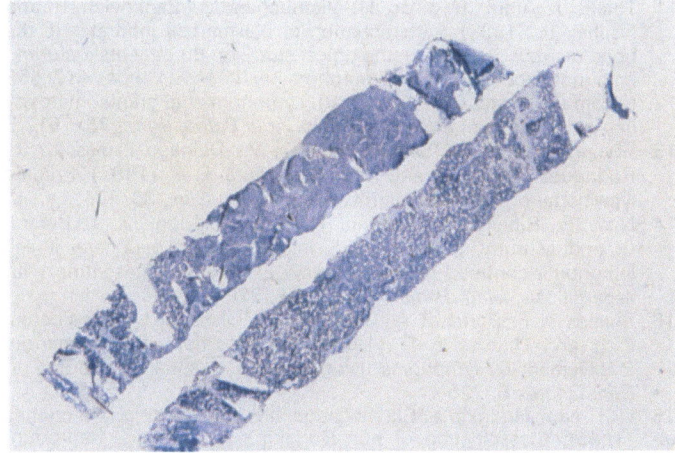

Fig. 8.189 Two biopsies taken from the same area, one with involvement and one without. HD diagnosed by this biopsy

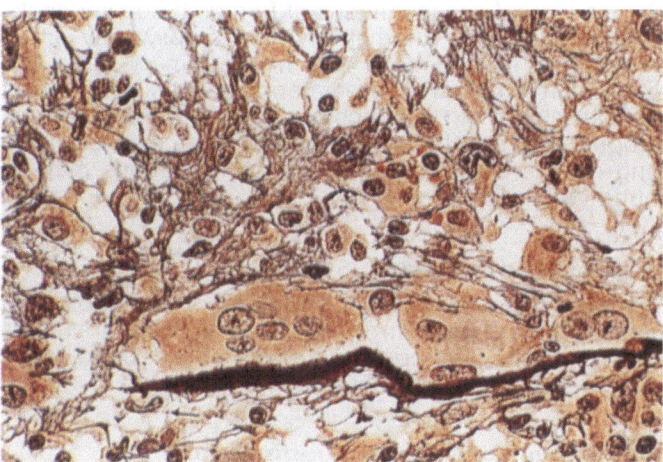

Fig. 8.190 Osteoclastic resorption of a trabecula within an area of HD infiltration. Gomori

When Hodgkin's disease has already been diagnosed elsewhere, mononuclear Hodgkin's cells within an appropriate setting are considered evidence of bone marrow involvement.

Subtyping of HD in the bone marrow

Three criteria are utilized: (1) a high content of lymphocytes, (2) a low content of lymphocytes and (3) a high content of epithelioid cells (Figs 8.191–8.195)[1,89]. Bone marrow involvement by definition indicates stage IV. The trabecular bone structure is usually affected when the involved areas are large: osteosclerosis, osteolysis or osteoporosis or combinations of these have all been described. Hypercalcaemia and elevated 1,25-dihydroxy-vitamin D levels have been found, presumably due to metabolism of vitamin D by the granulomas as in sarcoidosis and in tuberculosis.

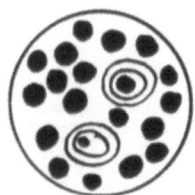 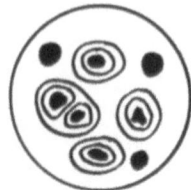 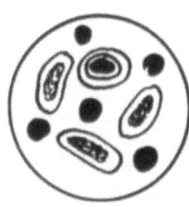

HIGH CONTENT OF LYMPHOCYTES   LOW CONTENT OF LYMPHOCYTES   HIGH CONTENT OF EPITHELIOID CELLS

Fig. 8.191 Histological types of bone marrow involvement in Hodgkin's disease

Epithelioid cell granulomata are foci of fibrous tissue or lymphocytic nodules without the presence of R-S or H cells. These may be found in the BMB of patients with HD documented elsewhere, but are not considered as evidence of bone marrow involvement.

Nodular lymphocyte predominance HD (in lymph node histology) has recently been shown to have important phenotypic as well as clinical differences from other forms of HD, including the possibility of late relapse[90].

Non-involved bone marrow biopsies in HD

Bone biopsies of many patients with histologically documented HD but without marrow involvement exhibit a variety of reactions. These include lymphoid cell nodules, epithelioid cell granulomas, increased phagocytic macrophages[91], focal accumulations of fibrous tissue and leukaemoid reactions. Alternatively, the biopsy may show infiltrations of lymphoid, plasma and mast cells and maturation inhibition of haematopoietic precursors. Areas of replacement of haematopoiesis by fat cells, or serous atrophy, may also be present and be quite extensive. If a long core is examined, different manifestations may be found within one biopsy.

Heavy Chain Diseases

Gamma, alpha and mu chain: no specific histopathological pattern in the bone marrow has been reported. Increases in plasma cells, lymphocytes, histiocytes may be found as well as some areas of trabecular osteolyses.

Additional Bone Biopsy Findings in LPD

Histological discordance, variability, conversion or transformation, concurrent neoplasias, development of other neoplasias have all been documented in the bone marrows of patients with lymphoproliferative disorders. For example malignant lymphoma centroblastic/centrocytic in the lymph node biopsy and malignant lymphoma immuno-cytic in the bone marrow; development of Richter's syndrome in CLL, development of a myeloproliferative disorder together with a pre-existing malignant lymphoma.

Complications such as phagocytic histiocytosis may also be found by examination of the bone marrow. Effects of therapy on both the malignant lymphomas in BMB of patients with involvement, as well as on the haematopoietic tissue, may be monitored by bone biopsy. In many cases, though a considerable reduction in amount of lymphomatous infiltration is achieved, some residual foci remain even when the marrow has become severely hypoplastic (Figs 8.196 and 8.197).

References

1. Clark, P., Normansell, D. E., Innes, D. J. and Hess, C. E. (1986). Lymphocyte subsets in normal bone marrow. *Blood*, **67**, 1600
2. Frisch, B., Lewis, S.M., Burkhardt, R. and Bartl, R. (1985). *Biopsy Pathology of Bone and Bone Marrow*. London: Chapman and Hall
3. Faulkner-Jones, B. E., Howie, A. J., Boughton, B. J. and Franklin, I. M. (1988). Lymphoid aggregates in bone marrow: study of eventual outcome. *J. Clin. Pathol.*, **41**, 768
4. Navone, R., Valpreda, M. and Pich, A. (1985). Lymphoid nodules and nodular lymphoid hyperplasia in bone marrow biopsies. *Acta Haematol.*, **74**, 19
5. Tin Han, Ozer, H., Gavignan, M., Gajera, R., Minowada, J., Bloom, M. L., Sadamori, N., Sandberg, A. A., Gomez, G. A. and Henderson, E. S. (1984). Benign monclonal B cell lympho-cytosis – a benign variant of CLL: clinical, immunologic, phenotypic, and cytogenic studies in 20 patients. *Blood*, **64**, 244
6. Preud'Homme, J. L. (1984). Monoclonality and malignancy in lymphoid tumours. *Lancet*, **2**, 48
7. Cleary, M. L. and Sklar, J. (1984). Lymphoproliferative disorders in cardiac transplant recipients are multiclonal lymphomas. *Lancet*, **2**, 489
8. Shearer, W. T., Ritz, J., Finegold, M. J., Geurra-Celine, I., Rosenblatt, H. M., Lewis, D. E., Pollack, M. S., Taber, L. H., Sumaya, C. V., Grumet, F. C., Clearly, M. L., Warnke, R. and Sklar, J. (1985). Epstein-Barr virus-associated B-cell proliferation of diverse clonal origins after bone marrow transplantation in a 12-year-old patient with severe combined immunodeficiency. *N. Engl. J. Med.*, **312**, 1151
9. Michaeli, J., Lugassy, G., Raz, I., Uzieli, B. and Polliack, A. (1987). Chronic lymphocytic leukaemia and malignant lymphoma developing in patients with auto-immunity or other Ill-defined immune stigmata: A review of the literature and report of additional 9 cases. *Haematol. Rev.*, **1**, 291
10. Peterson, L., Brown, B. A., Crosson, J. T. and Mladenovic, J. (1986). Application of the immunoperoxidase technic to bone marrow trephine biopsies in the classification of patients with monoclonal gammopathies. *Am. J. Clin. Pathol.*, **85**, 688
11. Thiele, J., Arenz, B., Klein, H., Vierbuchen, M., Zankovich, R. and Fischer, R. (1988). Differentiation of plasma cell infiltrates in the bone marrow. A clinicopathological study on 80 patients including immunohistochemistry and morphometry. *Virchows Arch.*, **412**, 553
12. Ninomura, A. and Ohta, G. (1986). Lymphomatoid granulomatosis-like lesions in malignant lymphoma. *Acta Pathol. Jpn.*, **36**, 1617
13. Romero-Garcia, F., Vazquez-Villegas, V., Delgado-Lamas, J. J., Rodriguez-Carrillo, J. and Rodriguez-Mora, E. A. (1987). Primary lymphoma of the bone marrow. *Rev. Invest. Clin.*, **39**, 171
14. Nuss, R., Ribeiro, R. C., Bunin, N., Behm, F., Jenkins, J., Berard, C. and Murphy, S. B. (1988). Immunoblastic peripheral T-cell lymphoma confined to bone marrow in an infant presenting with aspergillosis. *Med. Pediatr. Oncol.*, **16**, 220
15. Shields, A. F., Porter, B. A., Churchley, S., Olson, D. O., Appelbaum, F. R. and Thomas, E. D. (1987). The detection of bone marrow involvement by lymphoma using magnetic resonance imaging. *J. Clin. Oncol.*, **5**, 225
16. NCI Non-Hodgkin's Classification Project Writing Committee (1985). Classification of non-Hodgkin's lymphomas. Reproducibility of major classification systems. *Cancer*, **55**, 91
17. Waldmann, T. A., Davis, M. M., Bongiovanni, K. F. and Korsmeyer, S. J. (1985). Rearrangement of genes for the antigen receptor on T cells as markers of lineage and clonality in human lymphoid neoplasms. *N. Engl. J. Med.*, **313**, 776
18. Ersboll, J., Schultz, H. B. and Hougaard, P. (1985). Comparison of the working formulation of non-Hodgkin's lymphoma with the

(Continued on p. 164)

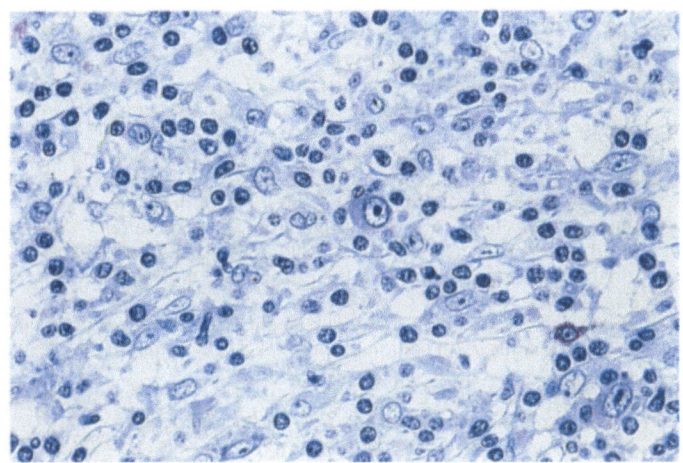

Fig. 8.192 HD with high content of lymphocytes in the bone marrow

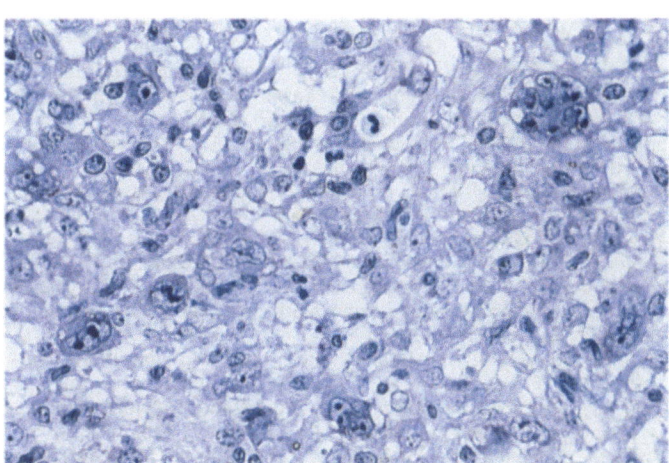

Fig. 8.193 HD with low content of lymphocytes in the bone marrow

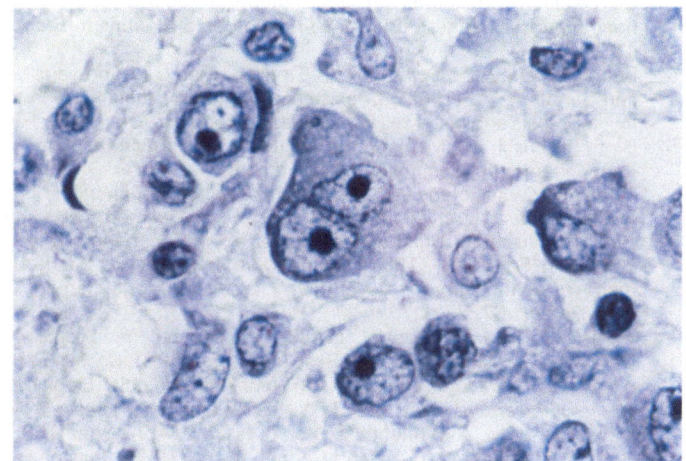

Fig. 8.194 Higher magnification to show classic binucleate Reed–Sternberg cell and Hodgkin's cell

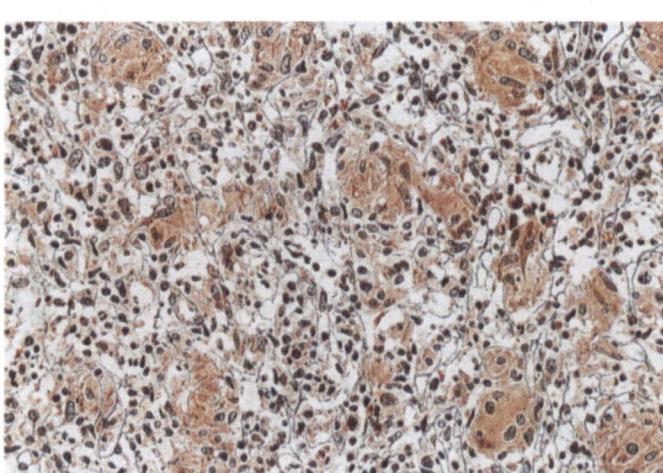

Fig. 8.195 Multiple small epithelioid cell aggregates in involved area in bone marrow in HD. Gomori

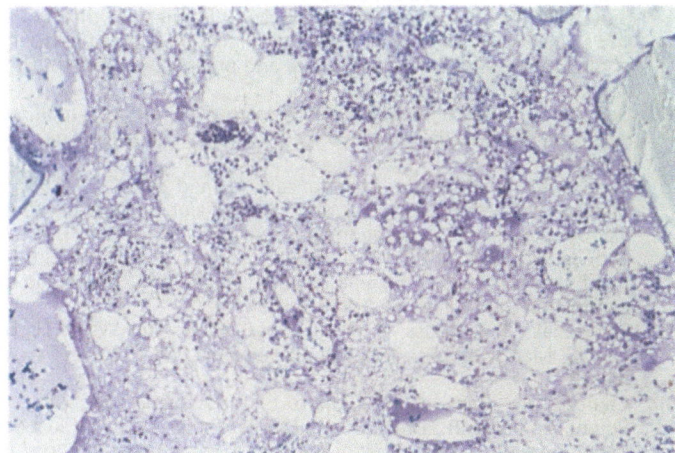

Fig. 8.196 Extensive serous atrophy in non-involved area of bone biopsy in HD

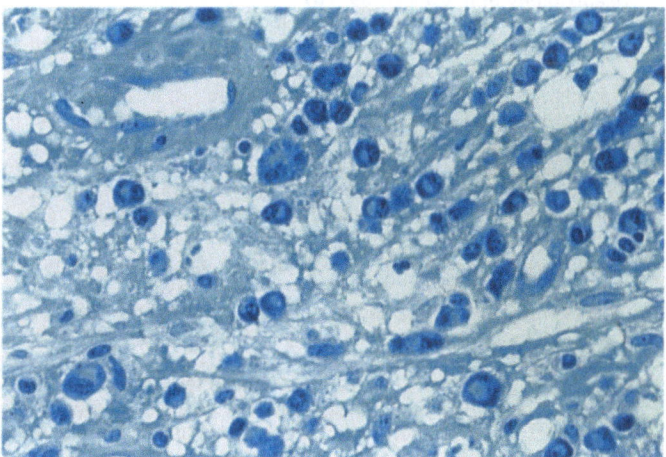

Fig. 8.197 Section of bone biopsy of patient with HD after chemotherapy. Serous atrophy and reactive plasmacytosis

Rapaport, Kiel, and Lukes & Collins classifications. Translational value and prognostic significance based on review of 658 patients treated at a single institution. *Cancer,* **55**, 2442

19. Jaffe, E. S. (1986). Relationship of classification to biologic behaviour of non-Hodgkin's lymphomas. *Sem. Oncol.,* **13**, 3

20. Foon, K. A. and Tood, R. F. (1986). Immunologic classification of leukaemia and lymphoma. *Blood,* **68**,1

21. Mazza, P., Gherlinzoni, F., Kemna, G., Poletti, G., Zanzani, P. L., Verlicchi, F., Lauria, F., Fiacchini, M., Pileri, S., Rivano, M. T., Gobbi, M., Bandini, G., Emiliani, E., Babini, L. and Tura, S. (1987). Clinicopathological study on non-Hodgkin's lymphomas. *Haematologica,* **72**, 351

22. Schuurman, H-J., van Baarlen, J., Huppes, W., Lam, B. W., Verdonck, L. F. and van Unnik, J. A. M. (1987). Immunophenotyping of non-Hodgkin's lymphoma. Lack of correlation between immunophenotype and cell morphology. *Am. J. Pathol.,* **129**, 140

23. Suchi, T., Lennert, K., Ly, T., Kikuchi, M., Sato, E., Stansfeld, A. G. and Feller, A. C. (1987). Histopathology and immunohistochemistry of peripheral T cell lymphomas: a proposal for their classification. *J. Clin. Pathol.,* **409**, 995

24. Stansfeld, A. G., Diebold, J., Kapanci, Y., Kelenyi, G., Lennert, K., Mioduszewska, O., Noel, H., Rilke, F., Sundstrom, C., van Unnik, J. A. M. and Wright, D. H. (1988). Updated Kiel classification for lymphomas. *Lancet,* **1**, 292

25. Bartl, R., Hansmann, M. L., Frisch, B. and Burkhardt, R. (1988). Comparative histology of malignant lymphomas in lymph node and bone marrow. *Br. J. Haematol.,* **69**, 229

26. McKenna, R. W. and Hernandez, J. A. (1988). Bone marrow in malignant lymphomas. In Hyun, B. H. (ed.), *Hematology/Oncology of North America. 'Bone Marrow Examination'.* Philadelphia: W. B. Saunders, Vol. 2

27. Thaler, J., Danz, H., Gattringer, C., Glassl, H., Leichleitner, M., Dietze, O. and Huber, H. (1987). Diagnostic and prognostic value of immuno-histological bone marrow examination: results in 212 patients with lymphoproliferative disorders. *Blut,* **54**, 213

28. Freedman, A. S. and Nadler, L. M. (1987). B cell development in chronic lymphocytic leukaemia. *Sem. Hematol.,* **24**, 230

29. Gale, R. P. and Foon, K. A. (1987). Biology of chronic lymphocytic leukaemia. *Sem. Hematol.,* **24**, 209

30. Fermand, J. P., James, J. M., Herait, P. and Brouet, J. C. (1985). Associated chronic lymphocytic leukaemia and multiple myeloma: origin from a single clone. *Blood,* **66**, 291

31. Gingold, N., Dosius, L. and Berceanu, S. (1985). Bone marrow patterns in chronic lymphocytic leukaemia related to various clinical and haematological findings. A preliminary report. *Haematologia,* **18**, 115

32. Geisler, C., Ralfklaer, E., Hansen, M. M., Hou-Jensen, K. and Olesen-Larsen, S. (1986). The bone marrow histological pattern has independent prognostic value in early stage chronic lymphocytic leukaemia. *Br. J. Haematol.,* **62**, 47

33. Pangalis, G. A., Roussou, P. A., Kittas, C., Kokkinou, S. and Fessas, P. (1987). B-chronic lymphocytic leukaemia. Prognostic implication of bone marrow histology in 120 patients. Experience from a single haematology unit. *Cancer,* **59**, 767

34. Frisch, B. and Bartl, R. (1988). Histologic classification and staging of chronic lymphocytic leukaemia. A retrospective and prospective study of 503 cases,. *Acta Haematol.,* **79**, 140

35. Hamblin, T. J., Stevens, O. J. R. and Smith, J. L. (1987). Long survival in B-CLL correlates with surface IgMk phenotype. *Br. J. Haematol.,* **66**, 21

36. Lerma-Puertas, E., Gonzalez-Campora, R., Amerigo-Navarro, J., Rubi-Uria, J. Galera-Davidson, H. (1988). Morphometric study of bone marrow in chronic lymphocytic leukaemia. *Anal. Quant. Cytol. Histol.,* **10**, 28

37. Foon, K. A. and Gale, R. P. (1987). Staging and therapy of chronic lymphocytic leukaemia. *Sem. Haematol.,* **24**, 264

38. Montserrat, E. and Rozman, C. (1987). Bone marrow biopsy in chronic lymphocytic leukaemia: a review of its prognostic importance. *Blood-Cells,* **12**; 315

39. Bernhards, J., Dohler, U., Freund, M., Rastetter, J. and Georgii, A. (1988). The significance of histopathology of bone marrow for the life expectancy of patients with chronic lymphatic leukaemia. *Med. Klin.,* **83**, 637

40. Vashi, P., Patel, B., Musson, P., Fahrner, J. and Rosenbaum, R., (1987). Corticosteroid-responsive pure red cell aplasia in chronic lymphatic leukaemia. *Am. J. Haematol.,* **26**, 279

41. Zanke, B. W., Johnston, J. B. and Israels, L. G. (1988). Erythemic myelosis in chronic lymphocytic leukaemia. *Cancer,* **62**, 954

42. Anderson, K. C., Boyd, A. W., Fisher, D. C., Leslie, C., Schlossman, S. F. and Nadler, L. M. (1985). Hairy cell leukaemia: a tumor of pre-

plasma cells. *Blood,* **65**, 620

43. De Panfilis, G., Manara, G. C., Ferrari, C., Torresani, C. and Sansoni, P. (1988). Hairy cell leukaemia cells express CDIa antigen. *Cancer,* **61**, 52

44. Katayama, I. (1988). Bone marrow in hairy cell leukaemia. In Hyun, B. H. (ed.), *Hematology/Oncology Clinics of North America. Bone Marrow Examination.* Philadelphia: W. B. Saunders, Vol. 2

45. Bartl, R., Frisch, B., Hill, W., Burkhardt, R., Sommerfeld, W. and Sund, M. (1983). Bone marrow histology in hairy cell leukaemia. Identification of subtypes and their prognostic significance. *Am. J. Clin. Pathol.,* **79**, 531

46. Zimmerman, K. G., Payne, C. M. and Nagle, R. B. (1984). Ribosome—lamellae complexes in benign plasma cells accompanying neoplastic infiltrates. *Am. J. Clin. Pathol.,* **81**, 364

47. Diez Martin, J. L., Cy, L. I. and Banka, P. M. (1987). Blastic variant of hairy-cell leukaemia. *Am. J. Clin. Pathol.,* **87**, 576

48. Agnarsson, B. A. and Kadlin, M. E. (1987). An unusual B-cell lymphoma simulating hairy cell leukaemia. *Am. J. Clin. Pathol.,* **88**, 752

49. Melo, J. V., Robinson, D. S., Gregory, C. and Catovsky, D. (1987). Splenic B cell lymphoma with 'villous' lymphocytes in the peripheral blood: a disorder distinct from hairy cell leukaemia. *Leukaemia,* **1**, 294

50. Flandrin, G., Sigaux, F., Castaigne, S., Billard, C., Aguet, M., Boiron, M., Falcoff, E. and Degos, L. (1986). Treatment of hairy cell leukaemia with recombinant alpha interferon: quantitive study of bone marrow changes during the first months of treatment. *Blood,* **67**, 817

51. Subramanian, V. P., Gomez, G. A., Tin Han, Kim, U., Minowada, J. and Sandberg, A. (1985). Coexistence of myeloid metaplasia with myelofibrosis and hairy-cell leukaemia. *Arch. Intern. Med.,* **145**, 164

52. Bartl, R., Frisch, B., Mahl, G., Burkhardt, R., Fateh-Moghadam, A., Pappenberger, R., Sommerfeld, W. and Hoffmann-Fezer, G. (1983). Bone marrow histology in Waldenström's macroglobulinemia. Clinical relevance of subtype recognition. *Scand. J. Haematol.,* **31**, 359

53. Bartl, R., Frisch, B., Burkhardt, R., Jäger, K., Pappenberger, R. and Hoffmann-Fezer, G. (1984). Lymphoproliferations in the bone marrow: identification and evolution, classification and staging. *J. Clin. Pathol.,* **37**, 233

54. Bergsagel, D. and Rider, W. (1985). Plasma cell neoplasms. In DeVita, V. T., Hellman, K. S. and Rosenberg, S. A. (eds), *Cancer, Principles and Practice of Oncology,* 2nd edn. Philadelphia: Lippincott

55. *Hematological Oncology.* Eds J. W. Parker and R. J. Lukes, G. P. Cancellos, J. M. A. Whitehouse. Vol. 6, Issue 2, April–June 1988.

56. Buss, D. H., Prichard, R. W. and Cooper, M. R. (1988). Plasma cell dyscrasia. In Hyun, B. H. (ed.), *Hematology/Oncology of North America, Bone Marrow Examination.* Philadelphia: W. B. Saunders, Vol. 2

57. Paule, B. and Quillard, J. (1988). Prognostic and therapeutic impact of the cellular morphology and type of bone marrow invasiveness in multiple myeloma. *Bull. Cancer-(Paris),* **75**, 567

58. Greipp, P. R., Raymond, N. M., Kyle, R. A. and O'Fallon, W. M. (1985). Multiple myeloma: Significance of plasmablastic subtype in morphological classification. *Blood,* **65**, 305

59. Bartl, R., Frisch, B., Fateh-Moghadam, A., Kettner, G., Jaeger, K. and Sommerfeld, W. (1987). Histological classification and staging of multiple myeloma. A retrospective and prospective study of 674 cases. *Am. J. Clin. Pathol.,* **87**, 342

60. Bartl, R. and Frisch, B. (1989). Bone marrow histology in multiple myeloma. Prognostic relevance of histologic characteristics. (In press)

61. Boccadoro, M., Massala, M., Dianzani, U. and Pileri, A. (1987). Multiple myeloma: biological and clinical significance of bone marrow plasma cell labelling index. *Haematologica,* **72**, 171

62. Ludwig, H., Fruhwald, F., Tscholakoff, D., Rasoul, S., Neuhold, A. and Fritz, E. (1987). Magnetic resonance imaging of the spine in multiple myeloma. *Lancet,* **2**(8555), 364

63. Krzyzaniak, R. L., Buss, D. H., Cooper, M. R. and Wells, H. B. (1988). Marrow fibrosis and multiple myeloma. *Am. J. Clin. Pathol.,* **89**, 63

64. Carbone, A., Manconi, R., Sulfaro, S., Vaccher, E., Zogonel, V., Poletti, A., Volpe, R., Tirelli, U. and Monfardini, S. (1987). Practical importance of routine paraffin-embedded bone marrow biopsy in multiple myeloma. *Tumori,* **73**, 315

65. Aghai, E., Avni, G., Lurie, M., Quitt, M., Hornstein, L. and Froom, P. (1988). Bone marrow biopsy in multiple myeloma: a clinical pathological study. *Isr. J. Med. sci.,* **24**, 298

66. Canfield, R. E., Siris, E. S. and Jacobs, T. P. (1987). Dichloromethylene disphosphonate action in hematologic and other malignancies. *Bone,* **8**(Suppl. 1), S57

67. Smith, D. B., Harris, M., Gowland, E., Chang, J. and Scarffe, J. H. (1986). Non-secretory multiple myeloma: a report of 13 cases with a review of the literature. *Hematol. Oncol.*, **4**, 307

68. Rubio-Felix, D., Giralt, M., Giraldo, P., Martinez-Penuela, J. M., Oyarzabal, F., Sala, F. and Raichs, A. (1987). Nonsecretory multiple myeloma. *Cancer*, **59**, 1847

69. Pettersson, T., Koivunen, E., Ilvonen, M., Jouppila, J., Aalto, E. and Wasastjerna, C. (1987). Sarcoidosis and multiple myeloma: and association. *Br. Med. J.*, **295**, 958

70. Frizzera, G. (1985). Castleman's disease: more questions than answers. *Human Pathol.*, **16**, 202

71. Levo, Y., Behar, A. J., Blum, I. and Frisch, B. (1987). A benign course of multicentric Castleman's disease with involvement of the spleen and bone marrow. *Eur. J. Haematol.*, **39**, 471

72. Lowenthal, D. A., Filippa, D. A., Richardson, M. E., Bertoni, M. and Straus, D. J. (1987). Generalized lymphadenopathy with morphologic features of Castleman's disease in an HIV-positive man. *Cancer*, **60**, 2454

73. Case Records of the Massachusetts General Hospital (1987). Case 10-1987. *N. Engl. J. Med.*, **316**, 605

74. Weiss, L. M. and Warnke, R. A. (1985). Follicular lymphoma with blastic conversion: a report of two cases with confirmation by immunoperoxidase studies on bone marrow sections. *Am. J. Clin. Pathol.*, **83**, 681

75. De Jong, D., Voetdjik, B. M. H. and Beverstock, G. C. (1988). Activation of the c-myc oncogene in a precursor B-cell blast crisis of follicular lymphoma, presenting as composite lymphoma. *N. Engl. J. Med.*, **318**, 1373

76. Patsouris, E., Noel, H. and Lennert, K. (1988). Histological findings in lymphoepithelioid cell lymphoma (Lennert's lymphoma). *Am. J. Surg. Pathol.*, **12**, 341

77. Spier, C. M., Lippman, S. M., Miller, T. P. and Grogan, T. M. (1988). Lennert's lymphoma. A clinicopathologic study with emphasis on phenotype and its relationship to survival. *Cancer*, **61**, 517

78. Steinberg, A. D., Seldin, M. F., Jaffe, E. S., Smith, H. R., Klinman, D. M., Krieg, A. M. and Cossman, J. (1988). Angioimmunoblastic lymphadenopathy with dysproteinemia. *Ann. Intern. Med.*, **108**, 575

79. Ghani, A. M. and Krause, J. R. (1985). Bone marrow biopsy findings in angioimmunoblastic lymphadenopathy. *Br. J. Haematol.*, **61**, 203

80. Knecht, H., Odermatt, B. F., Maureir, R. and Ruttner, J. (1987). Diagnostic and prognostic value of monoclonal antibodies in immunophenotyping of angioimmunoblastic lymphadenopathy/lymphogranulomatosis X. *Br. J. Haematol.*, **67**, 19

81. Matthews, J. H., Smith, N. A. and Foroni, L. (1988). A case of angioimmunoblastic lymphadenopathy associated with a long spontaneous remission, retrobulbar neuritis, a clonal rearrangement of the T-cell receptor gamma chain gene and an unusual marrow infiltration. *Eur. J. Haematol.*, **41**, 295

82. Hanson, C. A., Brunning, R. D., Gajl-Peczalska, K. K., Frizzera, G. and McKenna, R. W. (1986). Bone marrow manifestations of peripheral T-cell lymphoma. A study of 30 cases. *Am. J. Clin. Pathol.*, **86**, 449

83. Horning, S. J., Weiss, L. M., Crabtree, G. S. and Warnke, R. A. (1986). Clinical and phenotypic diversity of T cell lymphomas. *Blood*, **67**, 1578

84. Drexler, H. G., Amlot, P. L. and Minowada, J. (1987). Hodgkin's disease-derived cell lines – conflicting clues for the origin of Hodgkin's disease? *Leukaemia*, **1**, 629

85. Weiss, L. M., Movahed, L. A., Warnke, R. A. and Sklar, J. (1989). Detection of Epstein-Barr viral genomes in Reed-Sternberg cells of Hodgkin's disease. *N. Engl. J. Med.*, **320**, 502

86. Jaffe, E. S. (1989). The elusive Reed–Sternberg cell. *N. Engl. J. Med.*, **320**, 529

87. Linch, D. C., Berliner, N., O'Flynn, K., Kay, L. A., Jones, H. M., MacLennan, K., Huehns, E. R. and Goff, L. (1985). Hodgkin-cell leukaemia of B-cell origin. *Lancet*, **1**(8420), 78

88. MacIntyre, E. A., Vaughan-Hudson, B., Linch, D. C., Vaughan-Hudson, G. and Jelliffe, A. M. (1987). The value of staging bone marrow trephine biopsy in Hodgkin's disease. *Eur. J. Haematol.*, **39**, 66

89. Kinney, M. C., Greer, J. P., Stein, R. S., Collins, R. D. and Cousar, J. B. (1986). Lymphocyte-depletion Hodgkin's disease. Histopathology diagnosis of marrow involvement. *Am. J. Surg. Pathol.*, **10**, 219

90. Regula, D. P. Jr, Hoppe, R. T. and Weiss, L. M. (1988). Nodular and diffuse types of lymphocyte predominance Hodgkin's disease. *N. Engl. J. Med.*, **318**, 214

91. Penchansky, L. and Krause, J. P. (1986). Phagocytic macrophages in the bone marrow biopsies of children with Hodgkin's disease. *Pediatr. Pathol.*, **6**, 369

The designation 'mononuclear phagocyte system' has replaced the previous more comprehensive name of 'reticuloendothelial system', as this included non-phagocytic cells, such as fibroblast and endothelial cells, and cells which did not arise from the monocyte–macrophage progenitor, which also produces the granulocytic cell line. Recent studies have provided additional support for earlier conclusions on the derivation and function of monocytes and macrophages[1,2]. The bone marrow stem cells produce the committed progenitor which gives rise to the monoblast, promonocyte and monocyte in the bone marrow. The monocytes leave the bone marrow after their maturation, remain only a short time in the peripheral blood, migrate out into the tissues where they become macrophages. In previous sections, mention has been made of bone marrow macrophages – their number is increased in various conditions, such as infections by any of numerous agents; or disorders involving ineffective haematopoiesis with intramedullary cell destruction and subsequent accumulation of numerous haemosiderin-containing macrophages in the bone marrow stroma. Thus, the bone marrow produces monocytes which become macrophages in the tissues of the body, but monocytes can also become macrophages and perform their phagocytic functions within the bone marrow itself. Moreover, scavenging and phagocytosis are not their only activities: the mononuclear phagocyte produces a variety of secretions; it participates in regulation of the immune response and macrophages function as antigen-presenting cells. Activated monocytes act in concert with other cells in various biological processes, for example bone resorption. The inflammatory reactions which occur in the bone marrow, and the agents which evoke them, have been dealt with in a previous chapter. It should be emphasized that epithelioid and multinucleated giant cells are all derived from the mononuclear phagocyte system[3].

Inherited Disorders of the Mononuclear Phagocyte System

Storage diseases

These are the consequence of inherited enzyme deficiencies which lead to accumulation of the substances that are incompletely catabolized in the cells of the mononuclear phagocyte system in organs such as liver, spleen and bone marrow[4] (Figs 9.1–9.3).

Gaucher's disease

This is due to a defective lysosomal glucosidase which splits beta-glucosecerebrosides[5] (Figs 9.4–9.6). There are different levels of enzymic activity in the mononuclear phagocyte system and these in turn influence the time of appearance of the disease so that three types are recognized – infantile, juvenile and adult.

Macrophages containing cerebroside accumulate in the liver, spleen and bone marrow. Subsequently, there may be pancytopenia due to replacement of the bone marrow and increased splenic destruction. Lytic bone lesions and aseptic necrosis may lead to pathological fractures.

Within the bone marrow the aggregates of macrophages with the typical wrinkled silk or tissue-paper appearance of Gaucher cells, alternate with areas of normal haematopoietic tissue. Fat cells are decreased, macrophages in all stages of development to Gaucher cells are found in the marrow. In some cases, patches of fat cells remain and haematopoiesis is decreased in spite of the occupation of large areas of the marrow by Gaucher cells. Immunoglobin production in Gaucher's disease is increased due to chronic stimulation of the immune system which eventually may lead to development of a lymphoproliferative disorder in both adults and children[6].

Nieman–Pick disease

This is also a heterogeneous group of diseases. Large foamy cells with small eccentric nuclei accumulate in bone marrow. Most cases are diagnosed in infancy and childhood as the disease is rapidly fatal.

Fabry's disease

This is due to lack of the enzyme galactosidase, resulting in a storage disease affecting not only the mononuclear phagocyte system but also parenchymal cells of other organs. The macrophages have a foamy whorled appearance (Figs 9.7 and 9.8).

Farquhar's disease (lymphohistiocytosis)

This was originally called familial haemophagocytic reticulosis[7]; it is possibly an acute variant of the Letterer–Siwe syndrome. There is widespread histiocytosis, in some cases also involving the meninges. The disease affects infants and young children and is rapidly fatal.

Lipid storage diseases

In these conditions, also known as the hyperlipidaemias (such as alpha-lipoprotein deficiency), macrophages containing cholesterol or cholesterol esters may be found in the bone marrow (Fig. 9.9). However, in sections of the bone marrow the cholesterol is dissolved out during the histological processing, so that empty spaces are left. Similar macrophages may be large and multiloculated. Such macrophages are also found in other conditions such as diabetes, hyperthyroidism and in hypercholesterolaemia.

Hermansky–Pudlak syndrome

This is one variant of oculocutaneous albinism, characterized by hypo-pigmentation of the skin, hair and eyes (Figs 9.10 and 9.11)[8,9]. The following features are found in the Hermansky–Pudlak variant: it is autosomal recessive; tyrosinase positive; there is an enzyme defect leading to deposition of a ceroid-lipofuchsin-like material in macrophages; there is a storage-pool defect in platelets which causes functional disturbances and hence bleeding complications, especially in females (reproductive system) and during and after surgical interventions. The macrophages in the bone marrow are dispersed singly or in clusters among the haematopoietic cells, are large, may

(Continued on p. 169)

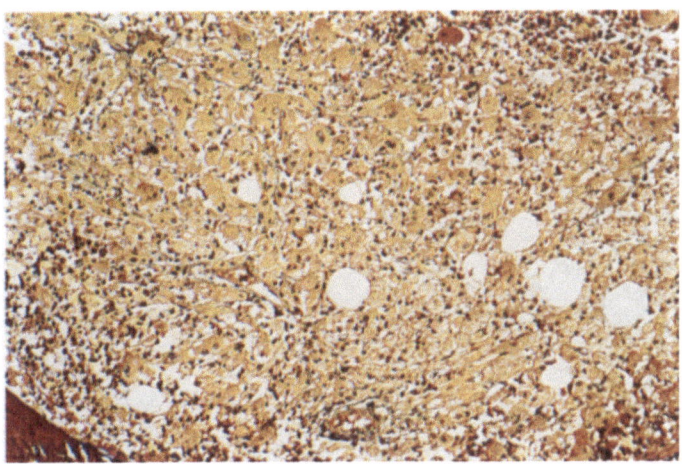

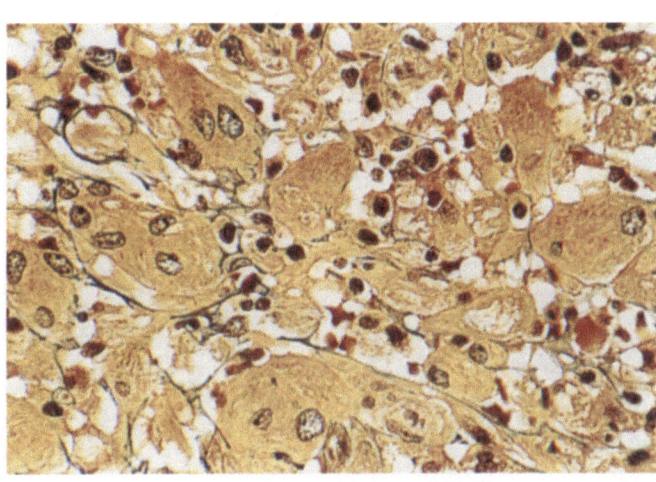

Figs 9.1–9.3 Sections of a bone biopsy of a patient with a storage disease

Fig. 9.1 Large aggregate of macrophages with abundant cytoplasm; note haematopoietic precursors around the aggregate; Gomori

Fig. 9.2 Higher magnification of the aggregate of monomorphic macrophages with one or several nuclei

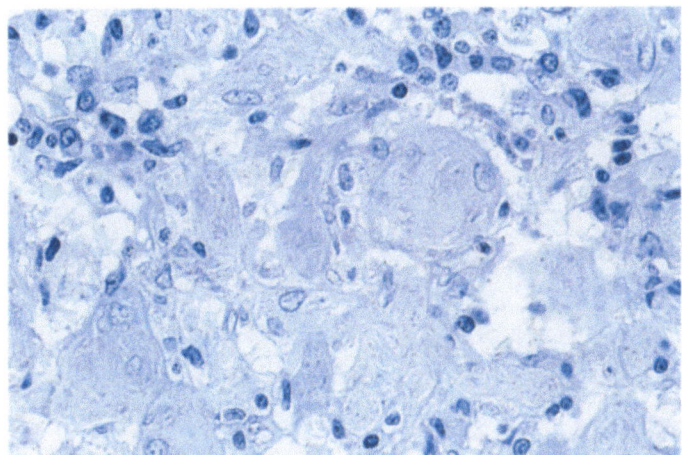

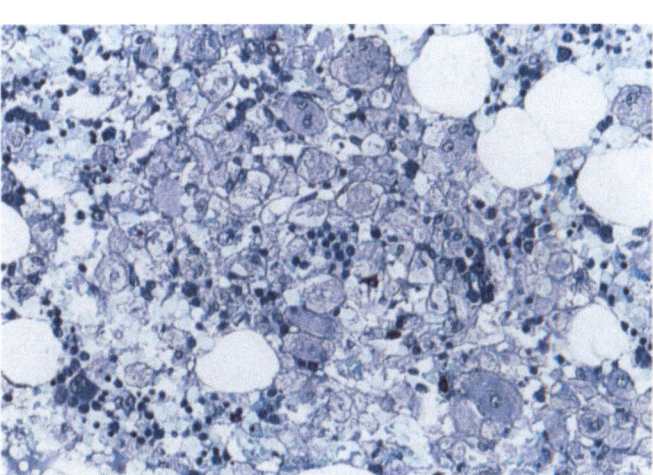

Fig. 9.3 Higher magnification of area in Fig. 9.1, showing storage cells at different stages of development, and lymphocytes and erythroblasts between them. In spite of intensive investigation, a definite diagnosis was not made in this case

Figs 9.4–9.6 Bone biopsy sections of a 38-year-old patient with Gaucher's disease

Fig. 9.4 Clusters of macrophages with the typical wrinkled tissue-paper appearance of the cytoplasm

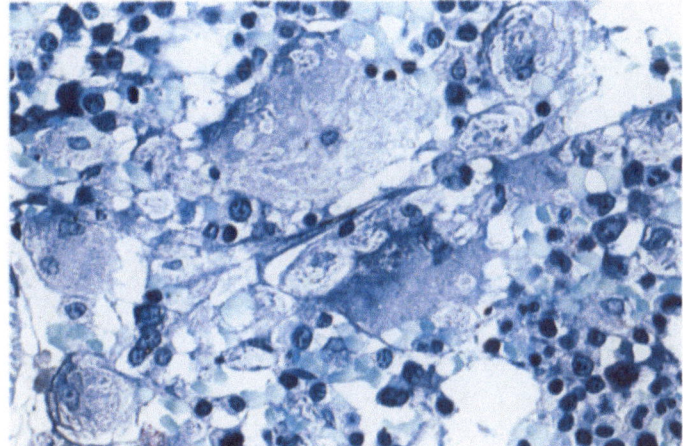

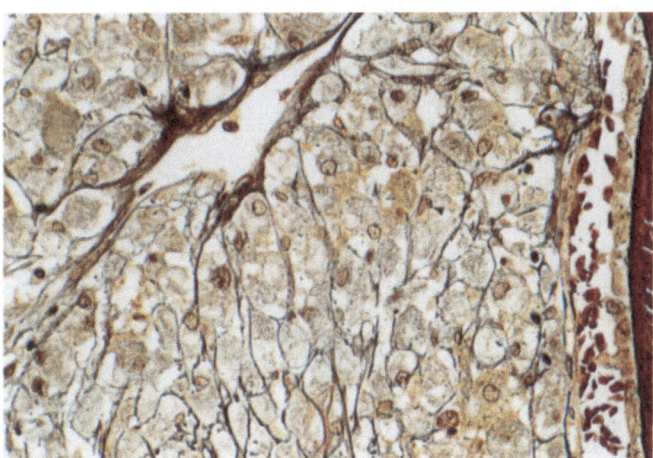

Fig. 9.5 Higher magnification of part of Fig. 9.4, showing the typical Gaucher cells dispersed among haematopoietic cells

Fig. 9.6 Gaucher cells within a network of fibers. Gomori.

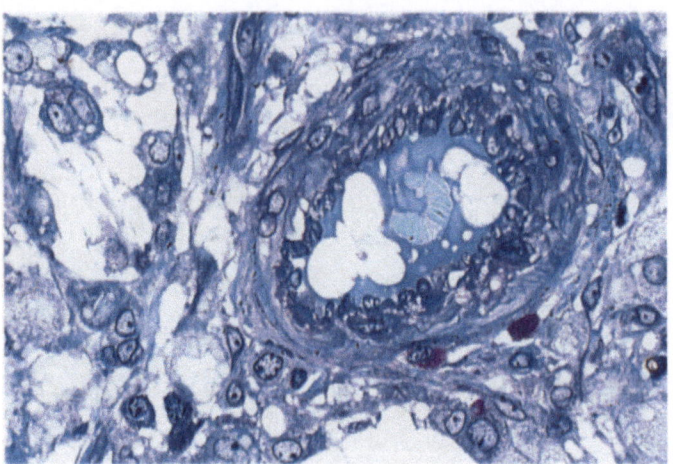

Fig. 9.7 Section of bone biopsy of patient with Fabry's disease, showing macrophages around a blood vessel

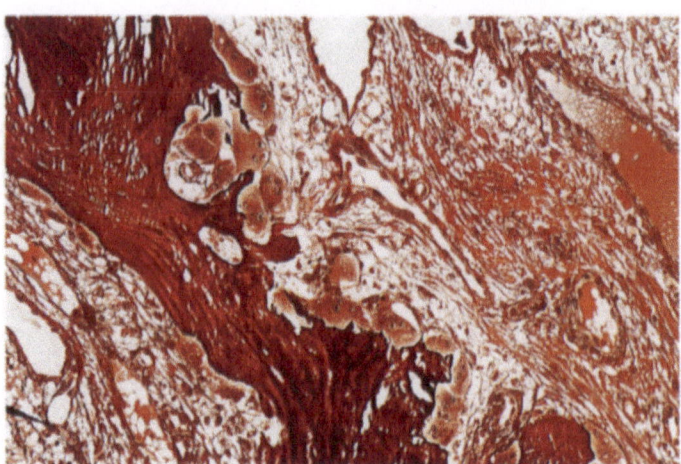

Fig. 9.8 Section of bone biopsy of patient with Fabry's disease showing increased osteoclastic remodelling, Gomori

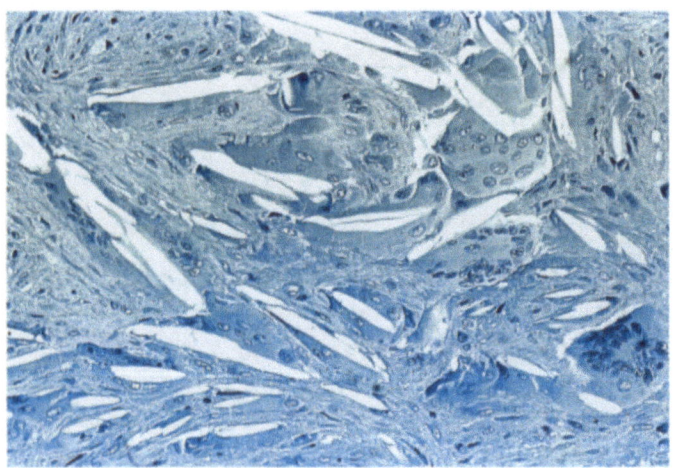

Fig. 9.9 Section of bone biopsy of patient with lipid storage disease illustrating empty spaces left by extraction of the lipid

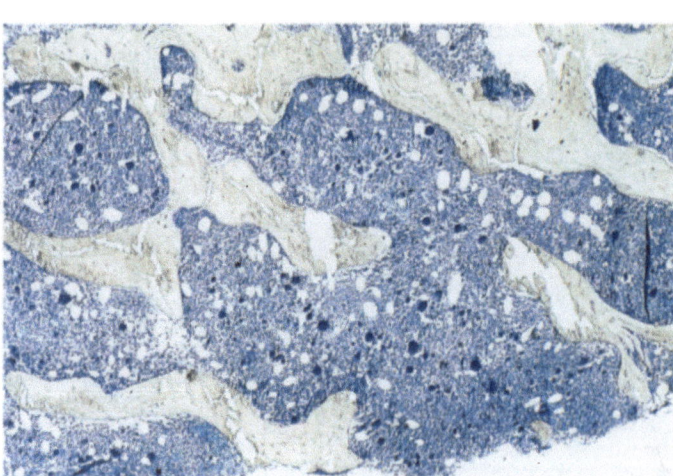

Fig. 9.10 Bone biopsy section of 42-year-old female patient with Hermansky–Pudlak syndrome, showing cellular bone marrow

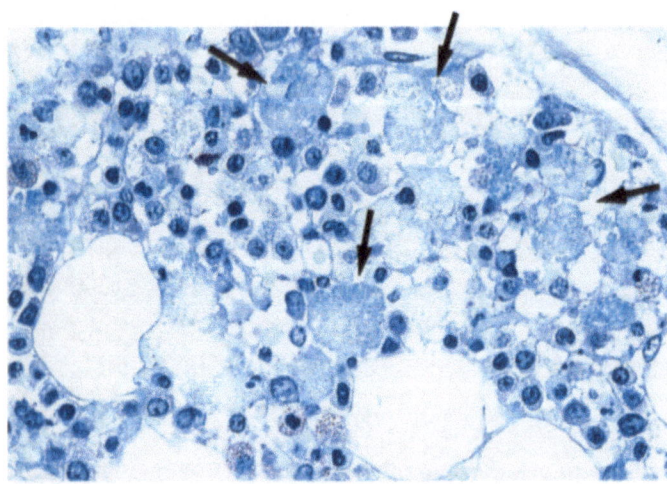

Fig. 9.11 As Fig. 9.10 showing the large, usually mononuclear macrophages (arrows) often situated near the endosteal surface

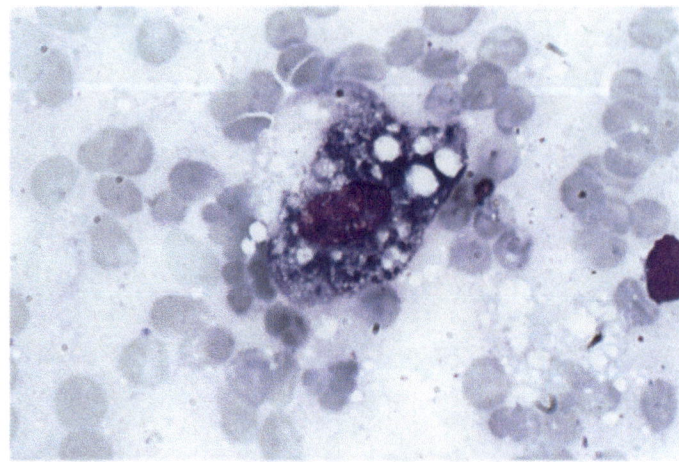

Figs 9.12–9.15 Cells and sections of bone biopsies of patients with histiocytosis X – the Hans–Schüller–Christian variant
Fig. 9.12 Large vacuolated macrophage in smear of aspirate

contain vacuoles and pigment which is negative in stains for iron.

Sea-blue histiocytosis

Macrophages containing sea-blue-coloured inclusions may be found in the bone marrow in many different conditions including thalassaemias, myeloproliferative disorders, chronic granulomatous conditions and others. Whether it occurs as an independent entity has not yet been settled.

Pseudo-Gaucher (or pseudo-storage disease)

Many congenital or acquired conditions involve ineffective haematopoiesis with a consequently high turnover rate. This may lead to the development of Gaucher-like macrophages in the bone marrow, for example in CML. But the large multiple aggregates with replacement of the marrow seen in Gaucher's disease do not occur in these conditions.

Histiocytosis X

This designation comprises eosinophilic granuloma, Hand–Schüller–Christian disease, and Letterer–Siwe disease. The cause is unknown, though a disturbance of immune regulation has been postulated. This group of diseases has now been re-named Langerhans-cell histiocytosis, and specific criteria established for the definitive diagnosis[10].

Eosinophilic granuloma of bone

Though occurring more often in males and young people, females and any age group may be affected. The lesions may be single or multiple and consist of aggregates of macrophages and eosinophils; foam cells, giant cells and fibres may also be present.

Hand–Schüller–Christian disease

This occurs mainly in children and involves the bone as well as many other organs (Figs 9.12–9.15). The lesions consist of monomorphic infiltrations of histiocytes, and include lymphocytes, plasma cells, eosinophils, fibroblasts and fibres. The histiocytes have irregular nuclei, and abundant, well-demarcated cytoplasm.

Letterer–Siwe

Infiltrates similar to those described above are found. The diagnoses of these variants are made on clinical grounds and not only on a purely histopathological basis.

Malignant histiocytosis (also known as histiocytic medullary reticulosis HMR)

This is considered a malignancy of the mononuclear phagocyte system with neoplastic proliferation of histiocytes in the bone marrow, liver and spleen (Figs 9.16–9.19)[11]. Nevertheless, there is still some uncertainty about the aetiology of the disease and the nature of the histiocytes. An association between HMR and EBV infection has been demonstrated, supporting previous suggestions that HMR may be a fatal form of infectious mononucleosis. The differential diagnosis includes viral-associated haemophagocytic syndrome (VAHS), and haemophagocytosis in other infections[12–16]. Histiocytic proliferations with haemophagocytosis may accompany diseases such as lymphoproliferative disorders, especially in their terminal phases, or gastric carcinoma; sinus histiocytosis with massive lymphadenopathy; and erythrophagocytic T-cell lymphoma. Increase in bone marrow histiocytes with erythrophagocytosis is also found in Kawasaki's disease.

Viral-associated Haemophagocytic Syndrome (VAHS)

This resembles malignant histiocytosis both clinically and histologically (Fig. 9.20). There is hyperplasia of the mononuclear phagocyte system in the bone marrow with striking haemophagocytosis; multinucleated giant cells may also be present. The marrow architecture is disrupted and haematopoiesis is decreased. The morphological distinction between the two conditions (ie. HMR and VAHS) may be very difficult. A relationship between histiocytic medullary reticulosis and T-cell lymphomas has recently been proposed.

True Histiocytic 'Lymphoma'

'Lymphomas' derived from the mononuclear phagocyte system are rare, and special techniques are required for their identification. These include immunological and enzymic markers and electron microscopy[17].

The Bone Marrow in Acquired Immune Deficiency Syndrome (AIDS)

Over the past few years, bone marrow histopathology in AIDS has been extensively studied[18,19]. The results of even the early investigations led to the speculation that the bone marrow is a target organ in AIDS, though to date no direct evidence has been put forward to support this claim, as retroviral infection of bone marrow progenitors has not been demonstrated. AIDS virus has been detected in macrophages from brain tissue of AIDS patients with encephalopathy[20]. Presumably these macrophages were infected at the portal of entry and migrated. Therefore, the bone marrow could become infected in a similar fashion. Since the macrophage is directly and initially involved in AIDS, it was considered appropriate to consider the bone marrow manifestations of AIDS in this section.

With the increase in the number of patients suffering from AIDS has come the recognition that AIDS patients are especially susceptible, and that disease manifestations in these patients may differ from those in the general population. This applies to a variety of infections, as well as to the development of malignant lymphomas, Kaposi's sarcoma, and other neoplasms. For example, the gastrointestinal tract, the brain, and the heart as predominant sites for malignant lymphomas, the incidence of which has been steadily increasing in AIDS patients[21–29]. Haematological abnormalities are also common in AIDS patients, who therefore frequently undergo examination of the bone marrow during investigation for cytopenias, opportunistic infections, malignancies and fever of unknown origin[30–34].

A wide spectrum of findings has been reported in the bone marrow[35–41], ranging from marked hypocellularity to normocellularity and hypercellularity with disappearance of fat cells (Figs 9.21–9.25). An 'AIDS pattern' has been described[36], characterized by separation of fat cells by haematopoietic elements, in contrast to normal marrow where small groups of fat cells are closely apposed without intervening haematopoietic elements. However, this finding was not confirmed by other workers in subsequent reports[40,19]. Other features (Figs 9.26–9.42) include marrow damage, areas of serous or gelatinous atrophy, or even necrosis with or without haemophagocytosis, lymphoplasmacytic aggregates, histiocytosis, plasmacytosis, uni-, bi-, or tri-linear myelodysplasias and hypoplasias, granulomas, an increase or decrease of stainable iron, reticulin fibrosis and demonstrable organisms, especially *Mycobacterium avium intracellulare*. They have been found in granulomas, as well as in macrophages dispersed in the marrow, and some of these macrophages may resemble

(Continued on p. 175)

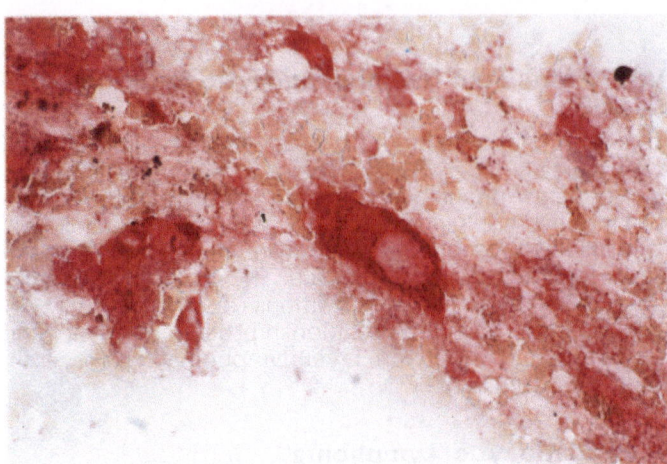

Fig. 9.13 Imprint of biopsy, α-naphthylesterase activity in macrophage

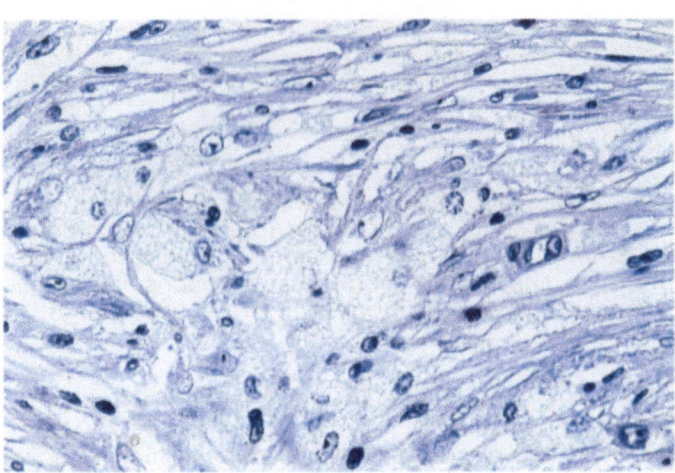

Fig. 9.14 Section of bone biopsy, there was replacement of the marrow by histiocytes.

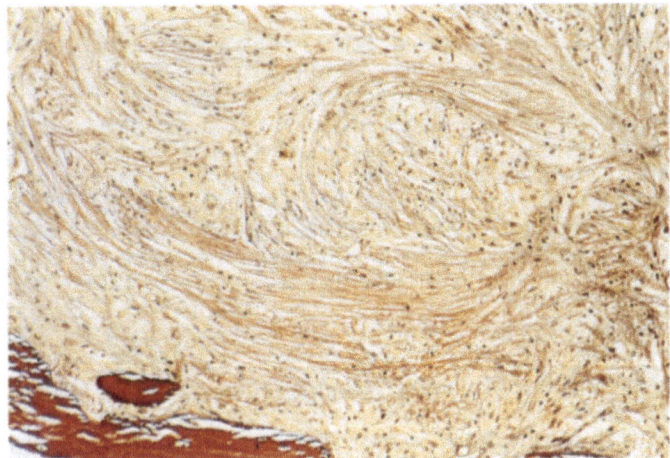

Fig. 9.15 Parallel section stained by Gomori. Note extensive fibrosis between the histiocytes

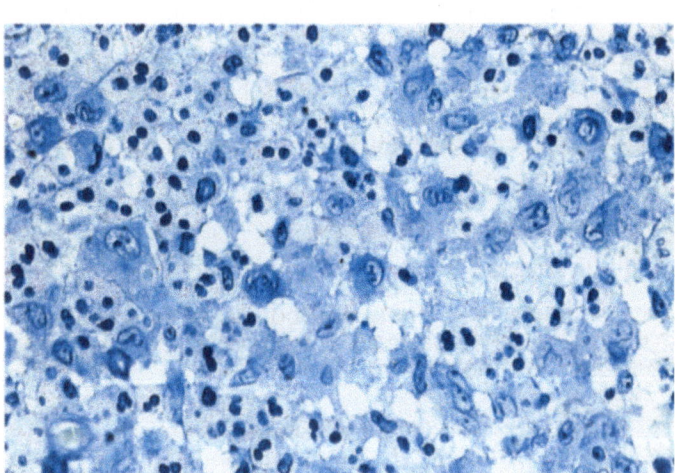

Fig. 9.16 Section of bone biopsy of patient with malignant histiocytosis; the marrow cavities are completely occupied; only isolated haematopoietic precursors remain

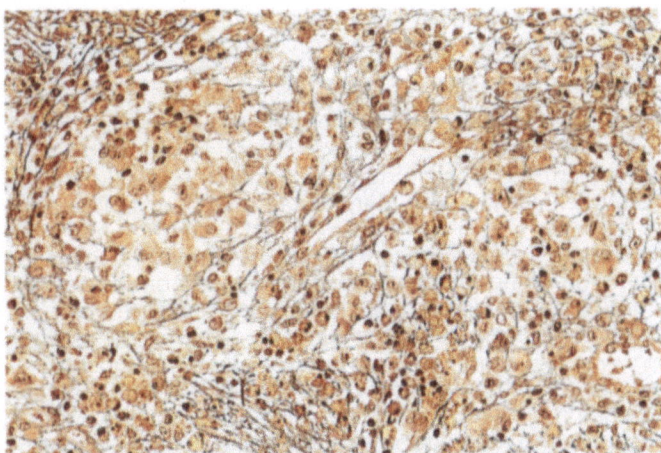

Fig. 9.17 As Fig. 9.16. There is a variable fibrosis in the infiltrated areas, stained by Gomori's stain

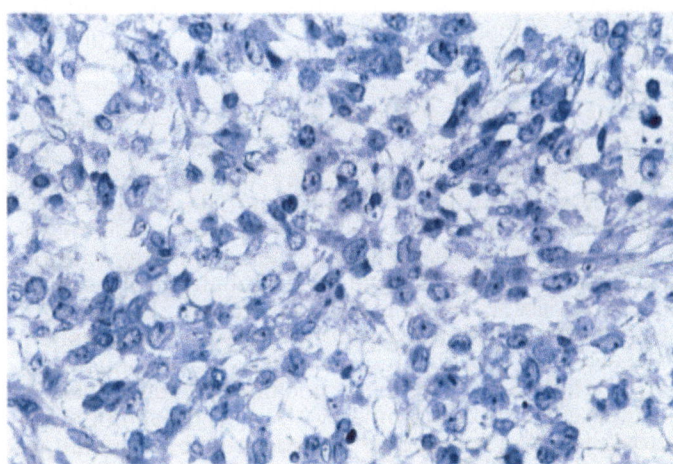

Fig. 9.18 Bone biopsy section of another case of malignant histiocytosis, the cytoplasmic boundaries of these histiocytes are less well demarcated

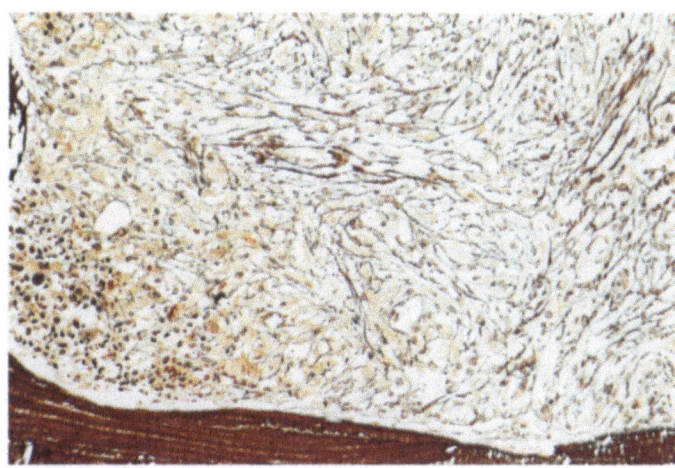

Fig. 9.19 As Fig. 9.18. There is marked coarse fibrosis in the affected areas of the bone marrow. Gomori

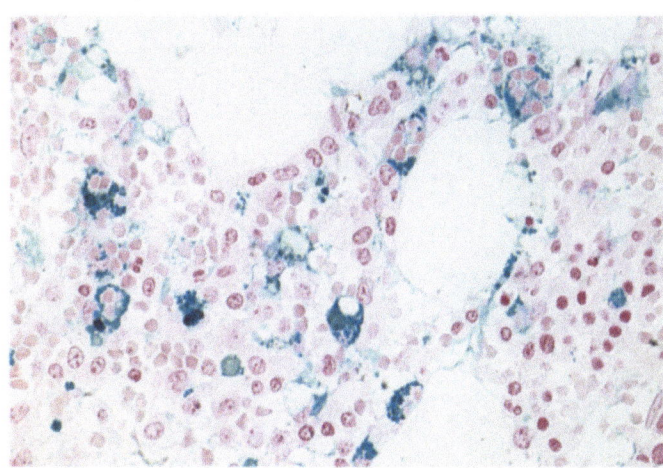

Fig. 9.20 Section of bone biopsy of patient with VAHS. Note numerous histiocytes engorged with erythrocytes; section stained with Berlin blue

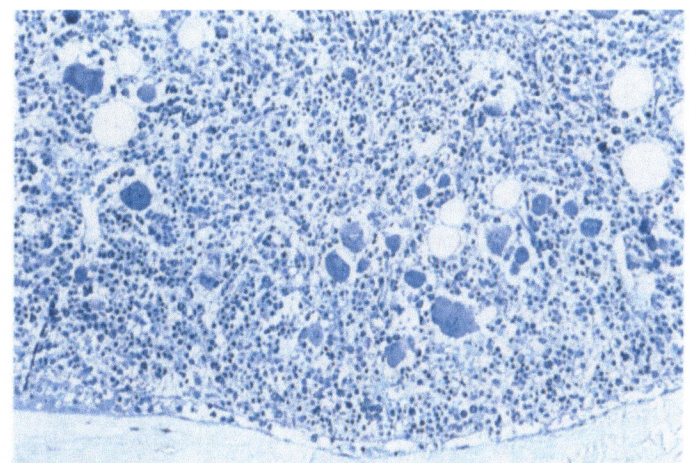

Figs 9.21–9.40 Sections of bone biopsies of patients with AIDS. The bone marrow cellularity varies from hyper- to hypocellular. Parts of the biopsy may show exudative myelitis or serous atrophy. There was no consistent relationship between peripheral blood values and marrow cellularity

Fig. 9.21 Hypercellular bone marrow. Note uneven distribution of megakaryocytes, and range in their size

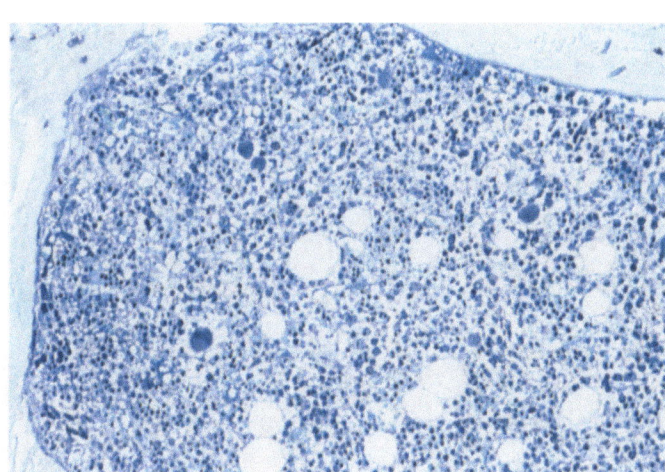

Fig. 9.22 Hypercellular bone marrow with disorganization of the normal marrow architecture

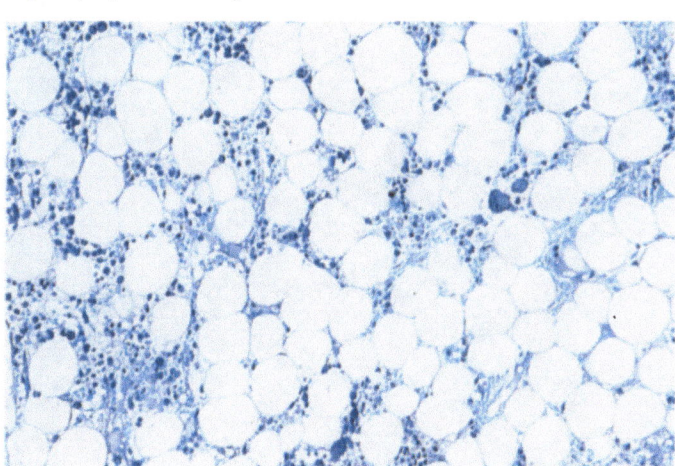

Fig. 9.23 Hypocellular bone marrow

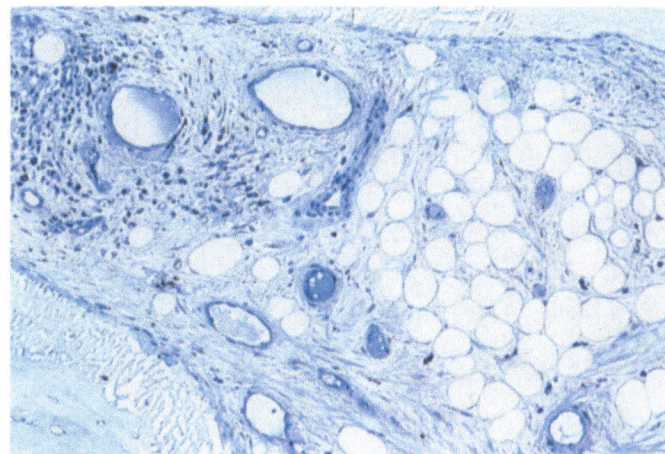

Fig. 9.24 Bone marrow showing atrophy and fibrosis

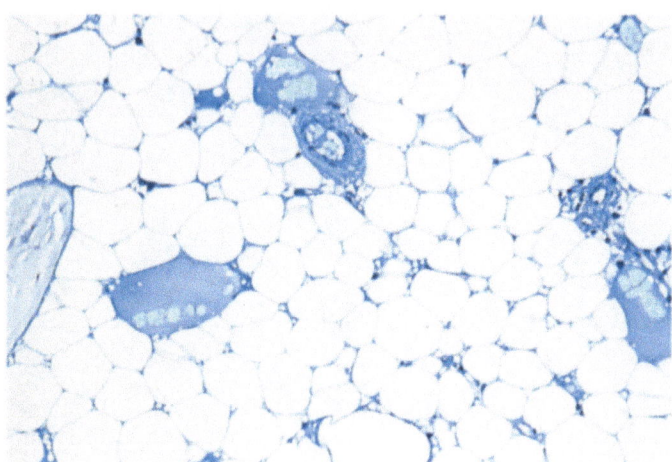

Fig. 9.25   Bone marrow showing virtual replacement of haematopoietic tissue by fat cells

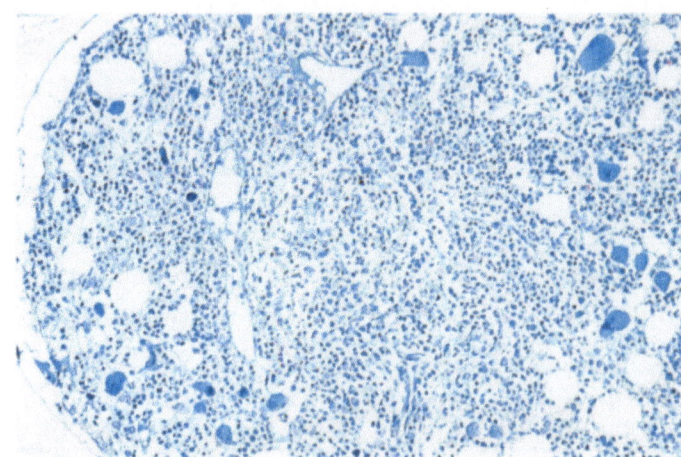

Fig. 9.26   Large lymphoid nodule in cellular bone marrow

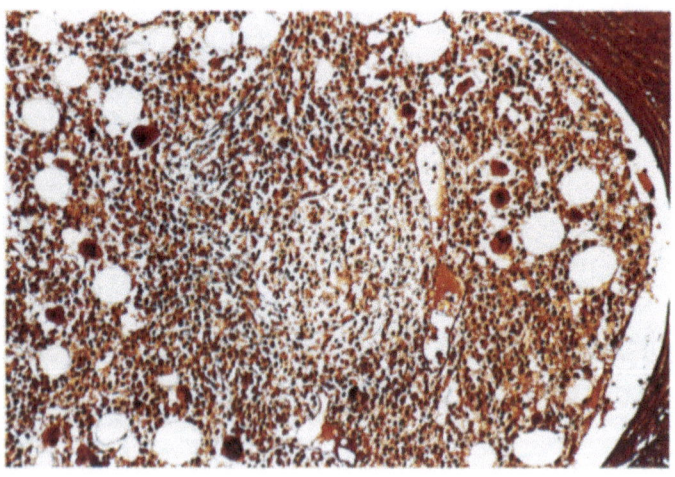

Fig. 9.27   Large lymphoid follicle with germinal centre in cellular bone marrow. Gomori

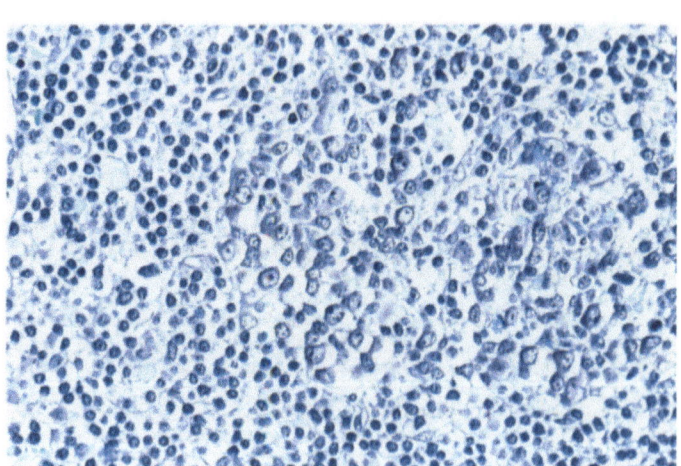

Fig. 9.28   Higher magnification of the follicle in Fig. 19.27, showing germinal centre

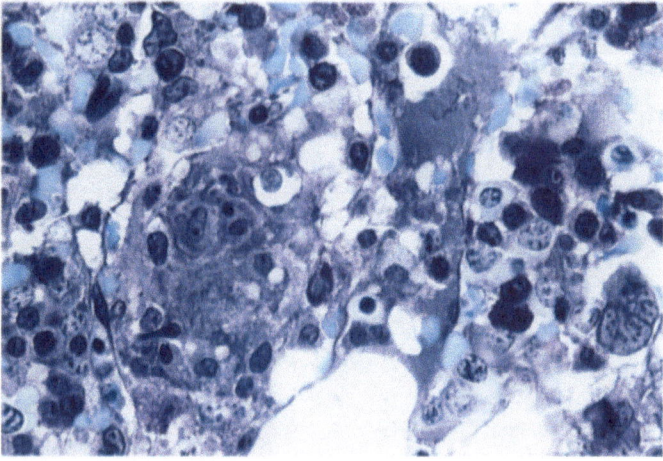

Fig. 9.29   Poorly demarcated granuloma

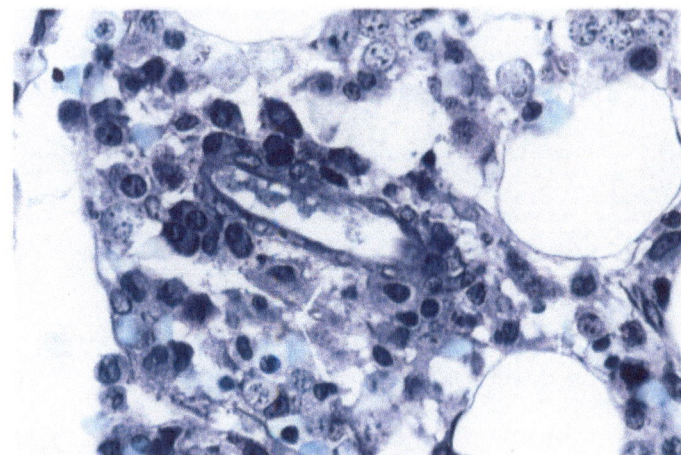

Fig. 9.30   Perivascular plasmacytosis

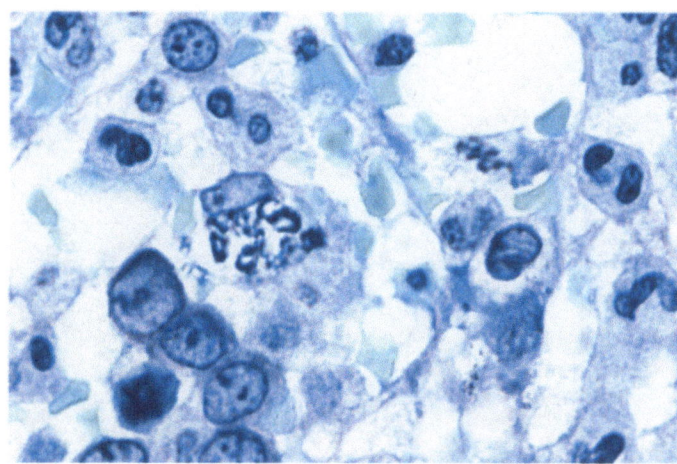

Fig. 9.31 Macrophages with cellular debris – haemophagocytosis

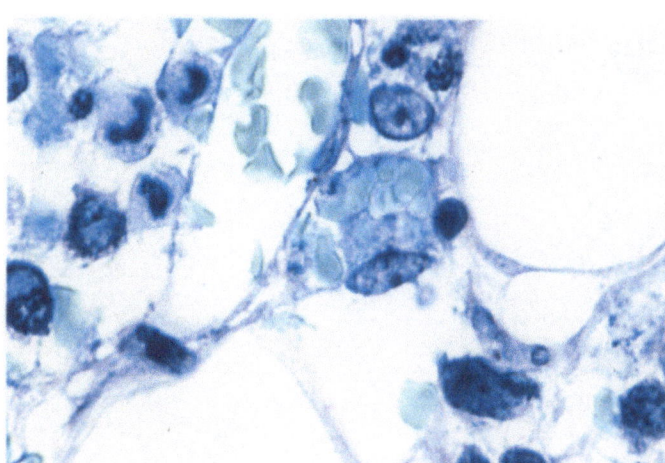

Fig. 9.32 Erythrophagocytosis

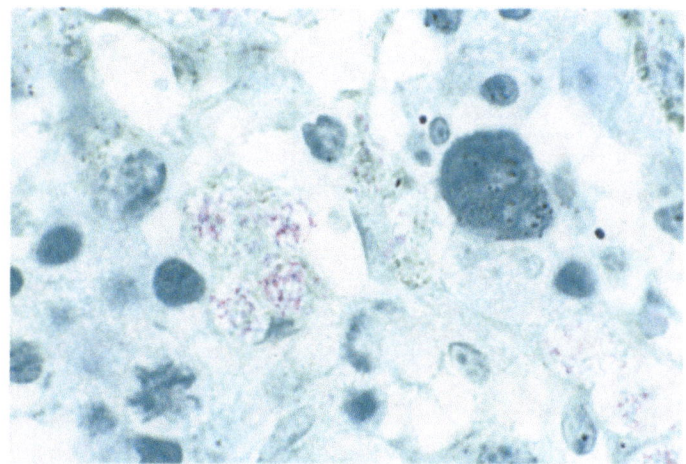

Fig. 9.33 A positive Ziehl–Nielsen stain: demonstration of acid-fast organisms; most appear to be intracellular

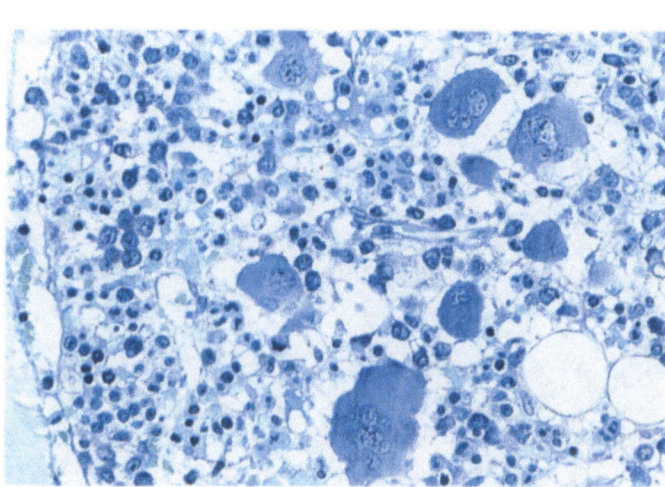

Fig. 9.34 Effacement of the normal marrow architecture with topographic disorganization (i.e. mylodysplasia) is shown in this section. Note also fine fibrosis, marked left shifted megaloblastic erythropoiesis, and micromegakaryocytes with single small nuclei

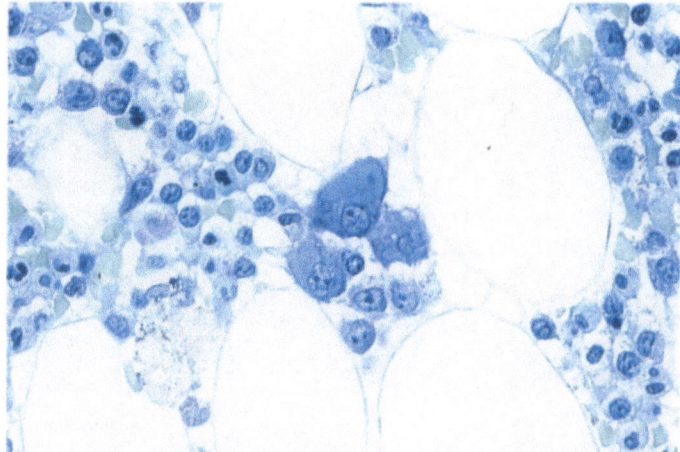

Fig. 9.36 Moderate reticulin fibrosis in cellular marrow, section stained by Gomori's stain

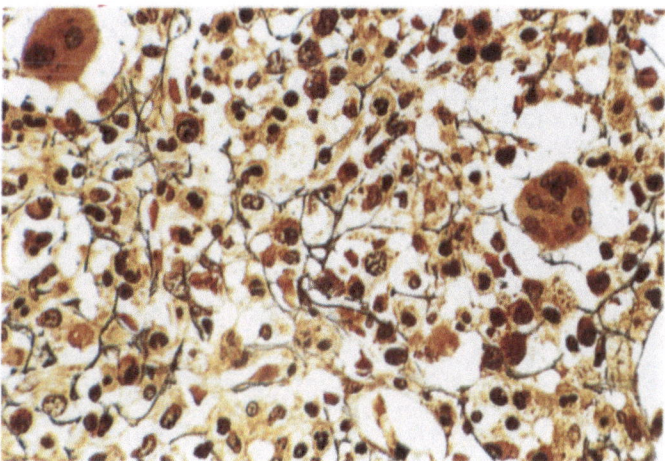

Fig. 9.35 Higher magnification to show micromegakaryocytes – similar to those seen in MDS

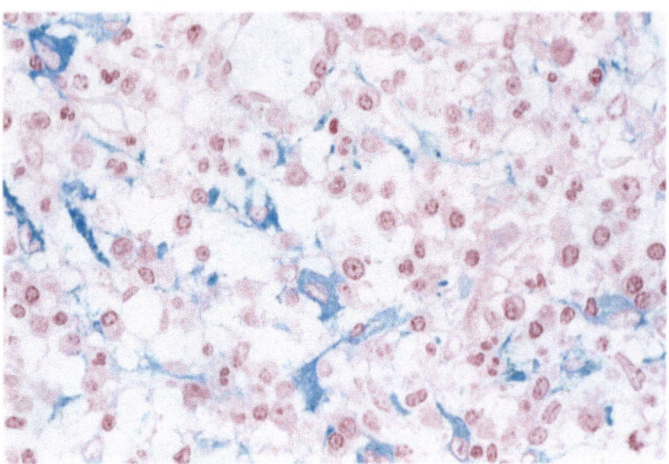

Fig. 9.37 Section stained by Prussian blue for demonstration of iron; there is increased iron in the stromal cells

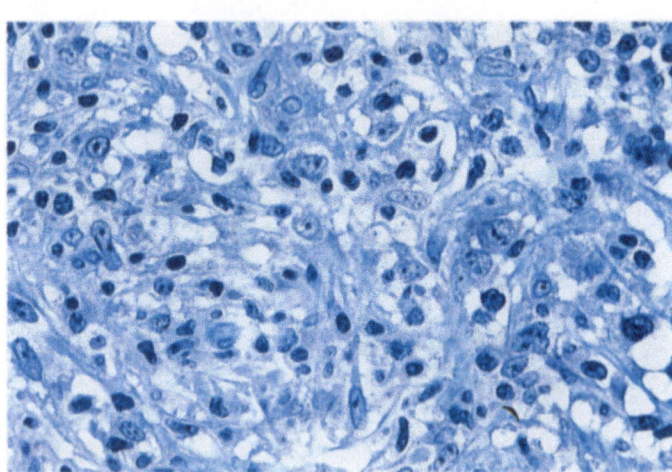

Figs 9.38–9.40 Lesions similar to those seen in bone marrow involvement in AILD in bone biopsy sections of patients with AIDS

Fig. 9.38 Note epithelioid and lymphoid cells

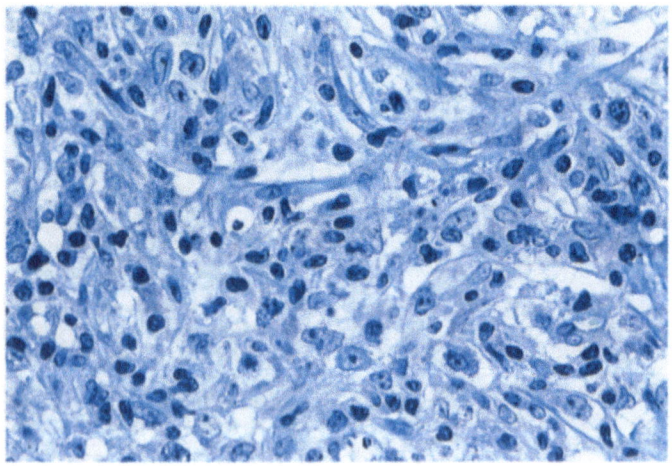

Fig. 9.39 Note arborizing vascular network

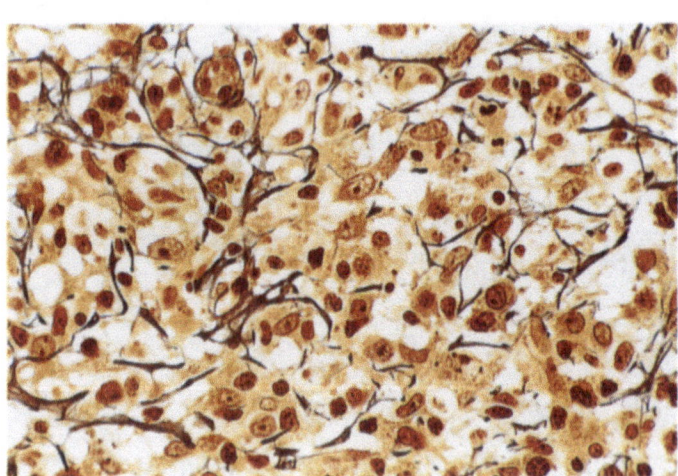

Fig. 9.40 Thick connective issue fibres between the cells; section parallel to that shown in Fig. 9.39. Gomori

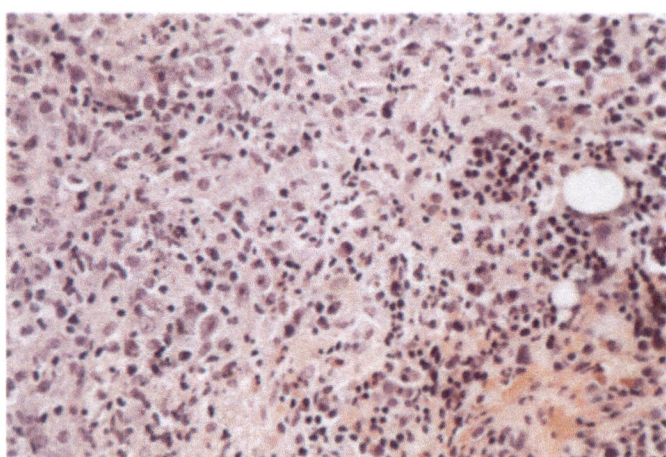

Fig. 9.41 Paraffin-embedded bone biopsy of patient with AIDS who developed Hodgkin's disease with bone marrow involvement

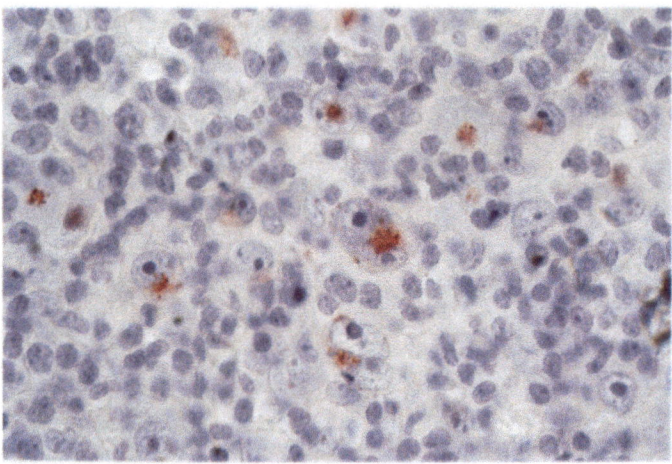

Fig. 9.42 As Fig. 9.41; section reacted with antibody Leu M1 to Reed–Sternberg and mononuclear Hodgkin's cells

the storage cells in Gaucher's disease. The lymphohistiocytic aggregates may be accompanied by vascular proliferations, and may be indistinguishable (by morphology alone) from bone marrow involvement by peripheral T-cell lymphoma or AILD. Diffuse bone marrow lymphocytosis, as well as lymphocytic aggregates, nodules and follicles, have been observed.

The pathogenesis of the bone marrow findings is undoubtedly multifactorial: (1) possibly involving direct retroviral infection of haematopoietic precursors, (2) abnormal regulation of haematopoiesis, (3) a variety of immune phenomena and (4) the response of the bone marrow to the infections or (5) the direct effects of the infections on the marrow. It is of interest that a case of transmission of HIV through transplantation of bone has recently been reported[42].

Bone marrow in the primary immunodeficiency syndromes

The diagnosis is made on the basis of the clinical findings, laboratory tests and peripheral blood examinations. A bone marrow biopsy is generally not taken.

References

1. Johnston, R. B. Jr (1988). Monocytes and macrophages. *N. Engl. J. Med.*, **318**, 747
2. Auger, M. J. (1989). Mononuclear phagocytes. Recent research suggests a large repertoire of actions. *Br. Med. J.*, **298**, 546
3. James, D. G. and Williams, W. J. (1985). Sarcoidosis and other granulomatous disorders. In Smith, L. A. (ed.), *Major Problems In Internal Medicine*. Philadelphia: W. B. Saunders, Vol. 24
4. Burchell, A., Lang, C. C., Jung, R. T., Bennet, W. and Shepherd, A. N. (1987). Diagnosis of type Ia and type Ic glycogen storage diseases in adults. *Lancet*, **1**, 1059.
5. Blandet, A. L. (1987). Gaucher's disease. *N. Engl. J. Med.*, **316**, 619
6. Burstein, Y., Rechavi, G., Rausen, A. R., Frisch, A. and Spirer, Z. (1985). Association of Gaucher's disease and lymphoid malignancy in 2 children. *Scand. J. Haematol.*, **35**, 445
7. Marrian, V. J. and Sanerkin, N. G. (1963). Familial histiocytic reticulosis (familial haemophagocytic reticulosis). *J. Clin. Pathol.*, **16**, 65
8. Hermansky, F. and Pudlak, A. (1959). Albinism associated with hemorrhage diathesis and unusual pigmented reticular cells in the bone marrow: report of two cases with histochemical studies. *Blood*, **14**, 162
9. Schinella, R. A., Greco, M. A., Garay, S. M., Lackner, H., Wolman, S. R. and Fazzini, E. P. (1985). Hermansky–Pudlak syndrome, a clinicopathological study. *Hum. Pathol.*, **16**, 366
10. The Writing Group of the Histiocyte Society (1987). Histiocytosis syndromes in children. *Lancet*, **1**, 208
11. Favara, B. E., McCarthy, R. C. and Mierau, G. W. (1983). Histiocytosis. *Hum. Pathol.*, **14**, 663
12. Auerbach, M., Haubenstock, A. and Soloman, G. (1986). Systemic Babesiosis. Another cause of the haemophagocytic syndrome. *Am. J. Med.*, **80**, 301
13. Horny, H. P., Inniger, R., Kaiserling, E. and Busch, F. W. (1988). Hemophagocytic syndrome. Differential diagnostic aspects in case of well differentiated malignant histiocytosis. *Pathol. Res. Pract.*, **183**, 80
14. Lee, R. E. (1988). Histiocytic diseases of bone marrow. In Hyun, B. H. (ed.), *Haematology/Oncology Clinics of North America*. Philadelphia: W. B. Saunders, Vol. 2
15. Trends in lymphoma diagnosis. Editorial (1989). *Lancet*, **1**, 249
16. Su, I. J., Hsieh, H. J. and Lee, C. Y. (1989). Histiocytic medullary reticulosis: a lethal form of primary EBV infection in young children in Taiwan. *Lancet*, **1**(8634), 389
17. Thomas, P., Said, J. W., Rosenfelt, F. P. and Heifetz, L. J. (1984). True histiocytic lymphoma: an immunohistochemical and ultrastructural study of two cases. *Am. J. Clin. Pathol.*, **81**, 243
18. Duggan, M. J., Weisenburger, D. D., Sun, N. C. J. and Purtilo, D. T. (1988). Bone marrow findings in immunodeficiency syndromes. In Hyun, B. A. (ed.), *Haematology/Oncology Clinics of North America*. Philadelphia: W. B. Saunders, Vol. 2
19. Frisch, B. and Bartl, R. (1989). Bone marrow manifestations in the acquired immune deficiency syndrome (AIDS). A study of 40

20. Koenig, S., Gendelman, H. E., Orenstein, J. M., Dal Canto, M. C., Pezeshkpour, G. H., Yungbluth, M., Janotta, F., Aksamit, A., Martin, M. A. and Fauci, A. S. (1986). Detection of AIDS virus in macrophages in brain tissue from AIDS patients with encephalopathy. *Science*, **233**, 1089
21. Ioachim, H. L., Cooper, M. C. and Hellman, G. C. (1985). Lymphomas in men at risk for acquired immune deficiency syndrome (AIDS). A study of 21 cases. *Cancer*, **56**, 2831
22. Levine, A. M., Gill, P. S., Meyer, P. R., Burkes, R. L., Ross, R., Dworsky, R. D., Krailo, M., Parker, J. W., Lukes, R. J. and Rasheed, S. (1985). Retrovirus and malignant lymphoma in homosexual men. *J. Am. Med. Assoc.*, **254**, 1921
23. Di Carlo, E. F., Amberson, J. B., Metroka, C. E. *et al.* (1986). Malignant lymphomas and the acquired immunodeficiency syndrome. *Arch. Pathol. Lab. Med.*, **110**, 1012
24. Constantino, A., West, T. E., Gupta, M. and Loghmanee, F. (1987). Primary cardiac lymphoma in a patient with acquired immune deficiency syndrome. *Cancer*, **60**, 2081
25. Presant, C. A., Gala, K., Wiseman, Ch., Kennedy, P., Blaney, D., Sheibani, K., Winberg, C. D. and Rasheed, S. (1987). Human immunodeficiency virus-associated T-cell lymphoblastic lymphoma in AIDS. *Cancer*, **60**, 1459
26. Ahmed, K., Wormser, G. P., Stahl, R. E., Mamtani, R., Cimino, J., Glasser, M., Mittelman, A., Friedland, M. and Arlin, Z. (1987). Malignant lymphomas in a population at risk for acquired immune deficiency syndrome. *Cancer*, **60**, 719
27. Ioachim, H. L., Weinstein, M. A., Robbins, R. D., Sohn, N., Lugo, P. N. (1987). Primary anorectal lymphoma. A new manifestation of the acquired immune deficiency syndrome (AIDS). *Cancer*, **60**, 1449
28. Lane, H. C., Feinberg, J., Davey, V., Deyton, L., Baseler, M., Manischewitz, J., Masur, H., Kovacs, J. A., Herpin, B., Walker, R., Metcalf, J. A., Salzman, N., Quinnan, G. and Fauci, A. S. (1988). Anti-retroviral effects of Interferon-a in AIDS-associated Kaposi's sarcoma. *Lancet*, **2**, 1218
29. Ng, V. L., Jacobson, M. A., Khayam-Bashi, H., and McGarth, M. W. (1988). Lymphoma in HIG-positive man after disappearance of a paraprotein. *N. Engl. J. Med.*, **318**, 1761
30. Spivak, J. L., Bender, B. S. and Quinn, T. C. (1984). Hematologic abnormalities in the acquired immune deficiency syndrome. *Am. J. Med.*, **77**, 224
31. Rothenberg, R., Woelfei, M., Stonenburner, R., Milberg, J., Parker, R. and Truman, B. (1987). Survival with the acquired immunodeficiency syndrome. Experience with 5833 cases in New York City. *N. Engl. J. Med.*, **317**, 1297
32. Zon, L. I., Arkin, Ch., Groopman, J. E. (1987). Haematologic manifestations of the human immune deficiency virus (HIV). *Brit. J. Haematol.*, **66**, 251
33. Glatt, A. E., Chirgwin, K., and Landesman, S. (1988). Treatment of infections associated with human immunodeficiency virus. *N. Engl. J. Med.*, **318**, 1439
34. Cattaneo, R., Rossi, G., Carella, G., Gloria, R., Bettinziolli, M. and Stellini, R. (1988). HLA antigens and thrombocytopenia in HIV seropositive subjects. *Br. J. Haematol.*, **68**, 268
35. Osborne, B. M., Guarda, L. A. and Butler, J. J. (1984). Bone marrow biopsies in patients with the acquired immunodeficiency syndrome. *Hum. Pathol.*, **15**, 1048
36. Geller, S. A., Muller, R., Greenberg, M. L. and Siegal, F. P. (1985). Acquired immunodeficiency syndrome. Distinctive features of bone marrow biopsies. *Arch. Pathol. Lab. Med.*, **109**, 138
37. Castella, A., Croxson, Th. S., Mildvan, D., Witt, D. H. and Zalusky, R. (1985). The bone marrow in AIDS. A histologic, hematologic, and microbiologic study. *Am. J. Clin. Pathol.*, **84**, 425
38. Shenoy, C. M. and Lin, J. H. (1986). Bone marrow findings in acquired immunodeficiency syndrome (AIDS). *Am. J. Med., Sci.*, **292**, 372
39. Namiki, T. S., Boone, D. C. and Meyer, P. R. (1987). A comparison of bone marrow findings in patients with acquired immunodeficiency syndrome (AIDS) and AIDS related conditions. *Haematol. Oncol.*, **5**, 99
40. Delacretaz, F., Perey, L., Schmidt, P. M., Chave, J. P. and Costa, J. (1987). Histopathology of bone marrow in human immunodeficiency virus infection. *Virchows Arch. A.*, **411**, 543
41. Treacy, M., Lai, L., Costello, Ch. and Clark, A. (1987). Peripheral blood and bone marrow abnormalities in patients with HIV related disease. *Br. J. Haematol.*, **65**, 289
42. Transmission of HIV through bone transplantation: Case report and public health recommendations (1988). *Morbid. Mortal. Weekly Rep.*, **37**, 597

Metastases in the Bone Marrow

10

The introduction of advanced technology for obtaining biopsies under radiological guidance, improvements in biopsy needles, the development of specific monoclonal antibodies and tumour markers, and the progress in histological techniques have led to a widespread upsurge of interest in examination of the bone marrow for detection of metastases[1-11]. Moreover, evidence has now accumulated that any primary tumour has the ability to spread as soon as it is established and has access to lymphatic or blood vessels. Metastatic potential is also related to the cellular heterogeneity of the primary tumour[12].

It has been estimated that about 30 divisions are needed for a developing neoplastic growth to reach a size of 1 cm^3, which is considered a minimum for clinical detection. This may take 2–3 years and, since most tumours are larger when first suspected and detected, a longer interval will have passed during which metastases could have been disseminated (Figs 10.1–10.11)[6]. Metastases in turn also require a certain period of time before they are clinically detectable, and there are as yet no reliable methods available for their detection in the initial stages of development.

The sinusoidal system of the red haematopoietic marrow, lined by a thin endothelial layer and without tight junctions, has a slow perfusion rate but a large blood flow, thus facilitating passage of the tumour cell emboli into the extravascular spaces[13]. In addition, the bone marrow sinusoids are an ideal location for the formation of tumour-cell-platelet thrombi. Moreover, the cells of the haematopoietic system probably provide the neoplastic cells with growth and other factors required for their survival, establishment and expansion. Once the tumour cell emboli have settled in the bone marrow the surrounding bone is also affected in the majority of cases. Extensive occupation of the intertrabecular spaces by metastases without an effect on the cancellous bone structure is relatively rare.

Incidence of Skeletal Metastases

The rates of detection reported in the literature differ widely; these differences are due to one or more of the following factors: (1) which primary tumour is involved, (2) the stage of the disease at which the bone biopsy is taken, (3) the size of the biopsy core, (4) the quality of the histological preparation.

In a recent study of 1725 patients with solid carcinomas the overall bone marrow involvement was 33%. Metastases of unknown primary tumours, of prostate, of breast and of lung comprised 78% of the positive cases. However, in a survey of skeletal metastases in autopsy cases the rate of occurrence was over 75% for cancer of breast and prostate; 30–60% for thyroid; up to 50% for kidney, uterus and bladder; 40% for lungs; while metastases of all other tumours were listed as infrequent or rare[3,14,15].

Indications for Bone Biopsy

The indications for bone biopsies in recent years have broadened and now include:

1. Part of the initial investigation for staging and prognostic factors, and decisions on therapy.
2. Clinical suspicion of metastases.
3. Anaemia, other cytopenia, weakness or fatigue.
4. Follow-up and monitoring of therapy.
5. Unexplained pyrexia.
6. Hypercalcaemia.
7. Raised osseous alkaline phosphatase levels.
8. Suspicious areas on X-ray or bone scan.
9. Differentiation of therapy-induced hypoplasia or aplasia from replacement of the bone marrow by metastases.
10. Investigation of the effects of the malignancy on the marrow and the bone, and investigation of tumour–host interactions.

Histology of Metastases in the Bone Marrow

The four major types of bone marrow involvement by metastatic cancer are demonstrated in Figs 10.12–10.22. Tumours in the bone marrow, as elsewhere, are composed of parenchyme and stroma in various proportions. The following histological types are recognized: solid, adenomatous, scirrhous, squamous, small cell and mixed (Figs 10.23–10.40). Though a system employing four grades of tumour differentiation is widely used, a system employing only three grades has recently been advocated[16]. A thin connective tissue layer may be interposed between the tumour cells and their stroma. The stromal components have been divided into four main groups in primary tumours: (1) new blood vessels; (2) inflammatory cells, e.g. lymphocytes, macrophages; (3) connective tissue – which includes matrix components such as fibronectin, collagens, elastins and glycosaminoglycans and cells such as fibroblasts and myofibroblasts; (4) the fibrin–gel matrix which traps extravasated proteins and water and forms a provisional matrix which is later replaced by connective tissue (Figs 10.41–10.46). Thus the extravascular deposition of fibrin is closely linked to the formation of new connective tissue. These processes in the formation of the stroma of tumours are similar to those of wound healing[17,18].

Rarely, metastases in the bone marrow biopsy sections are confined to the vascular system; these are composed of tumour masses with little stroma. In all other cases the stimulation of new blood vessels – neo-angiogenesis – from host vessels occurs, and may be especially prominent at the margins of the metastases. Such vessels rarely have the anatomical structure of their normal counterparts. They are often irregular channels with scanty perivascular tissue, or incomplete endothelium, or even lined by tumour cells. The degree of vascularity varies greatly. Together with the blood vessels, fibroblasts and fibres, mast cells and various other infiltrating cells enter the metastases. Mast cells play a role in tumour angiogenesis and vascularization, as well as having the capacity to stimulate proliferation of tumours – at least *in vitro*[19,20]. The stroma of all tumours, and of the metastases, depends partly on the neoplastic cells' ability to organize themselves, and

(Continued on p. 185)

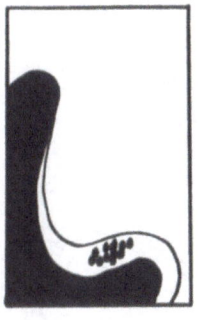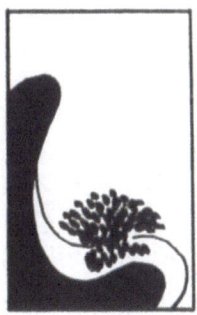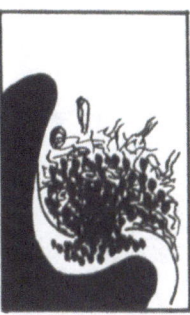

INTRA-
SINUSOIDAL

TRANS-
SINUSOIDAL

STROMAL
INDUCTION

Fig. 10.1 Establishment of metastasis in the bone marrow: passage of the tumour cells through the sinusoidal endothelium, and stimulation of host cells to produce the stroma for neoplastic cells

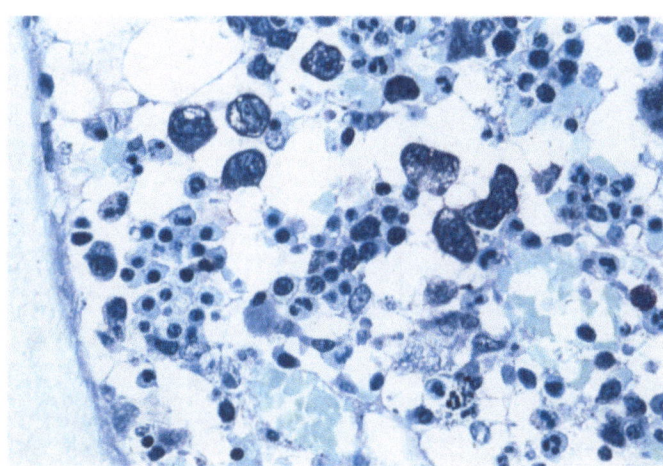

Fig. 10.2 Single tumour cells among haematopoietic cells. Bone marrow biopsy of patient with tumour of unknown primary

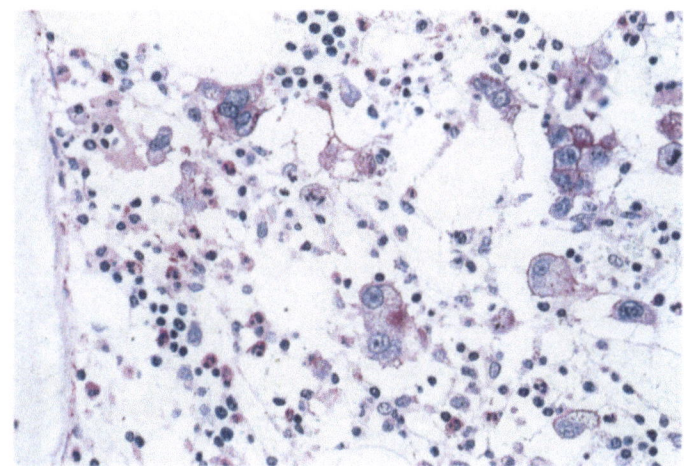

Fig. 10.3 PAS-positive tumour cells scattered in bone marrow; mammary carcinoma. PAS

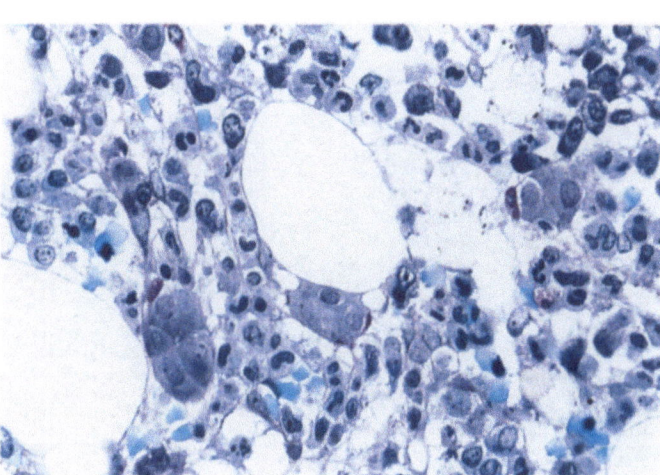

Fig. 10.4 Several tumour cell clusters in bone marrow interstitium; metastases of unknown primary

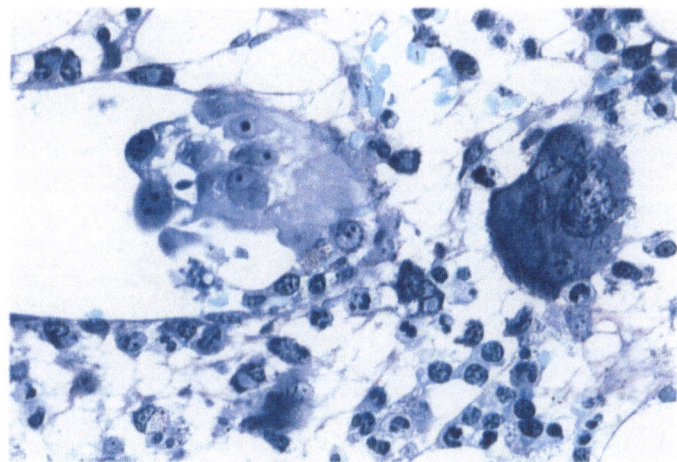

Fig. 10.5 Intravascular tumour cell embolus attached to endothelium; mammary carcinoma

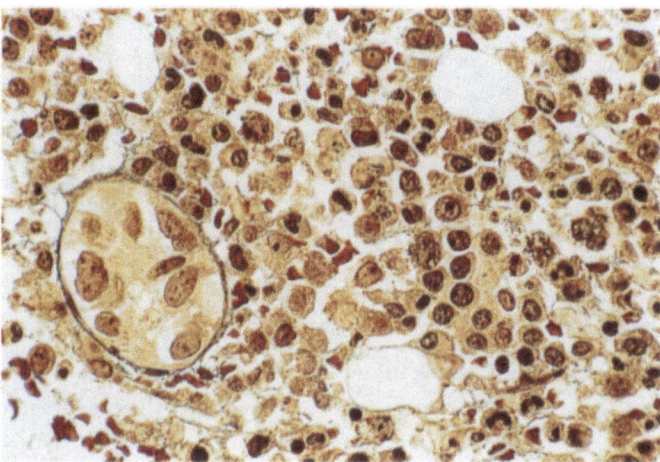

Fig. 10.6 Intravascular tumour cell embolus in cellular bone marrow; mammary carcinoma, Gomori

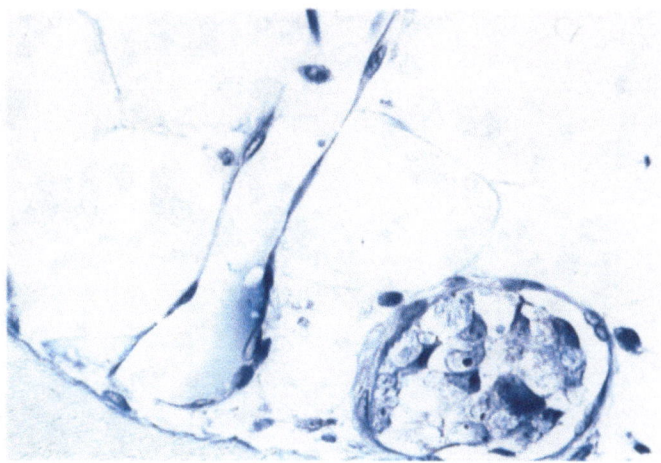

Fig. 10.7 Intravascular tumour cell embolus in atrophic marrow; carcinoma of prostate

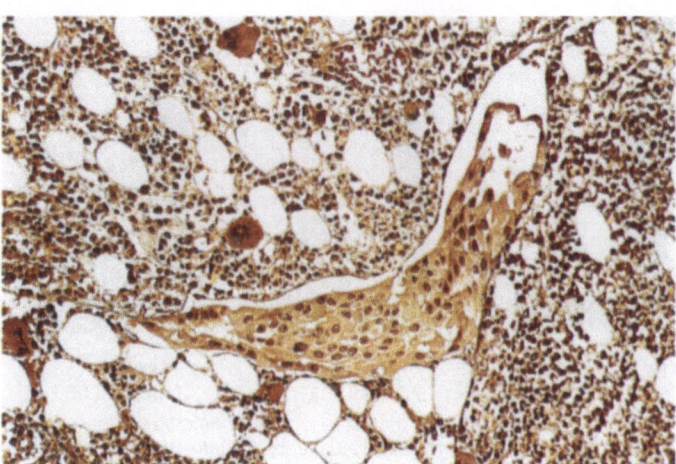

Fig. 10.8 Large intravascular tumour cell embolus without reaction in adjacent marrow, carcinoma of lung. Gomori

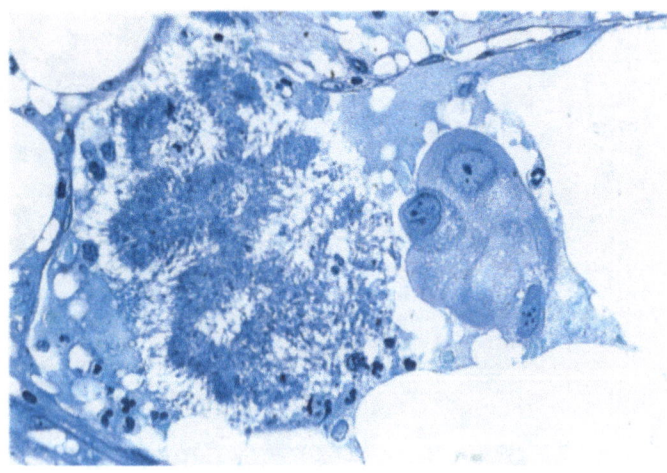

Fig. 10.9 Tumour cell embolus in sinus with clumps of platelets, metastases of unknown primary

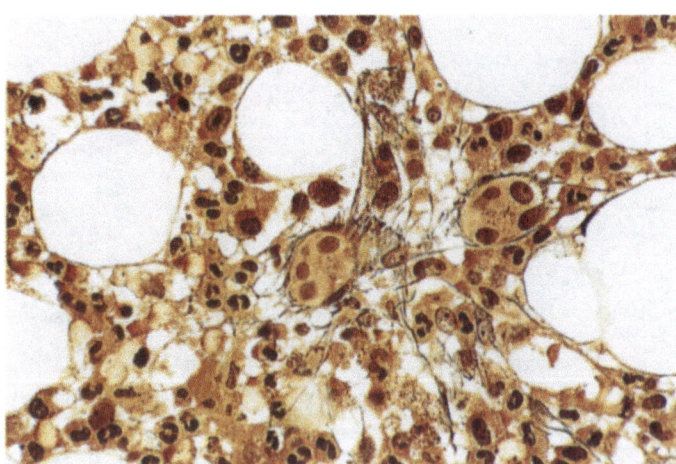

Fig. 10.10 Two interstitial tumour cell emboli with incipient fibrosis; metastases of unknown primary. Gomori. The tumour cells in Figs 10.2–10.10 might have been overlooked without high-quality histology

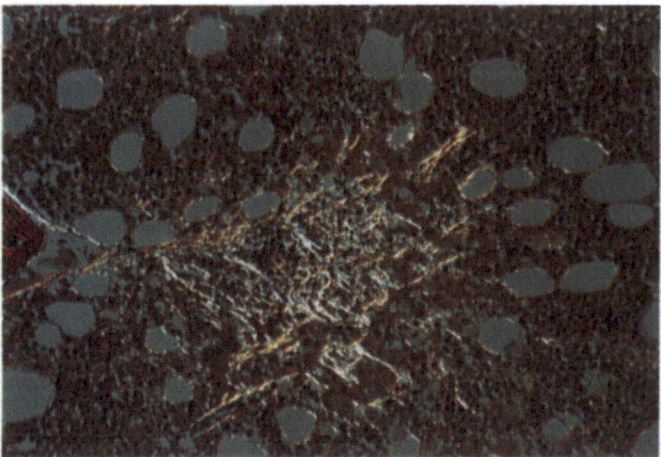

Fig. 10.11 Micrometastasis with stromal induction as shown in section stained by Gomori and viewed by polarized light; mammary carcinoma

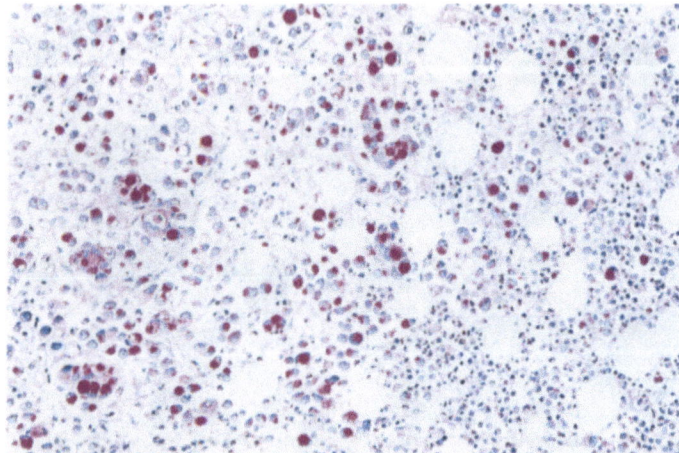

Fig. 10.13 Microcolonies dispersed in bone marrow; carcinoma of intestinal tract. PAS

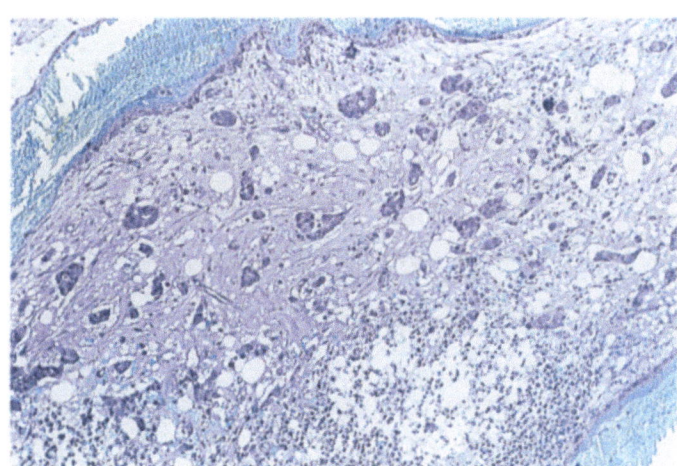

Fig. 10.14 Multiple foci within oedematous fibrotic stroma. Note osteoblastic reactions; carcinoma of prostate

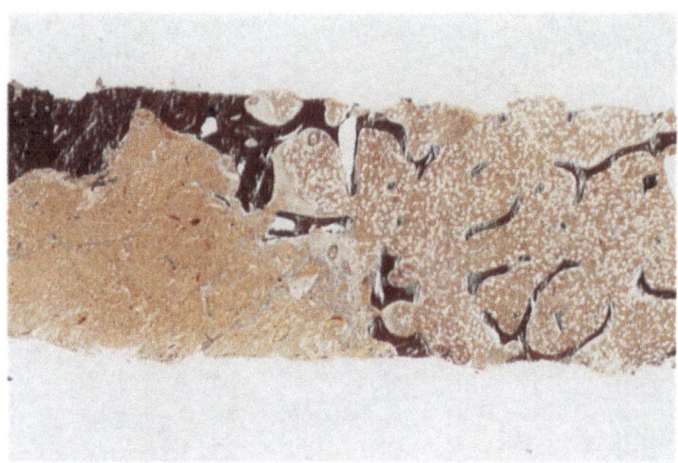

Fig. 10.15 Large metastatic mass replacing bone marrow; metastases of unknown primary. Gomori

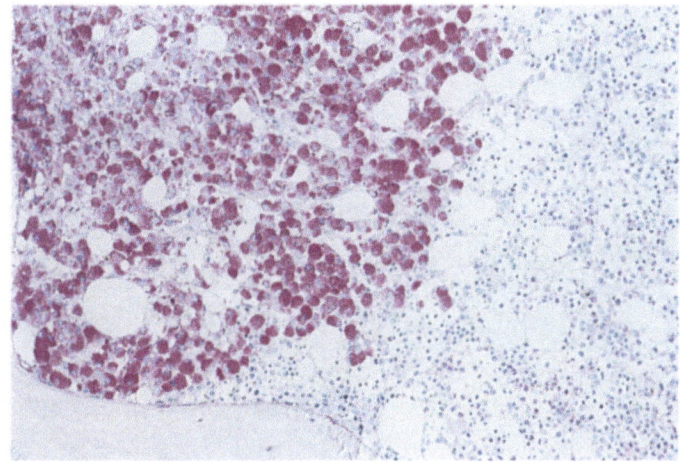

Fig. 10.16 Paratrabecular mass of tumour cells; metastases of gastric carcinoma. PAS

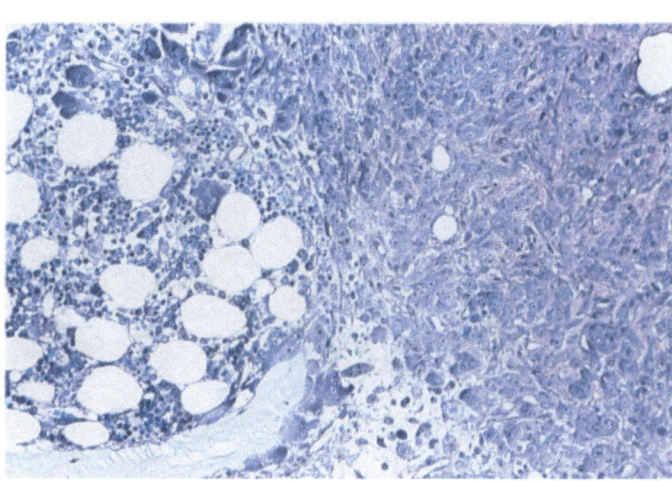

Fig. 10.17 Large tumour mass with marginal reaction and osteoblastic activity; mammary carcinoma

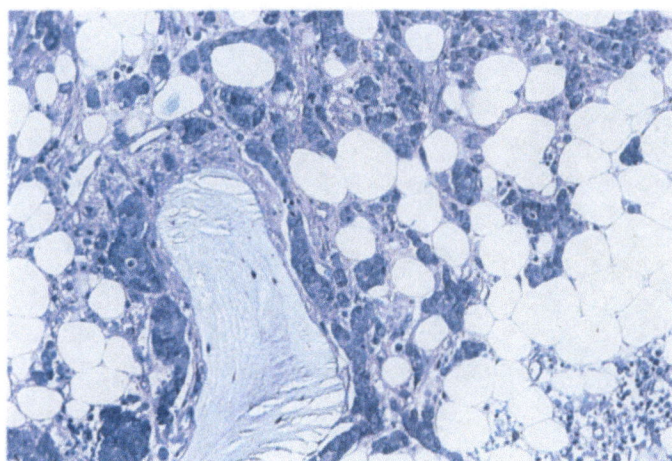

Fig. 10.18 Tumour cells in paratrabecular sinus and infiltrating between fat cells; mammary carcinoma

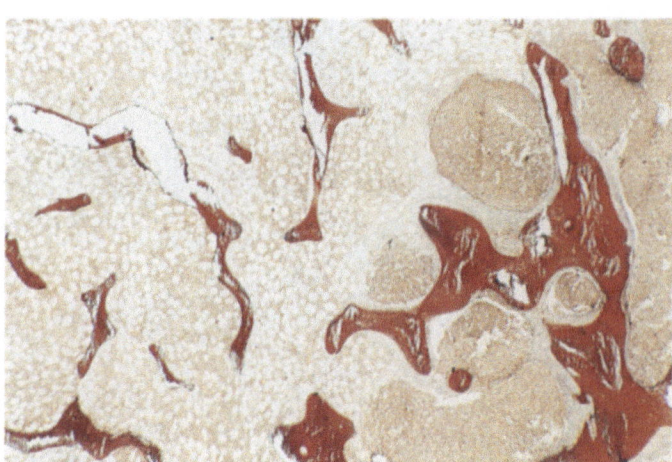

Fig. 10.19 Focal, sharply delineated tumour masses with osteosclerosis; mammary carcinoma. Gomori

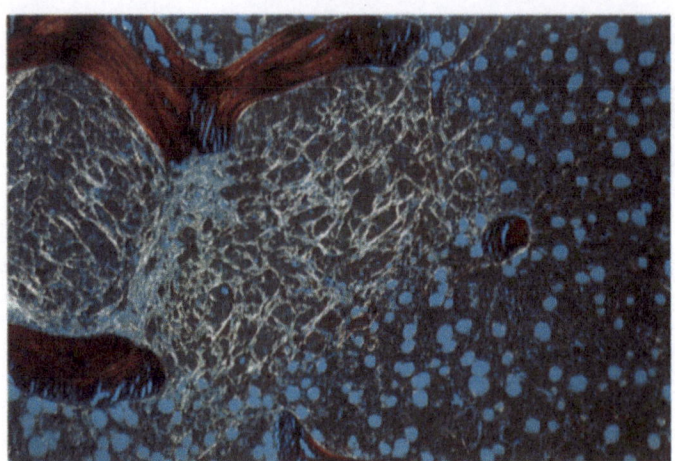

Fig. 10.20 Fibrosis within metastases; carcinoma of prostate. Gomori, polarized light

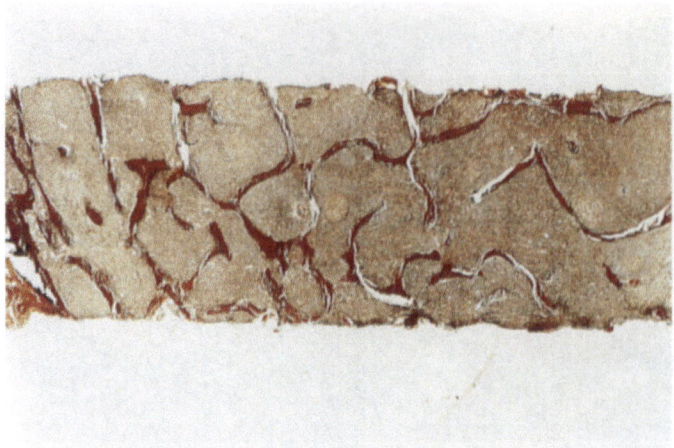

Fig. 10.21 Complete replacement of bone marrow by metastasis, but no alteration of trabecular bone structure; carcinoma of lung. Gomori

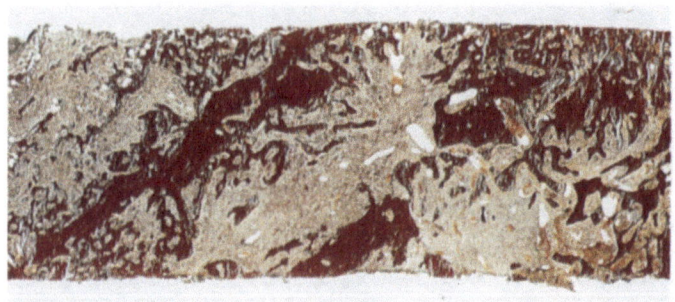

Fig. 10.22 Bone biopsy with complete replacement of marrow and both osteolysis and osteosclerosis of trabecular bone; unknown primary tumour. Gomori

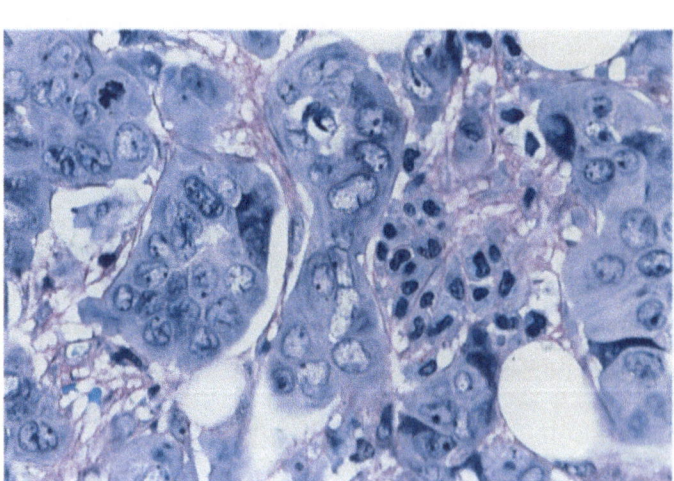

Fig. 10.24 Metastasis showing gland-like structures; mammary carcinoma

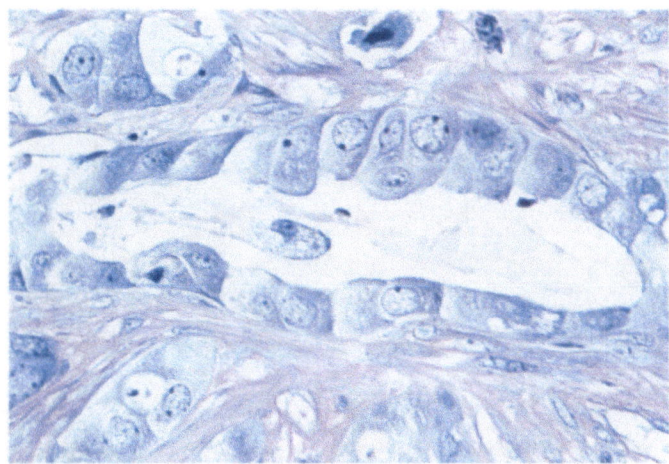

Fig. 10.25 Metastasis of adenocarcinoma showing wide lumen; mammary carcinoma

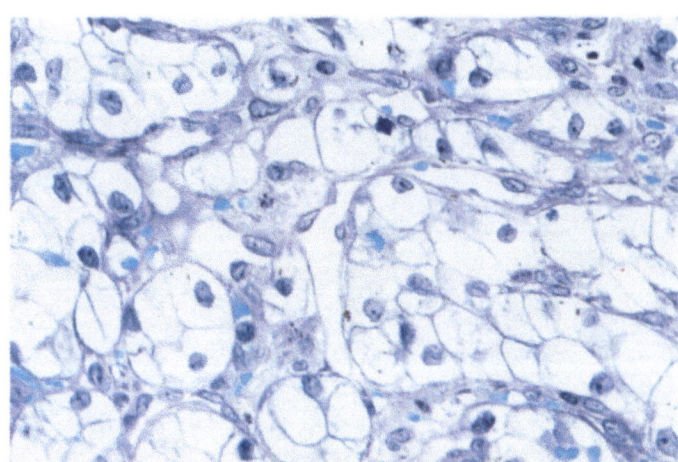

Fig. 10.26 Clear cell adenocarcinoma; renal carcinoma

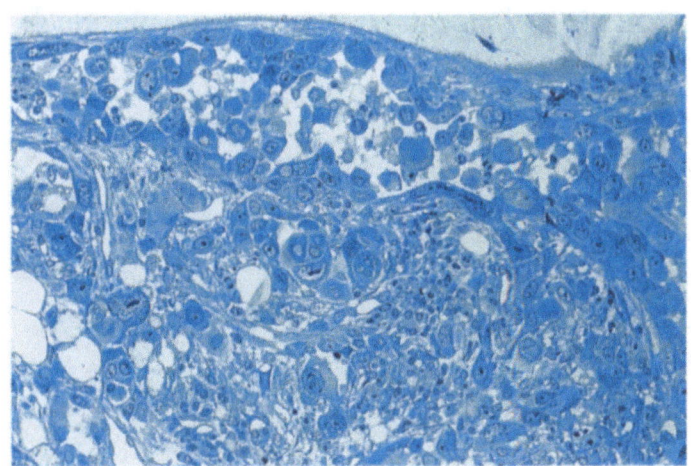

Fig. 10.27 Bone marrow metastasis of squamous cell carcinoma; unknown primary tumour

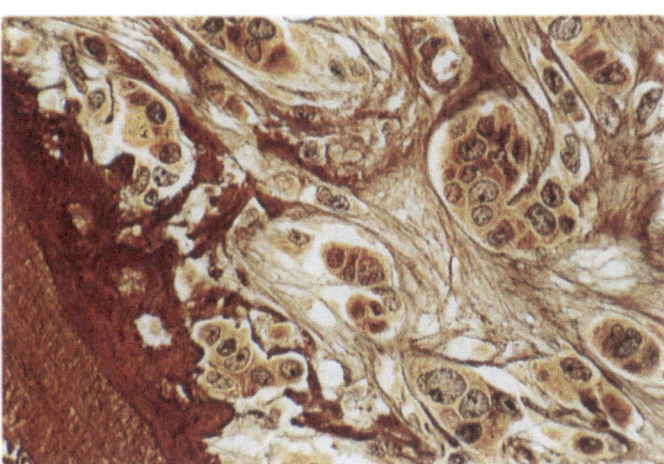

Fig. 10.28 Coarse fibrosis with osteoblastic reaction in involved area; mammary carcinoma. Gomori

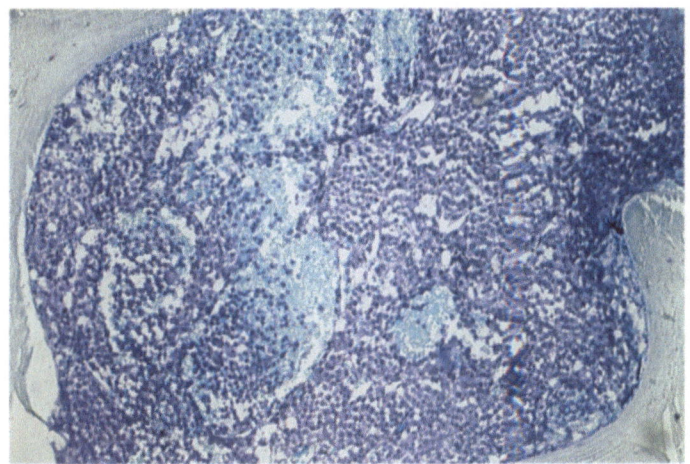

Fig. 10.29 Metastasis composed of masses of tumour cells, virtually no stroma. There is no osseous reaction, in spite of complete occupation of the bone marrow throughout the whole biopsy; metastases of malignant melanoma

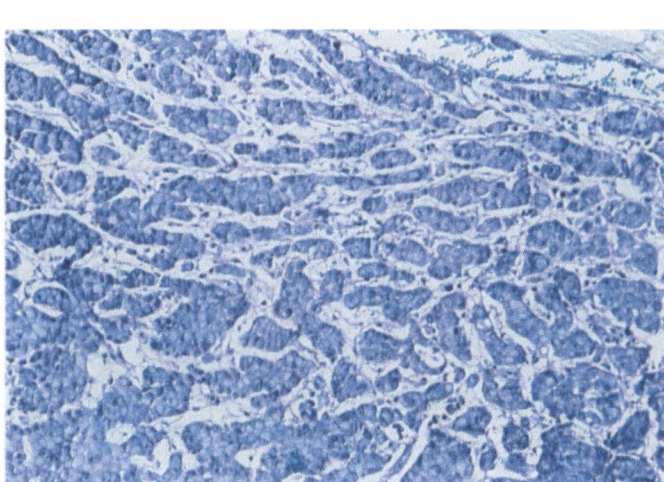

Fig. 10.30 Metastasis composed of tumour cell clusters with little connective tissue between them; mammary carcinoma

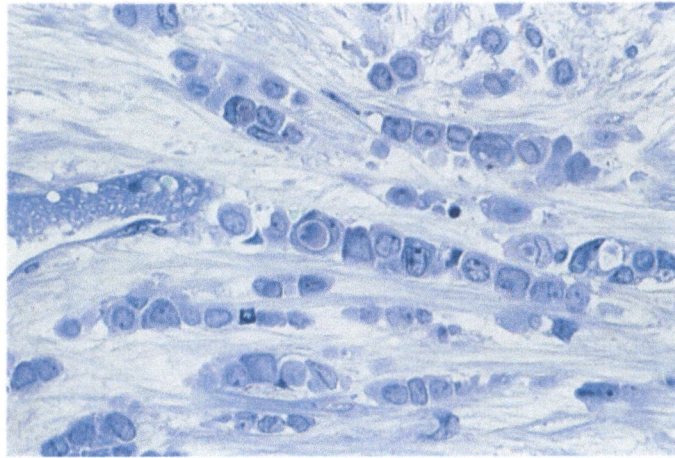

Fig. 10.31 'Indian file' formation of tumour cells between wide bands of connective tissue; mammary carcinoma

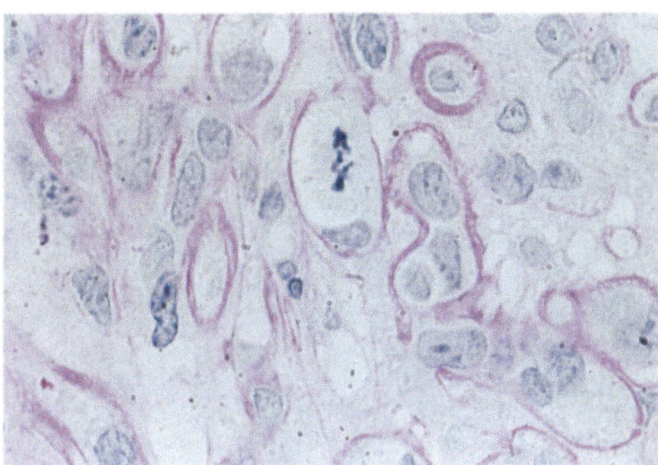

Fig. 10.32 A thin PAS-positive layer encircles tumour cell clusters, or even single tumour cells; prostatic carcinoma

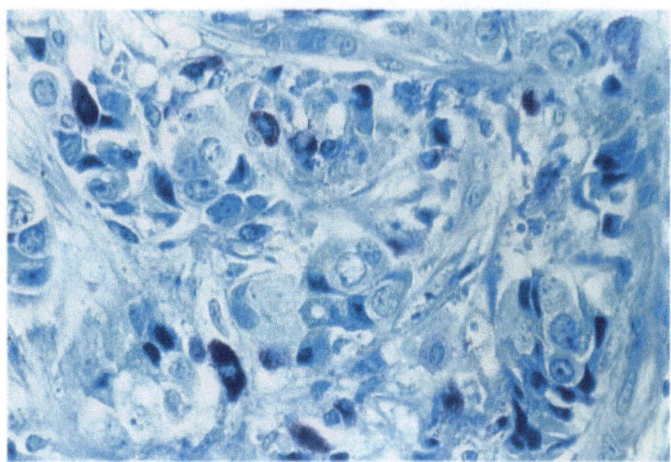

Fig. 10.33 Tumour and mast cells in a network of connective tissue fibres; mammary carcinoma

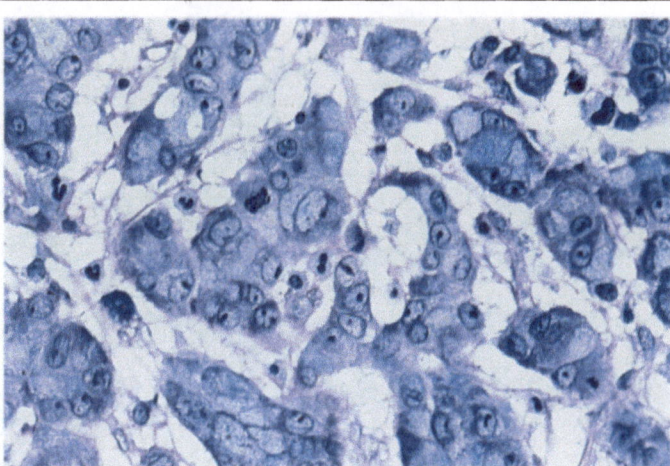

Fig. 10.34 Polymorphic clusters of tumour cells; metastases of gastric carcinoma

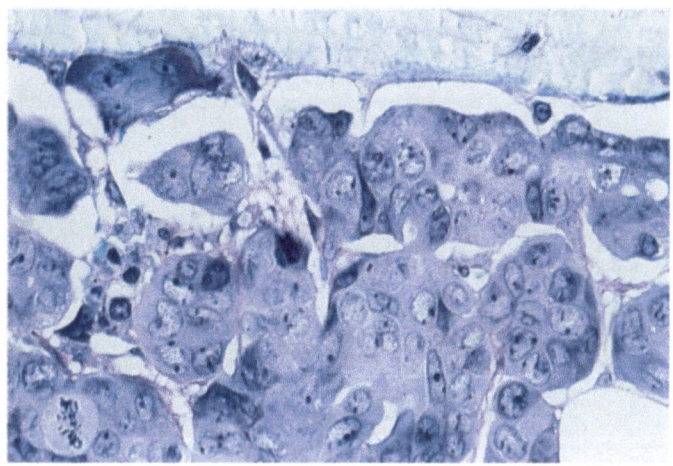

Fig. 10.35 Clusters of pleomorphic tumour cells with active osteoclast on bone; mammary carcinoma

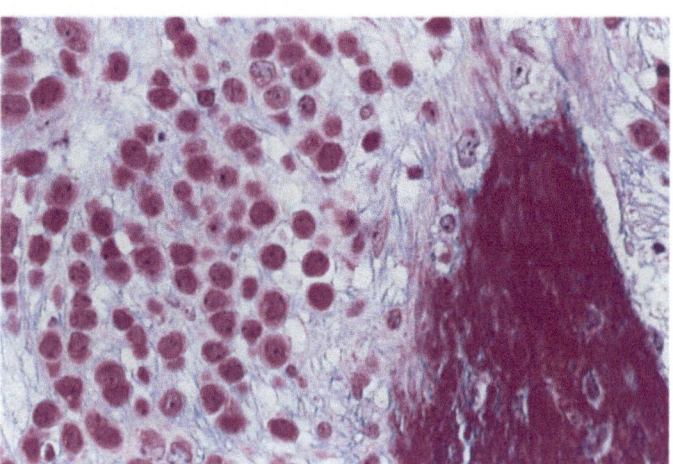

Fig. 10.36 Primitive bone formation within metastatic focus, with fibres radiating out from surface of osteoid; mammary carcinoma. Ladewig

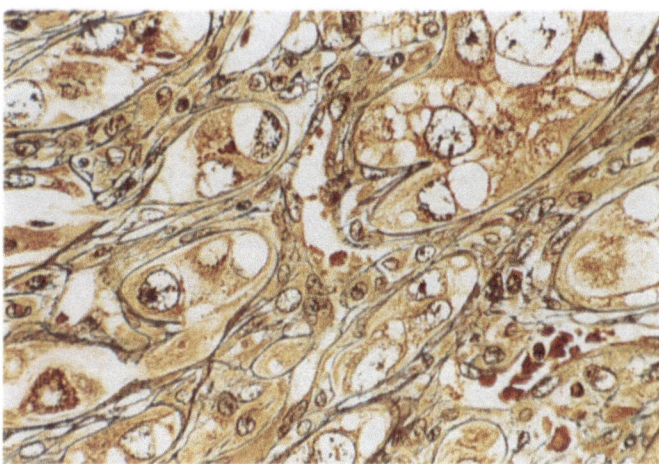

Fig. 10.37 Small pleomorphic tumour cell clusters separated by bands of connective tissue; renal carcinoma. Gomori

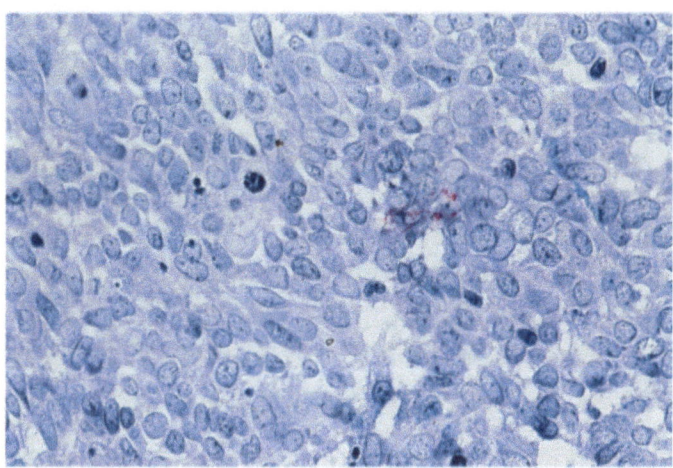

Fig. 10.38 Solid mass of tumour cells, metastasis of oat cell carcinoma of lung

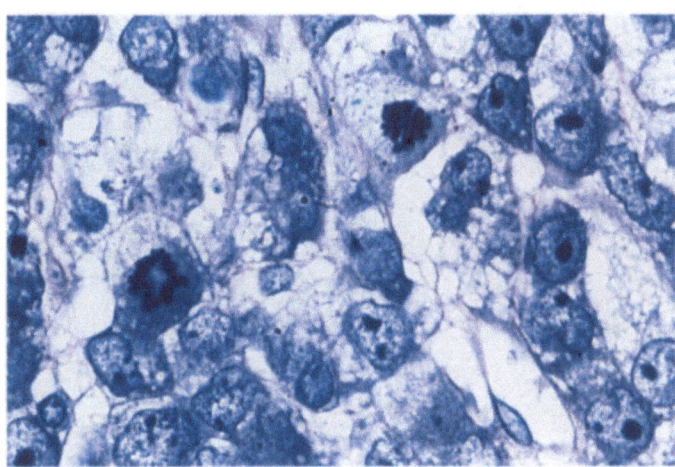

Fig. 10.39 Large, anaplastic metastatic cells of prostatic carcinoma. Note mitotic figures

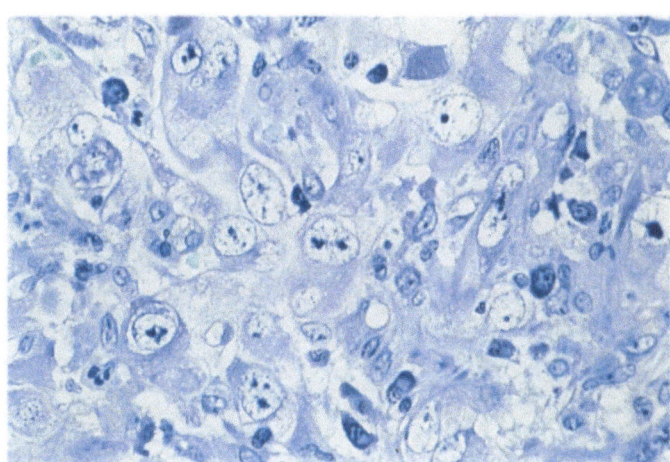

Fig. 10.40 Anaplastic metastasis of renal carcinoma. Note infiltrating plasma cells

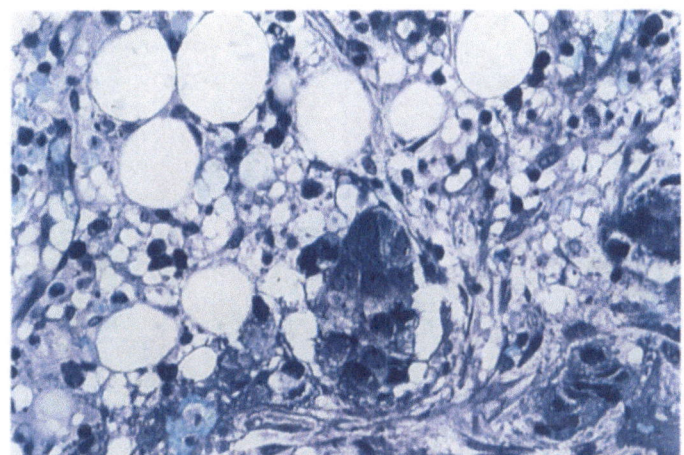

Fig. 10.41 Tumour cell cluster in marginal zone of metastases: carcinoma of prostate

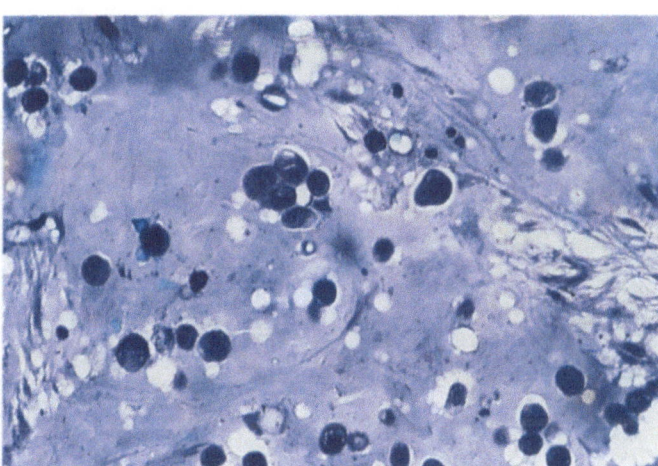

Fig. 10.42 Single tumour cells in gelatinous matrix in bone biopsy with no residual haematopoiesis; mammary carcinoma

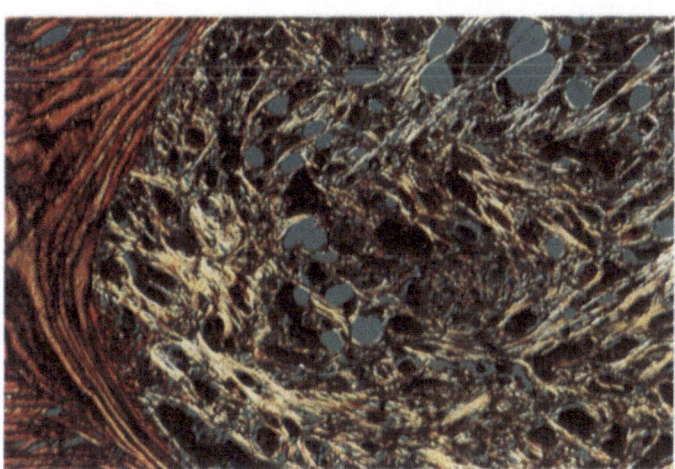

Fig. 10.43 Coarse fibrosis without alteration of trabecular bone structure. There were few residual tumour cells; mammary carcinoma. Gomori, polarized light

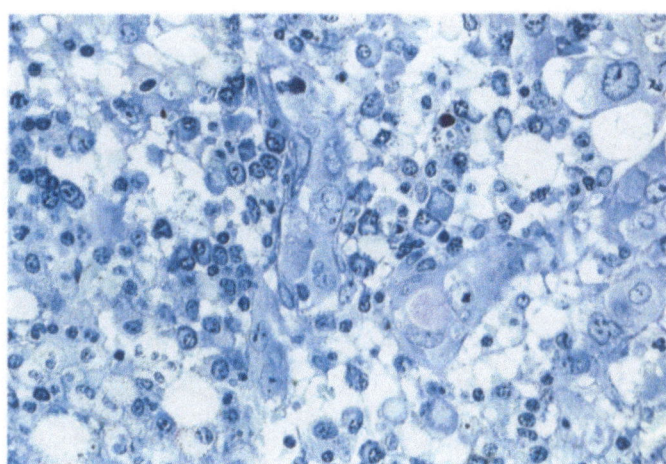

Fig. 10.44 Plasmacytic infiltration around tumour cells: metastases of unknown primary

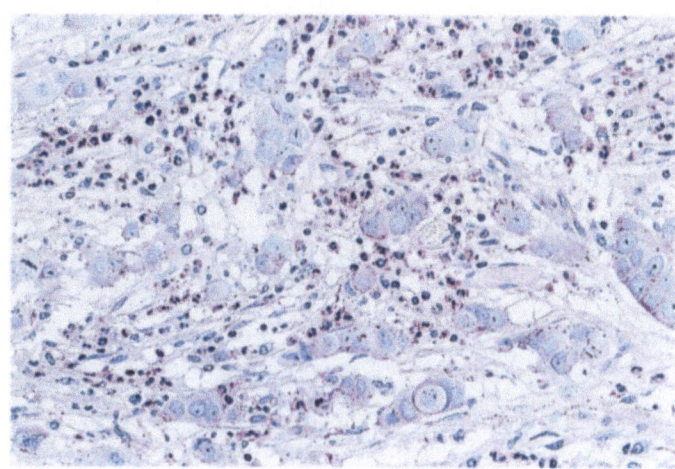

Fig. 10.45 Intense granulocytic infiltration around tumour cells; metastases of unknown primary tumour. PAS

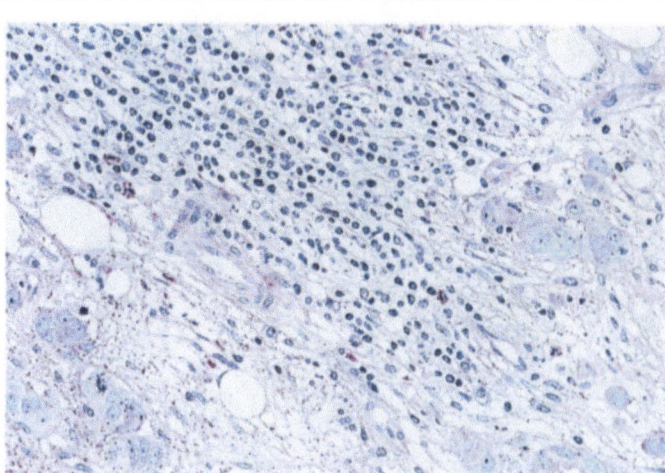

Fig. 10.46 Lymphoid infiltration within metastasis; metastases of unknown primary tumour. PAS

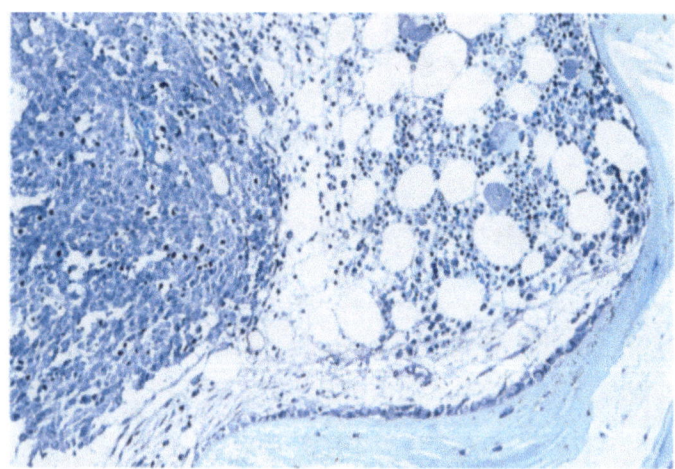

Fig. 10.47 Marginal zone around metastasis of carcinoma of lung. Note residual haematopoiesis, paratrabecular fibrosis, osteoblasts and osteoid

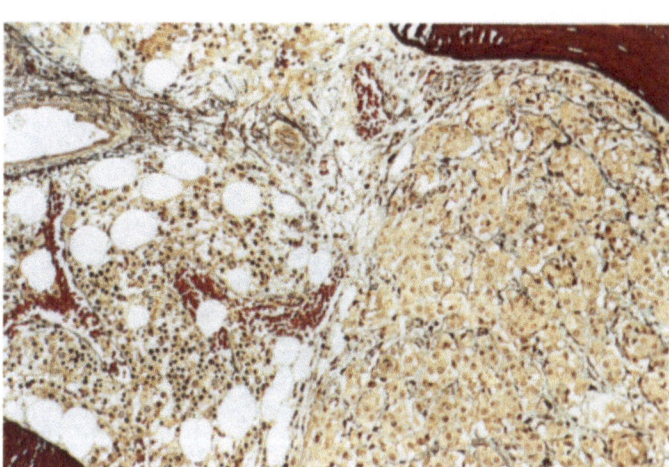

Fig. 10.48 Sharply demarcated metastasis; carcinoma of lung. No osseous reaction. Gomori

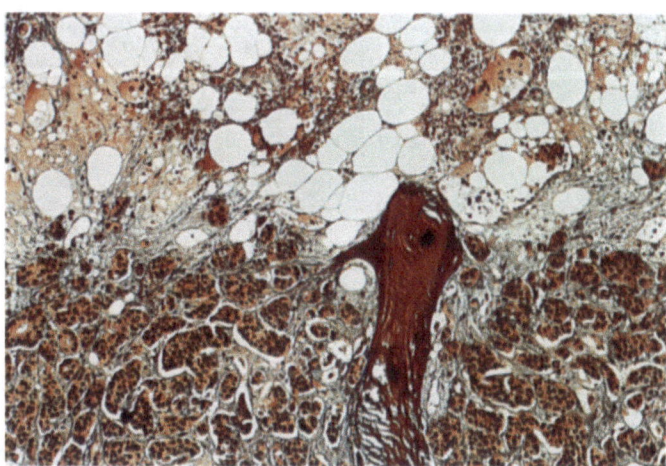

Fig. 10.49 Large metastasis separated by zone of degeneration, oedema and fibrosis from residual bone marrow; carcinoma of prostate. Gomori

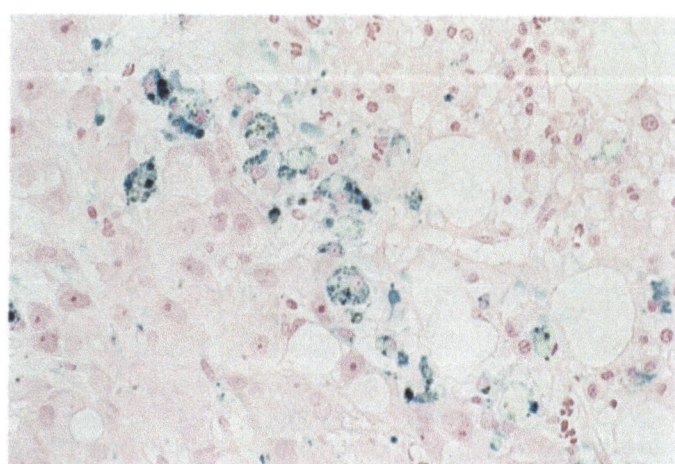

Fig. 10.50 Bone marrow metastasis surrounded by macrophages containing iron; carcinoma of prostate. Berlin blue

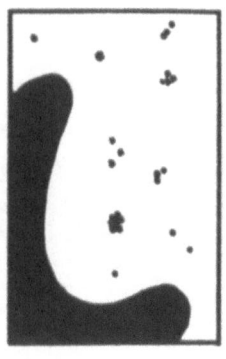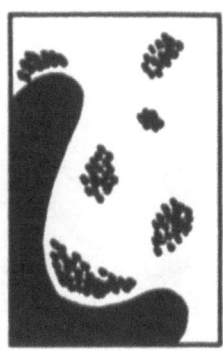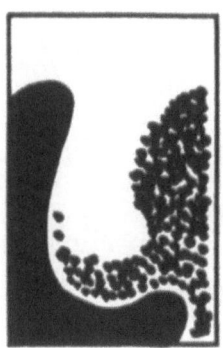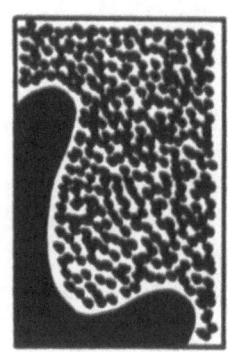

MICRO-
COLONIES
MULTIPLE
FOCI
LARGE
MASSES
TOTAL
REPLACEMENT

Fig. 10.12 Histological aspects of bone marrow involvement by metastases: multiple microemboli or colonies; multiple extravascular foci; large masses and complete replacement of the normal marrow

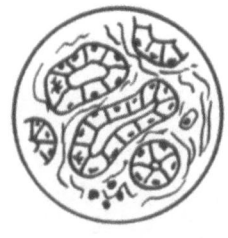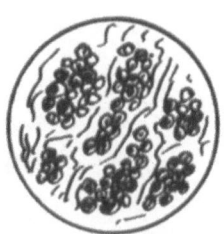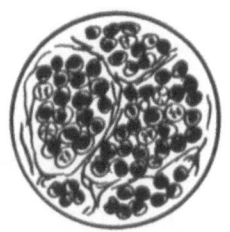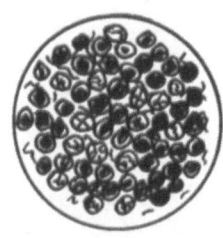

GRADE I   GRADE II   GRADE III   GRADE IV

Fig. 10.23 Histological grades of metastases in the bone marrow

also on their capacity to produce factors which elicit the cellular and stromal reactions of the host: this may vary in different parts of the same metastases. The effects of angiogenic, osteoblast and osteoclast activating factors are often striking, even with very small metastases. Other tumour factors stimulate erythropoiesis, granulopoiesis or thrombopoiesis, or are chemotactic for lymphocytes, eosinophils, monocytes or macrophages, whose possible functions around and within metastases still remain to be clarified.

Reactions to the metastases may be found: (1) within the marrow near them, (2) at the margin or interface between the tumour cells and bone marrow, (3) within the metastases – all three are highly variable (Figs 10.47– 10.51). The residual marrow in biopsies (with or without involvement) may be hypo-, normo- or hypercellular, erythropoiesis may be selectively decreased (or increased in the event of bleeding or haemolysis), macrophages and megakaryocytes increased. The tumour–marrow interface may rarely show an abrupt transition from metastases to normal haematopoiesis. Mostly, however, there is a zone of variable width separating the two which consists of oedema, a loose network of fibres, a few fibroblasts, sprouting blood vessels and an assortment of infiltrating cells and possibly a few haematopoietic precursors.

Within the metastases themselves – except when there are multiple foci within the biopsy – usually no haemato-poietic tissue remains. The quantity of stroma and its composition, as well as the quantity and type of infiltrating cells, vary greatly. In addition to lymphocytes, monocytes, macrophages, mast and plasma cells, neutrophils may be prominent in and around metastases, possibly due to degeneration of the tumour cells and accumulation of breakdown products, other tumour factors or infection. Necrosis of bone marrow and of the metastases may also be found, especially when their rate of multiplication outstrips their blood supply[21].

Metastases and Bone

In the great majority of cases the trabecular bone is affected very early on in the metastatic process so that the normal trabecular bone structure is destroyed (Figs 10.52–10.67). The process is rarely purely osteolytic or osteosclerotic; mostly there is both resorption and formation. However, due to the altered architecture, mech-anical strength and resilience are decreased so that patho-logical fractures may ensue, even when the total amount of bone is not greatly reduced. In early stages the bone is resorbed by osteoclasts activated by the tumour cells; subsequently when no haematopoietic tissue remains, and the metastases lie directly on the bone, other mechan-isms are involved, possibly a direct action of the tumour cells on bone. New bone formation may likewise be accomplished by at least two mechanisms – appositional new bone formation by osteoblasts on pre-existing ossicles, or sprouts of new bone jutting out from them; or by the formation of woven bone – mineralization of a dense collagenous connective tissue stroma. In addition to the local bone resorption mediated by malignant cells in proximity to bone, a second mechanism has for some time been postulated: the humoral hypercalcaemia of cancer resulting from osteoclastic activity mediated by factor(s) secreted by neoplastic cells not located within the skeleton[22,23]. Examples are cancers of the kidney, bladder and ovary. A parathyroid hormone-like peptide secreted by neoplastic cells has now been identified in patients with the humoral hypercalcaemia of cancer. Recently, inhibition of osteoclasts and sclerosis of oste-olytic bone lesions has been achieved with phosphon-ates[24-26]. Hence, an early bone biopsy may provide infor-mation required for decisions on therapy.

Cancer of the Prostate

Skeletal metastases may already be present at diagnosis in 50–80% of the patients, or will develop in most cases,

(Continued on p. 189)

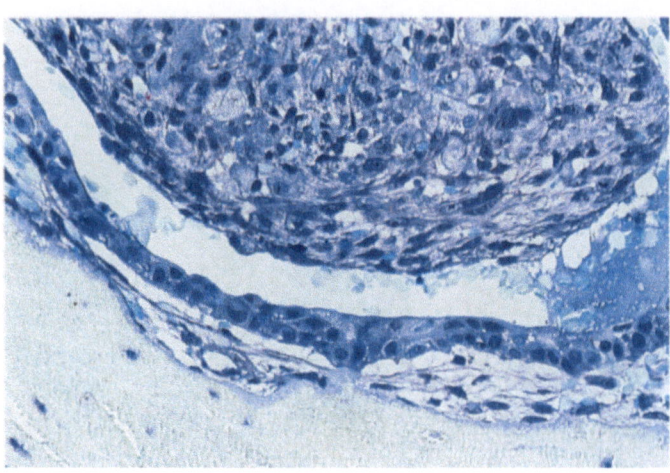

Fig. 10.51 Metastasis of transitional cell carcinoma of bladder. Note tumour cell layer on endothelium of paratrabecular sinus and large tumour mass within its lumen

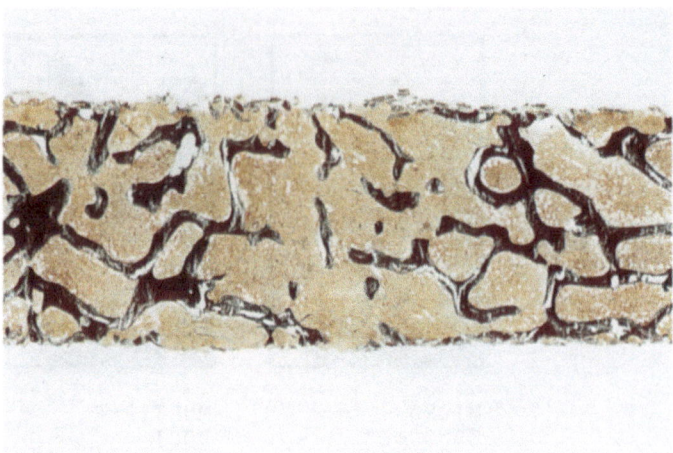

Fig. 10.52 Complete occupation of marrow cavities without alteration of trabecular bone structure; carcinoma of lung. Gomori

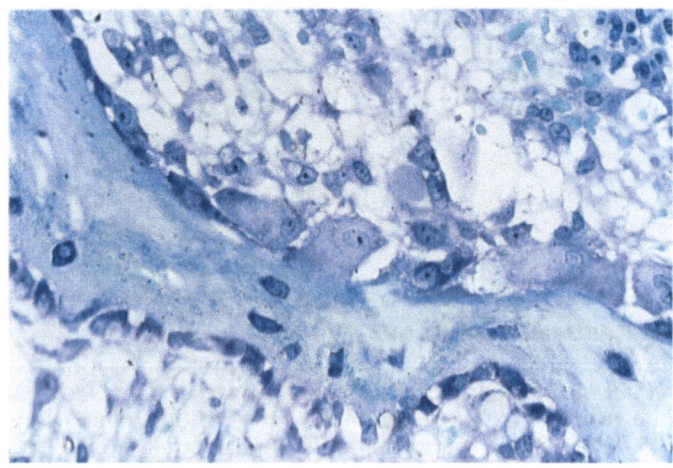

Fig. 10.53 Metastasis evoking unco-ordinated osseous resorption and formation. Note contiguous osteoblasts and osteoclasts; mammary carcinoma

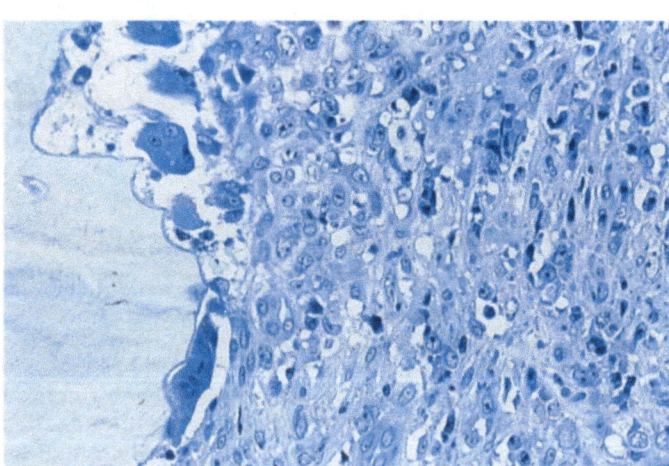

Fig. 10.54 Metastasis inducing unopposed osteoclastic resorption; mammary carcinoma

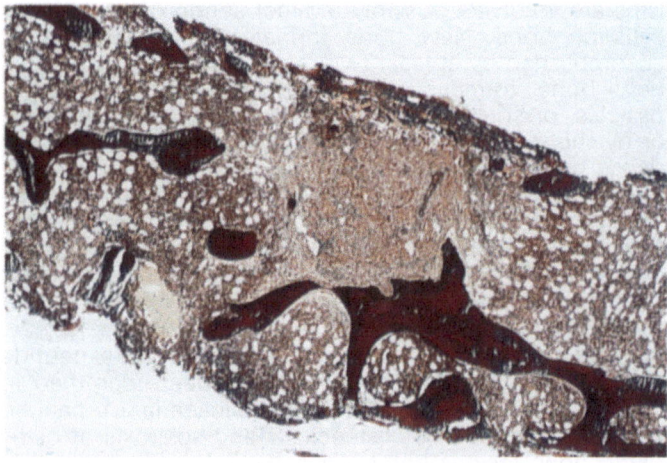

Fig. 10.55 Bone biopsy with one osteolytic metastatic focus, as well as incipient sclerosis; mammary carcinoma

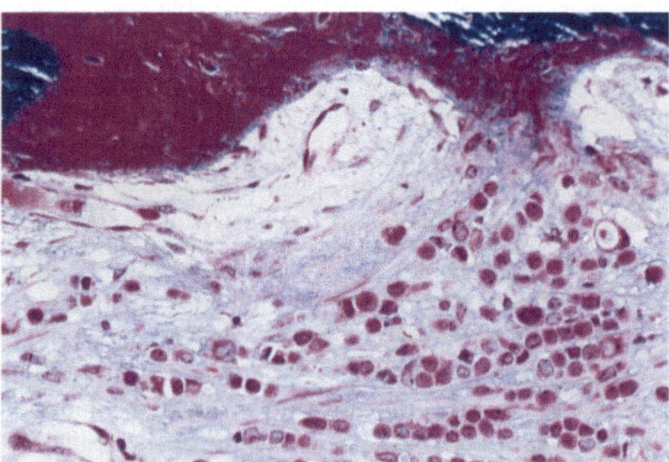

Fig. 10.56 Metastasis inducing bone formation. Note broad osteoid seam (red), osteoblasts, and connective tissue attached to bone; mammary carcinoma

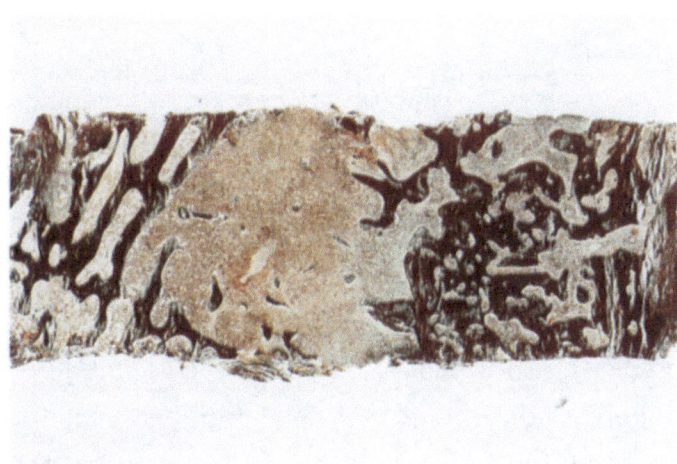

Fig. 10.57 Bone biopsy showing both osteolysis and osteosclerosis. Metastasis of mammary carcinoma. Gomori

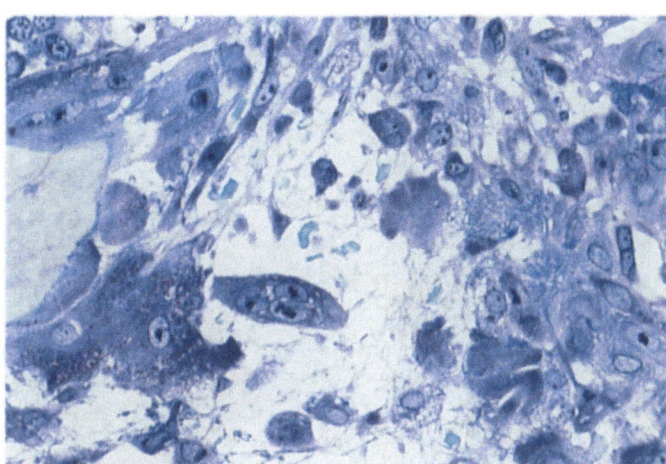

Fig. 10.58 Area from edge of osteolytic metastasis in Fig. 10.57, showing marked osteoclastic activation

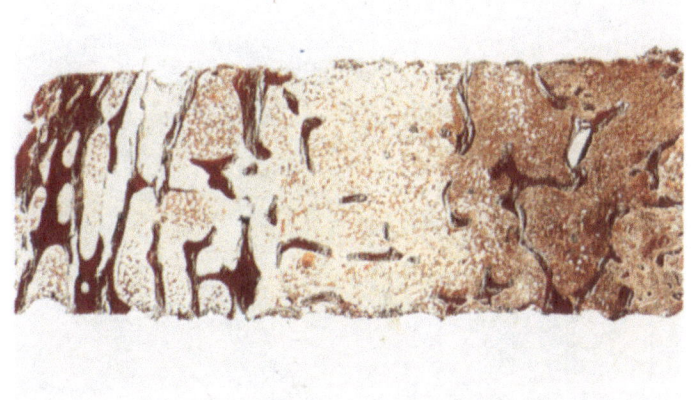

Fig. 10.59 Bone biopsy showing normal trabecular bone within the metastasis and osteopenia in adjacent area of fatty marrow; carcinoma of lung. Gomori

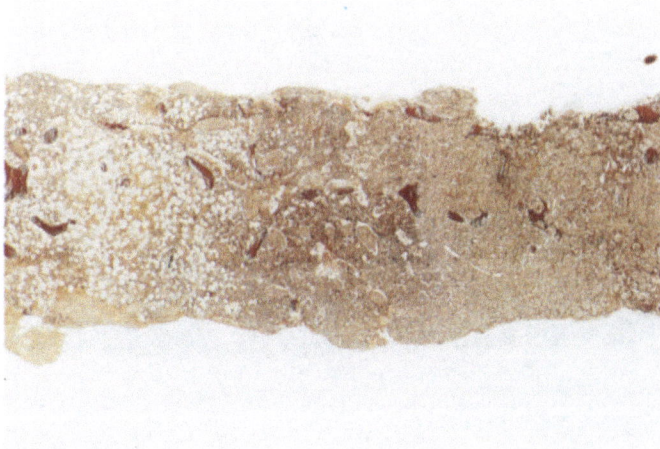

Fig. 10.60 Massive reduction of trabecular bone in biopsy of patient with widespread skeletal metastasis of unknown primary tumours. Gomori

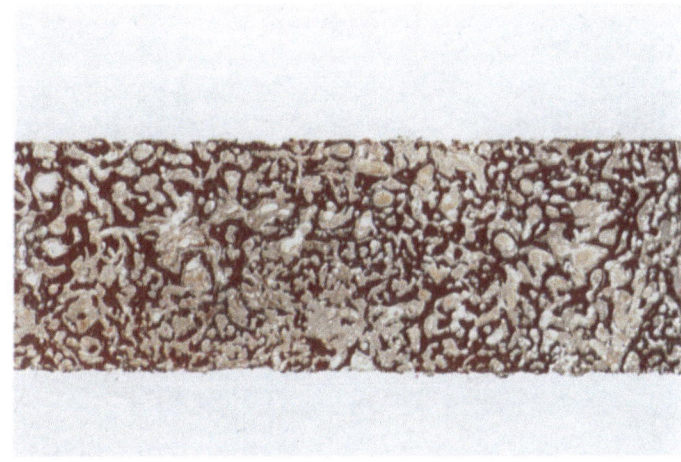

Fig. 10.61 Dense network of primitive bone in metastatic carcinoma of prostate. Gomori

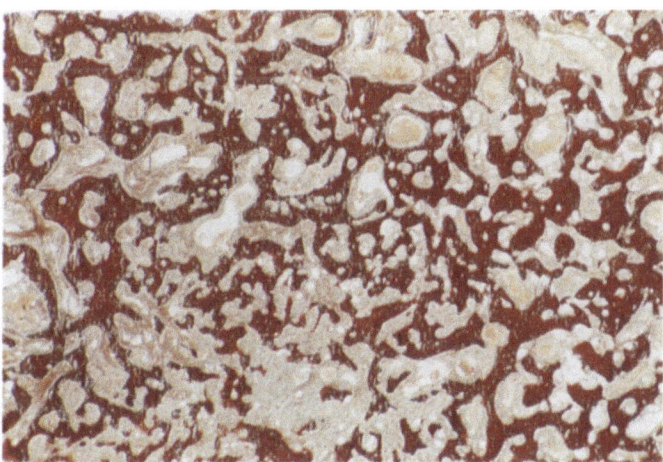

Fig. 10.62 Higher magnification of Fig. 10.61; replacement of marrow by fibrosis. Gomori

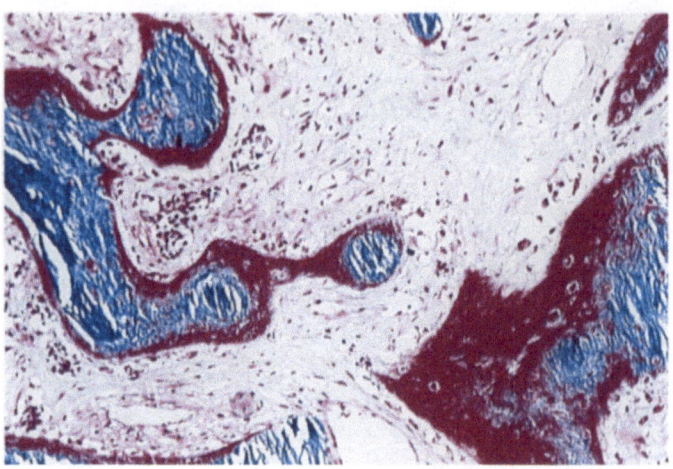

Fig. 10.63 Section from the same biopsy as in Fig. 10.61, showing uncalcified bone (red) and connective tissue with few tumour or haematopoietic cells. Ladewig

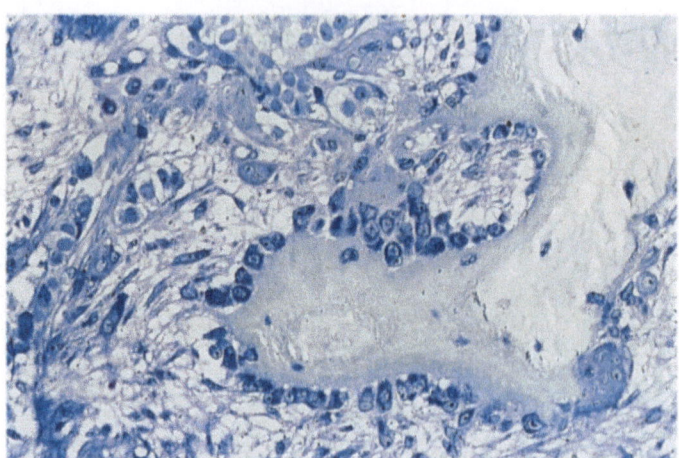

Fig. 10.64 Another area from Fig. 10.61, demonstrating appositional bone formation, osteoclastic resorption and both osteoblasts and osteoclast in the surrounding mesenchyme. Again no tumour cells in the vicinity

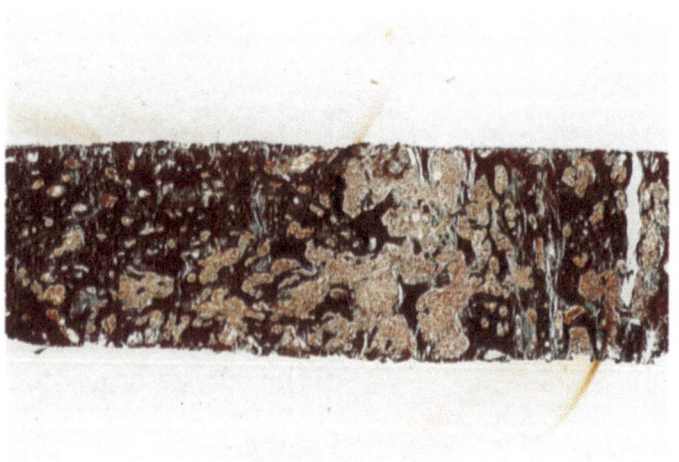

Fig. 10.65 Marked osteosclerosis in metastasis of prostatic carcinoma. Gomori

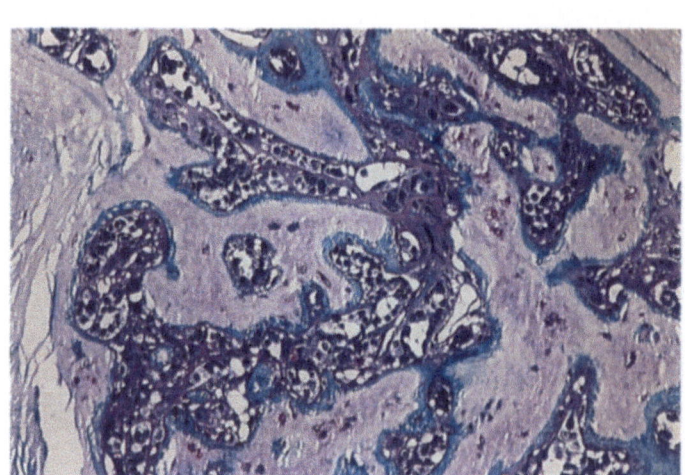

Fig. 10.66 Area from Fig. 10.65. Interosseous areas occupied by tumour cells

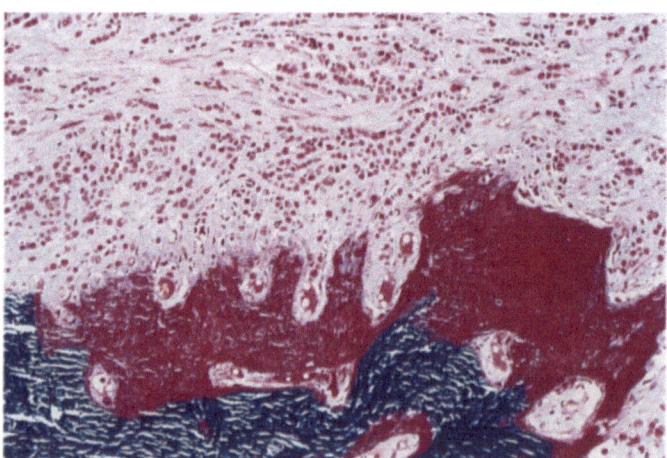

Fig. 10.67 New bone formation in metastasis of mammary carcinoma. Tumour cells within the osteoid (red). Ladewig

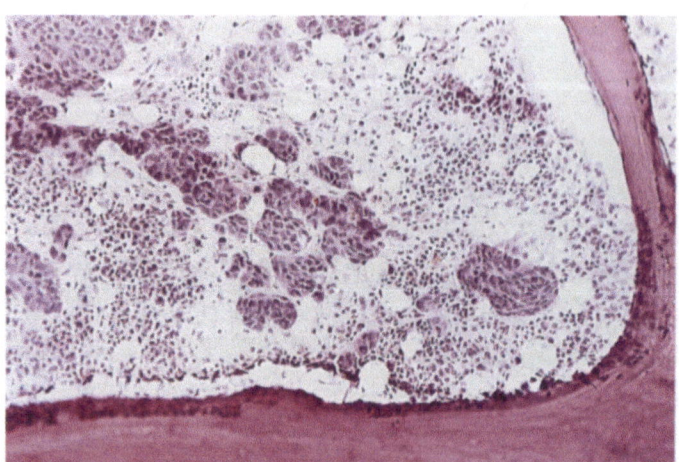

Fig. 10.68 Cryostat section for rapid diagnosis in patient with back pain, suspected metastasis and inconclusive finding on X-ray and bone scan. Multiple tumour clusters in bone marrow, no osseous reaction; carcinoma of lung

especially with involvement of the pelvic lymph nodes (Figs 10.68–10.80)[27–29]. Perineural lymphatic spread, dissemination via the vertebral venous plexus and a vascular route by way of the systemic circulation from secondary deposits in the lungs have all been implicated.

The histological appearance of metastases of prostatic cancer shows a striking variability[12]. Frequently they appear as lobules separated by bands of connective tissue. The lobules may be solid masses or have some glandular structure. The alveolar type is usually composed of small to medium-sized cells, while the medullary type may have pleomorphic anaplastic cells with prominent nuclei. All types have the ability to evoke an osteoblastic reaction, which may lead to marked osteosclerosis with osteomalacia if the newly formed bone is not mineralized. In a few cases, intravascular metastases may be found in an atrophic marrow. Occasionally, the metastases may contain large areas of necrosis.

Breast Cancer

The natural history of breast cancer shows that it encompasses a heterogeneous group of diseases with variable time courses, and although there is undoubtedly a relation between histological classification, including presence or absence of tumour cell markers, grade and 'malignant potential' of breast cancer, clinical trials and therapeutic protocols make no distinction between the different types, and the results are assessed as though 'breast cancer' were a single entity[30]. Some aspect of the histological heterogeneity is reflected in the bone marrow metastases, illustrated in Figs 10.81–10.94.

Breast cancer also has a high incidence of skeletal metastases[31,32]. Metastases of breast cancer may become manifest from one month to many years after surgical removal of the primary tumour, whether or not radio- and/or chemotherapy had been given. This raises the intriguing question of 'dormant metastases' which appear to be kept in check by host defence mechanisms until some event upsets the equilibrium. In experimental animals dormant metastases may be triggered into growth by changes in hormonal or immune status of the host or by surgery.

There is as yet no consensus on the relative merits of X-rays, bone scans or examination of the bone marrow by aspirates from multiple sites, or by bone biopsies, without or with the use of monoclonal antibodies[33–37]. Recent studies indicate that radioimmunoimaging may be a more sensitive method than the conventional bone scan[38]. The distribution of skeletal metastases in advanced breast cancer reflects the distribution of red haematopoietic marrow in the adult skeleton[39].

Pulmonary Cancer

Primary cancer of the lungs is divided into four major groups (each of which has subtypes and variants): (1) squamous cell carcinoma, (2) small cell carcinoma, (3) adenocarcinoma, (4) large cell carcinoma (Figs 10.95–10.99). Metastases, especially of small cell (oat cell) carcinoma, occur in the bones, even from clinically silent primary tumours. Their detection may be facilitated by monoclonal antibodies. Altogether, about 20% of patients are estimated to have bone marrow metastases at diagnosis; this figure rises to 30% with bilateral iliac crest biopsies and to over 40% in anaplastic carcinoma[7,40,41]. On purely histological grounds there may be difficulty in distinguishing involvement by oat-cell carcinoma from a malignant lymphoma. In such cases, immuno-histochemistry may be decisive[42]. Pulmonary cancer is still the cause of about a third of cancer deaths in men, while the incidence in women is increasing, especially in those who smoke.

Gastrointestinal Tumours

Skeletal metastases of gastric and colorectal tumours are probably more frequent than the 20% reported, but no large series have been published (Figs 10.100–10.103).

Carcinoid may metastasize to bones and the tumour cells have a signet-ring-like appearance[43] (Fig. 10.104).

Renal Tumours

Metastases of renal carcinoma (hypernephroma) in the bone marrow often consist of large clear cells with relatively abundant cytoplasm; but other types are encountered also (Figs 10.105 and 10.106). In children skeletal metastases of renal tumours are rare; when present they may cause hypercalcaemia[44].

Malignant Melanoma

If the melanotic granules are present there is no difficulty in recognition of the cells (Figs 10.107–10.109). If not, some cells may still be positive in the Masson Fontana stain. These positive cells do not reveal blue granules in the Prussian blue or other method for demonstration of intracellular iron granules, or haemosiderin. Should the Masson Fontana stain also be negative, demonstration of the presence of a tumour marker such as S100 may be helpful.

Neuroblastoma

A rosette-like arrangement is characteristic for metastases of this tumour. Metastatic neuroblastoma has been described after 52 years of dormancy[45–48].

Medulloblastomas

Metastases may consist of small undifferentiated cells which mimic leukaemic infiltrations in the bone marrow.

Malignant Meningioma

There is complete replacement of the bone marrow, as shown in Figs 10.110 and 10.111.

Haemangiopericytoma

Metastases of this tumour – a form of angioblastic meningioma – may also be found in the pelvic bones. They may look like signet-ring cells, with PAS+ intracellular material.

Rhabdomyosarcoma

Bone marrow metastases were detected in 29% of 103 patients at diagnosis, and this constituted a poor prognostic sign (Figs 10.112–10.114)[49,50].

Kaposi's Sarcoma

This may also involve the bone marrow. It has been reported in patients with AIDS (Fig. 10.115)[51,52].

Metastases in the Bone Marrow of Unknown Primary Tumours and Others

In some cases, the origin of these metastases may be deduced from the clinical picture; in others, if conventional histology is insufficient, the use of monoclonal antibodies may be helpful[53–56]. Bone marrow metastases have also been described in nasopharyngeal carcinoma, intracranial astrocytoma and epithelioid sarcoma[57,58], as well as in many other more common primary tumours (Figs 10.116–10.122).

(Continued on p. 199)

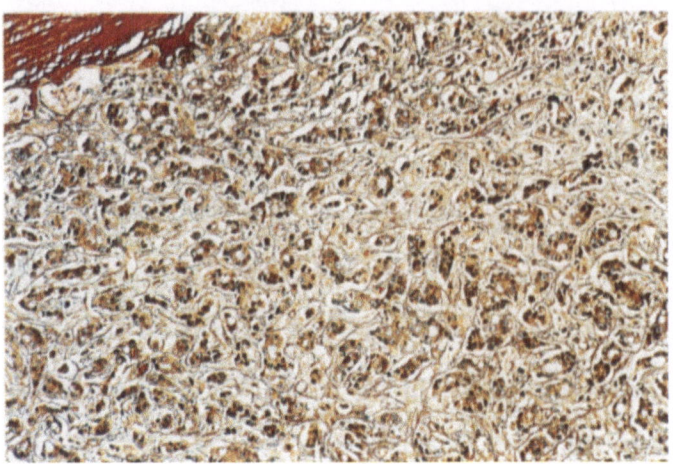

Figs 10.69 to 10.76 Aspects of bone marrow metastasis of prostatic carcinoma

Fig. 10.69 Metastasis consisting of multiple small gland-like structures separated by loose connective tissue stroma. Gomori

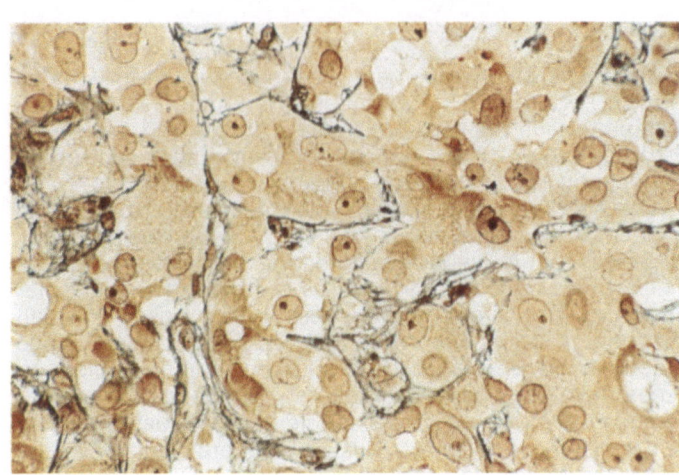

Fig. 10.70 Metastasis with densely packed gland-like structures. Gomori

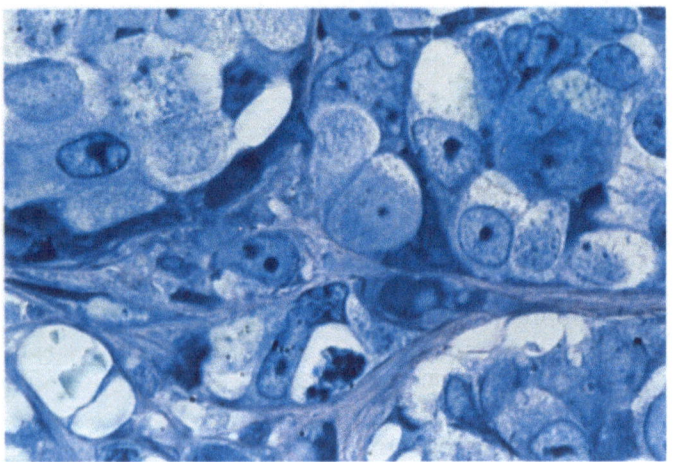

Fig. 10.71 Clusters of large tumour cells with little indication of glandular formation

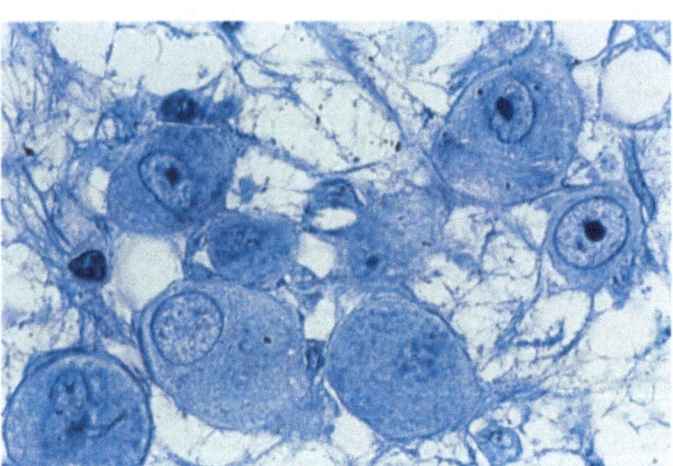

Fig. 10.72 Large anaplastic cell metastasis of prostatic carcinoma. Note prominent nucleoli. This metastasis showed no organization

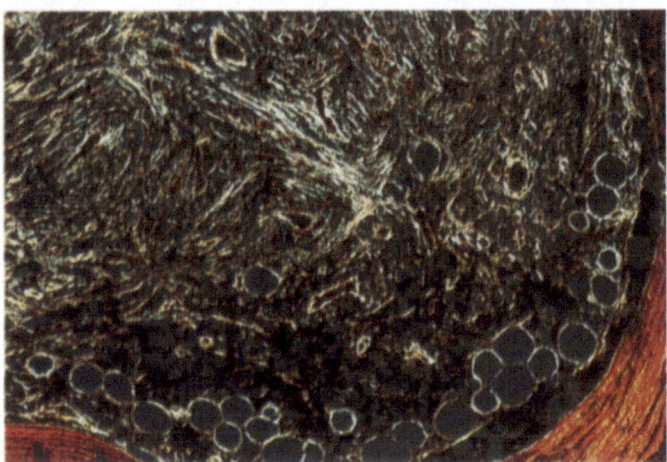

Fig. 10.73 Fibrosis of marrow cavity, residual paratrabecular fat cells, no osseous reaction, no tumour cells identified in this area of bone biopsy. Gomori, polarized light

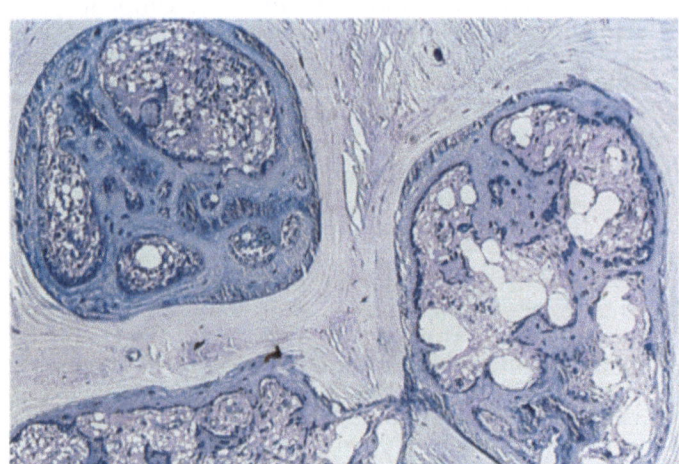

Fig. 10.74 Metastasis of prostatic carcinoma, replacement of marrow cavity by new bone and fibrosis with numerous small clusters of tumour cells

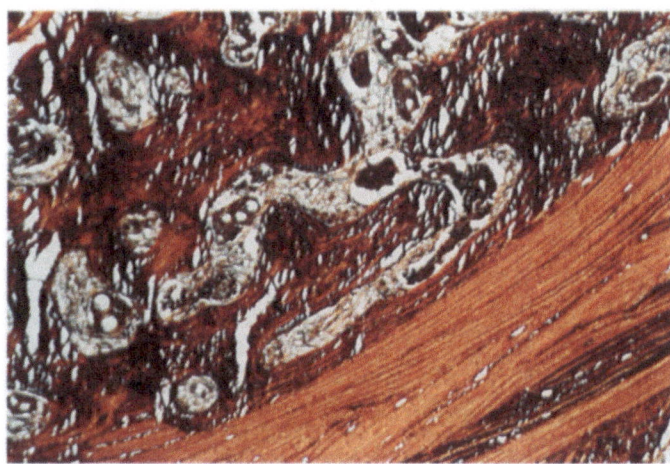

Fig. 10.75 Intravascular tumour cell emboli, marrow cavity replaced by primitive bone and connective tissue. Gomori, polarized light

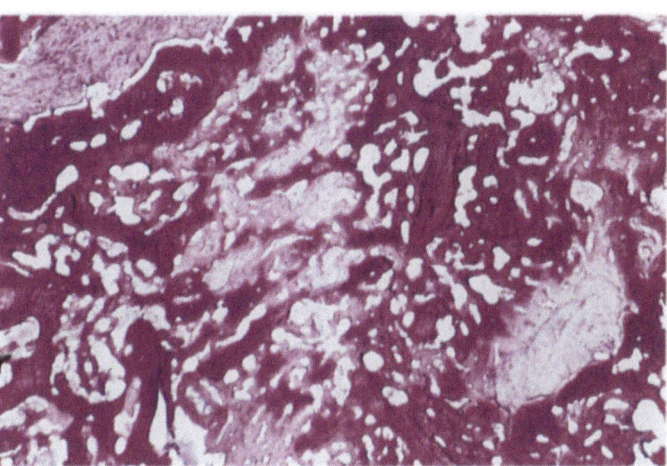

Fig. 10.76 Cryostat section of bone biopsy of elderly patient who presented with pancytopenia. Replacement of bone marrow by osteoblastic metastasis of prostatic carcinoma. H&E

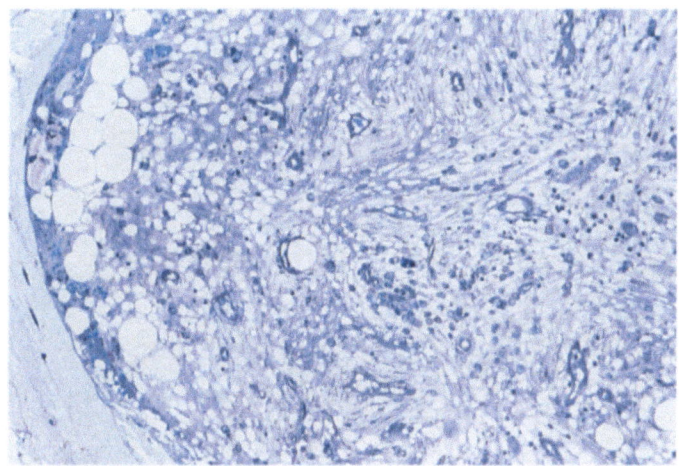

Fig. 10.77 Bone biopsy of patient with prostatic carcinoma after therapy. Oedematous, fibrotic bone marrow with plasmacytic infiltration

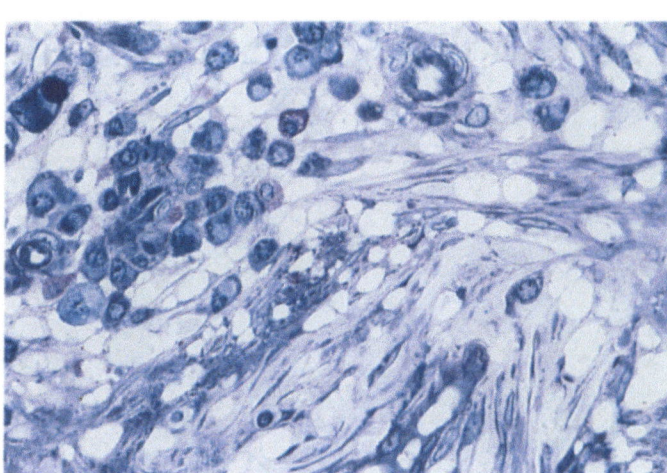

Fig. 10.78 Higher magnification of Fig. 10.77, no tumour cells found in the section, plasmacytic infiltration and mast cells

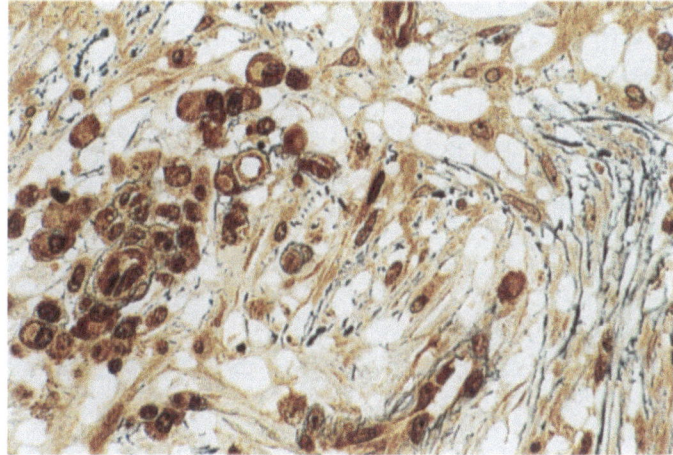

Fig. 10.79 Biopsy section of Fig. 10.77 stained with Gomori, showing fine and coarse fibrosis

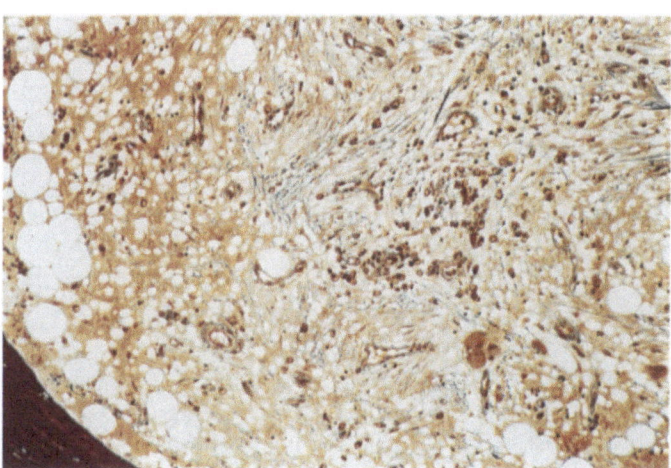

Fig. 10.80 Another section of the same patient as in Fig. 10.77, with similar bone marrow picture but containing isolated residual tumour cells. Gomori

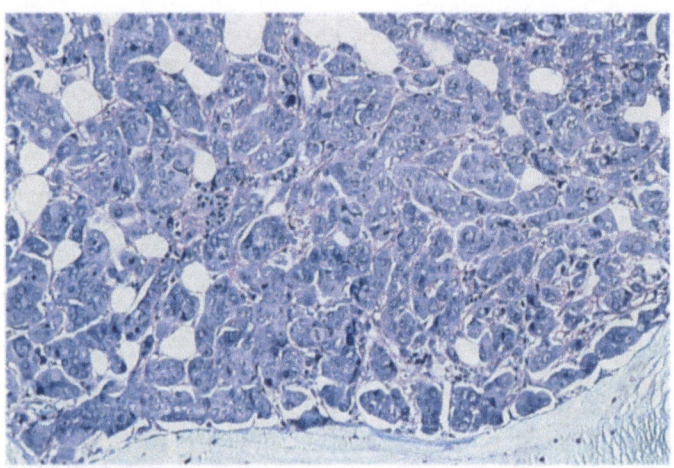

Figs 10.81–10.87 Sections of bone biopsies of patients with mammary carcinoma

Fig. 10.81 Mass of tumour cell clusters, some with gland-like structure, little osseous reaction

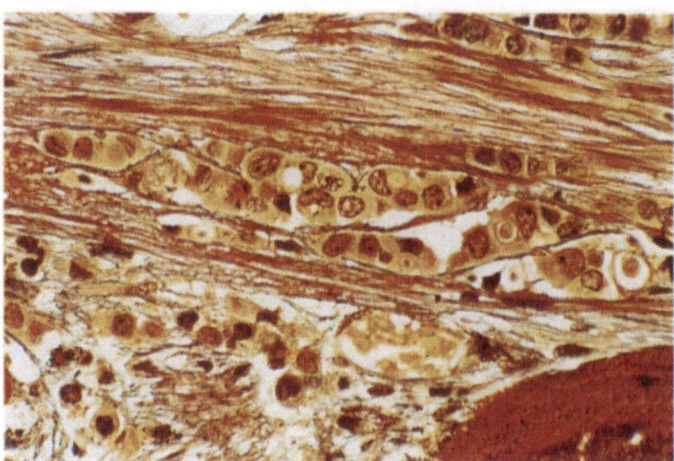

Fig. 10.82 Scirrhous metastasis of mammary carcinoma

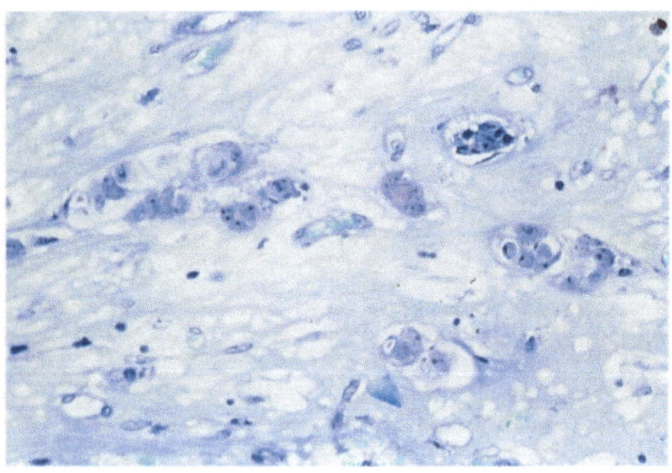

Fig. 10.83 Isolated tumour cells in dense stroma

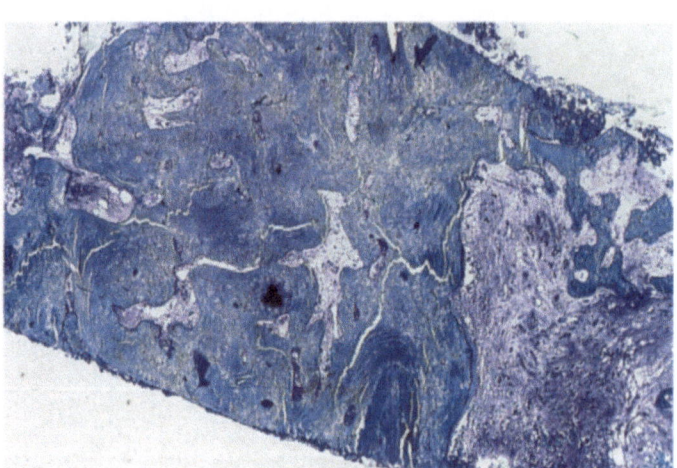

Fig. 10.84 Cortical bone and fibrotic bone marrow

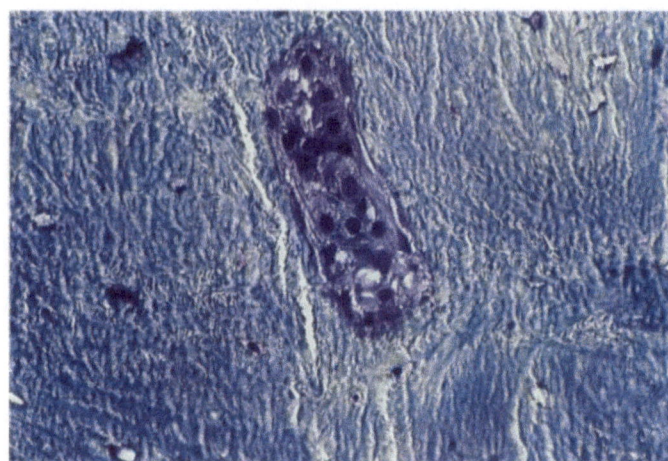

Fig. 10.85 Higher magnification of area of cortical bone in Fig. 10.84, showing metastatic tumour cells in Haversian canal in cortex

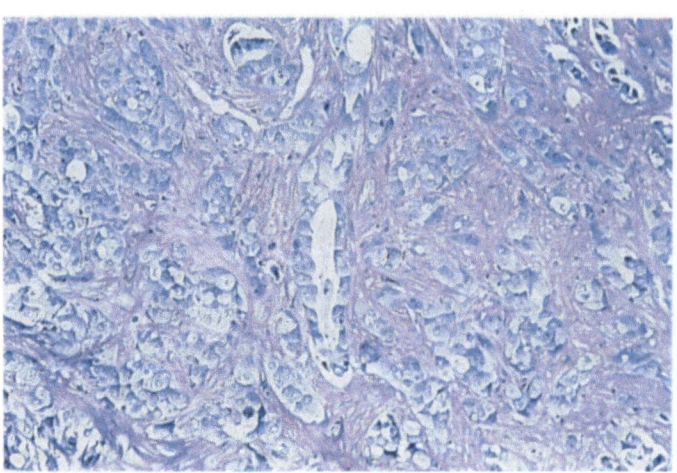

Fig. 10.86 Broad bands of connective tissue separating gland-like structures

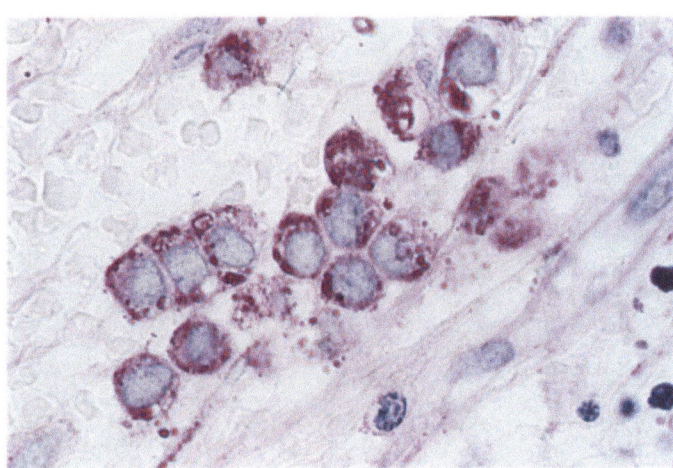

Fig. 10.87 Tumour cells containing PAS-positive secretion. PAS

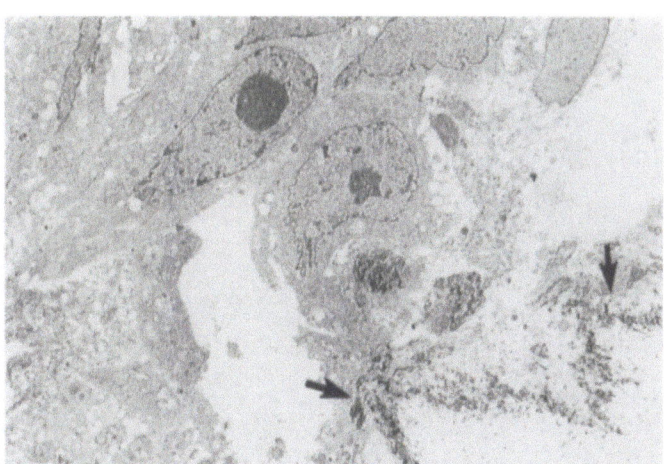

Fig. 10.88 Tumour cells at trabecular surface (arrowed) in bone biopsy of patient with mammary carcinoma. EM × 20 000

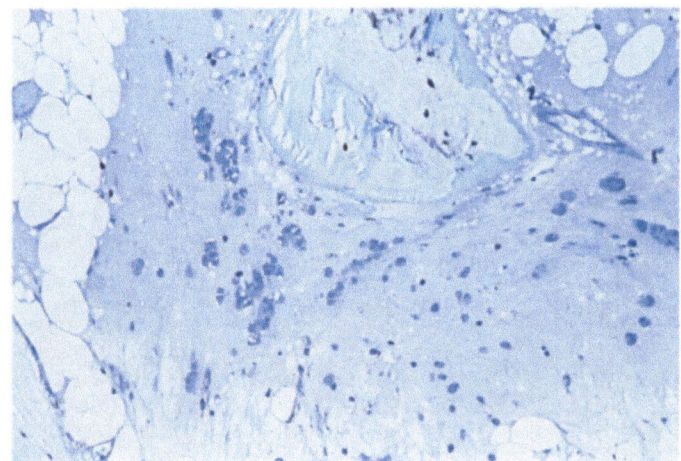

Fig. 10.89 Residual tumour cells in oedematous fibrotic stroma, post-therapy

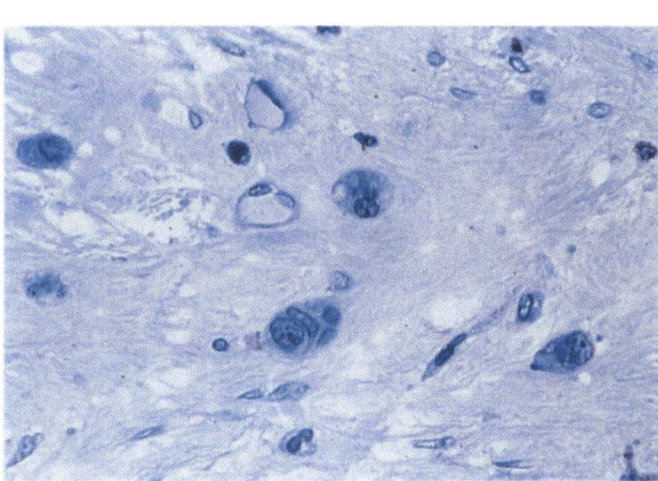

Fig. 10.90 Higher magnification of Fig. 10.88, showing single residual tumour cells

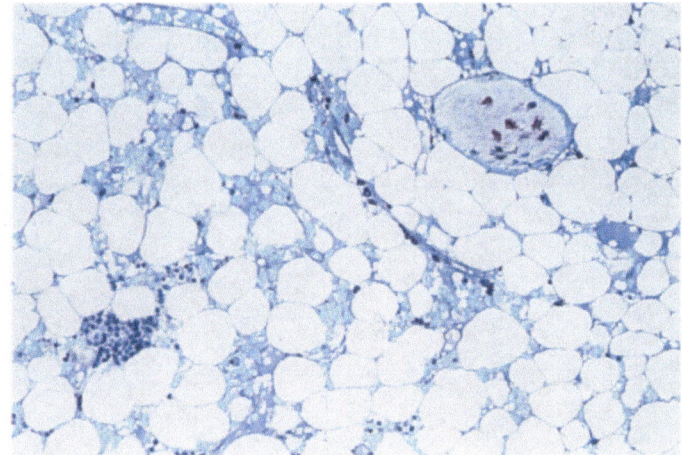

Fig. 10.91 Hypoplastic bone marrow post-therapy, showing neither haematopoiesis nor tumour cells

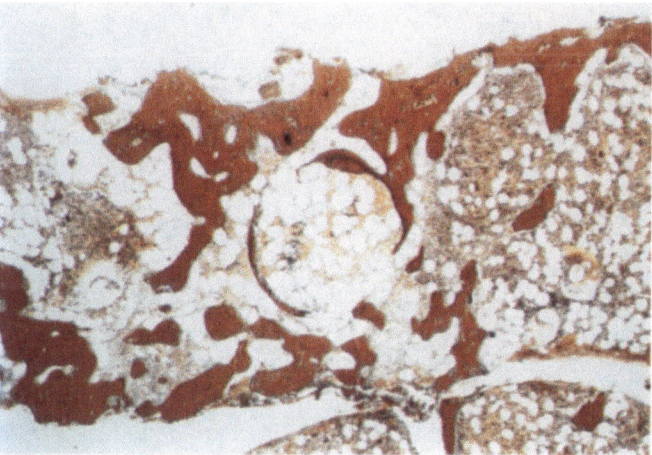

Fig. 10.92 Post-therapy bone marrow of patient with mammary carcinoma, showing fatty tissue in area of previous metastasis as indicated by altered trabecular bone structure. Gomori

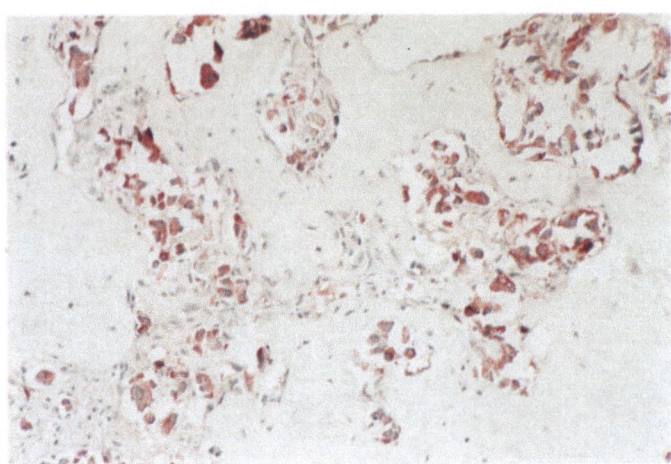

Fig. 10.93 Section of paraffin-embedded bone biopsy of patient with mammary carcinoma. Mainly intravascular tumour cells stained by 'epithelial membrane antigen' (EMA)

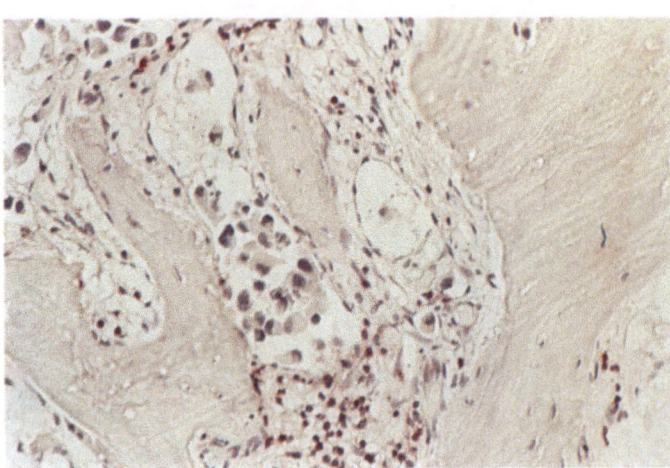

Fig. 10.94 Parallel section to Fig. 10.93 stained with 'common leukocyte antigen' (CLA). Cancer cells are negative, while infiltrating lymphoid cells are positive

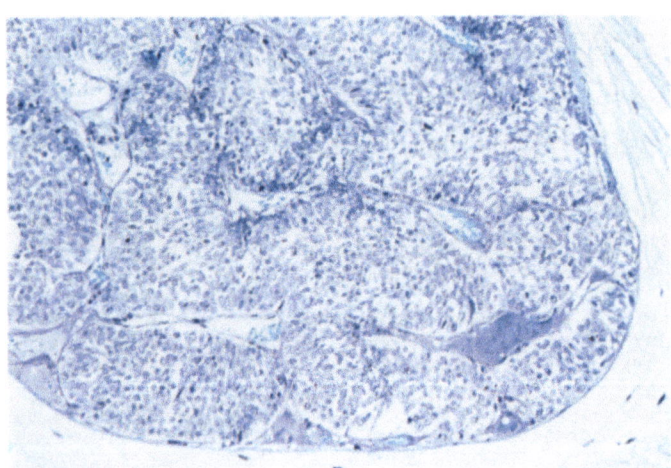

Fig. 10.95 Complete occupation of marrow cavity by oat-cell carcinoma of lung

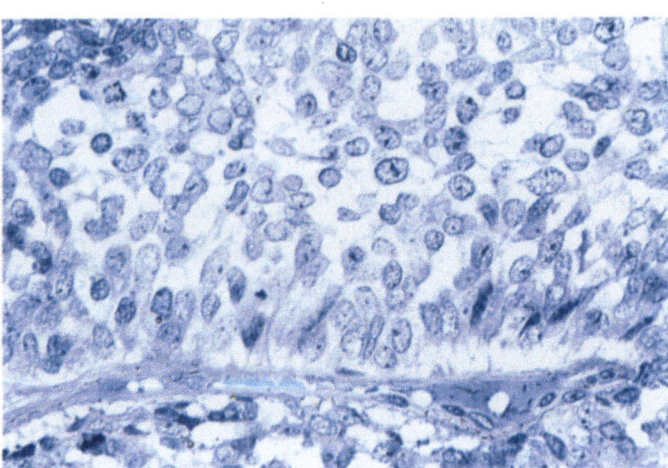

Fig. 10.96 Higher magnification of Fig. 10.95 to show the tumour cells. Note nuclei with very little cytoplasm

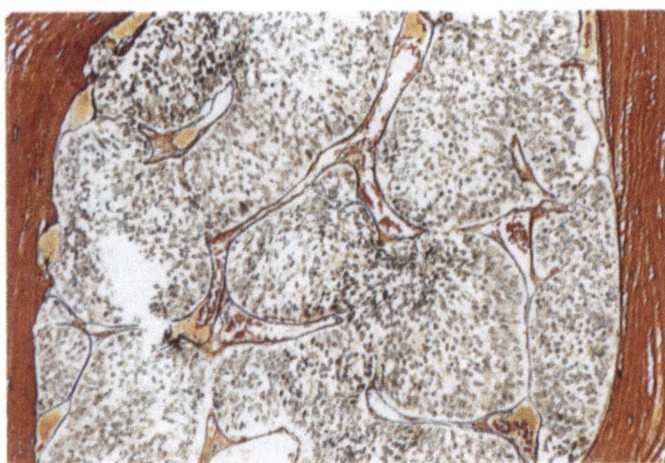

Fig. 10.97 Parallel section to Fig. 10.95 stained by Gomori. Fibres surrounding blood vessels which form septa between tumour cell masses

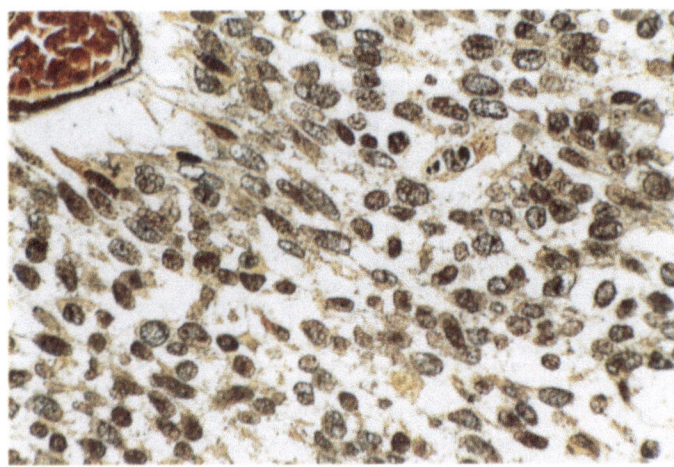

Fig. 10.98 Higher magnification of Fig. 10.97 demonstrating virtual absence of connective tissue within the metastasis. Gomori

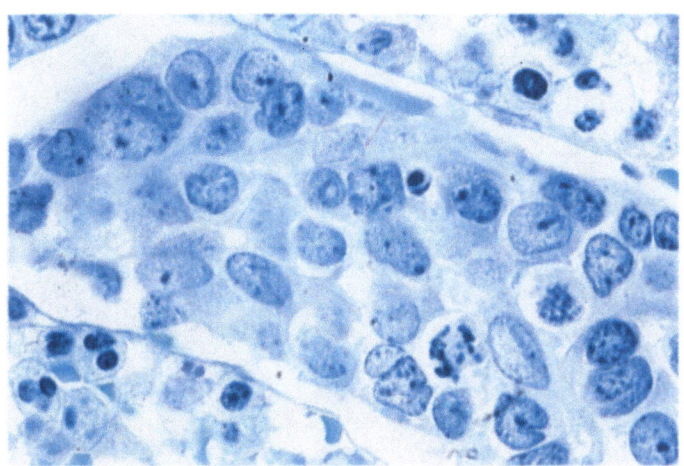

Fig. 10.99 Intravascular metastasis of large cell carcinoma of lung

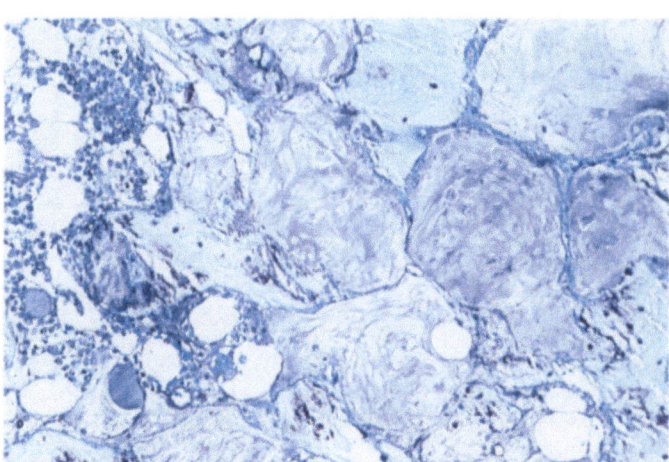

Fig. 10.100 Mucin-secreting metastasis of gastric carcinoma

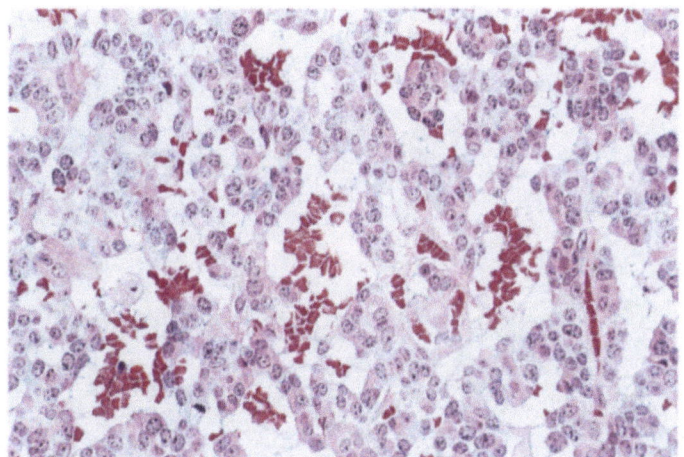

Fig. 10.101 Metastases of gastric carcinoma in bone marrow; little organization or stroma. Ladewig

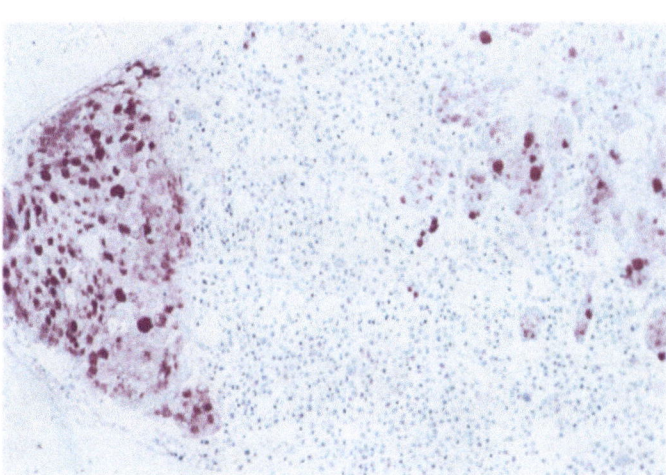

Fig. 10.102 Large and small clusters of tumour cells in bone marrow, many with abundant cytoplasmic PAS-positive secretion; gastric carcinoma. PAS

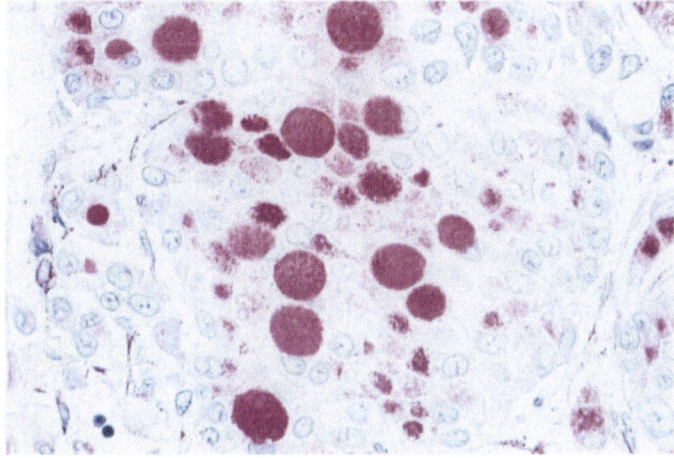

Fig. 10.103 Higher magnification of Fig. 10.102 to show large cytoplasmic droplets of PAS-positive secretion. PAS

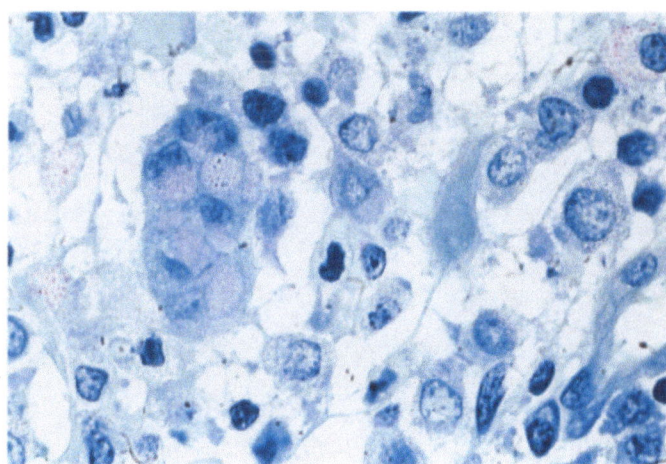

Fig. 10.104 Tumour cell embolus in bone marrow of patient with carcinoid

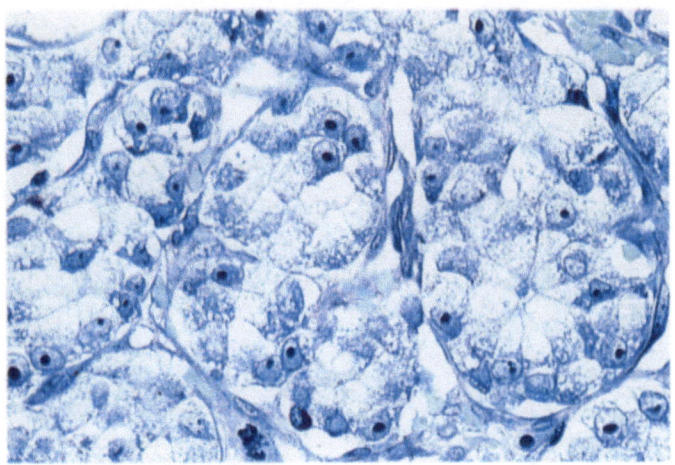

Fig. 10.105 Bone marrow metastasis of renal clear cell carcinoma

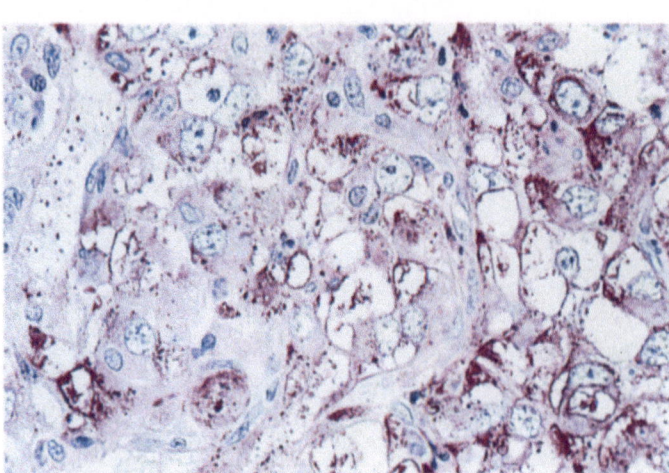

Fig. 10.106 Metastasis of large cell renal carcinoma with PAS-positive inclusions. PAS

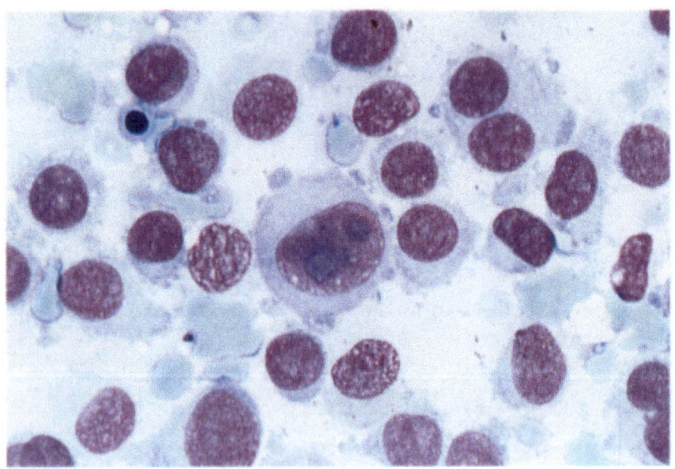

Fig. 10.107 Aspirate smear of patient with malignant melanoma

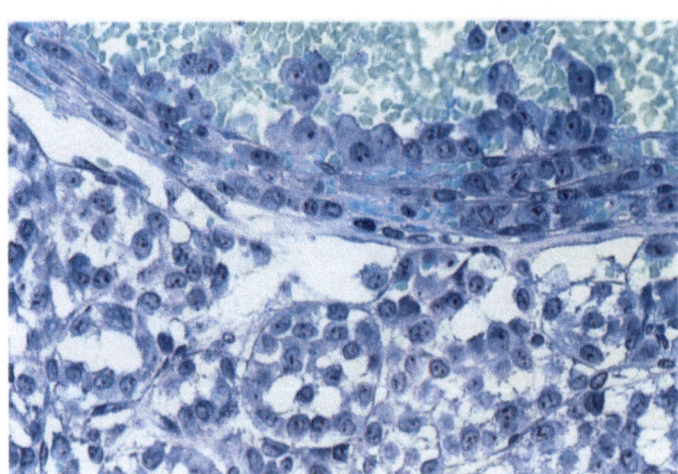

Fig. 10.108 Part of bone biopsy section showing replacement of marrow by the malignant cells. Vascular channel lined by malignant cells

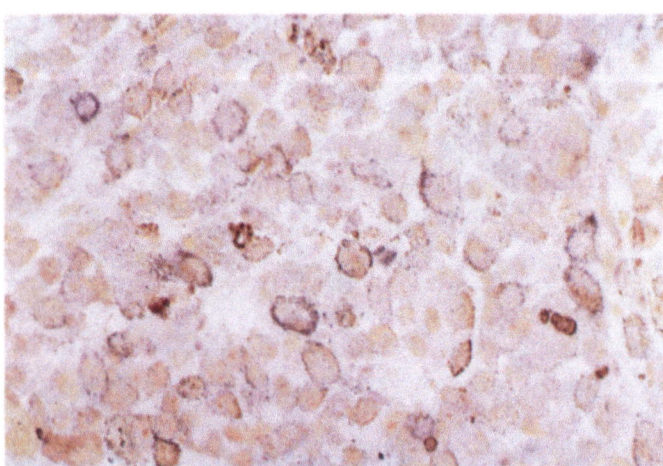

Fig. 10.109 Parallel section to that shown in Fig. 10.108, stained by Fontana stain for demonstration of melanin granules

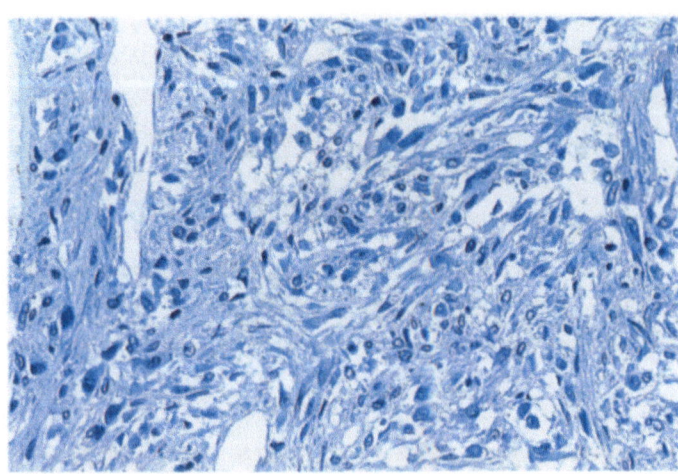

Fig. 10.110 Bone biopsy of patient with malignant meningioma; complete replacement of the marrow

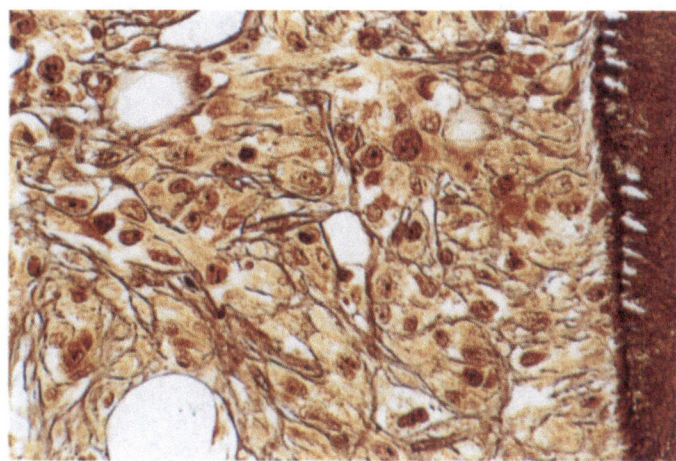

Fig. 10.111 Parallel section to that shown in Fig. 10.110, stained by Gomori, showing clusters of tumour cells surrounded by fibres

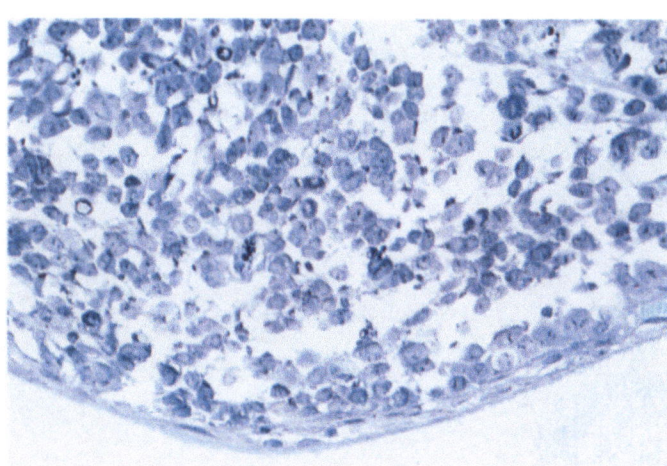

Fig. 10.112 Bone biopsy of patient with rhabdomyosarcoma. Bone marrow replacement with solid masses of tumour cells

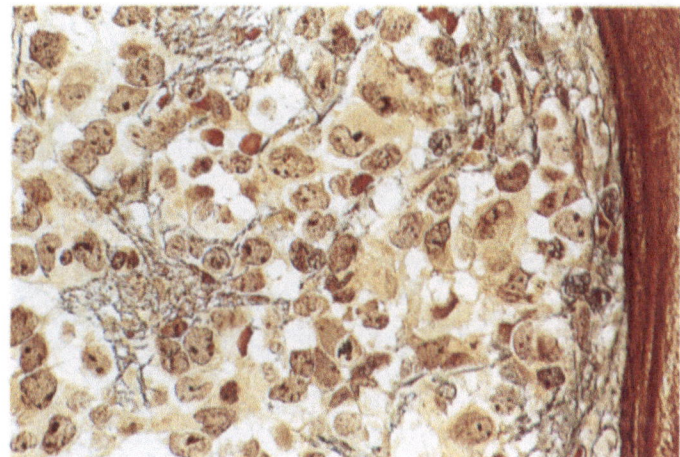

Fig. 10.113 Higher magnification of Fig. 10.112, demonstrating polymorphic tumour cell nuclei and little intercellular connective tissue. Gomori

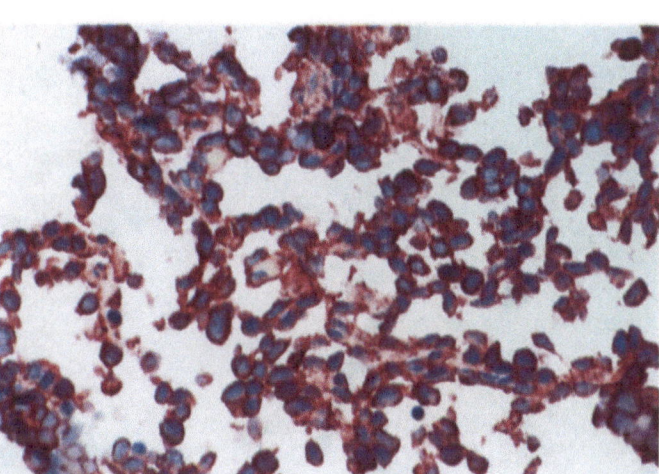

Fig. 10.114 Cryostat section of bone biopsy of patient with rhabdomyosarcoma, stained with antibody to desmin

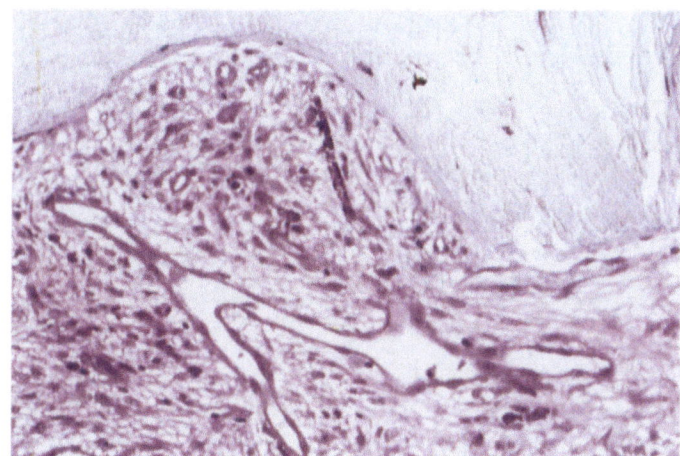

Fig. 10.115 Bone biopsy of patient with Kaposi's sarcoma. There was complete replacement of the marrow

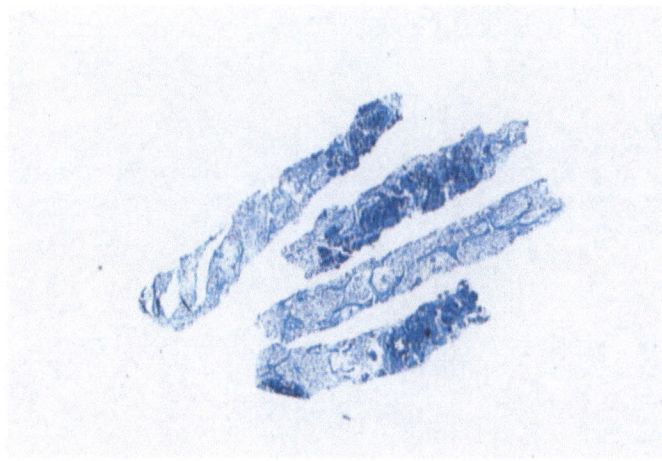

Fig. 10.116 Bone biopsy of patient with unknown primary tumour. Two cylinders which were cut in half, partial involvement in three pieces and none in one

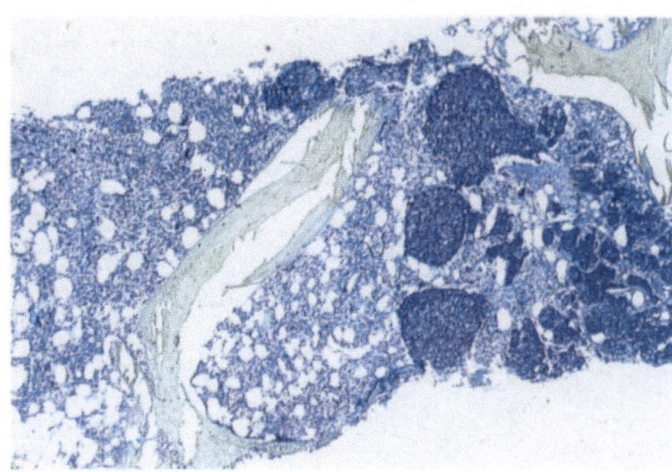

Fig. 10.117 Higher magnification of Fig. 10.116, showing tumour cells in marrow

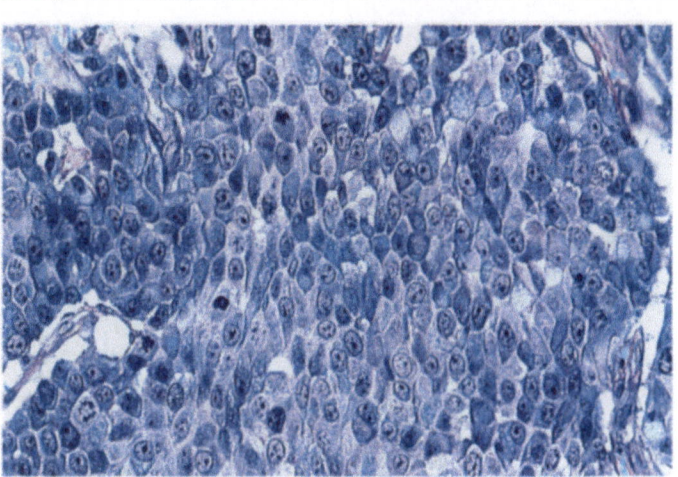

Fig. 10.118 Higher magnification of Fig. 10.116, demonstrating solid mass of monomorphic tumour cells. Note mitotic figures

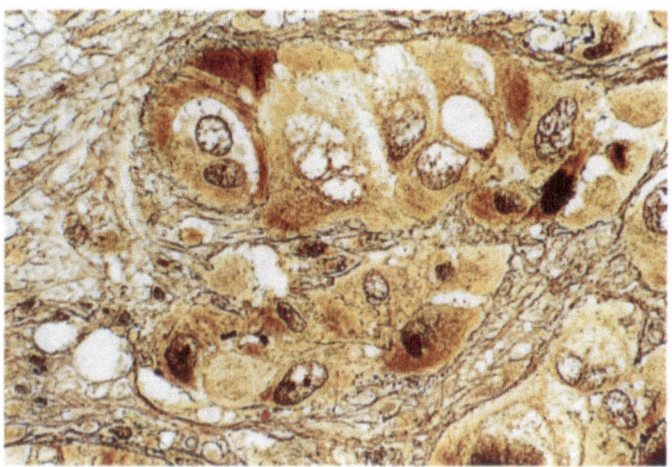

Fig. 10.119 Anaplastic metastasis in bone biopsy of patient with unknown primary tumour. Gomori

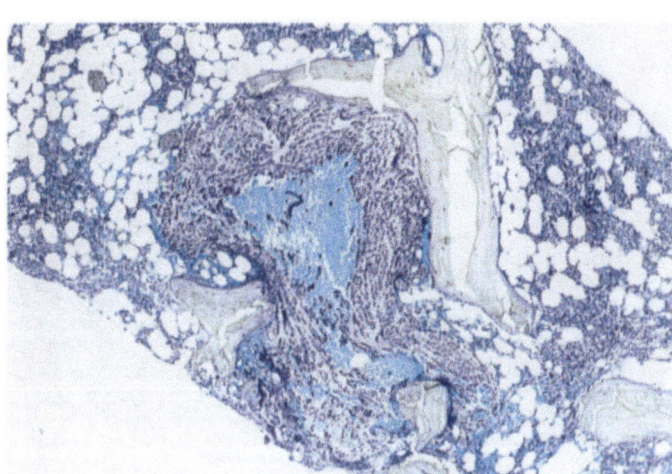

Fig. 10.120 Bone marrow involvement by metastasis of neuroectodermal tumour, initially diagnosed as of unknown primary tumour. The metastasis forms a wide vascular channel lined by the neoplastic cells

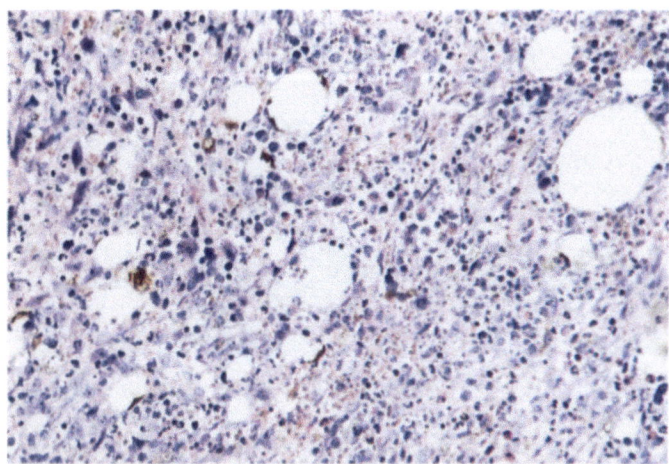

Fig. 10.121 Section of paraffin-embedded bone biopsy of 47-year-old patient with low back pain and multiple osteolytic lesions on X-ray. Found to have multicentre haemangiosarcoma; section showing bone marrow involvement

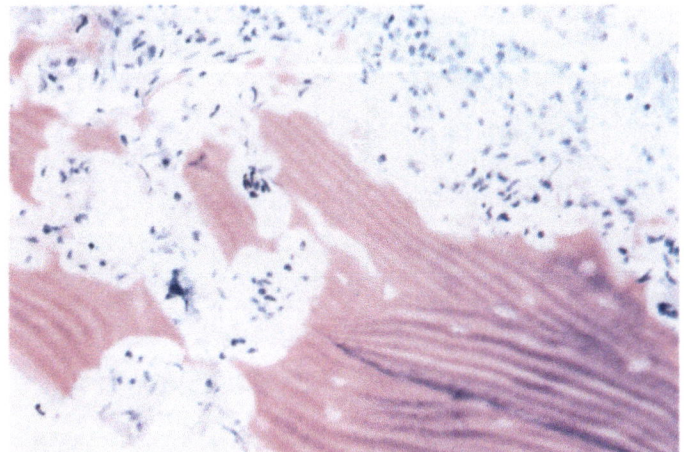

Fig. 10.122 As Fig. 10.121, showing osetolytic lesion. H&E

References

1. Weiss, L. and Gilbert, H. A. (eds) (1981). *Bone Metastasis*, Boston: G. K. Hall Medical Publishers
2. Frisch, B., Bartl, R., Burkhardt, R. (1982). Bone marrow biopsy in clinical medicine: an overview. *Haematologia*, **3**, 245
3. Frisch, B., Bartl, R., Mahl, G. and Burkhardt, R. (1984). Scope and value of bone marrow biopsies in metastatic cancer. *Invasion Metastasis*, **4**, (Suppl. 1), 12
4. Frisch, B., Lewis, S. M., Burkhardt, R. and Bartl, R. (1985). *Biopsy Pathology of Bone and Bone Marrow*. London: Chapman and Hall
5. Scanlon, E. F. (1985). The process of metastasis. *Cancer*, **55**, 1166
6. Poste, G. (1986). Pathogenesis of metastatic disease: implications for current therapy and for the development of new therapeutic strategies. *Cancer Treat. Reports*, **70**, 183
7. Schlimok, G., Funke, I., Holzmann, B., Gottlinger, G., Schmidt, G., Hauser, H., Swierkot, S., Warnecke, H. H., Scheider, B., Koprowski, H. *et al.* (1987). Micrometastatic cancer cells in bone marrow: in vitro detection with anti-cytokeratin and in vivo labeling with anti-17-1A monoclonal antibodies. *Proc. Natl. Acad. Sci. USA*, **84**, 8672
8. Pignon, T., Ralantoarimihanta, M., Vicens, R. and Coulanges, P. (1987). Bone marrow examination in cancerology. Apropos of 92 marrow biopsies performed at the Antananarivo Hemato-cancerology Service. *Arch. Inst. Pasteur-Madagascar*, **53**, 157
9. Wang, J. M., Shih, L. Y., Lai, G. M. and Ng, K. T. (1987). Bone marrow metastases from solid tumours – clinical analysis of 96 cases. *Chang. Keng. I. Hseuh*, **10**, 283
10. Favrot, M. C. and Herve, P. (1987). Detection of minimal malignant cell infiltration in the bone marrow of patients with solid tumours, non-Hodgkin lymphomas and leukaemias. *Bone Marrow Transplant*, **2**, 117
11. Im, T., Yamane, T., Sagawa, H., Hiyoshi, M., Kishida, T., Sasaki, A., Yokomatsu, Y., Kojima, K., Sannomiya, Y., Yoshikawa, T. *et al.* (1987). Clinicopathological study of cancer metastasis to bone marrow by bone marrow biopsy. *Rinsho. Byori*, **35**, 1292
12. Schnippen, L. E. (1986). Clinical implications of tumour-cell heterogeneity. *N. Engl. J. Med.*, **314**, 1423
13. Al-Mondhiry, H. and McGarvey, V. (1987). Tumour interaction with vascular endothelium. *Haemostasis*, **17**, 245
14. Castello, A., Coci, A., Magnini, U. and Ascari, E. (1986). Histopathology of bone marrow metastases. Considerations on 104 cases. *Haematologia*, **71**, 369
15. Willis, R. A. (1973). *The Spread of Tumours in the Human Body*, London: Butterworths
16. Henson, D. E. (1988). The histological grading of neoplasms. *Arch. Pathol., Lab. Med.*, **112**, 1091
17. Dvorak, H. F. (1986). Tumours: wounds that do not heal. Similarities between tumor stroma generation and wound healing. *N. Engl. J. Med.*, **315**, 1650
18. Sporn, M. B. and Roberts, A. B. (1986). Peptide growth factors and inflammation, tissue repair, and cancer. *J. Clin. Invest.*, **78**, 329
19. Roche, W. R. (1985). Mast cells and tumours. The specific enhancement of tumour proliferation in vitro. *Am. J. Pathol.*, **119**, 57
20. Roche, W. R. (1985). Mast cells and tumour angiogenesis: the tumour-mediated release of an endothelial growth factor from mast cells. *Int. J. Cancer*, **36**, 721
21. Knupp, C., Pekala, P. H. and Cornelius, P. (1988). Extensive bone marrow necrosis in patients with cancer and tumor necrosis factor activity in plasma. *Am. J. Haematol.*, **29**, 215
22. Burtis, W. J., Wu, R. L., Insogna, K. L. and Stewart, A. F. (1988). Humoral hypercalcemia of malignancy. *Ann. Intern. Med.*, **108**, 454
23. Broadus, A. E., Mangin, M., Ikeda, K., Insogna, K. L., Weir, E. C., Burtis, W. J. and Stewart, A. F. (1988). Humoral hypercalcemia of cancer. Identification of a novel parathyroid hormone-like peptide. *N. Engl. J. Med.*, **318**, 556
24. Elomas, I., Blomqvist, C., Porkka, L., Lamberg-Allandt, C. and Borgstrom, G. H. (1987). Treatment of skeletal disease in breast cancer: a controlled clodronate trial. *Bone*, **8**, (Suppl. 1), S53
25. Canfield, R. E., Sirus, E. S. and Jacobs, T. P. (1987). Dichloromethylene disphosphonate action in hematological and other malignancies. *Bone*, **8**, (Suppl. 1), S57
26. Morton, A. R., Cantrill, J. A., Pillai, G. V., McMahon, A., Anderson, D. C. and Howell, A. (1988). Sclerosis of lytic bone metastases after disodium aminohydroxypropylidene bisphosphonate (ADP) in patients with breast carcinoma. *Br. Med. J.*, **297**, 772
27. Editorial, anonymous (1985). Dilemmas in the management of prostatic carcinoma. *Lancet*, **2**, 1219
28. Patenson, A. H. G. (1987). Bone metastases in breast cancer, prostate cancer and myeloma. *Bone*, **8** (Suppl. 1), S17
29. Soloway, M. S., Hardeman, S. W., Hickey, D., Raymond, J., Todd, B., Soloway, S. and Moinuddin, M. (1988). Stratification of patients with metastatic prostate cancer based on extent of disease on initial bone scan. *Cancer*, **61**, 195
30. Berger, U., Bettelheim, R., Mansi, J. L., Easton, D., Coombes, R. C. and Munro Neville, A. (1988). The relationship between micrometastases in the bone marrow, histopathologic features of the primary tumor in breast cancer and prognosis. *Am. J. Clin. Pathol.*, **90**, 1
31. Mansi, J. L., Berger, U., Easton, D., McDonnell, T., Redding, W. H., Gazet, J.-C., McKinna, A., Powles, T. J. and Coombes, F. C. (1987). Micrometastases in bone marrow in patients with primary breast cancer: evaluation as an early prediction of bone metastases. *Br. Med. J.*, **295**, 1093
32. Zajicek, G. (1987). Long survival with micrometastasis. At least 9% of breast cancer patients carry metastases for more than 10 years. *Cancer J.*, **1**, 381
33. Ceci, G., Franciosi, V., Nizzoli, R., De Lisi, V., Lottici, R., Boni, C., Di Blasio, B., Passalacqua, R., Guazzi, A. and Cocconi, G. (1988). The value of bone marrow biopsy in breast cancer at time of diagnosis. A prospective study. *Cancer*, **61**, 96
34. Untch, M., Harbeck, N. and Eiermann, W. (1988). Micrometastases in bone marrow in patients with breast cancer. *Br. Med. J.*, **296**, 290
35. Kamby, C., Guldhamer, B., Vejborg, I., Rossing, N., Dirksen, H., Daugaard, S. and Mouridsen, H. T. (1987). The presence of tumor cells in bone marrow at the time of first recurrence of breast cancer. *Cancer*, **60**, 1306
36. Manegold, C., Krempien, B., Kaufmann, M., Schwechheimer, K. and Schettler, G. (1988). The value of bone marrow examination for tumor staging in breast cancer. *J. Cancer Res. Clin. Oncol.*, **114**, 425
37. Porro, G., Menard, S., Tagliabue, E., Orefice, S., Salvadori, B., Squicciarini, P., Amdreola, S., Rilke, F. and Colnaghi, M. I. (1988). Monoclonal antibody detection of carcinoma cells in bone marrow biopsy specimens from breast cancer patients. *Cancer*, **61**, 2407
38. Reske, S. N., Gloekner, W., Schwarz, A., Karstens, J. H., Steinstrasser, A. and Ammon, J. (1989). Radioimmunoimaging for diagnosis of bone marrow involvement in breast cancer and malignant lymphoma. *Lancet*, **1**(8633), 299
39. Coleman, R. E. and Rubens, R. D. (1985). Bone metastases and breast cancer. *Cancer Treat. Rev.*, **12**, 251
40. Clamon, G. H., Edwards, W. R., Hamous, J. E. and Scupham, R. K. (1984). Patterns of bone marrow involvement with small cell lung cancer. *Cancer*, **54**, 100
41. Stahel, R. A., Mabry, M., Skarin, A. T., Speak, J. and Bernal, S. D. (1985). Detection of bone marrow metastasis in small-cell lung cancer by monoclonal antibody. *J. Clin. Oncol.*, **3**, 455
42. Battifora, H. and Silva, E. G. (1986). The use of antikeratin antibodies in the immunohistochemical distinction between neuroendocrine (Merkel Cell) carcinoma of the skin, lymphoma, and oat cell carcinoma. *Cancer*, **58**, 1040
43. Ariza, A., Bitterman, P. and Nash, I. (1986). Diagnosis of intestinal carcinoid tumor by bone marrow biopsy. *Connecticut Med.*, **50**, 307
44. Jayabose, S., Iqbal, K., Newman, L., San Filippo, J. A., Davidian, M. M., Noto, R. and Sagel, I. (1988). Hypercalcemia in childhood renal tumors. *Cancer*, **61**, 788
45. Bostrom, B., Nesbit, M. E. Jr and Brunning, R. D. (1985). The value of bone marrow trephine biopsy in the diagnosis of metastatic neuroblastoma. *Am. J. Pediatr. Hematol. Oncol.*, **7**, 303
46. Kushner, B. H., Helson, L., Lane, J. M. and Hadju, S. L. (1986). Metastatic neuroblastoma after 52 years of apparent dormancy. *N. Engl. J. Med.*, **315**, 196
47. Favrot, M. C., Frappaz, D., Maritaz, O., Philip, I., Fontaniere, B., Gentihomme, O., Bailly, C., Zucker, J. M., Gentet, J. C., Kemshead, J. *et al.* (1986). Histological, cytological and immunological analyses are complementary for the detection of neuroblastoma cells in bone marrow. *Br. J. Cancer*, **54**, 637
48. Reid, M. M. and Hamilton, P. J. (1988). Histology of neuroblastoma involving bone marrow: the problem of detecting residual tumour after initiation of chemotherapy. *Br. J. Haematol.*, **69**, 487
49. Javier de la Serna, F., Matrinez, M. A., Valdes, M. D., Hornedo, J., Mestre, M. J. and Morales, J. M. (1988). Rhabdomyosarcoma presenting with diffuse bone marrow involvement, hypercalcemia and renal failure. *Med. Pediat. Oncol.*, **16**, 123
50. Ruymann, F. B., Newton, W. A., Ragab, A. H., Donaldson, M. H. and Foulkes, M. (1984). Bone marrow metastases at diagnosis in children and adolescents with rhabdomyosarcoma. A report from the Intergroup Rhabdomyocarcoma Study. *Cancer*, **53**, 368
51. Conran, R. M., Granger, E. and Reddy, V. B. (1986). Koposi's sarcoma of the bone marrow. *Arch. Pathol. Lab. Med.*, **110**, 1083
52. Little, B. J., Spivak, J. L., Quinn, T. C. and Mann, R. B. (1986).

Kaposi's sarcoma with bone marrow involvement: occurrence in a patient with acquired immunodeficiency syndrome. *Am. J. Med. Sci.,* **292**, 44

53. Gatten, K. C., Heryet, A., Alcok, C. and Mason, D. Y. (1985). Clinical importance of analysing malignant tumours of uncertain origin with immunohistological technique. *Lancet,* **1**(8441), 1302

54. Simon, M. A. and Bartucci, E. J. (1986). The search for the primary tumor in patients with skeletal metastases of unknown origin. *Cancer,* **58**, 1088

55. Ringenberg, Q. S., Doll, D. C., Yarbro, J. W. and Perry, M. C. (1986). Tumors of unknown origin in the bone marrow. *Arch. Intern. Med.,* **146**, 2027

56. Micheau, C., Boussen, H., Klinjanienko, J., Cvikovic, E., Stosic, S., Schwaab, G., Eschwege, F. and Armand, J. P. (1987). Bone marrow biopsies in patients with undifferentiated carcinoma of the nasopharyngeal type. *Cancer,* **60**, 2459

57. LoRusso, P. M., Tapazoglou, E., Zarbo, R. J., Cullis, P. A., Austin, D. and Al-Sarraf, M. (1988). Intracranial astrocytoma with diffuse bone marrow metastasis: a case report and review of the literature. *J. Neurooncol.,* **6**, 53

58. Rosenberg, A. E., Garber, J. E., Bennett, W., Bhan, A. K., Antman, K. H. and Mark, E. J. (1988). Epithelioid sarcoma with diffuse bone marrow metastases and associated leukemoid reaction. A case report and brief literature review. *Am. J. Clin. Pathol.,* **90**, 723

Bone Marrow in Osteopathies

11

Bone marrow and bone are closely interrelated, and disorders of the one invariably affect the other to a lesser or greater degree: for example osteolysis in multiple myeloma or anaemia in osteopetrosis[1]. However, it is beyond the scope of this atlas to deal extensively with osteopathies, only a few examples in which bone marrow changes are prominent will be mentioned briefly.

Osteoporotic Syndromes

Physiological or age-related osteoporosis; i.e. post-menopausal in females and senile in both sexes (Figures 11.1–11.13)[2-10]. These syndromes are characterized by trabecular osteopenia, and in iliac crest biopsies may be accompanied by a reduction in haematopoietic marrow and an increase in fat cells, especially in older individuals[11]. Three types of histological osteopenia (osteoporosis) have been described[12]: Type I – trabecular osteopenia with decreased osteoblasts, osteoclasts and osteoid seams; Type II – trabecular osteopenia with increased osteoclasts; usually flat acid-phosphatase-positive cells closely apposed to the surface of attenuated trabeculae, without the presence of erosions or Howship's lacunae. Type III is the so-called poromalacia, in which the osteopenic trabecular bone is lined by thin extensive osteoid seams. Whatever the putative mechanisms of age-related decrease of trabecular bone may be, the results reflect the inability of bone formation to replace bone lost by resorption. This has been underlined by the efficacy of calcitonin in preventing post-menopausal bone loss by its inhibitory effect on osteoclasts[13]. The replacement by fat cells of haematopoietic marrow in skeletal regions which are prone to fractures in the elderly may also be a contributory pathogenic factor[14]. Osteoporosis is a major, but not the sole, cause of fractures in the elderly. However, trabecular osteopenia also occurs in many other situations and the state of the bone marrow depends on the condition with which the osteopenia is associated, for example, hyper- or hypothyroidism, and increased production or administration of steroids as in patients with asthma or rheumatoid arthritis. The latter itself may give rise to osteolytic lesions[15,16].

Osteodystrophies

In these there is a lack of balance between bone resorption and bone formation which results in alterations of the normal trabecular architecture (Figures 11.14–11.29). Some degree of osteomalacia – i.e. increased osteoid – is present in nearly all cases of osteodystrophy. Increased osseous remodelling and activation of osteoclasts and osteoblasts is accompanied by paratrabecular fibrosis and vascular proliferation in the affected areas. This fibrosis may be extensive and may partly replace the haematopoietic elements. Classic examples are primary and secondary hyperparathyroidism. If a bone biopsy is taken from a focus of osseous remodelling during an active phase of the disease, there may be no residual haematopoiesis, the intertrabecular areas being filled with vascular connective tissue, infiltrated by lymphocytes, plasma cells, macro-

phages and mast cells. In primary hyperparathyroidism brown tumours may be found: aggregates of osteoclasts and haemosiderin-laden macrophages within a fibrotic stroma. In renal osteodystrophy the reduction in haematopoiesis and the inhibition of erythropoiesis contribute to the anaemia of chronic renal disease.

Paget's Disease of Bone

This occurs mainly in adults, with the incidence rising in the older age groups (Figures 11.30–11.35). There is focal involvement of the skeleton, with great variability in extension. Monostotic and polyostotic forms have been described. Recent evidence suggests that 'familial chronic hyper-phosphatasemia' represents the childhood form of Paget's disease. A disease of osteoclasts, it is characterized by greatly increased osteoclastic and osteoblastic remodelling accompanied by paratrabecular fibrosis, reduction of the marrow cavities and of haematopoiesis in the affected areas, and frequently associated with anaemia. Paget's disease of bone is now thought to be due to a slow viral infection of osteoclasts[18]. In 72% of patients there is involvement of the pelvic bones.[19]

Osteopetrosis

Three forms have been described – the early congenital, the intermediate and the late (Figures 11.36 and 11.37)[20]. Osteopetrosis results from a congenital defect of osteoclasts which cannot resorb bone. Hence there is progressive thickening of both cancellous and cortical bone leading to progressive diminution of the marrow cavities, with resulting reduction in haematopoiesis as well as neurological and other complications. Of the three forms described, that occurring in infancy is rapidly fatal, though recently patients have had repopulation and restoration of normal osteoclast function by means of compatible bone marrow transplantation and development of donor osteoclasts. The other two forms are relatively benign. The osteosclerosis that occurs in the course of other conditions – for example in Paget's disease, in the myeloproliferative disorders, in osteosclerotic metastases – are dealt with in the appropriate sections.

Fibrous Dysplasia

This occurs in three forms: monostotic, polyostotic and as part of Albright's syndrome together with skin pigmentation and endocrinopathies (Figures 11.38 and 11.39). The bone marrow is replaced in the affected areas by connective tissue, and though both trabeculae and compact bone are affected, few osteoclasts and osteoblasts are found in the lesions. Recently, oestrogen receptors have been demonstrated in bone in a patient with polyostotic fibrous dysplasia[21].

Gorham's Vanishing Bone Disease

This involves abnormal and unopposed activity of osteoclasts resulting in extensive erosion of bone (Fig. 11.40).

(Continued on p. 209)

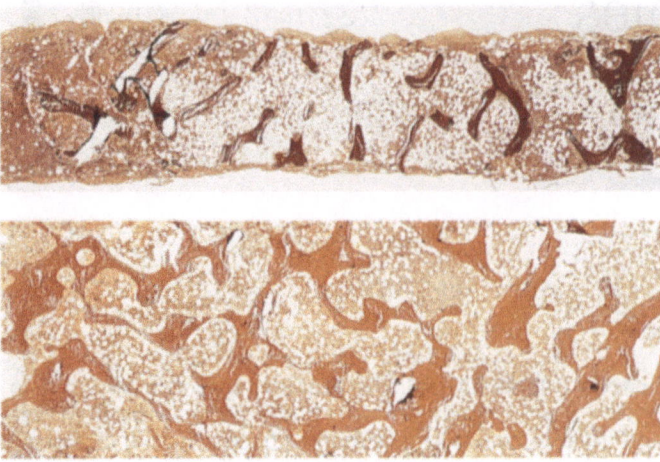

Fig. 11.1 Low-power view of sections of two bone biopsies (one 2 mm and one 4 mm wide) illustrating normal trabecular bone structure. Gomori

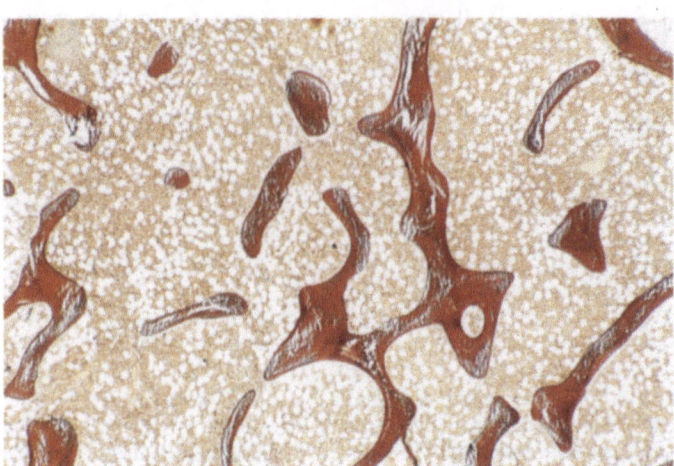

Fig. 11.2 Higher magnification showing trabecular network and normocellular bone marrow. There are few 'disconnected' or isolated trabecular profiles

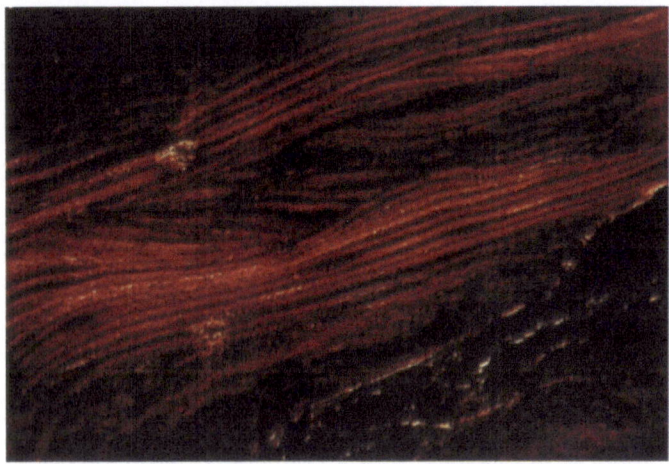

Fig. 11.3 Normal lamellar bone structure. Gomori's stain, viewed in polarized light

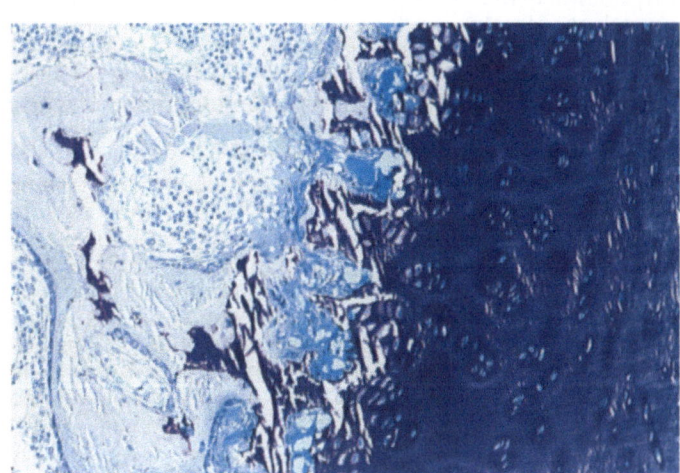

Figs 11.4–11.6 Sections of bone biopsy of child.
Fig. 11.4 Epiphyseal plate, and trabecular bone with layer of osteoblasts

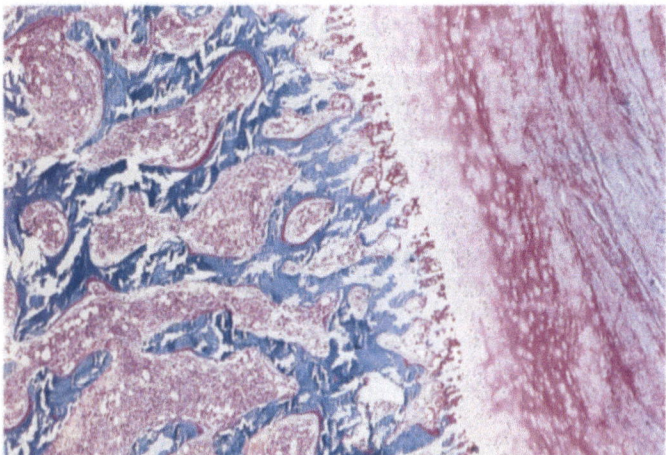

Fig. 11.5 Section stained by Ladewig's stain. Note osteoid seam on trabecular bone; and cellular bone marrow with few fat cells

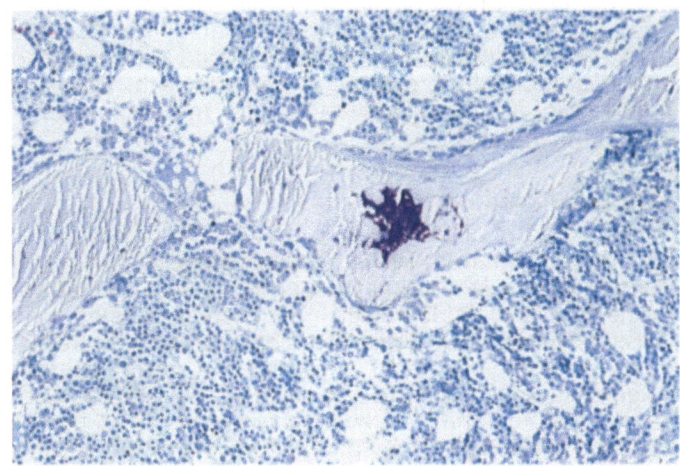

Fig. 11.6 Trabecular bone from area near cortical bone. Note uncalcified focus, osteoid seams and osteoblasts

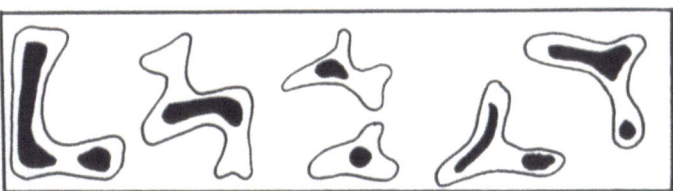

OSTEOPOROSIS

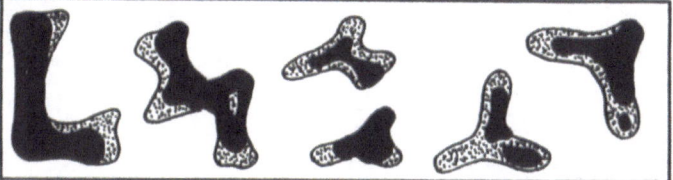

OSTEOMALACIA

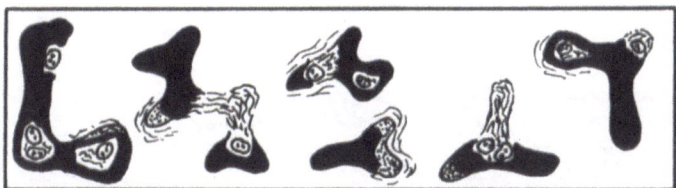

HYPERPARATHYROIDISM

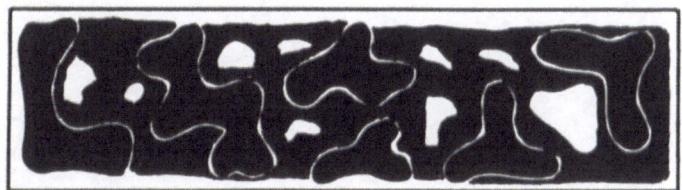

OSTEOSCLEROSIS

Fig. 11.7 Cancellous bone in four main types of osteopathy: reduction in trabecular bone in osteoporosis; increased osteoid seams in osteomalacia; excavating osteoclastosis with paratrabecular fibrosis in primary and secondary hyperparathyroidism; greatly increased quantity of trabecular bone in osteosclerosis

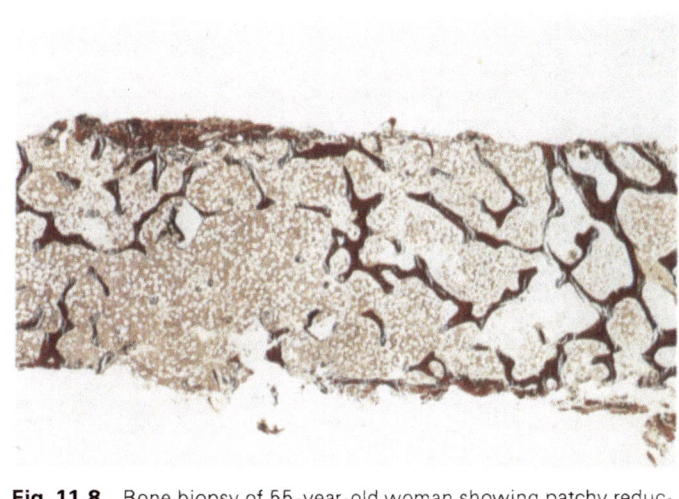

Fig. 11.8 Bone biopsy of 55-year-old woman showing patchy reduction in trabecular bone. Gomori

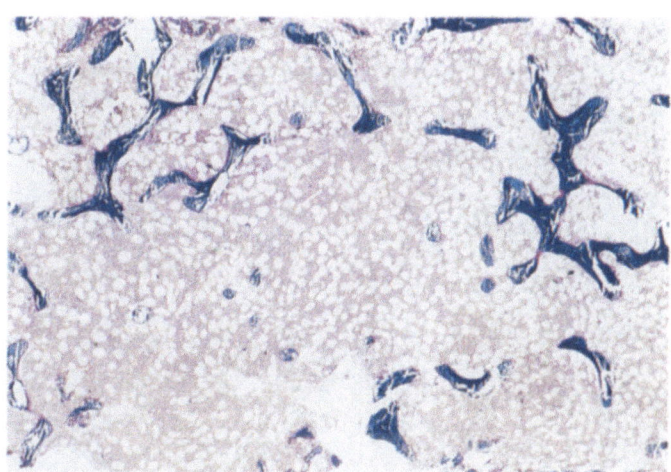

Fig. 11.9 Higher magnification of osteopenic area in Fig. 11.8. Note that there is very little osteoid

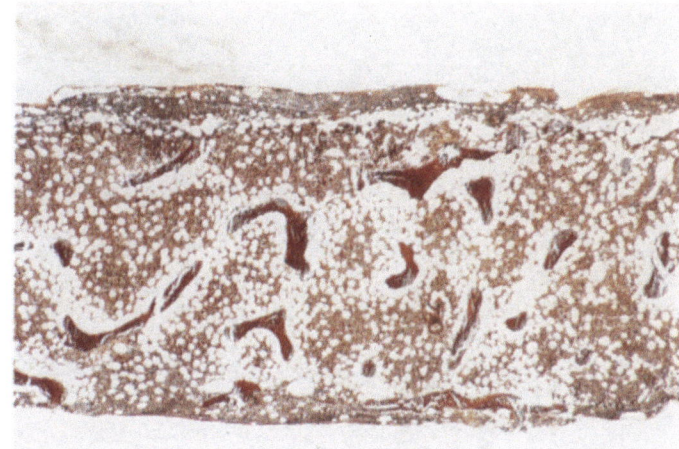

Fig. 11.10 Section of bone biopsy of 60-year-old woman showing ossicles surrounded by layer of fat cells, and reduction in trabecular bone. Gomori

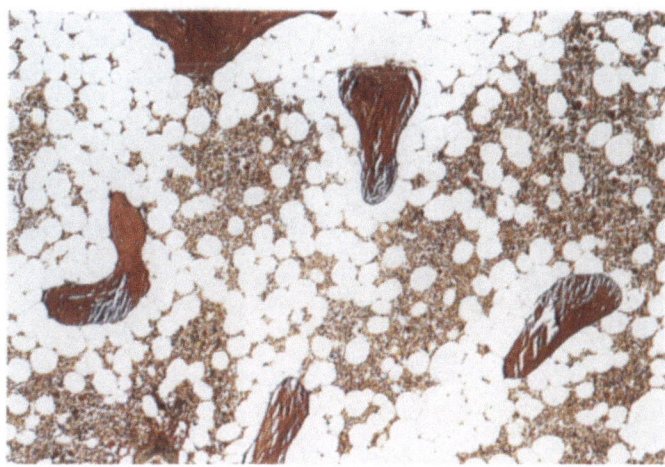

Fig. 11.11 Higher magnification of area from Fig. 11.10. Trabecular network enveloped by a layer of fat cells, no osteoblasts or osteoclasts present

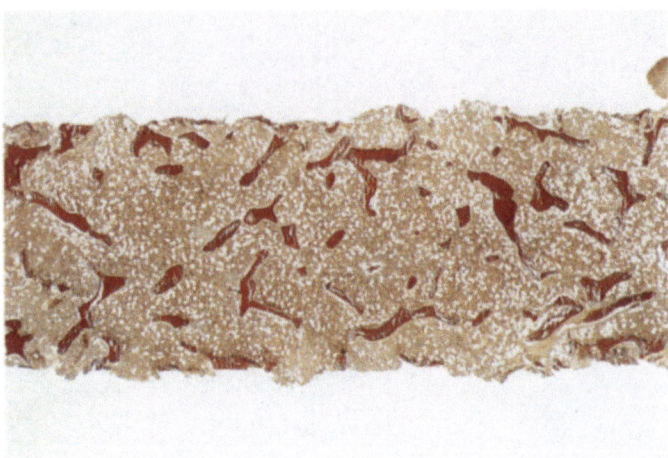

Fig. 11.12 Osteoporosis with normocellular bone marrow. Gomori

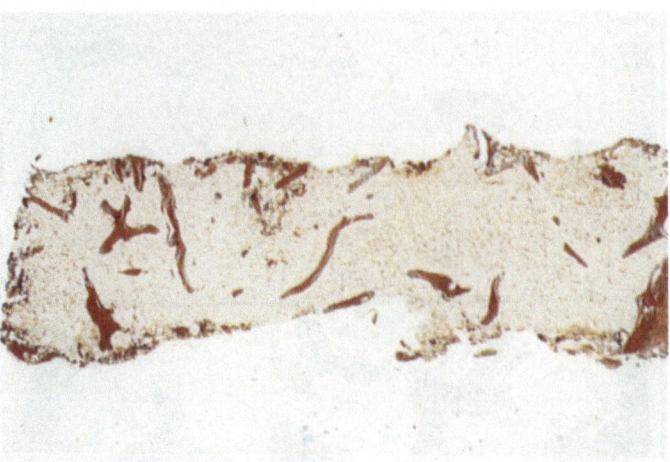

Fig. 11.13 Sections of bone biopsy of 70-year-old male patient with aplasia and osteoporosis. The peripheral blood count was normal and he had not had cytotoxic therapy or radiation to the pelvis

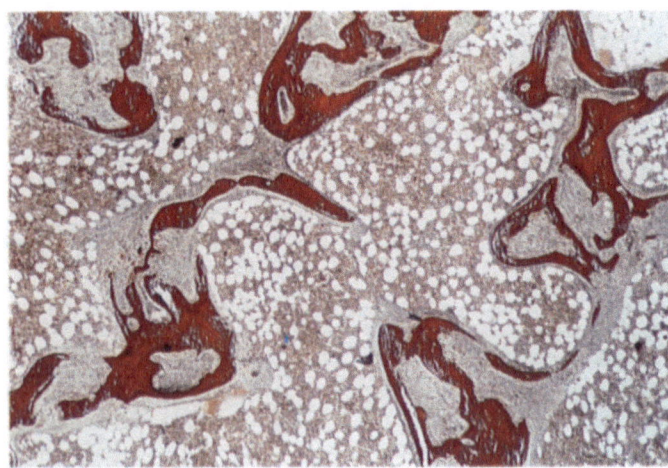

Figs 11.14–11.16 These sections illustrate aspects of the altered trabecular structure and of osseous remodelling in primary hyperparathyroidism; stained by Gomori

Fig. 11.14 Excavating osteoclastosis with little paratrabecular fibrosis and cellular bone marrow. Note numerous trabecular erosions all filled with and encased in fibrous tissue

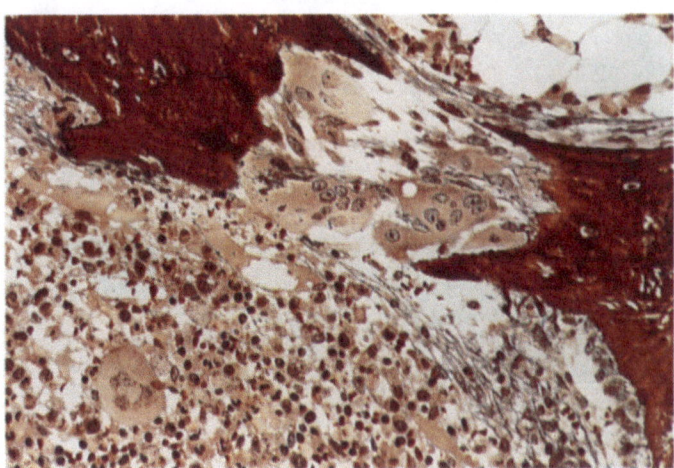

Fig. 11.15 Higher magnification of a trabecula from Fig. 11.14. Note close association between the bone cells, blood vessels and fibres, and no osteoblasts in the erosion cavity

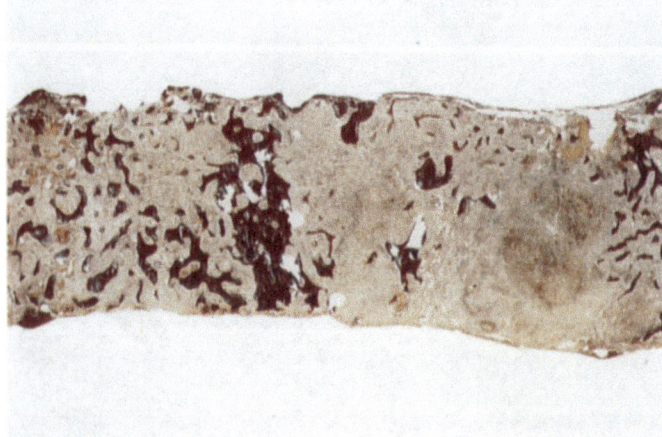

Fig. 11.16 Low magnification of bone biopsy section illustrating complete effacement of the trabecular network in half of the biopsy with altered structure in the other half

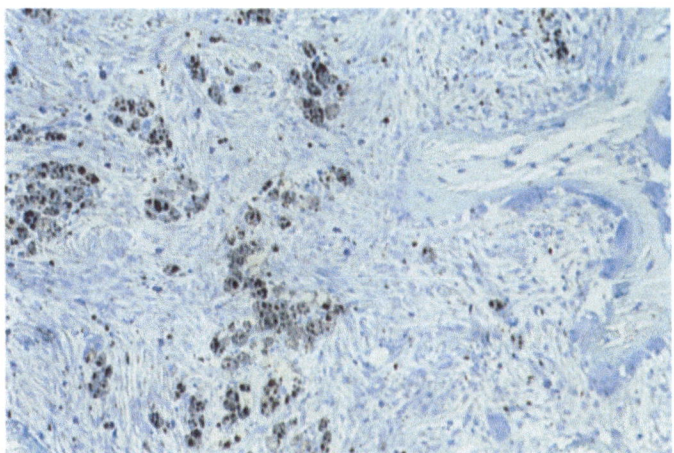

Fig. 11.17 Section of bone biopsy of patient with primary hyperparathyroidism. Note accumulation of haemosiderin-loaded macrophages – the so-called brown tumours; and replacement of normal marrow by connective tissue

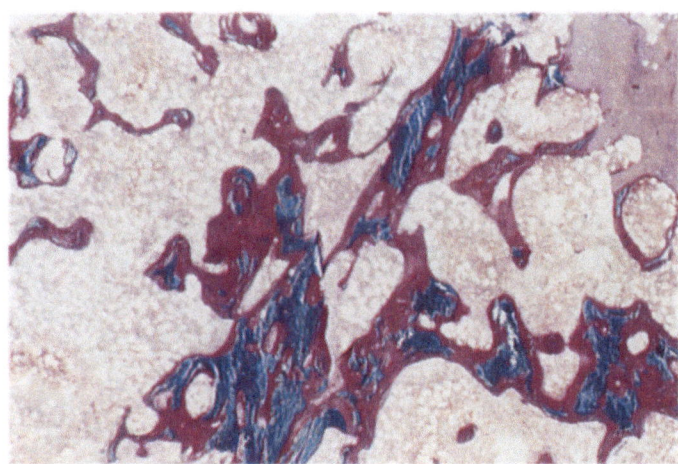

Figs 11.18–11.24 Aspects of secondary (renal) osteodystrophy

Fig. 11.18 Low-power view to show destruction of the normal trabecular network, and the high proportion of osteoid (red). Ladewig

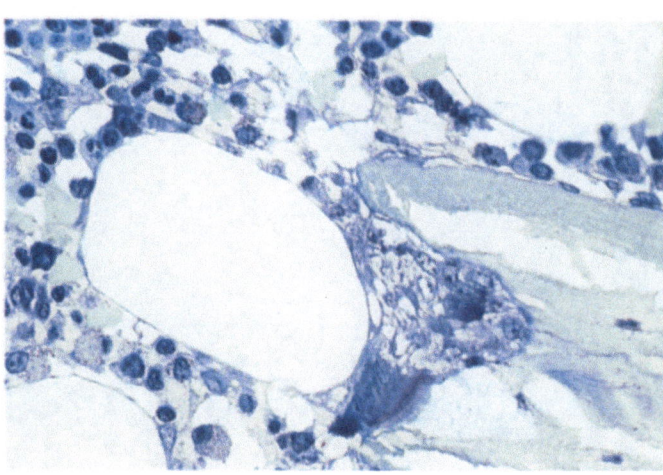

Fig. 11.19 Small erosion cavity filled with fibres. Note osteoclasts in the cavity under the osteoid seam

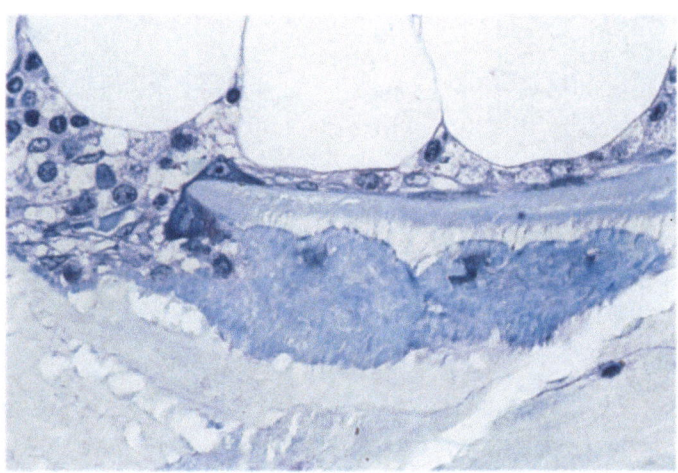

Fig. 11.20 Osteoclasts resorbing both calcified bone and osteoid

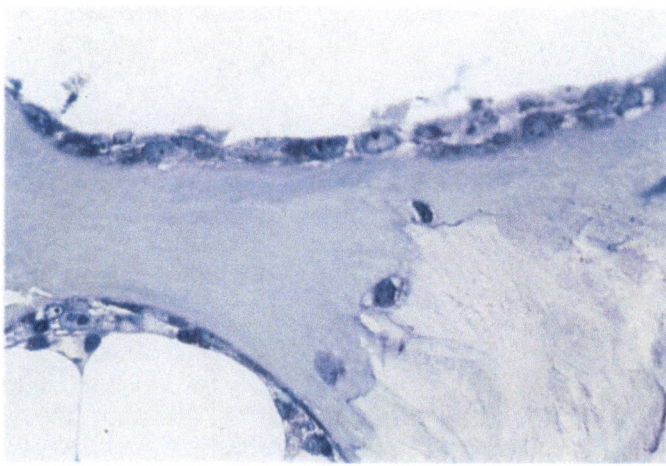

Fig. 11.21 Osteoid forming junction between two trabeculae, with layer of osteoblasts at the surface

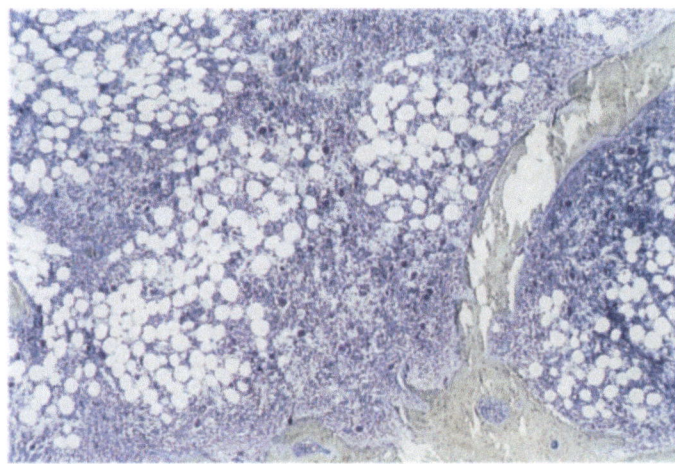

Figs 11.22–11.24 Sections of bone biopsy of 38-year-old patient with renal failure on haemodialysis

Fig. 11.22 Low-power view showing paratrabecular fibrosis and patchy cellularity

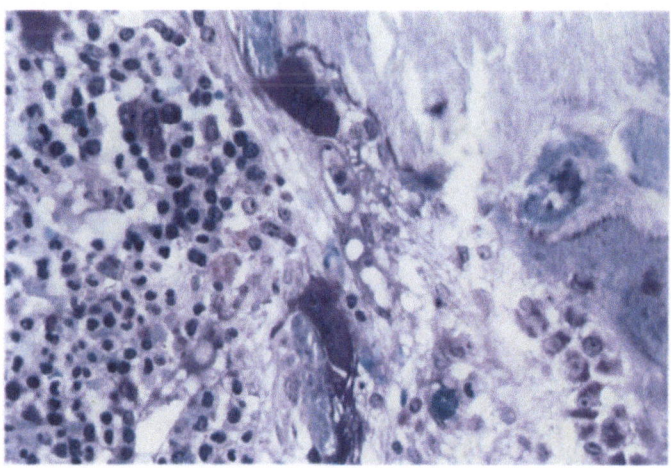

Fig. 11.23 Higher magnification of area of osseous remodelling from Fig. 11.22, showing both osteoclasts and osteoblasts

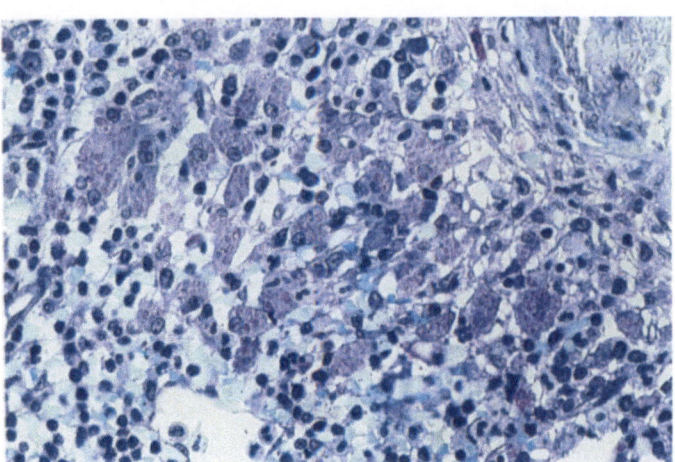

Fig. 11.24   A different area from the same biopsy, showing an aggregate of macrophages and lymphoid cells. Toluidine blue. This patient developed a malignant lymphoma approximately 2 years after this biopsy was taken

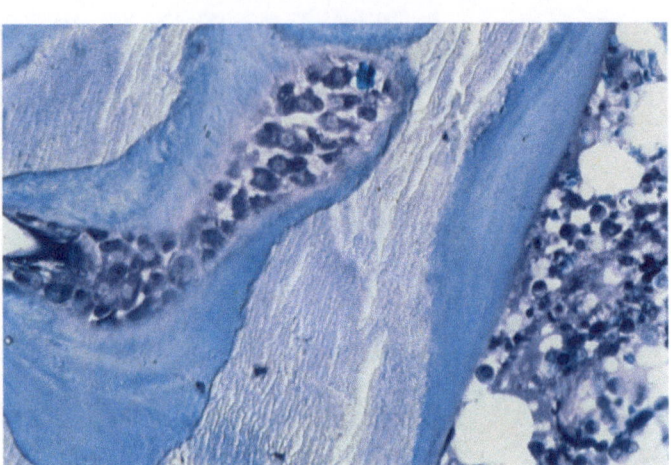

Figs 11.25–11.28   Bone biopsy sections in cases of vitamin D deficiency

Fig. 11.25   Bone biopsy section of 74-year-old male patient with bone pains and muscular weakness; malignancy was suspected. Section stained by toluidine blue. Note broad osteoid seams, osteomalacia

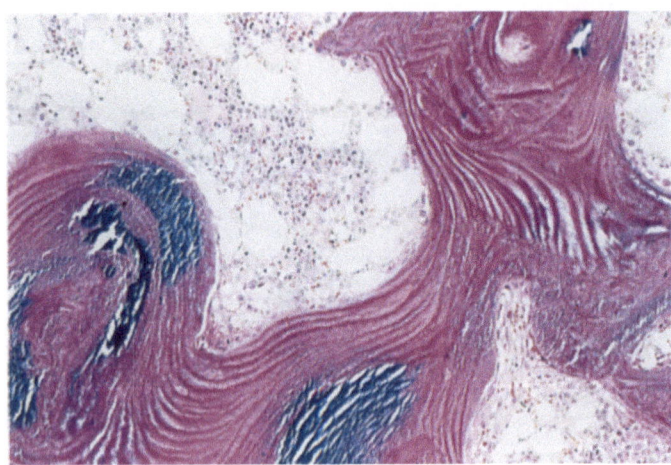

Fig. 11.26   Section stained by Ladewig's stain for demonstration of osteoid (red) and calcified bone (blue). Note demineralization of the trabeculae

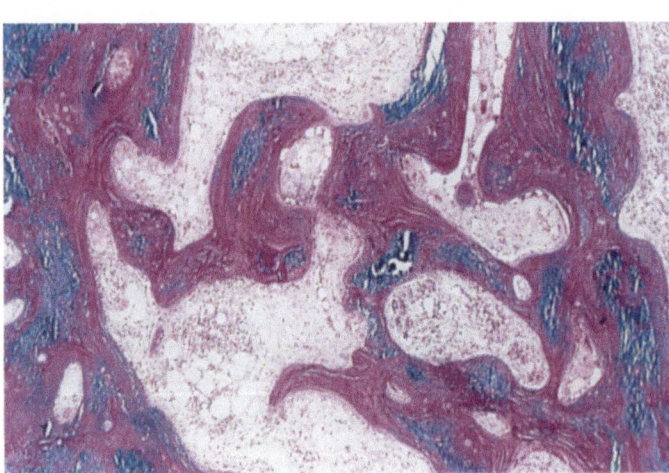

Fig. 11.27   A different area from the same biopsy, showing alteration of the trabecular bone structure. Ladewig

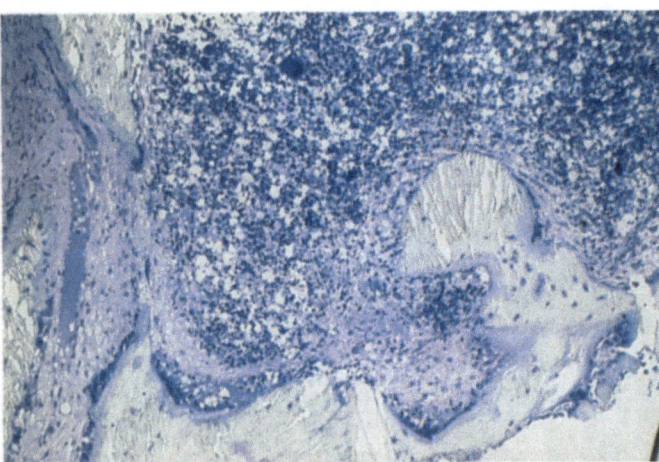

Fig. 11.28   Bone biopsy section of 6-month-old baby with vitamin D deficiency and myelofibrosis. There is osteoblastic remodelling. Note osteoid seams and paratrabecular fibrosis. This biopsy was from a cellular area

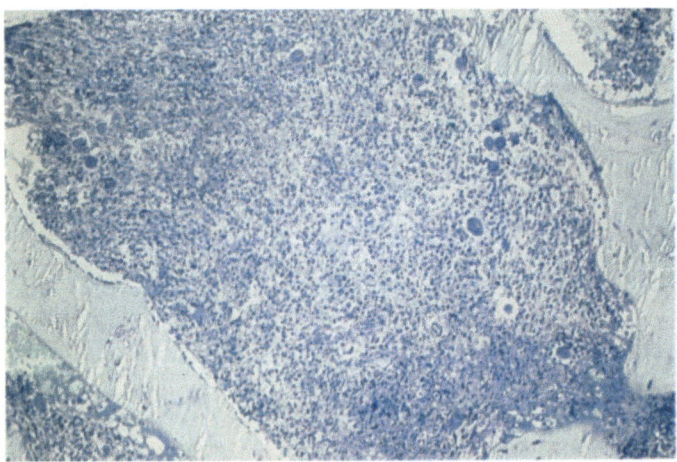

Fig. 11.29   Bone biopsy (see Fig. 11.28) taken after several months of therapy – no sign of increased osseous remodelling or fibrosis

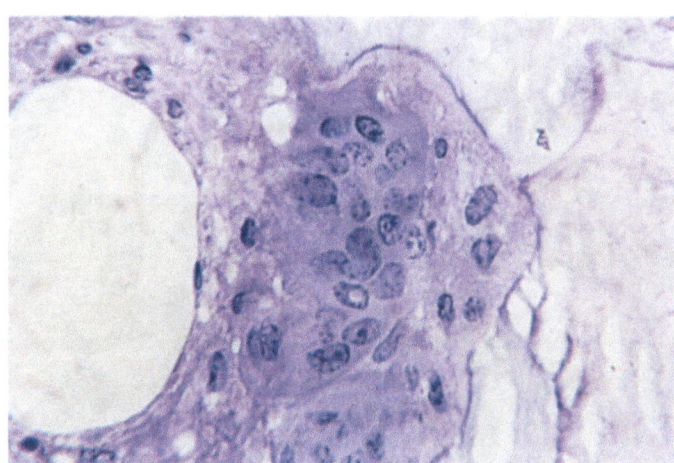

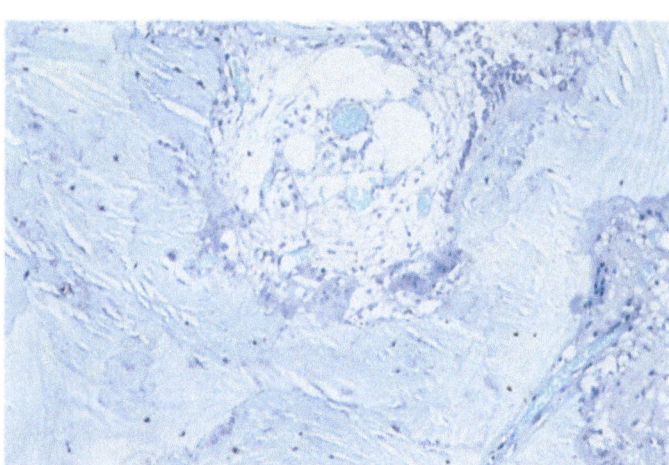

Figs 11.30–11.36 Sections of bone biopsies of patients with Paget's disease of bone

Fig. 11.30 Large multinucleated osteoclast in erosion cavity; the number of nuclei per cell may reach a hundred. H&E

Fig. 11.31 Relatively small osteoclasts in deep cavity in trabecular bone, filled with vascular connective tissue. Note osteoblasts at one side

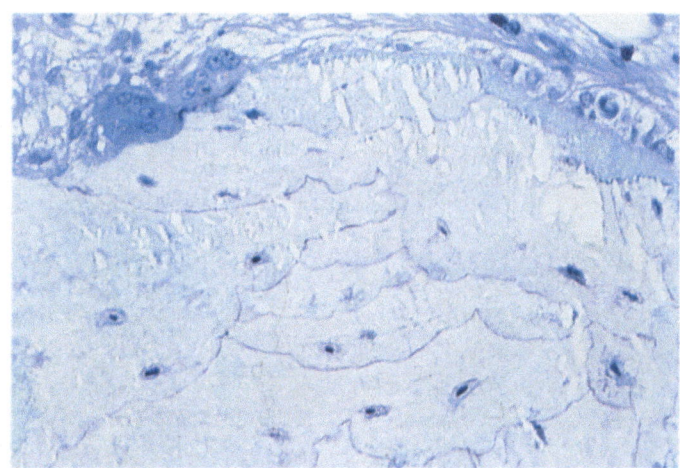

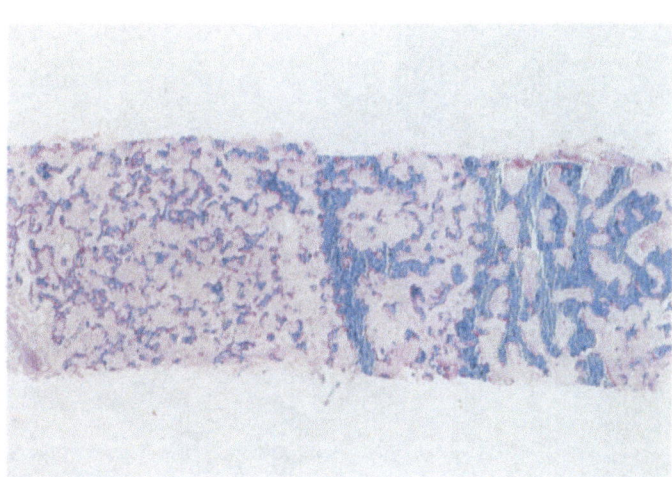

Fig. 11.32 Typical cement lines – the mosaic pattern characteristic of Paget's disease

Fig. 11.33 Alteration of the normal trabecular network. Note that one half of the biopsy is more affected than the other. Ladewig

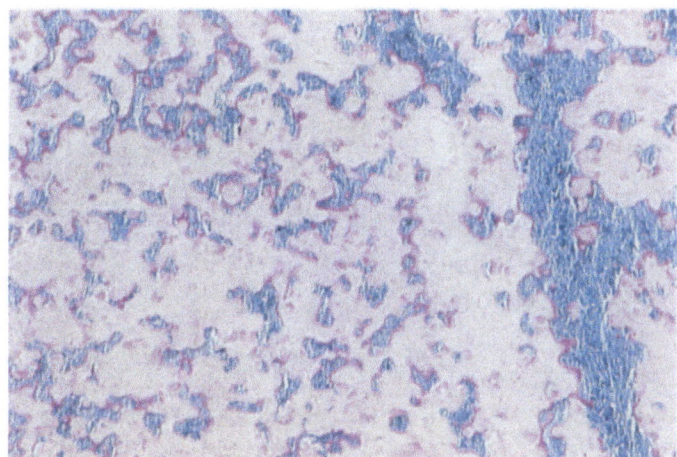

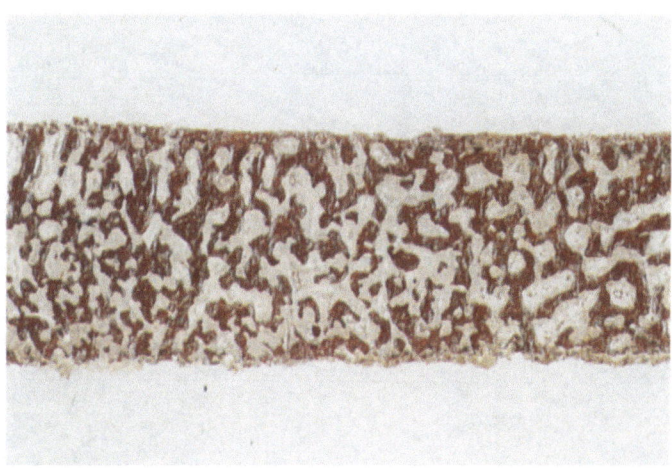

Fig. 11.34 Higher magnification of part of Fig. 11.3. There is replacement of the haematopoietic tissue by fibrosis

Fig. 11.35 Low-power view of bone biopsy of patient with Paget's disease, showing a dense network of bone and no residual haematopoietic tissue. Gomori

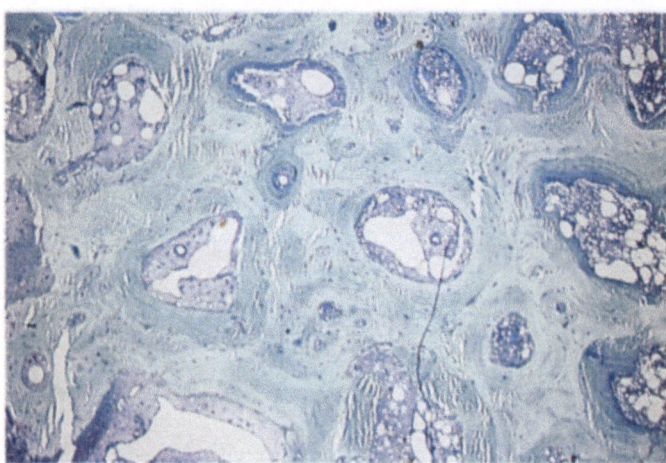

Fig. 11.36 Section of bone biopsy of patient with osteosclerosis. Note extensive patchy osteoid and progressive encroachment of bone on the marrow cavities which contain dense connective tissue

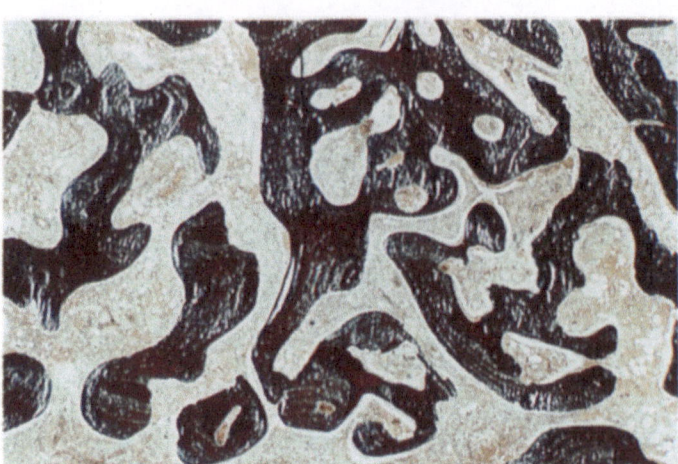

Fig. 11.37 Bone biopsy of an 8-year-old child with osteopetrosis. There is a dense trabecular network; the spaces in between are occupied by loose connective tissue. Gomori

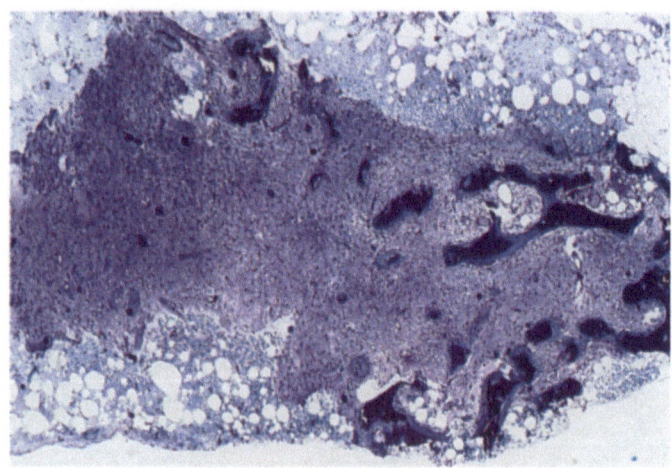

Fig. 11.38 Bone biopsy section of patient with Albright's disease showing fibrous dysplasia. Part of the marrow is replaced by dense fibrous tissue. Toluidine blue

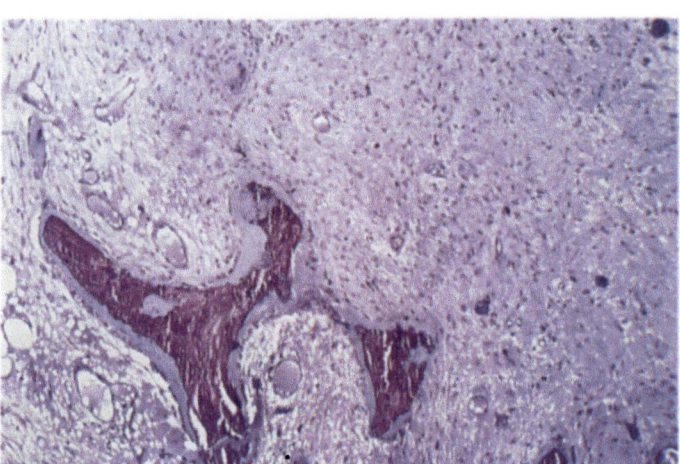

Fig. 11.39 Higher magnification of area from Fig. 11.38, showing trabecular bone with osteoid seam, and fibrous tissue containing fibroblasts and mast cells. Toluidine blue

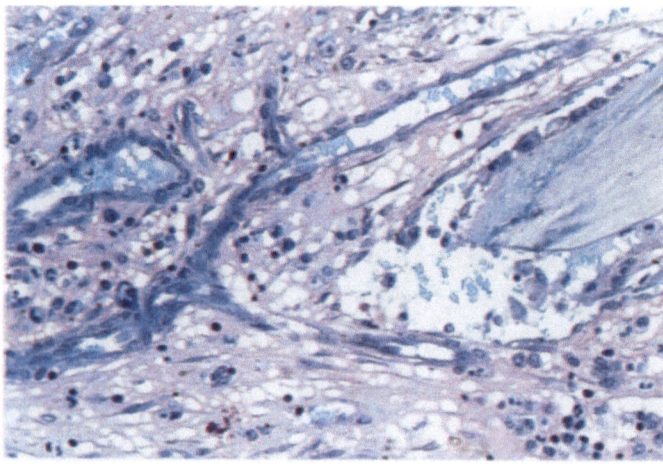

Fig. 11.40 Section of bone biopsy of patient with Gorham's vanishing bone disease. Note replacement of bone marrow by fibrous tissue with inflammatory infiltration

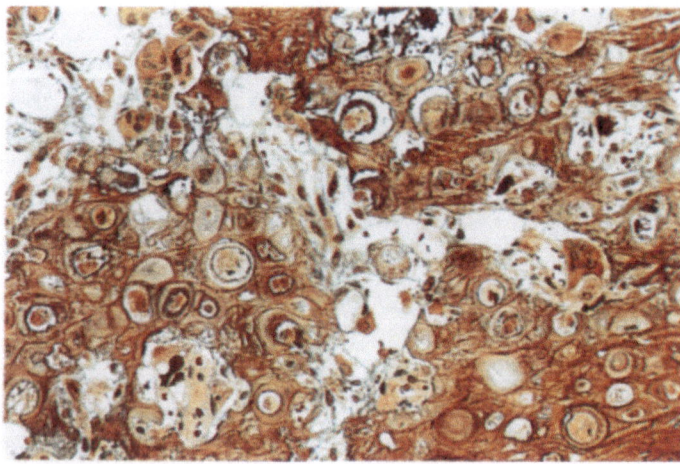

Fig. 11.41 Section of bone biopsy of 17-year-old patient with osteochondrosarcoma; replacement of bone marrow by cartilage with abnormal chondrocytes; note osteoclasts (upper left). Gomori

Osteochondrosarcoma

There is replacement of the haematopoietic tissue in the affected areas (Fig. 11.41).

Myelogenous Osteopathies

As mentioned previously, alterations in trabecular bone structure have been observed in most conditions affecting the bone marrow: in haematological malignancies as well as in non-neoplastic changes in bone marrow cellularity. Most of these are referred to in the appropriate sections. Changes in trabecular bone structure caused by metastases are dealt with in the section on metastatic involvement of the bone marrow.

References

1. Nisbet, N. W. (1987). Bone marrow transplantation in precocious osteopetrosis. *Br. Med. J.*, **294**, 463
2. Riggs, B. L. and Melton, L. J. III (1986). Involutional osteoporosis. *N. Engl. J. Med.*, **314**, 1676
3. Smith, R. (1987). Osteoporosis: cause and management. *Br. Med. J.*, **294**, 329
4. Consensus Development Conference: prophylaxis and treatment of osteoporosis (1987). Conference Report. *Br. Med. J.*, **295**, 914
5. Meuleman, J. (1987). Beliefs about osteoporosis. A critical appraisal. *Arch. Intern. Med.*, **147**, 762
6. Peck, W. A., Riggs, B. L., Bell, N. H., Wallace, R. B., Johnston, C. C., Gordon, S. L. and Shulman, L. E. (1988). Research directions in osteoporosis. *Am. J. Med.*, **84**, 275
7. Savvas, M., Studd, J. W. W., Fogelman, I., Dooley, M., Montgomery, J. and Murby, B. (1988). Skeletal effects of oral oestrogen compared with subcutaneous oestrogen and testosterone in postmenopausal women. *Br. Med., J.*, **297**, 331
8. Raisz, F. H. (1988). Local and systemic factors in the pathogenesis of osteoporosis. *N. Engl. J. Med.*, **318**, 818
9. Kanis, J. A. and Passmore, R. (1989). Calcium supplementation of the diet – I. Not justified by present evidence. *Br. Med. J.*, **298**, 137
10. Kanis, J. A. and Passmore, R. (1989). Calcium supplementation of the diet – II. Not justified by present evidence. *Br. Med. J.*, **298**, 205
11. Burkhardt, R., Kettner, G., Böhm, W., Schmidmeier, M., Schlag, R., Frisch, B., Mallmann, B., Eisenmenger, W. and Gilg, Th. (1987). Changes in trabecular bone, haematopoiesis and bone marrow vessels in aplastic anaemia, primary osteoporosis, and old age: a comparative histomorphometric study. *Bone*, **8**, 157
12. Schaefer, H. E. (1985). Beckenkammbioptische Diagnostik. Osteologie – Haematologie – Onkologie – Metabolische störungen. *Internist*, **26**, 453
13. MacIntyre, I., Whitehead, M. I., Banks, L. M., Stevenson, J. C., Wimalawansa, S. J. and Healy, M. J. R. (1988). Calcitonin for prevention of postmenopausal bone loss. *Lancet*, **1**, 900
14. Frisch, B. and Eventov, I. (1986). Hematopoiesis in osteoporosis. Preliminary report comparing biopsies of the femoral neck and iliac crest. *Isr. J. Med. Sci.*, **22**, 380
15. Marcus, R. (1987). Normal and abnormal bone remodeling in man. *Ann. Rev. Med.*, **38**, 129
16. Bone erosions in rheumatic disease (1987). *Lancet*, **2**(8555), 375
17. Einhorn, T. A. (1988). Metabolic bone disease: diagnosis and treatment. *Orthopedics*, May/June, 45
18. Mirra, J. M. (1987). Pathogenesis of Paget's disease based on viral etiology. *Clin. Orthop.*, **217**, 162
19. Meunier, P. J., Salson, C., Mathieu, L., Chapuy, M. C., Delmas, P., Alexandre, C. and Charhon, S. (1987). Skeletal distribution and biochemical parameters of Paget's disease. *Clin. Orthop. Rel. Res.*, **217**, 37
20. Kaibara, N., Katsuki, I., Hotokebushi, I. and Takagishi, K. (1982). Intermediate form of osteopetrosis with recessive inheritance. *Skeletal Radiol.*, **9**, 47
21. Kaplan, F. S., Fallon, M. D., Boden, S. D., Schmidt, R., Senior, M. and Haddad, J. G. (1988). Estrogen receptors in bone in a patient with polyostotic fibrous dysplasia (McCune-Albright syndrome). *N. Engl. J. Med.*, **319**, 421

Index

Italic references are to figures